Fundamentals of Geriatric Pharmacotherapy:

An Evidence-Based Approach

Lisa C. Hutchison, Pharm.D., MPH, BCPS
Associate Professor
University of Arkansas for Medical Sciences
College of Pharmacy
Little Rock, Arkansas

Rebecca B. Sleeper, Pharm.D., FASCP, BCPS
Associate Professor and Division Head
Geriatrics Division, Department of Pharmacy Practice
Texas Tech University Health Sciences Center School of Pharmacy
Lubbock, Texas

American Society of Health-System Pharmacists®

Bethesda, Maryland

Any correspondence regarding this publication should be sent to the publisher, American Society of Health-System Pharmacists, 7272 Wisconsin Avenue, Bethesda, MD 20814, attention: Special Publishing.

The information presented herein reflects the opinions of the contributors and advisors. It should not be interpreted as an official policy of ASHP or as an endorsement of any product.

Director, Special Publishing: Jack Bruggeman
Acquisitions Editor: Rebecca Olson
Senior Editorial Project Manager: Dana A. Battaglia
Project Editor: Bill Fogle
Design Director/Page Layout: Carol A. Barrer
Page Design: David Wade

ISBN 978-1-58528-228-9

Dedication

We dedicate this textbook to those who have supported us and shown us the way:

- My grandmother, who lived independently until her mid-90s; my parents, who made my dream of becoming a pharmacist possible; my husband, whose love continues to support me; and my mentors, who encouraged me to be a pioneer in the practice of clinical pharmacy. (LCH)

- My father Kenneth, through whose career as a nursing facility administrator I was first exposed to long term care; my husband Brian, who is my greatest source of love and support and also a fellow pharmacist who well understands my passion for this subject; and to my students, who inspire me daily and who will one day care for us all. (RS)

- The senior patients who have taught us the most about the use of medications. They continue to inspire us through their lives and words.

Preface

The older population is growing. The U.S. Census bureau projects the worlds' 65 and older population will double by the year 2050, and the 85 and older population will increase fivefold in the same time period.[1] With elderly patients come special healthcare needs, and the health professions' workforce needs to be prepared. More and better focused information on geriatric health must be disseminated to health care providers.

For most patient populations, in order to provide the best pharmacotherapy for patients, health care providers refer to evidence-based guidelines and the studies that these recommendations are based upon. This practice assumes that elderly subjects are well-represented in the study populations; however, most trials exclude elderly participants, especially participants who have multiple disease states, are frail or are more susceptible to rare adverse effects. The risk-benefit may be skewed in these patients, particularly those who are nearing the century mark. This text is designed to build upon content that would be delivered in a general pharmacotherapy text. The learner's foundation knowledge of disease-specific pathophysiology and pharmacology is assumed, allowing this book to focus on evidence published in the elderly population, stressing the differences that are seen across the continuum of young-old, middle-old, and oldest old.

This textbook is divided into two sections. Section one provides general concepts with biomedical principles of aging, social/behavioral issues, ethical considerations, approaches to geriatric assessment, adverse drug events, and polypharmacy. This foundational material assures a knowledge base required for the general approach to caring for geriatric patients. The second section, which is the bulk of the book, covers disease states commonly encountered in the aging adult, reviewing age-specific epidemiology and evidence for treatment in the different senior populations. Common problems and clinical controversies encountered when treating elderly patients are described with suggested methods to minimize their occurrence. Every chapter includes key terms, learning objectives, key points, patient cases, clinical pearls, and self-assessment questions that help guide the student through the maze of information required in caring for an older patient. In addition, web-based materials such as course outlines or lesson plans are available to facilitate incorporation of the textbook into course delivery. As a contributed work, we have solicited the expertise of authors and reviewers who practice in the care of elderly patients or who mentor learners in pharmacy or other health professions in the mastery of geriatric pharmacotherapy content.

While designed primarily as a textbook for pharmacy students to use in an elective or required course focused on geriatric pharmacotherapy, this book would

---

[1] U.S. Census Bureau News, Press release, June 23, 2009.

also prove useful for practicing pharmacists and other healthcare providers who wish to learn more about pharmacotherapy in the elderly patient. The use of medications continues to be one of the most difficult aspects of geriatric practice, regardless of the professional discipline.

It is our fondest hope that this book will serve as a mechanism for pharmacists and other clinicians to improve the use of medications in their older adult patients so they may experience the longest life possible coupled with fullest quality of life in those golden years.

Lisa C. Hutchison
Rebecca B. Sleeper
February, 2010

Foreword

Beginning in January 2010 the U.S. sits on the cusp of a great social demographic change as the Baby Boomer generation begins to turn 65 years of age. Persons near to or who have already crossed this threshold are likely to claim that chronological age is not reflective of their true age and vitality. If being 50 is the new 35, what does that make 75? Aging or being "old" is not a well accepted or welcomed stage of life in our culture. Anti-aging therapies ranging from skin creams that affect cosmetic appearance to individualized hormone regimens that increase or maintain muscle mass, maintain vitality and diminish the appearance of age dominate the market and media spotlight, while shaping the national conscience of how we think about aging. It is unfortunate and damaging that such an industry can delude the public and tarnish the real champions of older adults. Pharmacists have a role in setting this record straight.

The golden age of geriatric clinical pharmacology took place in the 1970s and 1980s, when the basic age-associated pharmacokinetic and pharmacodynamics changes were identified. Since then information on the efficacy and safety of new drugs, and how to dose and monitor them, has been generated by pharmacoepidemiologic studies, pooled and secondary analyses of trials of persons above a certain age that met inclusion and exclusion criteria. The pearls of geriatric pharmacotherapy are not generated from such trials and findings, but by experienced and intellectually curious clinicians and scientists such as those fielded to contribute to this text.

To my knowledge the first recognized pharmacist-leaders in geriatrics were Ron Stewart and the late Peter Lamy. Their contributed works and mentorship directly impacted many of the authors of this textbook. That the field of geriatrics has been atrophying is well documented—training programs continue to decline in number, geriatrics continues to be underemphasized in curriculums, and practices cannot survive on Medicare alone. All workforce predictions conclude that the U.S. health care education system cannot train enough pharmacists, physicians, nurses, and other health professionals to meet the demand. Thus, all health care professionals, including pharmacists, must have working competencies in geriatrics to care for the nation's aging population. That is where this text can be of great value and contribution.

Divided into two sections "Social, Ethical, and Economic Issues of Aging" and "General Biomedical and Pharmacotherapy Issues," *Fundamentals of Geriatric Pharmacotherapy* provides a comprehensive knowledge and reference for both novice and experienced clinician. Each chapter includes learning objectives that will be useful for educators and self-learners. Geriatrics, like all specialties, has its own language and the key terms defined in each chapter compose a helpful glossary for understanding this language. Rather than a stand-alone chapter on demographics, the chapter "Challenges in Geriatric Care" nicely integrates terminology with demographic changes and puts chronological age into context with the other variables that must be considered when providing care for the older patient. The clinical pearls, key points, cases, and questions in each chapter provide the reader with clinical insight that is not found in clinical trials, meta-analyses, or systematic reviews. The case histories accurately represent the complexity and decision-making encountered when caring for geriatric patients in a variety of clinical settings; good exposure for the student reader. How to critique and interpret clinical trials for their geriatric content and implications for care are discussed in detail with examples in several of the chapters.

As crucial as knowing when to start a medication, knowing when to stop them can be just as crucial as the risk: benefit ratio shifts and goals of care change. In addition, as we age our heterogeneity increases, i.e., we become less like one another, our differences become magnified. These points are not lost in the text.

Medication management can be a complex and comprehensive task for patients, caregivers, and families. The medication management challenges for pharmacists, physicians, nurses, and others are similarly complex and time consuming and often require in-depth reviews of a patient's history; home visits; an understanding of the patient's and family's knowledge and belief about medications; and assessments of function, cognition, and social support as well as contacting multiple prescribers. These challenges and the tools to address them are presented throughout the text along with the pharmacotherapy for treating the diseases, conditions, and syndromes encountered when caring for geriatric patients.

The American Society of Health-System Pharmacists, editors Drs. Lisa Hutchison and Rebecca Sleeper, and all the authors are to be congratulated for their foresight in recognizing the need for a new text on geriatric pharmacotherapy. *Fundamentals of Geriatric Pharmacotherapy* is a welcomed addition to the library of texts on geriatrics and gerontology. The target audience should not be exclusively pharmacists, but all healthcare professionals who prescribe or have a desire to know more about this important component of geriatrics. Pharmacists, pharmacy educators, and students will find the text a beneficial tool in attaining or teaching geriatric competencies.

Where will future leaders in geriatric pharmacy come from? Hopefully this text will inspire, stimulate, and nurture them.

Todd P. Semla, M.S., Pharm.D., BCPS, FCCP, AGSF
Clinical Pharmacy Specialist
U.S. Department of Veterans Affairs
Associate Professor, Departments of Medicine and Psychiatry
Northwestern University, Chicago, IL
Past President and Chairman, American Geriatrics Society

Table of Contents

Section 1: Social, Ethical, and Economic Issues of Aging

Chapter 1

Rebecca B. Sleeper

Chapter 2

Susan W. Miller

Section 2: General Biomedical and Pharmacotherapy Issues

Chapter 3

Lisa C. Hutchison

Chapter 4

Sunny A. Linnebur

Chapter 5

Rebecca B. Sleeper

Chapter 6

Emily R. Hajjar, Joseph T. Hanlon

Chapter 7

Kristen Cook, James E. Tisdale

Contributors

Myra T. Belgeri, Pharm.D., CGP, BCPS
Clinical Pharmacist
HospiScript Services, LLC
Saint Louis, Missouri

Amie Taggart Blaszczyk, Pharm.D., CGP, BCPS, FASCP
Assistant Professor of Pharmacy Practice, Geriatrics
Texas Tech University Health Sciences Center School
   of Pharmacy
Dallas, Texas

Michael R. Brodeur, Pharm.D., CGP, FASCP
Associate Professor
Department of Pharmacy Practice
Albany College of Pharmacy and Health Sciences
Albany, New York

Angela Cheng-Lai, Pharm.D., BCPS
Clinical Pharmacy Manager
Montefiore Medical Center
Assistant Professor of Medicine
Albert Einstein College of Medicine
Bronx, New York

Lisa B. Cohen, Pharm.D., CDE, CDOE
Assistant Professor of Pharmacy
University of Rhode Island
Kingston, Rhode Island

Kristen Cook, Pharm.D., BCPS
Assistant Professor
University of Nebraska Medical Center College of
   Pharmacy
Clinical Pharmacist
Nebraska-Western Iowa Veteran's Hospital
Omaha, Nebraska

Erica L. Estus, Pharm.D., CGP
Clinical Assistant Professor
Department of Pharmacy Practice
University of Rhode Island College of Pharmacy
Kingston, Rhode Island

Michelle A. Fritsch, Pharm.D., CGP
Professor and Chair
Department of Clinical and Administrative Sciences
School of Pharmacy
College of Notre Dame of Maryland
Baltimore, Maryland

Emily R. Hajjar, Pharm.D., BCPS, CGP
Assistant Professor
Jefferson School of Pharmacy
Thomas Jefferson University
Philadelphia, Pennsylvania

Joseph T. Hanlon Pharm.D., MS
Professor, Department of Medicine (Geriatrics)
University of Pittsburgh
Health Scientist, Pittsburgh VAHS
Pittsburgh, Pennsylvania

Meri Hix, Pharm.D., CGP
Associate Professor of Pharmacy Practice
Midwestern University Chicago College of Pharmacy
Downers Grove, Illinois

Anne L. Hume, Pharm.D., FCCP, BCPS
Professor of Pharmacy
University of Rhode Island
Kingston, Rhode Island

Lisa C. Hutchison, Pharm.D., MPH, FCCP, BCPS
Associate Professor
University of Arkansas for Medical Sciences
College of Pharmacy
Little Rock, Arkansas

Sum Lam, Pharm.D., BCPS
Associate Clinical Professor
Department of Clinical Pharmacy Practice
College of Pharmacy and Allied Health Professions
St. John's University
Queens, New York

Jeannie Kim Lee, Pharm.D., BCPS
Clinical Assistant Professor
University of Arizona Colleges of Pharmacy and Medicine
Research Associate and Faculty
Geriatric Education Center
Arizona Center on Aging
Geriatric Clinical Pharmacist
Southern Arizona VA Health Care System
Tucson, Arizona

Sunny A. Linnebur, Pharm.D., FCCP, FASCP, BCPS, CGP
Associate Professor
University of Colorado Denver School of Pharmacy
Department of Clinical Pharmacy
Aurora, Colorado

Monica Mathys, Pharm.D.
Assistant Professor of Pharmacy Practice
Texas Tech Health Sciences Center School of Pharmacy
Dallas/Fort Worth Regional Campus
Dallas, Texas

Susan W. Miller, B.S. Pharm., Pharm.D.
Professor
Mercer University College of Pharmacy and Health Sciences
Atlanta, Georgia

Sean M. Mirk, Pharm.D.
Assistant Professor, Department of Pharmacy Practice
Albany College of Pharmacy and Health Sciences
Albany, New York

James Nawarskas, Pharm.D., BCPS
Associate Professor of Pharmacy
University of New Mexico
College of Pharmacy
Albuquerque, New Mexico

Mary Beth O'Connell, Pharm.D., BCPS, FASHP, FCCP
Associate Professor
Pharmacy Practice Department
Eugene Applebaum College of Pharmacy and Health Sciences
Wayne State University
Detroit, Michigan

Norma J. Owens, Pharm.D., BCPS, FCCP
Professor of Pharmacy
Department of Pharmacy Practice
University of Rhode Island College of Pharmacy
Kingston, Rhode Island

Rebecca B. Sleeper, Pharm.D., FASCP, BCPS
Associate Professor and Division Head
Geriatrics Division, Department of Pharmacy Practice
Texas Tech University Health Sciences Center School of Pharmacy
Lubbock, Texas

James E. Tisdale, Pharm.D.
Professor
School of Pharmacy & Pharmaceutical Sciences
Purdue University
Adjunct Professor
Indiana University School of Medicine
Indianapolis, Indiana

Reviewers

Nicole J. Brandt, Pharm.D., CGP, BCPP, FASCP
Associate Professor, Geriatric Pharmacotherapy, Pharmacy Practice and Science UMB School of Pharmacy
Director, Clinical and Educational Programs of Peter Lamy Center Drug Therapy and Aging
Baltimore, Maryland

Noll L. Campbell, Pharm.D., FASCP, BCPP, CGP
Wishard Health Services
Indianapolis, Indiana

Kelli L. Coover, Pharm.D., CGP
Assistant Professor of Pharmacy Practice
Creighton University
School of Pharmacy and Health Professions
Omaha, Nebraska

Ruth E. Emptage, Pharm.D, CGP
Clinical Assistant Professor of Pharmacy Practice and Administration
The Ohio State University
Columbus, Ohio

Sue Fosnight R.Ph., CGP, BCPS
Clinical Lead Pharmacist-Geriatrics
Summa Health System
Akron, Ohio
Assistant Professor of Pharmacy Practice
Northeastern Ohio Colleges of Medicine and Pharmacy
Rootstown, Ohio

Carol Fox, Pharm.D.
Assistant Professor, Geriatrics Division, Abilene
Texas Tech University Health Sciences Center
School of Pharmacy
Amarillo, Texas

Chris M. Herndon, Pharm.D., BCPS, CPE
Assistant Professor, School of Pharmacy
Southern Illinois University, Edwardsville School of Pharmacy
Edwardsville, Illinois

Peter D. Hurd, Ph.D.
Professor and Assistant to the Dean for Research
St. Louis College of Pharmacy
St. Louis, Missouri

Sean M. Jeffrey, Pharm.D., CGP, FASCP
Program Director
VA Connecticut Healthcare System
West Haven, Connecticut
Associate Clinical Professor of Pharmacy Practice
School of Pharmacy
University of Connecticut
Storrs, Connecticut

Susan W. Miller, Pharm.D.
Mercer University
College of Pharmacy and Health Sciences
Department of Pharmacy Practice
Atlanta, Georgia

Randolph E. Regal, B.S., Pharm.D.
Clinical Pharmacist
Clinical Associate Professor
Adult Internal Medicine
University of Michigan Hospitals and
College of Pharmacy
Ann Arbor, Michigan

Mark Ruscin, Pharm.D.
Professor of Pharmacy Practice
Southern Illinois University Edwardsville
School of Pharmacy
Edwardsville, Illinois

Melody Ryan, Pharm.D., MPH, CGP, BCPS
Associate Professor
Department of Pharmacy Practice and Science
Department of Neurology
University of Kentucky, School of Pharmacy
Lexington, Kentucky

Maha Saad, Pharm.D., CGP, BCPS
Assistant Clinical Professor
St. Johns University
College of Pharmacy and Allied Health Professions
Queens, New York

Jeffrey T. Sherer, Pharm.D., MPH, BCPS, CGP
Clinical Associate Professor
University of Houston College of Pharmacy
Houston, Texas

Patricia W. Slattum, Pharm.D., Ph.D., CGP
Director, Geriatric Pharmacotherapy Program
Associate Professor of Pharmacotherapy and
    Outcomes Science
Virginia Commonwealth University
Richmond, Virginia

Mark A. Stratton, Pharm.D., BCPS, CGP, FASHP
Professor of Pharmacy and Langsam Endowed Chair
    in Geriatric Pharmacy
Director, Institute for Geriatric Pharmacy
University of Oklahoma College of Pharmacy
Oklahoma City, Oklahoma

Angela Treadway, Pharm.D., BCPS
Assistant Professor of Pharmacy Practice, Texas Tech
    Health Sciences Center School of Pharmacy
Advanced Practice Pharmacist in Geriatrics, VA North
    Texas Health Care System
Dallas, Texas

Bradley R. Williams, Pharm.D., FASCP, CGP
Professor, Clinical Pharmacy & Clinical Gerontology
Titus Family Department of Clinical Pharmacy
    and Pharmaceutical Economics and Policy
USC School of Pharmacy
Los Angeles, California

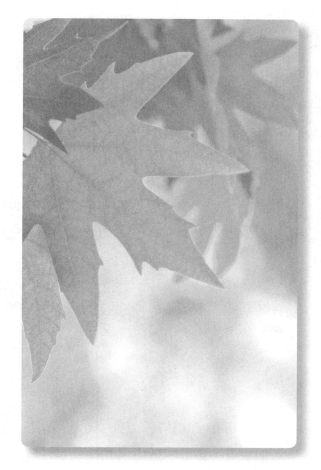

Social, Ethical, and Economic Issues of Aging

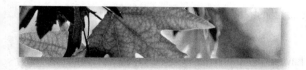

Challenges in Geriatric Care

REBECCA B. SLEEPER

Learning Objectives

1. Evaluate the applicability of clinical literature to the elderly patient using an approach that is tailored to specific subgroups of the geriatric population.

2. Differentiate the roles of health professionals and the various services and venues available in the care of geriatric patients.

3. Infer scenarios in which geriatric patients are at risk for suboptimal care and intervene when breakdowns in the continuum of care are identified.

4. Recognize the impact of caregiver burden on patient outcomes.

Key Terms

ASSISTED LIVING FACILITY: Living environment that can provide added services to the individual who is safe to live in the community environment but requires some assistance with various daily activities.

CAREGIVER BURDEN: Psychosocial and physical stress experienced by an individual who provides care to another person.

CERTIFIED GERIATRIC PHARMACIST: Pharmacist who has achieved certification by examination from the Commission for Certification in Geriatric Pharmacy.

CERTIFIED NURSE'S ASSISTANT (CNA): Individual who has earned a certificate to practice as a nurse's assistant and who may work in a wide variety of health care settings ranging from long term care facilities to private homes.

GERIATRIC: Adjective generally used to refer to an older individual.

GERIATRICIAN: Physician with expertise, as demonstrated by fellowship or other added qualifications, in the care of older persons.

GERONTOLOGICAL NURSE: Nurse with expertise, as demonstrated by exam or other added qualifications, in the care of older persons.

INFORMAL CAREGIVER: An individual who does not have formal training as a health care professional but who provides daily care to another individual, often unpaid.

INTERDISCIPLINARY TEAM: Health care team made up of multiple health professionals, which may include physicians, nurses, pharmacists, physical therapists, occupational therapists, speech therapists and other allied health professionals, dieticians, social services coordinators, psychologists, and others.

LONG TERM CARE FACILITY: 24-hour care environment for individuals who require significant assistance or supervision with daily activities.

SENIOR CARE PHARMACIST: Pharmacist who specializes in the care of older persons.

Introduction

The first challenge in addressing the health care needs of a **geriatric** population is in determining what the term *geriatric* actually means. There is not a universally accepted definition. In general terms, geriatric refers to an older person, but age is a relative descriptor, and it is one that may not always be applicable when describing the appropriateness of various health care interventions.

Social or legal definitions of older populations are often based on age. For instance, age 65 is commonly considered the threshold age for the geriatric population and most health care literature criteria will use this definition. Government statistics such as census data also define older populations based upon this age, and 65 is the age for eligibility for federal programs such as Medicare. The FDA also requires available clinical trial data for individuals over the age of 65 to be included as part of the required labeling for medications.[1] Manufacturers are required to report special considerations for dosage adjustment or avoidance in older patients based on age-related changes in drug metabolism or sensitivity. However, age-based definitions of what constitutes "older" populations vary. One of the nation's largest public action groups, the American Association of Retired Persons (AARP), uses a threshold age of 50 years,[2] and in contrast, full retirement age for the purposes of Social Security benefits

has increased to greater than age 65; up to age 67 for individual born after 1960.[3]

Aside from the fact that there is lack of agreement regarding a specific age threshold, there are drawbacks to assuming that all individuals over any age cut-off are the same, or have the same health care needs. Clinicians would not consider it appropriate to treat a 5-year-old child the same as a 40-year-old adult, as the 35-year span between these two ages are associated with significant developmental changes. Likewise, it would be inappropriate to treat a 65-year-old adult the same as a 100-year-old adult as they are also at the extremes of a 35-year span. The specific physiologic changes between the two adult patients are distinct from those that separate a child from an adult, but the principle is the same. Failing to recognize the potential for altered response to medication therapy across the age span can result in unwanted adverse outcomes.

Therefore, age is but one factor that must be considered within the context of overall health status and functional ability. In addition, despite age or health status, any given individual's health care needs are often addressed very differently depending on what environment that individual is living in or cared for in. Therefore, there are many avenues through which we can arrive at a description of the geriatric patient. This presents an inherent problem when it comes to medical decision making for the geriatric patient because it can be difficult to know if, or how, to best apply evidence-based strategies to those individuals who may not actually be represented in the population the evidence was derived from. While general treatment principles are important to understand, clinicians must also recognize the heterogenicity of the population we refer to as geriatric. This presents a tricky balance for our society and health care system: Providing optimal healthcare to a huge and growing population while recognizing the differing needs of subgroups.

The purpose of this chapter is to outline the distinctions within the geriatric population and present the many challenges faced by healthcare providers and caregivers in working with this diverse group. The chapter discusses the various roles of the healthcare team and the different care venues. And more importantly, it addresses the problems inherent in the health-care system that allows for suboptimal care in this very vulnerable population.

Subpopulations of Elderly Patients

For practical purposes, there is a need to classify subgroups so that the approach to the elderly patient can be structured and evidence based, yet as specific as possible to individual needs. Interpretation of clinical literature should be performed with these considerations in mind.

There are three primary angles from which to evaluate the applicability of the evidence base to an older patient. They are age strata, health or functional status, and living/care environment. Each of these can impact the way a health intervention is delivered, how safe or effective it is, or how it can be monitored or evaluated.

Age Strata

Sometimes cohorts of subjects in large studies or clinical trials are divided into age strata, and this can be one way of comparing and contrasting health outcomes or treatment effects in subgroups of geriatric patients. For instance, a subject population might be divided into groups by decades such as 60–70, 71–80, 81–90, or >90. Depending on the body of literature being evaluated, there is also terminology such as "young old" vs.

"old old" that suggests a similar, albeit more general, stratification of age.[4] The cut point between "young old" and "old old," while still somewhat arbitrary, is usually age 80 or 85 years. A focus on the "old old" population is becoming increasingly important given the rapid growth of this segment of the U.S. population.

The biggest challenge to evaluating differences in outcomes between groups is limitations in statistical power as a result of relatively low enrollment of subjects, particularly in the upper age strata. This can hamper the ability to detect a difference in outcomes for these patients. For this reason, sometimes the most useful information that comes from evaluating the age range of subjects in a study or clinical trial is the recognition of the upper age limit for which there is meaningful data. This can be determined by examining not just the average age of study subjects, but the upper end of the age range reported in a clinical study's subject characteristics. Based on this data "ceiling," a clinician must determine whether it is appropriate to assume that an outcome can be extrapolated to the oldest patients.

In addition, age is one of several considerations that are included in estimates of prognosis. The risk/benefit decision making that must occur when deciding whether to implement a medication intervention includes an assessment of how long it is expected for the treatment effect to be realized and whether the individual is likely to live long enough achieve that benefit, especially if there are risks associated with exposure to the medication.

Health or Functional Status

Sometimes, patients with certain co-morbidities or disabilities are excluded from research protocols, and therefore clinicians must make judgment calls about the risk benefit of employing "usual treatment" in patients with multiple co morbidities or functional deficits. In addition to concerns about how medication therapy outcomes may be altered by drug-disease interactions in an individual with complex comorbidities, there are multiple ways in which functional status can affect the likelihood of achieving healthy aging.[4] Cognitive function and physical function are two domains where deficits can significantly affect medication outcomes. In these cases, this may not be directly related to a drug's pharmacology, but to inappropriate medication administration or monitoring.

An individual with mild cognitive impairment who manages their own medication regimen may be vulnerable to poor adherence or medication self-administration errors. Such an individual may also be less able to self-monitor for efficacy and may not appropriately interpret or report potential side effects. Problematic medications may include those with narrow therapeutic windows, such as warfarin, or medications which require specific technique to administer, such as bisphosphonates. These may be the interventions of choice from a drug-disease standpoint, but their safe use requires consideration of logistical hurdles, which, if not overcome, can tip the balance of benefit to risk.

Similar concerns apply for individuals with deficits in physical function, as medication taking ability can be affected by altered vision, coordination, motor function, or swallowing function. Functional deficits may also affect decisions about the appropriateness of medication therapy as it relates to prognosis. For instance, bladder antispasmodics can provide a significant benefit for an individual with urge incontinence, but consider how the ratio of benefit to risk is altered in an individual who is functionally dependent for all their personal care, and who is dependent upon incontinence undergarments despite the use of the medication.

Living or Caregiving Environment

Living or caregiving environment can impact an individual's risk factors for certain illnesses, accessibility to diagnostic tests/procedures, ability to access, administer or receive treatment, and ability to undergo appropriate follow-up. Whether interpreting epidemiology data or clinical outcomes in clinical literature, it is important to consider the setting in which the research was conducted. For instance, studies that evaluate the risk of falls and related injury will identify different fall rates and risk factors in the community setting vs. the long term care setting. Likewise, a clinical

trial that demonstrated a treatment benefit of a medication in an independent-living community population may not achieve the same outcomes in a population of hospitalized patients. Lastly, the ability to insure that a clinical intervention can be implemented and monitored in the same manner as in a clinical trial depends upon the resources available to the individual in the environment where they live. Does the patient have to drive to an office or clinic to receive care by a health professional? Do they qualify for reimbursement to receive services in the home? Does the environment provide medication administration assistance? If so to what degree? Is there 24-hour supervision for assistance with daily activities and monitoring of health status?

 KEY POINT: Subgroups can be defined in numerous ways; three of the most common are age strata, health or functional status, and living environment.

When evaluating the applicability of the clinical literature to a geriatric subgroup, there are several factors to consider.

1. Are there any studies or clinical trials designed for, or conducted in, populations that mirror the characteristics of the sub-group in question?

2. If not, are there other types of publications involving geriatric patients that might shed light on the nature of medication response? (For example, there may be no clinical trials of a medication in elderly populations, but there may be case reports that describe either treatment response or adverse events in older patients.)

3. Failing this, broaden the search to literature in the general adult population. Evaluate the inclusion/exclusion criteria or baseline characteristics of the study population. Are there any subjects included that are representative of the sub-group in question? If so, how many?

It is also important to be careful about interpreting the applicability of consensus guidelines in the adult population for geriatric patients. It is important to consider whether the guideline is specific to older populations, or if not, if there is any elderly-specific language included. If recommendations are made for the older patient, it is imperative to determine whether the guideline identifies specific subgroups of the elderly population or if it suggests that the recommendation is universal to all older patients. Regardless, a good strategy for the clinician to employ is to evaluate the individual studies cited by the guideline as support for the recommendation. After evaluating the inclusion/exclusion criteria and baseline characteristics of the populations in those studies, it can be determined whether application or extrapolation is appropriate to all older patients.

KEY POINT: Clinical literature must be scrutinized to determine how elderly patients are represented.

Venues of Care
Who Provides Care?

Many individuals provide care to older patients. Formal health care services are provided by physicians, nurses, pharmacists and allied health professionals. Specific credentials are not required to care for older patients. In fact, with the exception of those who specialize in Pediatrics, almost all health professionals will provide care to older patients regardless of their discipline or practice setting. Based on the growth of the oldest strata of the population, competence in geriatric care will be imperative for virtually all health professionals. However, there is a growing need for health professionals with expertise in this area, and various training is available for health professionals wishing to specialize in geriatric care.

Physicians

Physicians in almost all areas of specialty will have significant interactions with older patients.

Many physicians who have practices largely comprised of older patients may have earned, through experience, significant practical knowledge about meeting the special needs of this population, however official recognition as a **geriatrician** implies additional training and certification.[5] There are two primary routes of such. This first is via examination, where a certificate in added qualifications in geriatric medicine is available to physicians in the areas of internal medicine or family medicine. Other added qualifications offered by examination include certification in osteopathic geriatrics or geriatric psychiatry.[6] The other route is through fellowship training in geriatrics. A fellowship of 1–3 years in the specialty area of geriatrics is usually completed after residency training in either internal medicine or family medicine.[5]

Nurses

Nurses of all levels of training provide care to older patients across a broad spectrum of care venues. There are four certification exams available for nurses in gerontology, at the associate degree/diploma level or baccalaureate level for registered nurses, and at the advanced practice level, for clinical nurse specialists in gerontological nursing or **gerontological nurse** practitioners.[7]

Although elderly patients make up 90% of long term care populations and 80% of home care visits[8] most of these individuals are not cared for by nurses with this level of training. In many environments, the majority of care is provided or supervised by licensed vocational nurses (LVNs) or **certified nurse's assistants (CNAs),** also called nurses aides. In long term care environments, the majority of staff is made up of nurses aides and these individuals provide the day-to-day hands on care required by facility residents. Supervision of this care is usually provided by LVNs in the role of charge nurse. Registered nurses usually serve in administrator roles, such as director of nursing, in these environments. Long term care regulations require facilities to have at least one full time RN but this requirement must often be waived, particularly in rural areas, due to lack of available workforce. Home health agencies or health clinics associated with **assisted living facilities** or senior housing centers are also staffed in a similar way.

Pharmacists

Pharmacists provide care to older patients in a variety of settings, and pharmacists in the community setting perhaps have the most frequent opportunities for interactions with older patients. However, one of the most prevalent areas of practice where the focus is geriatric pharmacotherapy is in long-term care facilities (LTCF). Every licensed LTCF must retain the services of a pharmacist to provide drug regimen review and consultation on other services related to drug acquisition, labeling, storage, security, administration, documentation, and destruction. The primary responsibility of the pharmacist is to identify medication-related problems and to formulate interventions to prevent or resolve them. Pharmacists often provide similar services in Assisted Living facilities, home based programs, hospices, and other specialized care settings that focus on the older individual. In the outpatient setting, such as a clinic, pharmacists may see patients in conjunction with a patient's primary care physician. Specific credentials in geriatrics are not required to practice in long-term care or other areas of geriatric practice, however, there are options for obtaining additional training or credentials in this area. Geriatric specialty residencies are available at many institutions, and the Commission for Certification in Geriatric Pharmacy has been offering credentials as a **certified geriatric pharmacist (CGP)** since 1997.[9] This certification is voluntary but has become increasingly popular among individuals with geriatric practice focuses. The process involves an evaluation of education and experience in the principles of geriatric pharmacotherapy and in the provision of pharmaceutical care to the elderly and an examination, and periodic recertification is required. The American Society of Consultant Pharmacists provides an educational programming that pharmacists can enroll in to prepare for this exam.

Other Health Professionals

Specialized care to address functional deficits associated with morbidity and functional decline are often provided by physical therapists, occupational therapists, and speech therapists. Their services are part of the skilled care that is provided to individuals during or after hospitalization, but can also be provided as outpatient or home based care. Physical therapists focus on motor function, range of motion, balance, strength and endurance. Occupational therapists differ from physical therapists, focusing on the performance of activities of daily living. Speech therapists not only address language/communication difficulties, but swallowing function and cognitive skills. Other professionals who provide care to older adults include dieticians, social workers, recreational therapists, or psychologists.

Interdisciplinary Teams

One of the most comprehensive forms of care for an older patient is by an **interdisciplinary team** of health professionals. Skilled nursing facilities, specialized clinics, hospital systems, or academic health sciences centers may offer the services of a geriatric Assessment team. Due to the interdisciplinary nature of such a team, patients can undergo comprehensive examination, screening, medication review and other evaluation. Such teams may either serve as the patient's primary source of health care follow-up, or may serve on a consultation basis to provide recommendations from an expert group to the patient's primary physician. The core disciplines in such a team usually include representatives from medicine, nursing, pharmacy, physical therapy, occupational therapy, speech therapy, and social services. Many teams also include broader participation of professionals such as dieticians, psychologists, recreational therapists, clergy or others based on the patient's needs. Depending on the institution's resources, these teams may also have access to consults or participation by specialists such as neurologists, cardiologists, psychiatrists, ophthalmologists, podiatrists, or dentists, to name a few.

Demographics of the Healthcare Force

The rapid growth in the geriatric population has been well described. In 2002 one in eight individuals were older than age 65, and this is expected to increase to one in five by the year 2030.[10] Unfortunately, the growth of the workforce that is trained to care for these individuals has not grown at a rate commensurate with this population's needs.

As of 2008, there were 7590 board-certified geriatricians in the United States.[6] This is less than 25% of the number estimated to be needed to meet the health care needs of today's population of elderly patients. Of the 468 first-year fellowship training slots open in 2006–2007, only 54% were filled. There has also been a decline in the number of United States medical school graduates entering geriatric fellowships with only about 0.5% currently entering this area of practice. Most physicians entering geriatric fellowships are from medical schools outside the U.S., with 184 of the 287 physicians entering fellowships in 2007 being international graduates.[11] Therefore, most elderly patients do not receive their primary physician care from an individual with these credentials.

In 2003, newly licensed nurses reported that older patients made up 62.5% of their patients.[12] However, less than one percent of Registered Nurses and less than three percent of advance practice nurses are certified in geriatric nursing.[13] In addition to the low numbers of nurses credentialed in geriatrics, there is a shortage of nurses in the health care workforce in general. There is also a shortage of nursing faculty, particularly in geriatric nursing, with 25% of nursing programs lacking a gerontological faculty member.[14] Nurses and nurses aids make up the "front line" of care for the huge population of older patients in almost every health care venue described in this chapter, and are in a position to either provide or oversee a significant proportion of the day-to-day hands on care that is delivered. Shortages in the workforce and in the training capacity, particularly in geriatrics, represents one of the most critical areas of weakness in the current health system.

Pharmacists' participation in senior care is a growing area of specialty focus. As with other health disciplines, most pharmacists will encounter older patients in their practice regardless of their practice setting, and there are no specialty credentials that are required. However, given the significant utilization of drug therapy by the older population and the rising concern with adverse drug outcomes, there is a growing need for pharmacists to serve as patient advocates in this area. Currently, the number of pharmacists who have

completed specialty residency training in geriatrics is small, but there is a growing number of pharmacists who have obtained certification in geriatric pharmacotherapy via the CGP examination.[9]

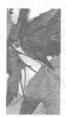

KEY POINT: One of the biggest challenges in providing tailored care to elderly patients is a lack of health care professionals who are specially trained in the principles of geriatrics.

Where Is Care Provided?

The continuum of care for elderly populations includes both chronic and acute care. Chronic care not only includes the day-to-day management of chronic disease states, but also may involve the maintenance of activities of daily living or provision of cognitive supervision. These services can be provided in the home, in assisted living facilities or other specialized senior housing, or in long term care facilities.

As for acute care, elderly patients also make up over 50% of hospitalized populations.[8] Compared to populations under age 65, patients have more frequent admissions to the hospital, have longer average lengths of stay, and have special needs in the emergency room or in the hospital.[8] They are particularly vulnerable to adverse outcomes such as delirium or residual disability after acute illness. Rehabilitation services, such as in a skilled nursing facility, are often required to assist a patient to regain strength and function before being discharged back to the living environment where they receive chronic care. As such, elderly patients are consumers of multiple venues of care.

Home-Based Care

Most individuals prefer to live in their own home for as long as possible, however, declining health status can result in disability that makes this difficult or unsafe. It may be possible to continue living in a private home in the community setting provided the proper support is available from either formal or **informal caregivers** or services.

Informal support is most often provided by a family member, usually a spouse or adult child, but depending on an individual's needs there are a variety of services for hire to assist an individual with day-to-day needs. This might include assistance with housekeeping, transportation, meal preparation, or other services for which no health care professional credentials are required. Individuals with more significant health needs may require assistance with personal care such as bathing, dressing, grooming, toileting, or ambulating. Assistance with medication management is also common. While it is very common for individuals to arrange services of this nature with individuals who are not health professionals, the front line of home based care is made up of home health agencies. Nurse aids may provide day-to-day personal care, but home health nurses are required to perform patient assessments and treatments such as intravenous therapy or PEG-tube or ostomy care. One of the biggest challenges to the provision of care by these agencies is the ability to achieve adequate staffing of trained caregivers, especially in rural areas, due to workforce shortages. In some instances, the Area Administration on Aging (AoA) can be a resource at the local/county level for locating available services.[15]

Physician visits in the home are possible in some areas, but these services are not wide spread. Typically, transportation must still be arranged to access physician care in an office or clinic. An alternative to this may be home visits by advance practice nurses such as nurse practitioners, who can extend the service range of the physician and can change medication therapy orders.

In this setting, access to both prescription and over the counter medications is generally through community pharmacies or mail order pharmacies. Home health agencies generally do not include consultant pharmacist services to provide drug regimen review, medication therapy interventions, or collaborative drug therapy management services, however entrepreneurial pharmacists have created unique practices of this nature in some outpatient settings.

Physical therapy, occupational therapy, speech therapy, or clinical lab services can also be arranged in the home setting.

Adjuncts and Alternatives to Home-Based Care

When an individual's lifelong home is not practical, options such as senior housing or life care communities present alternatives to placement in an institutional setting. Senior housing is often just a high-rise or campus of apartments, condominiums, or garden homes that cater to the needs of older individuals. Such settings may offer amenities such as housekeeping, laundry services, security, maintenance, fitness centers or social activities. Some may also provide transportation services or even have an on-site clinic with access to nursing staff. A life care community is based on the concept of "aging in place." It provides a continuum of private apartments, assisted living apartments, skilled nursing units and long term care units, all in one campus-style location. Individuals buy a residence in the community but also pay a monthly fee. For this investment, a community resident could move between any level of care as needed based on health status, while always paying the same monthly fee regardless of the extent of daily care required.[16]

For individuals who cannot be left alone but do not have a 24-hour caregiver, or for those whose primary caregiver is a family members who must work outside the home, adult day centers can provide a solution that allows the individual to continue to live in his or her home while providing socialization, supervision, or assistance during the day. Daytime meals, assistance with daily activities, or medication administration is often available.

A PACE program (Program of All-Inclusive Care for the Elderly) is an optional benefit under Medicare or Medicaid for individuals frail enough to be eligible for long-term care. In states that offer this benefit, this program bundles services in a comprehensive package that can be delivered at home or in adult day centers. PACE medical teams usually include primary care physicians, nurses, physician's assistants, occupational and recreational therapists, social workers, personal care attendants, dieticians, and drivers. Pharmacists are sometimes involved. The services must include all Medicare and Medicaid services provided by that state. Enrollees pay a premium each month and PACE receives a fixed monthly reimbursement from Medicare and Medicaid.[17]

Assisted Living Facilities

Individuals who require additional assistance with daily activities but who do not require the 24-hour care of a **long term care facility** may be a candidate for an assisted living facility (ALF). These environments are similar to senior housing but usually provide more structured services. In addition to those previously described, these setting usually provide all meals, on-site nursing services, medication administration assistance, and assistance with some activities of daily living. Although residents of an ALF may require some assistance with daily activities, they must be safe enough to remain unsupervised within their apartment and must have at least some ability to get around and transfer from bed to chair to commode. Residents may require adaptive equipment or assistive devices, but they must be able to accomplish these tasks under their own power.

While an ALF provides more formal services, it is not regulated in the same way as long term care. The LTCF requirements for frequency of physician follow-up, drug regimen review by a pharmacist, or specific patient assessment and monitoring by nursing staff are not mandated in the ALF setting at the federal level. This setting is regulated at the state level, so requirements may be more or less stringent based upon location.

Long Term Care Facilities

Individuals requiring the highest level of care may require long-term care placement. Long-term care may also be the only option for someone who does not require the highest level of care, but for whom proper caregiving resources in their own home are not available or affordable. These environments provide 24-hour care and there are strict state regulations under the Department of Health and Human Services (DHHS) that govern the day-to-day operations of licensed facilities. Facilities that receive reimbursement from Medicaid or Medicare must also comply with federal regulations under the Centers for Medicare and Medicaid Services (CMS). These regulations govern staffing requirements, the frequency of physician follow-up and the frequency and scope of consultant pharmacist activities. The facility operations manual and interpretive guidelines provide specific requirements for medication documentation, administration, monitoring, storage, labeling, and security.

Medicaid is the largest payer for long-term care, and facilities that receive reimbursement under Medicaid must dedicate a proportion of their facility beds to the care of individuals who quality for Medicaid based on income. Facility residents must expend available resources in a process commonly termed "spending down" until they qualify for Medicaid.

Facilities that receive reimbursement from Medicare are generally referred to as "skilled" nursing facilities (SNFs). Medicare does not pay for long term residential care but will provide reimbursement for short-term rehabilitation or other specialized care as a transitional step after hospital discharge.

An alternative to the traditional long term care setting is a Green House.[18] This is a small facility that is home to up to 10 residents with a 24 hour "universal worker," called a shabaz, who attends to daily needs. The concept is based upon the Eden Alternative, where the environment is home-like and centered around the individual and is intended to allow "aging in place" with a small group of residents and staff with whom close relationships can be formed. The Green House project began in 2005 and there are currently 20 Green Houses in 16 states. Depending on the location, the facilities vary in whether they are licensed as long-term care or skilled facilities, and therefore whether reimbursement is available from Medicaid or Medicare. Mechanisms for arranging formal health care services and regulations mandating the frequency of follow-up will also depend upon licensure status.

Emergency Rooms and Hospital Environments

In most acute care environments, elderly patients are cared for as part of the general adult population and the majority of hospitals and emergency rooms do not have specialized units or care teams for geriatric patients. Therefore all staff members need to be aware of the special needs of frailer patients in order to provide optimal care and to avoid iatrogenic problems. This includes, in part, an understanding of age-related changes in physiology that affect risk of disease, cause atypical clinical presentation, and alter medication response. Subsequent chapters of this text will describe the principles of geriatric Assessment, age-related changes in pharmacokinetics or dynamics, and an organ-system approach to pathophysiology and pharmaceutical care. In this chapter, it is also worth mentioning the specific aspects of the care environment that are not always conducive to an elderly patient's needs.

For instance, consider the care that is taken to prevent loss of a patient's personal effects upon admission to the emergency room. Personal clothing, glasses, hearing aids, dentures, and other belongings are usually removed, bagged, and labeled. Patients are provided with a hospital garment and though in most cases a patient may not need to be physically restrained, the placement of intravenous lines or catheters essentially restrict the patient to the bed. It is isolating and confusing for most individuals to feel, in addition to the illness or injury that caused the admission, cold and unable to see, hear, or speak well, or be able to move around. These processes are expedient and perhaps necessary given the specific circumstance, but consider the coping abilities of an individual in this circumstance if there is underlying cognitive impairment or in a patient who is at risk for mental status change or delirium due to their illness. If agitation results, either in the emergency room or in the hospital units, elderly hospitalized patients are vulnerable to the prescribing of chemical restraints, an intervention which may be crucial for the delivery of safe care in cases where the patient presents a danger to self or others, but which can be problematic if not used judiciously.

Elderly patients are also particularly vulnerable to the effects of immobility associated with hospitalization. Thromboembolism and infection are two of the most significant adverse outcomes often thought of as being related to immobility, but pressure ulcers, exacerbation of pain and constipation, increased vulnerability to orthostasis, deconditioning/muscle weakness, functional decline, and falls are common. Medication therapy can di-

rectly or indirectly exacerbate the risk of each of these. Last, elderly patients are vulnerable to iatrogenic harm caused by preventable adverse drug events, which will be discussed in Chapter 5.

The Continuum of Care

Challenges for Seniors Moving from One Care Venue to Another

The three most significant barriers to the assurance of good care are availability, cost, and coordination. The demographics of the geriatric population and the paucity of the healthcare workforce have already been discussed. The availability of assisted living apartments or long term care beds is also inadequate to meet population demands. The costs associated with specialized services can also be prohibitive for individuals on a fixed income, especially if savings are depleted by costs associated with chronic disease care. Residential care in a LTCF is generally financed on a private pay basis and in the United States the average cost per year ranges from $66,000.00–$76,000.00 ($187.00/day semi-private room, $209.00/day private room).[19]

Medicare benefits provide coverage for hospital or physician office visits and up to 100 days (per illness) of skilled nursing care after hospitalization under Parts A and B, and a prescription drug benefit under Part D, but Medicare does not pay for assisted living or long-term care. Medicaid does provide long-term care benefits to individuals who qualify based on income, but the biggest challenge is the availability, or lack thereof, of Medicaid beds in many long term care facilities where there may be extensive waiting lists. Unfortunately, for this reason selecting a long term care environment often becomes less a matter of choice and more often a matter of first-available spot. In the home based care environment, there are a variety of mechanisms for funding various services, but these are inconsistent from state to state in terms of who is eligible and what services are covered.

In addition to availability and cost considerations, another risk for elderly patients is the risk associated with moving from one care to another. Pharmacists are no doubt familiar with the concept of polypharmacy. The premise is that the more medications on the regimen, the more complex the pharmacological reactions between compounds and between disease states, increasing the vulnerability to increased cost, medication error, interaction, adverse reaction, morbidity, or even mortality. A similar concept in geriatric health care is "polyvenuism." The more an older patient, who may already be frail due to multiple co-morbidities or functional deficits, is shuttled between health care settings and health care providers, the higher the risk of miscommunication, gaps in information, medical or medication error, and adverse outcomes.

Current standards of care require health care institutions to employ safe medical practices and most employ some method of medication reconciliation upon admission or discharge. However, there is no requirement that each distinct environment employ uniform methods of carrying this out. Each health care environment will employ their own system of documentation and clinical records maintenance. Therefore, the same safeguards that exist within a health care environment may not exist between health care environments.

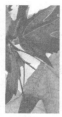 KEY POINT: Older patients are consumers of multiple care venues, and there are not always failsafe mechanisms to facilitate communication between these venues.

Once back in an out-patient environment there are also challenges to providing streamlined care. Coordinating the care provided by all of the care vendors is challenging. From physicians' offices (including primary care physicians, their mid-level practitioners, and any number of specialists), to home visits by nurses, therapists or other caretakers, to the community pharmacy, individuals not only receive care from multiple venues, but the documentation of that care is maintained in separate records sources. If a home health agency is involved, it may be possible to compile most relevant health information into a comprehensive medical record, as medical history data, treatment orders, medication orders, therapy orders, assessment data, and laboratory monitoring are generally ordered through the same agency. By contrast, an independent individual who coordinates their own health care and receives services in what could be described as an "a la carte" fashion would be the sole source of complete health care information, regardless of what data is maintained by each health professional involved in their care. Of note, it must be recognized that in either of the above scenarios, pharmacists are still "external vendors," as home health agencies do not have their own pharmacies and could not mandate use of a particular pharmacy even if they did. A patient will have the freedom of choice in pharmacy services, and may use more than one pharmacy. Therefore, it is important to remember that the medication lists maintained by other health professionals or by a home health agency is merely reflective of the current intent for medication orders, and specific (and repeated) "brown bag" medication and adherence review is often necessary to ascertain whether such medication list accurately mirrors what the patient is actually filling and taking. In such a review, the pharmacist would collect all available pill bottles, containers of over-the-counter or supplement products, and other materials related to medication taking or medication monitoring that the patient could provide and compile a complete medication history along with an assessment of patient adherence, level of understanding or health literacy, and to the extent possible, assessment of medication outcomes.

Access to Medication/Pharmacy Services Across the Continuum of Care

An individual's access to prescription and over the counter medications is usually through community or mail order pharmacies throughout most of the continuum of care. As such, it is the community pharmacist who has perhaps the greatest opportunity for interaction with geriatric patients.

In home based care, senior housing, and assisted living an individual will retain their choice of pharmacy provider(s). This is also true in long-term care. While long term care facilities with skilled nursing units will contract with a specific pharmacy vendor to provide medications under Medicare Part A, individuals receiving residential care may still choose from any pharmacy provider that will supply medications to a LTCF. The major difference, of course, between these settings has more to do with who controls medication acquisition, administration, and monitoring: the patient or a caregiver.

Independent community-dwelling individuals are responsible for their own medication purchases, refills, adherence, technique, self-monitoring, and self-reporting of outcome. The primary means of identifying efficacy outcomes or ADRs is through patient self-report. This means that there must be a mechanism for one or more health professionals to interact with patients on a regular basis to perform specific evaluations of medication therapy. The importance of medication review is widely accepted, and most health professionals perform this to some degree during their interactions with all patients, but it could be argued that there are barriers to the optimal performance of this task, and that recognizing and overcoming these barriers could help with the significant problem associated with adverse drug outcomes in elderly populations.

For instance, a thorough medication review should have the appropriate time dedicated to evaluating all indications, drugs, doses, intervals, durations, interactions, contraindications, adverse effects, efficacy endpoints, cost and adherence. This activity also must include all over the counter or herbal/supplement products. Time should also be spent in assuring that the patient understands the purpose of each medication, what to expect/how to monitor, and how to administer, especially for those medications requiring special technique. This often requires more time that can be afforded during a physician office visit or a home-care nurse visit. In addition, the frequency of patient encounters can vary. Some patients may see their doctor once a year or less, and in such situations the data from even a very thorough medication review can become outdated quickly.

Pharmacists can provide medication review and can bring a high level of expertise in drug therapy to this task, but there are also barriers to optimal review for these health professionals as well. In the community setting, pharmacists may be limited as to the data they have access to. Pharmacy databases are limited to the history of prescriptions filled or refilled within that pharmacy or pharmacy chain, or at least to those prescriptions filled under that individual's prescription drug plan. These databases also do not contain full medical history information. While history taking or basic patient assessment by the pharmacist can elicit some pertinent information related to indications for each medication and efficacy or side effect outcomes, these activities are often hindered by time constraints or reliability of patient report.

In settings where medication assistance or medication administration is provided by a nurse or nurses aide, patients may or may not be aware of what medications they take or why or how they should be administered and are vulnerable to medication error by the health professional. In these settings, such as in long-term care, a consultant pharmacist has access to the medical record and a more thorough evaluation of drug therapy outcomes may be possible, but such individuals often do not have the ability to intervene prospectively, at the time of prescription processing. A consultant pharmacist can periodically oversee a staff member passing medications and make recommendations about proper administration, but is usually not going to be able to do so before the first dose is administered. Periodic drug regimen review can also identify medication-related problems, but this is usually limited to the identification of problems associated with medications for which administration has already commenced, and in some cases, such as with antibiotics, the course of medication therapy may be initiated and completed in between chart reviews, making the ability to intervene in the case of inappropriate drug, dose, interval, route, duration, or monitoring very difficult.

By contrast, inpatient settings usually have on-site pharmacies that supply medications to patients during the time they are on the health care facility's service. In these environments the same department that has the prescription processing responsibilities also has the access to the complete medical record, perhaps making drug therapy intervention for medication related problems easier for all patients in that environment, not just older patients. Increasingly, pharmacy departments are staffed to provide pharmacist participation in both the pharmacy operations and medical team deliberations in the hospital units, but this is contingent upon whether an institution provides adequate allowances for budget and time to accommodate these services.

Another setting where the same institution can provide both types of services are Long-term care pharmacies that provide prescription processing, unit-dose packing, and delivery of product to long-term care facilities and also have a department of pharmacists that provide the required consultant services. Such pharmacies can provide bundled services at competitive costs, and skilled facilities or long term care facilities with skilled units can also contract with such pharmacies to provide medications to their residents under Medicare Part A. It should be recognized, however, that long term care facilities cannot mandate choice of pharmacy to residential-stay individuals, where choice of pharmacy vendor, much like the choice of personal physician, is a resident's right. That means that while a long-term care pharmacy may provide medications to all Part A recipients, they may not be the pharmacy vendor for all facility residents. Therefore, even if the long term care pharmacy is also the provider of consultant pharmacist services, there is still likely to be a proportion of patients for whom the consultant has no direct access to the order-entry portion of pharmaceutical care. In addition, the ability to intervene prospectively when a problematic drug is prescribed is not necessarily guaranteed in this setting as prescription processing data may not always be coordinated with the consultant pharmacists' practice. By contrast there are many consultant pharmacists who provide services freelance, either full- or part-time, who are not associated with a long term care pharmacy.

Long-term care is the only setting that is mandated to retain the services of a consultant pharmacist. [20] Consultant pharmacists must perform a drug regimen review for every resident of a LTCF every 30 days and submit recommendations about drug therapy problems to the director of nursing or the medical director. These recommendations do not have to be accepted and implemented, however they do have to be acted upon, meaning that a recommendation or request must be answered with either an "agree" or "disagree" and a rationale should be provided if the prescriber feels that implementing the change is not appropriate. Consultants will also advise the facility about appropriate procedures for medication ordering, labeling, storage, security (particularly for controlled substances), administration, monitoring, and record keeping. Therefore, in addition to review of the medical records, consultants will periodically audit these processes, by inspecting medication rooms and medication carts, by observing the nursing staff pass medications, through periodic controlled substance inventory counts, and through reconciliation and destruction of expired or discontinued medications. Consultant pharmacists also often participate in facility oversight activities such as medical director's meetings or quality assurance monitoring.

Prescription processing services and drug costs are reimbursed via direct consumer payment or through prescription drug plans, including Medicare Part D, and medication regimen review and patient counseling is an expected part of this. However, based on the above discussion it is clear that additional pharmaceutical care is often necessary beyond this, in the home, in the clinic, or within the interdisciplinary team. Such services are not formally reimbursed by Medicare, Medicaid, or most third party insurance plans. Most pharmacist services of this nature are provided on a fee-for-service basis, through independently negotiated contracts between the pharmacist (or pharmacy) and the institution. Because long-term care is mandated to retain the services of a consultant pharmacist, these institutions will set aside a portion of their budgets for the provision of this service. In assisted living facilities or other care venues, contracting for pharmacist services is voluntary. In light of the significant challenges associated with adverse drug outcomes in the geriatric population, it is important to critically evaluate the potential cost savings of additional pharmaceutical care interventions in the various health care environments so as to determine how to design, provide, and budget for services of this nature.

Summary of Pharmacy Services

Whether the site of practice is the community pharmacy, the long-term care pharmacy, a hospital, a clinic, an interdisciplinary team, or a consultant practice, there are a few key areas for which the pharmacist provides vital input and expertise:

- Drug regimen review and identification of medication related problems

- Drug therapy interventions to prevent or resolve medication related problems

- Assessment of medication history or medication administration

- Assurance of continued drug therapy monitoring for safety and efficacy

- Advice about proper storage, handling and disposal of drug products

- Drug information and education

Pharmacist Contributions to the Health Care Team

There is a long way to go to improve the quality chasm described by the Institute of Medicine in our current health care system.[21] Older patients, especially those with complex medical histories, are vulnerable to the fragmentation of care that often results from healthcare that is delivered across multiple venues by multiple individuals with varying levels of geriatrics expertise. The IOM proposes the ability to work in interdisciplinary teams as one of five core competencies essential to meet the needs of the 21st century health care system.[21] The IOM states that "all health professionals should be educated to deliver patient-centered care as members of an inter-disciplinary team, emphasizing evidence-based practice, quality improvement approaches, and informatics" but the specific role of pharmacists in this team is currently being defined. There is a compelling need for pharmacists with geriatrics training to be a part of the emerging landscape of team care. However, the hope for reforms tomorrow does not help the patient seen in practice today. At this time, whether a formal team exists or not, there is no substitute for the health professional who is knowledgeable enough about where the current system is broken to recognize how their patients are likely to be vulnerable and to advocate or intervene on their behalf. In addition to understanding the age related changes in physiology that affect pharmacokinetics, pharmacodynamics, and quality of drug outcomes, today's pharmacists must be familiar with the logistical barriers to pharmaceutical care such as polyvenuism, inconsistent, incomplete or out of date medical records data, and asynchronous communication with other health professionals. Skill sets not only include knowledge of pathophysiology and drug therapy, but the ability to audit, investigate, reconcile or verify patient history or medication data, and to facilitate communication, education, and recommendations to patients and their caregivers about drug therapy concerns.

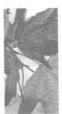

KEY POINT: Health professionals who understand the potential areas of vulnerability for an older patient in the health care system are in a better position to advocate for their patients.

Caregiver Burden

Who Is a Caregiver?

A general definition of a caregiver is an individual who assists with or performs functions for another who cannot perform them independently. The activities or functions referred to could be anything from assistance with home maintenance, meal preparation transportation or finances, all the way to personal care, such as personal hygiene/grooming dressing, eating, or ambulating. Based on such a definition almost all of us may find ourselves in the role of caregiver in some way during our lives. In healthcare, the definition of a caregiver is often divided into "formal" and "informal" categories. Formal caregivers are individuals who provide their services professionally, for a fee. Nurses and nurses aids in the long-term care, assisted living, or home health care industries usually come to mind when most people think of this group of caregivers, and it is often assumed that formal caregivers have training as a healthcare professional. However, "professional" caregivers are often hired in the role of "sitter" or "personal companion" and there is no specific training requirement to fulfill such a role. Informal caregiving is more often taken on by family members, whether a parent, child, spouse, or other relation, and in some instances by a friend or volunteer. While the American Red Cross can serve as a resource to provide basic training for informal caregivers,[22] this is voluntary and based upon availability. Informal caregivers are not paid for their time, and must balance caregiving responsibilities with other work or family commitments. In fact, the majority of adults who receive long-term care at home receive almost all of their care from unpaid family and friends.[23]

Caregiver and Care-Recipient Characteristics

It is estimated that 21% of the U.S. population over the age of 18 (approximately 44,443,800 individuals or 22,901,800 households) serves as a caregiver in some capacity for relatives or friends: 16% to individuals >50 years and 5% to individuals age 18–49.[23] Almost 79% of caregivers provide care to someone age 50 or older. Sixty one percent of caregivers are female, of an average age of 46, who provides an average of 20 hours or more per week in the caregiver role. These individuals are caring for mothers (34%), grandmothers (11%), or fathers (10%) with the average age of care recipients being 75 years. One in four of these caregivers report that the person they care for has Alzheimer's disease or other cognitive impairment.[23]

What Is Caregiver Burden?

Caregiver burden is defined as the caregiver's appraisal of the balance between care demands, resources, and the quality of the caregiver/care-recipient relationship, and may be a better predictor of the use of formal health care services than measures of the care recipient's mental or physical health or functional abilities.[24] There are two types of burden: that affecting personal decisions or activities, and those that affect the relationship between the caregiver and the care-recipient. There are also several levels of burden based upon the intensity of caregiving activities required. These levels range from Level 1, where caregivers perform no ADLs and spend only a few hours per week in caregiving activities, up to Level 5, where caregivers assist with at least two ADLs and provide care more than 40 hours per week.

Caregiver burden has a significant impact on both the physical and emotional health of the individual providing care. After controlling for age, gender, education, and other factors, there is a relationship between the level of care provided and the impact caregiving has on the caregivers perceived health. Higher caregiver burden levels also correlate with higher rates of unmet patient needs.

There has also been a "widower effect" described as a consequence of caregiver burden. A large study of married couples demonstrated the effect of hospitalization or death of one spouse on the health of another. After an individual is hospitalized, their spouse's risk of death increases and remains elevated for up to 2 years, with the greatest risk occurring within 30 days of the partner's hospitalization or death. During this initial 30 days, hospitalization of a spouse confers just as much risk of dying as the death of a spouse.[25]

Measuring Caregiver Burden

One of the most common instruments to quantify caregiver burden is the Zarit Index. This instrument evaluates strain by assessing time to self, feelings of stress or anger, strained relations with others, lack of privacy, effects on personal health, impedance on personal life, loss of control or choice. It also assesses whether caregivers feel guilt over not doing enough, or not knowing how best to provide care.[26]

Other instruments include the Caregiver Strain Index, Caregiver Burden Inventory, Caregiver's Burden Scale in End-of-Life Care, the Screen for Caregiver Burden, and the Caregiver Activity Survey.[27-31] They vary in their assessment of time, behavioral, physical, social, and emotional factors, as well as in the specific population of caregivers/care recipients tested. The utility in quantifying caregiver burden is several fold. First, a tool that allows recognition of caregivers at risk for poor outcomes as a result of significant burden can facilitate coordination of resources. In addition, assessments of caregiver burden have been employed in clinical trials evaluating the efficacy of interventions for frail elderly patients. For instance, the Resource Utilization in Dementia scale was included among the battery of tests administered in the evaluation of memantine for Alzheimer's disease.[32] Lastly, the ability to accurately quantify caregiver burden may have implications for public policy, especially as it relates to funding for elder care services. This is perhaps the most challenging aspect of caregiver burden assessment. Even scales that evaluate cost of care via estimates of time lost from wage earning employment or value of informal services provided do not completely quantify the total cost associated with informal care. This is a critical area that warrants further research due to the significant need to reduce the strain associated with informal caregiving.

Caregiver Resources and Strategies to Alleviate Caregiver Burden

Of the resources currently available to caregivers, most home and community based services programs are administered via State Units on Aging, with Area Agencies on Aging (AAAs) being the most common.[15] State programs use a variety of methods to track health care expenditures for the various services provided; therefore, there is no uniform method to assess costs nationwide. In general, funding for state programs comes from the National Family Caregiver Support Program, Medicaid waivers, the state's general funds, and individual contributions from recipients.

The most common service provided, available in all 50 states, is respite to family members. All but six states provide payment to families to provide care in at least one of their programs.[33] However, there is significant variability in the scope of services available form state to state. Differing eligibility requirements, service complexity, and fragmentation of services (even within a single state) have been cited as the most significant barriers to coordinating caregiver support. In addition, it is difficult to pinpoint how well state programs meet the needs of the populations they serve. Only 25% of states use a uniform assessment tool to evaluate home and community based care of the elderly, and in only five states does that assessment include a component related to family caregiving.[33]

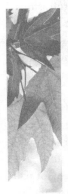

KEY POINT: A significant amount of the care for older individuals is provided by informal caregivers. While there are resources available to informal caregivers, they are not uniform across the country and there is not always a reliable mechanism for coordination or communication between formal and informal care.

Caregivers are essential keys to coordinating seamless care for frail patients. They are gatekeepers of information, coordinators of schedules, supervisors of treatment regimens, and often, the voice of the patient. When there are gaps in documentation, they often know the history that may not be found in the clinical record. When the clinician is struggling to determine whether a clinical presentation represents a significant change from a patient's baseline status, the caregiver knows the day-to-day norm. They can provide the personal details that remind us their loved one is an individual and not just a patient case. It is a position of power and vulnerability at the same time, as the caregivers themselves are vulnerable to stress, fatigue, and poor health outcomes. Health professional need to seek their input when evaluating a frail patient and when designing a care plan, not only to insure that the patient's needs are met, but to do so in a way that is appropriate based on the caregiver's abilities and needs.

CASE 1: USING A SUBGROUP PERSPECTIVE TO APPROACH THE LITERATURE

Setting:

Outpatient geriatric assessment clinic

Subjective:

95-year-old white female is brought to clinic by a family caregiver for a routine visit

Past Medical History:

Hypertension, mild Alzheimer's disease, osteoarthritis

Medications:

Donepezil 10 mg HS, acetaminophen 500 mg 1 tablet four times daily, multivitamin daily

Allergies:

NKDA

Social History:

Widowed, lives with daughter in daughter's home

Family History:

Non-contributory

Objective:

Physical exam unremarkable, vitals: BP 148/84 mmHg, HR 82, RR 20, T 97.8

Assessment:

The medical resident wishes to aggressively lower the blood pressure. He cites reduced risk of cardiovascular outcomes such as myocardial infarction with the attainment of a goal blood pressure of less than 140/90 per the Joint National Commission Guidelines, Seventh Report (JNC VII).[34] The guideline does, in fact, state that individuals over the age of 50 years should be treated the same as the general adult population, and indicates the same goal blood pressure. Is this guideline being appropriately applied to this patient?

Plan:

To answer the question posed in this case, it must be determined whether the adult treatment principles should be extrapolated to an elderly patient. The JNC VII guideline[34] is a well-respected, evidence based guideline, but does a recommendation for treatment of adults over 50 years apply to *all* geriatric patients? The first step in answering this question is to look at the references cited as support for this recommendation. Looking at the inclusion/exclusion criteria and baseline characteristics of subjects in the four major clinical trials evaluated, there does in fact appear to be evidence to support treatment of hypertension in an older population with at least stage II hypertension (baseline systolic pressure >160 mmHg) and a mean age of about 72 years, with the primary benefits being reduction in the risk of stroke and cardiovascular mortality. However, there are very few subjects included that were as old as the subject in this case, and none with the same stage of hypertension. This patient belongs to a subgroup that is not well represented by this guideline. To better decide if blood pressure lowing is appropriate, an additional literature search must be performed to identify data more pertinent to her subgroup. Data from meta-analysis such as INDANA or prospective trials such as the Hypertension in the Elderly Trial (HYVET), which evaluated treatment outcomes in the subgroup age 80 years and old may more closely represent this patient.[35-36] In addition, the literature search might yield studies that shed light on how drug therapy for hypertension affects her co-morbidities such as Alzheimer's disease.

Rationale:

The question posed in this case is not about whether or not to treat her hypertension (Chapter 7 will address the specific therapeutic issues related to hypertension in elderly patients) but whether a general adult treatment guideline applies to the patient in this scenario. Identification of the studies cited by the guideline and scrutiny of their baseline characteristics and inclusion/exclusion criteria are steps in ascertaining whether the data was derived from a population representative of this patient, or if a more tailored literature search is required.

Case Summary:

When the evidence is limited, choices about initiation of drug therapy will often become a judgment call, simply because an evidence-based treatment decision cannot be made for a patient who is not represented in the evidence base. This case illustrates but one disease state for which the clinician must question whether the adult treatment recommendation is the best course of action for this elderly patient.

CASE 2: COORDINATION OF CARE ACROSS MULTIPLE VENUES AND CAREGIVERS

Setting:

Private home of community dwelling individual

Subjective:

An 88-year-old African American man has just had two new prescriptions for ophthalmic eye drops presented to the pharmacist in a community pharmacy by way of a neighbor. He has called upon his friend to do this errand for him because he cannot drive due to poor vision. The friend declines medication counseling by the pharmacist stating "these aren't for me anyway" and reports that the patient has a home health nurse that visits each week who can help him.

Past Medical History:

Hypertension, hyperlipidemia, history of myocardial infarction 2003, and glaucoma

Medications:

Enalapril 10 mg twice daily, metoprolol 50 mg twice daily, pravastatin 40 mg at bedtime, aspirin 162 mg daily, timolol 0.25% solution, 1 drop each eye twice daily, latanoprost 0.005% solution, 1 drop each eye at bedtime (eye drops prescribed by ophthalmologist, not primary care physician)

Allergies:

PCN

Social History:

Lives alone, no close family

Family History:

Not known

Objective:

Physical exam not performed; vitals: last recorded vitals from a blood pressure check in the pharmacy include BP of 110/60 and pulse of 54 BPM.

Assessment:

This patient is receiving both formal and informal assistance from more than one venue or caregiver, and there are multiple ways in which this patient is vulnerable to a suboptimal outcome. They include:

At the pharmacy: The pharmacist filling the prescription has likely performed a drug regimen review and has offered counsel, but this has been declined.

Home health: The home health nurse who visits once weekly would not be able to assist with daily administration of the drops.

Physician: The prescriptions have been prescribed by an ophthalmologist, not the patient's regular doctor.

Plan:

To prevent a medication-related problem, this patient scenario must be assessed for opportunities to coordinate care. In optimal circumstances, communication would occur not only between the pharmacist and the patient or his caregiver, but could also occur between the pharmacist and the home health agency and physicians involved. Each health professional has data or information that the others don't. The pharmacist could provide medication counseling to the home health nurse, and can provide updated information about the current medication list and refills to the primary care doctor. The home health nurse can reinforce drug information about administration and self-monitoring to the patient, perform weekly vitals assessments and regularly ascertain medication understanding and inquire about adherence.

Rationale:

Coordination of care is necessary because this patient is vulnerable to potentially preventable adverse outcomes. In the pharmacy setting, even if medication counseling had been provided it would have to have been relayed through the patient's friend. Although the provision of written prescription information is required, this resident's poor vision may hinder the utility of this method of instruction. This is especially problematic due to the nature of the prescriptions that were filled. Ophthalmic drops require specific technique for proper instillation, and the administration of two eye drops requires adequate time be allowed in between drops for optimal absorption. Although the systemic effect of an ophthalmologic beta blocker preparation is likely small, this patient has had blood pressure and heart rate at the lower end of the desired range and there is a need to monitor any changes to these parameters. The home health nurse will not be able to administer these medications for him, but perhaps could provide education and evaluate weekly vitals, especially if there were communication from the pharmacist to alert the nurse why this was needed. In order to do this, there must be a mechanism for the pharmacist to ascertain which home health agency is providing care. With the dispensing of these two new prescriptions, the pharmacist would now have a more up-to-date medication list than would be available to the primary care physician, but by contrast, the pharmacist has no direct access to the medical record with a complete medical history, so while the pharmacist likely performed a drug-drug interaction check against the prescription history in the pharmacy database, the completeness of this check may be limited as pharmacist may not be aware if there are other medications that have been prescribed and filled elsewhere. The office of the primary care physician would maintain records about medical history and prescriptions ordered by that doctor but would not be aware of any potential interactions with the new medications until/if the patient returns to the office and provides a complete medication history, which may not occur until after the patient experiences a problem.

Case Summary:

Each health professional performs one aspect of the care of this patient, but all the parts do not equal a whole unless they are knitted together. Without coordination, this patient is vulnerable to subtherapeutic effect of the ophthalmic medications if not administered properly, or potential exacerbation of bradycardia if continuous monitoring of vitals is not insured while on both his antihypertensive regimen and his eye drops. Without communication between health professionals, there is no way for each member of the health care team to be aware that a potential problem exists. In traditional practices, the biggest barrier is a lack of a habitual or comfortable mechanism for each caregiver to communicate with one another. Is the relationship between pharmacist and doctor one that would facilitate notifications about updates, changes or concerns with drug therapy, either by phone or by fax? Does the home health agency maintain contact information for the patient's pharmacy of choice so as to have access to the pharmacist when drug therapy questions arise? If so, is such contact regularly made? Is the workflow in the pharmacy conducive to the performance of pharmaceutical care activities such as telephoning the patient and offering verbal counsel, or offering to coordinate counsel with the home health nurse if the patient is hard of hearing or would like a hands on demonstration of medication administration? For each answer of "no" to these questions, there is perhaps a hole in the safety net that is intended to knit this patient's care services together.

Clinical Pearls

Hospital Documentation vs. Long-term Care Facility Documentation

- *Upon transfer between the hospital and long-term care, the hospital's history and physical or discharge summary is often used as the admission history and physical in the long term care facility. Regulations allow this provided the document is authenticated as accurate and current by the resident's physician. However, it may not always be complete. Nursing facility regulations require that all medications, acute or chronic, must have a supporting indication for use, but hospital documentation may often be limited in scope to the primary medical conditions/medications pertinent to the inpatient admission, and the hospital's medication reconciliation may not always include data about history prior to admission or documentation of the rationale behind medication changes. Understanding that it can take up to 6 weeks to observe an adverse outcome resulting from a change in drug therapy made in the hospital, it is likely that many patients have been discharged to another care venue, such as a SNF or long-term care facility by the time before such a problem is realized. Therefore, decisions about medication continuation/discontinuation or duration of therapy are perhaps some of the most critical at the time of transfer, yet this is decision making that is often hampered by lack of complete data.*

Formulary Management

- *Formularies are common strategies to control costs and to standardize medication interventions for various clinical scenarios. These strategies work best in health care facilities where 1) there is a single pharmacy vendor, 2) there is one (or very few) third party payers, or 3) prescribers' clinical privileges are bound to the policies and procedures of the institution. The hospital setting is an example where a single formulary may apply, but in most other settings, there is no single vendor for medical or pharmacy services so there are any number of formularies that could be dictating choice of medication within the facility's population. As a patient moves from the hospital to skilled care to long-term care, formularies may change with each transition. For consultant pharmacists in long-term care, it is often difficult to know exactly which medications are on which formularies as these transitions occur. Therefore, it may be valuable for the consultant to record contact information for each individual patient's pharmacy vendor. In the event that questions arise about which product to recommend as part of a drug therapy intervention, the consultant could ascertain the appropriate options through that route.*

Chapter Summary

Based on what we know about the heterogenicity of the geriatric population, it is easy to understand why a health care force must include a strong group of professionals well-versed in the needs of this population. This introductory chapter has not only outlined the diversity of the geriatric population, but also of the available work force, care venues, services and programs. Subsequent chapters will provide further depth regarding the social, financial, physiological, and psychological vulnerabilities of this population, but the pertinent message of this chapter is that a thin and fragmented care and support network fundamentally exacerbates such vulnerabilities. Health care professionals who understand the cracks and deficits in our current health system may be in a better position to advocate for their patients. Recognizing different populations of elderly patients and using a subgroup perspective in the approach to the clinical literature allows for clinical decision making that is more tailored. Recognizing the type and availability of health care services, including the health care professionals who are providing them, can assist with the development of services to better meet the population's needs. On behalf of the geriatric population of today, as well as that of which we may each one day count ourselves a member, health care professionals must rise to meet the challenges described in this text.

Self-Assessment Questions

1. A health care diagnostics company has conducted a study of a new home machine that will allow patients who take warfarin to test and monitor their INR at home. The study demonstrated that regular home monitoring reduced the incidence of adverse events related to supratherapeutic INRs. Which of the following subgroups of elderly patients may present the greatest concern in applying this data?

   A. Individuals over the age of 85 years

   B. Individuals with cognitive impairment

   C. Individuals enrolled in home health care

   D. Individuals with recurrent antibiotic use for UTI

2. An assisted living facility offers a medication reminder service that entails assistance with the set-up of pill boxes and a daily visit by a nurse aide who will remind patients to take each dose and assess adherence via pill count. This individual can also take blood pressure and heart rate prior to the administration of any medication, if required. Which of the following medications would be most likely to be administered safely with the use of such a service?

   A. Atenolol 50 mg tablets, 1 tablet by mouth every morning

B. Alendronate 70 mg tablets, 1 tablet by mouth once weekly

C. Nitroglycerin 0.4 mg tablets, 1 tablet sublingually PRN chest pain

D. Zolpidem 5 mg tablets, 1 tablet at bedtime PRN insomnia

3. A 42-year-old woman who works outside the home and has school aged children has recently taken her mother into her home after hospitalization for hip fracture. Her mother has mild dementia and is currently mobile at a wheelchair level only. She requires supervision and assistance with activities of daily living, and she is eligible for Medicaid. Which of the following resources is most widely available to caregivers in this type of situation?

A. A long term care facility with a dedicated dementia-care unit and an open Medicaid bed

B. A life-care community where her mother could move between levels of care as needed

C. Respite care, such as an adult day center, identified through the Area Agency on Aging

D. A privately funded full time personal care attendant who will provide care in the home

References

1. Code of Federal Regulations, Title 21, Volume 4, Part 201. (21: CFR 201.57)

2. American Association of Retired Persons. Available at: http://www.aarp.org

3. Social Security online full retirement age calculator. Available at: http://www.ssa.gov/retirement/1960.html.

4. Depp CA, Jeste DV. Definitions and predictors of successful aging: a comprehensive review of larger quantitative studies. *Am J Geriatr Psychiatry*. 2006;14(1):6–20.

5. Stall RS. What is a geriatrician? Available at: http://stallgeriatrics.com. Accessed June 26, 2009.

6. Association of Directors of Geriatric Academic Programs (ADGAP) Longitudinal Study of Training and Practice in Geriatric Medicine. Training and Practice Update 2003;1(2):1–4.

7. American Association of Colleges of Nursing, The John A. Hartford Institute for Geriatric Nursing. *Older Adults: Recommended Core Competencies and Curricular Guidelines for Geriatric Nursing Care.* Washington, DC; 2000.

8. National Center for Health Care Statistics (2004). Home Health Care Patients: Data from the 2000 National Home and Hospice Care Survey. Available at: www.cdc.gov/nchs/releases/04facts/patients.htm

9. Commission for Certification in Geriatric Pharmacotherapy (CCGP). Available at: http://www.ccgp.org

10. Administration on Aging, U.S. Department of Health and Human Services. Available at: http://www.aoa.gov/AoARoot/Aging_Statistics/future_growth/future_growth.aspx

11. Association of Directors of Geriatric Academic Programs. Status of Geriatrics Workforce Study. Available at: http://www.adgapstudy.uc.edu

12. Wendt A. Mapping gerontological nursing competencies to the 2001 NCLEX–RN test plan. *Nurs Outlook.* 2003;51(4):152–57.

13. American Nurses Credentialing Center 2002. Available at: www.nursingworld.org/ancc

14. Berman A, Thornlow D. Your bright future in geriatric nursing. *NSNA Imprint* 2005;January:24–6.

15. Area Agencies on Aging, Available at: http://www.eldercare.gov/Eldercare.NET/Public/Network/AAA.aspx

16. What is a life care retirement community? Available at: http://www.lifecare.org/life_care_retirement.html

17. Program of All Inclusive Care for the Elderly (PACE) Overview. Available at: http://www.cms.hhs.gov/pace/

18. The Green House Project. Available at: http://www.ncbcapitalimpact.org/default.aspx?id=146

19. National Clearing House for Long Term Care Information. Available at: http://www.longtermcare.gov/LTC/Main_Site/Paying_LTC/Costs_Of_Care/Costs_Of_Care.aspx#What

20. State Operations Manual. Appendix PP—Guidance to surveyors of long term care facilities. Available at: http://cms.hhs.gov/manuals/Downloads/som107ap_pp_guidelines_ltcf.pdf

21. Greiner AC, Knebel E. Health Professions Education: A Bridge to Quality. Committee on the Health Professions Education Summit. Institute of Medicine. Washington, DC: National Academy of Sciences; 2003.

22. The American Red Cross. Preparing and Getting Trained, Family Caregiving. Available at: http://www.redcross.org/

23. National Alliance for Caregiving and AARP. Caregiving in the U.S.: Findings from the National Caregiver Survey 2004. Available at: http://www.caregiving.org/data/04finalreport.pdf

24. Potter JF. Comprehensive geriatric assessment in the outpatient setting: population characteristics and factors influencing outcome. *Exp Gerontol.* 1993;28(4–5):447–57.

25. Christakis NA, Allison PD. Mortality after the hospitalization of a spouse. *N Engl J Med.* 2006;354(7):719–30.

26. Zarit SH, Reever KE, Bach-Peterson J. Relatives of the impaired elderly: correlates of feelings of burden. *Gerontologist.* 1980;20:649–55.

27. Onega LL. Helping those who help others: the Modified Caregiver Strain Index. *Am J Nurs.* 2008;108(9):62–9.

28. Novak M, Guest C. 1989. Application of a multidimensional caregiver burden inventory. *Gerontologist.* 29;(6):798–803.

29. Dumont S, Fillion L, Gagnon P, Bernier N. A new tool to assess family caregivers' burden during end-of-life care. *J Palliat Care.* 2008;24(3):151–61.

30. Hirschman KB, Shea JA, Xie SX, Karlawish JS. The development of a rapid screen for caregiver burden. *J Am Geriatr Soc.* 2004;52:1724–9.

31. Davis KL, Marin DB, Kane R, Patrick D, Peskind ER, Raskind MA, Puder KL. The Caregiver Activity Survey (CAS): development and validation of a new measure for caregivers of persons with Alzheimer's disease. *Int J Geriatr Psychiatry.* 1997;12(10):978–88.

32. Reisberg B, Doody R, Stoffler A, Schmitt F, Ferris S, Mobius HJ. Memantine for moderate-to-severe Alzheimer's disease. *N Engl J Med.* 2003;348(14):1333–41.

33. The state of the states in family caregiver support: A 50-state study. Caregiver Alliance. National Center on Caregiving. Available at: http://www.caregiver.orgFamily

34. Chobanian AV, Bakris GL, Black HR, et al. The Seventh Report of the Joint National Committee on Prevention, Detection, Evaluation, and Treatment of High Blood Pressure: the JNC 7 report. *JAMA.* 2003;289:2560–72.

35. Gueyffier F, Bulpitt C, Boissel JP, et al. Antihypertensive drugs in very old people: a subgroup meta-analysis of randomized controlled trials. INDANA Group. *Lancet.* 1999;353(9155):793–6.

36. Beckett NS, Peters R, Fletcher AE, Staessen JA, Liu L, Dumitrascu D. HYVET study group treatment of hypertension in patients 80 years or older. *N Engl J Med.* 2008;358:1.

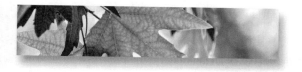

2

Ethical and Socioeconomic Considerations

SUSAN W. MILLER

Learning Objectives

1. Apply the tenets of biomedical ethics to ethical dilemmas commonly encountered in providing pharmaceutical care to geriatric patients.

2. Explain issues related to communication in the care of the geriatric patient, including informed consent, privacy and confidentiality, and surrogate decision making.

3. Describe patient, caregiver, family, and legal issues associated with end-of-life decisions.

4. Explain the effects of socioeconomic issues on access to pharmacy care by geriatric patients.

5. Describe medication financing options (including affordable medications) available for geriatric patients.

Key Terms

AUTONOMY: Respect for autonomy obliges health care professionals to honor the choices of adults with decision-making capacity; allows for a patient's right to self-determination, avoids paternalism, allows for the acceptance of the free choice of the patient, and ultimately permits the patient to make final decisions relating to his or her health care.

BENEFICENCE: Obliges health care professionals to help others and promote their welfare.

BLACK BOX WARNING: A notice in the prescribing information of a prescription medication that alerts prescribers and patients of severe or fatal side effects of the medication; often added retrospectively following the uncovering of the side effect in the routine use of the medication.

CULTURE: The group to which one belongs; extends beyond race and ethnicity to include age, gender, religion, and health beliefs.

DNR: Do not resuscitate; an order that states cardiopulmonary resuscitation (CPR) is not to be performed in the event of cardiac or respiratory arrest.

INFORMED CONSENT: A process in which a person learns key facts about a health care treatment, including potential risks and benefits, before deciding whether or not to accept the treatment.

JUSTICE: Obligation to treat patients who are equal, in relevant respects, in the same manner; giving what is due to patients.

LIVING WILL: A written, legal document that conveys the wishes of an individual in the event of a terminal illness; can convey the wishes of a one who is no longer able to communicate.

MANAGED CARE: A system created with the intent to control the cost of health care that uses financial incentives and management controls to direct patients to providers who are responsible for giving appropriate care in cost-effective treatment settings; financial risk is shared among the providers.

NONMALEFICENCE: An obligation to not inflict harm on others intentionally nor to engage in actions with foreseeable harmful effects; "At least, do no harm."

PROXY: A person authorized to act for another.

Introduction

Ethical and socioeconomic considerations are integral components in the delivery of health care to geriatric patients. Often the care of the geriatric patient centers on important decisions regarding health care choices and end-of-life issues for those who lack the mental capacity or physical ability to effectively communicate their personal choices. Access to health care, health care disparities, and financing health care are vital socioeconomic issues for older citizens. This chapter will describe ethical issues and socioeconomic considerations related to geriatric patients.

Ethics and Biomedical Ethics

Biomedical ethics is the branch of ethics concerned with the life of the patient and at the core of biomedical ethics are issues regarding the protection of life.[1] Table 2-1 provides examples of these issues. The promise to adhere to the principles of biomedical ethics is contained in the various oaths affirmed by health care professionals, including pharmacists. Of the various tenets of biomedical ethics four are particularly applicable in geriatric pharmacy practice. They are respect for (patient) **autonomy, nonmaleficence, beneficence**, and **justice**. Ethical dilemmas arise when these tenets are in conflict and a choice between two "rights" must be made. Biomedical ethics of-

ten involves situational ethics in which a particular situation may influence how one's reactions and values evolve in order to cope with changing circumstances. Caring for older adults provides frequent opportunity to apply these tenets as treatment choices are rarely straightforward.

Pharmacists are obligated to apply the tenets of biomedical ethics when providing pharmaceutical care for geriatric patients. For example, by providing full disclosure regarding the risk-benefit profile of medications, thus allowing the patient to make a personal choice as to whether to consume a particular medication, the pharmacist is providing patient care, as well as respecting autonomy, and acting with beneficence and nonmaleficence. The use of medications with a **black box warning** in the prescribing information can be a particularly difficult ethical dilemma for the pharmacist providing care for geriatric patients. Recently approved drugs may be more likely to have unrecognized adverse drug reactions (ADRs) than established drugs, especially in older frail patients. Serious ADRs commonly emerge after Food and Drug Administration approval and the safety of new agents cannot be known with certainty until a drug has been on the market for several years; yet physicians often prescribe new pharmacotherapeutic agents with the promise of improved efficacy and ease of dosing compared to older agents.[2] For example, the use of the newer classes of pharmacotherapeutic agents such as biguanides and thiazolidinediones can be prob-

Table 2-1. Issues in Biomedical Ethics

Biomedical Issue	Geriatric Specific Example(s)
Health care	Quality of life, public health issues
Patient rights	Privacy issues, decision-making regarding care options
Research in humans	Geriatric patients enrolled in clinical trials, translating research from younger cohorts into geriatric cohorts, obtaining informed consent
Organ transplants	Qualifications for receiving an organ transplant
Stem cell research	Cures for disease
Addiction	Treatment alternatives
Mental health	Use of psychotropic medications, involuntary treatment
Aging	Rationing of health care resources
Death and dying	ACDs, dying with dignity

lematic in the geriatric diabetic patient. Toxic metabolites of the biguanides can accumulate in patients with renal damage and heart failure and the thiazolidinediones can cause or exacerbate congestive heart failure. Both the biguanides and thiazolidinediones contain a black box warning in the prescribing information. Pharmacists have an ethical responsibility to inform patients of these potential effects and suggest the use of alternative oral antidiabetic agents (i.e., the sulfonylureas) that may be less potent, have less convenient dosing schedules, but fewer adverse effects. However, it is difficult for the community pharmacist who may lack detailed information about the patient's history, physical findings and laboratory results to know when the risk outweighs the benefit for an individual patient. Thus an ethical dilemma must be resolved.

Another example involves the use of atypical antipsychotic agents such as risperidone, ziprasidone, and quetiapine that are often prescribed off label to manage behaviors in elderly patients with dementia. The use of atypical antipsychotic agents is associated with increased mortality when used in elderly patients with dementia-related psychosis, mostly due to cardiovascular events or infectious diseases. The prescribing information for atypical antipsychotic agents contains this information in a black box warning. Pharmacists have the ethical responsibility to provide complete drug information to patients and/or surrogate decision makers

regarding potential nonpharmacologic and alternative pharmacotherapeutic options for behavior management. This particular situation is fraught with ethical issues as the patient with dementia may have difficulty providing input for his/her preferences, nursing home staff and family are frequently frustrated with behavior problems and busy physicians may not adequately evaluate all components driving the behaviors. The ideal scenario is for the pharmacist to participate in patient assessment meetings with other health care providers and including patients and surrogate decision makers, having each participant explain the problems objectively and discuss potential solutions. These interprofessional interactions result in a carefully chosen treatment plan devised with consideration of risk and benefit to the patient.

Pharmacists practicing as consultant pharmacists for institutionalized geriatric residents of skilled nursing facilities have a responsibility to make recommendations to add, modify, or discontinue pharmacotherapies in these patients following evidence-based medicine, disease management practice guidelines, algorithms or sound clinical judgment. The pharmacist should strive for a balance between beneficence and nonmaleficence in adhering to practice guidelines and making recommendations regarding drug therapy. Prior to the pharmacist making a recommendation to prescribe an antihyperlipidemic agent such as a statin for prevention and/or management of hypercholesterolemia in a specific geriatric patient, the life expectancy, effectiveness of therapy, adverse effects, and time to benefit should be taken into consideration. At issue is the general lack of high-quality evidence to use in assessing the risk/benefit in patients over the age of 80 years for most practice guidelines.

When individuals are unequal, in relevant respects, the obligation is to treat them in a fair manner and acting with justice means that those who have a greater need may rightly receive more of a particular resource than those with less need.[3] Pharmacists who immunize patients should follow the guidelines for administration of these vaccines. During the vaccination period prior to influenza season, pharmacists should apply the tenet of justice to provide protection for the most susceptible patients and prevent vaccine shortages. Justice, when applied to resource allocation in the provision of health care, is central to the debates over rationing of health care and whether health care is a right or a privilege.

Principles of Ethical Decision Making

Three principles of thinking that frame ethical decision making and are applicable in the patient care setting have been described by Kidder: ends-based thinking, rules-based thinking, and care-based thinking.[4] Ends-based thinking follows the maxim, "do whatever produces the greatest good for the greatest number." Decisions regarding the allocation of pharmacotherapy resources, as in cost-benefit analysis, are often rooted in ends-based thinking. Practical examples of ends-based thinking include implementation of therapeutic substitution within a formulary and the use of tiered copays in pharmacy benefit programs. Administration of influenza vaccine in all institutionalized patients will provide the best protection for that population against the disease. However, some patients may object or may be allergic to components of the vaccine, causing a fallacy in this line of thinking.

Rules-based thinking follows the maxim, "stick to your principles (the rules) and let the consequences follow." Decisions involving the obligation that the pharmacist owes to the patient follow rules-based thinking. An example of rules-based thinking is the provision of complete factual drug information to patients during counseling, including the most severe, albeit rare, adverse effects of the medication. Finally, care-based thinking follows the maxim, "do unto others as you would have them do unto you." The pharmacist's feeling of empathy for the patient is the result of care-based thinking. Examples of care-based thinking in the practice of pharmacy include providing drug information to patients receiving sample medications or whose insurance plan requires them to obtain their medications from mail-order pharmacies. The pharmacist who does not charge for this information will also not see a profit from sales of a prescription.

Respecting Choices

In the process of providing health care and pharmaceutical care to the geriatric patient, multiple opportunities exist for making choices relative to this care. Choices regarding the types of care necessitate full disclosure on the risks and benefits of each type; choices regarding privacy and confidentiality affect the delivery of care and personal heath information; a patient's **culture** can affect their health care beliefs and choices; and caregivers and family may take part in the shared responsibilities of the decision making. The tenets of biomedical ethics can be applied to the resolution of dilemmas that are central to the provision of health care for geriatric patients. The dependent nature of many geriatric patients can complicate the issues as the older patient may require assistance in making choices relative to health care. As a result of cognitive impairment or communication disorders, geriatric patients are often unable to express a preference for their health care matters. Publicized cases involving ethical issues have provided guidance for patients, family, and health care providers in the areas of establishing patient preference regarding health care decision-making and the right to die.[5] These cases have dealt with issues related to the persistent vegetative state,[6] physician-assisted suicide[7] and an individual patient's request for the right to die[8] as examples.

Communication between the pharmacist and the older patient is an additional factor involved in resolving ethical dilemmas and respecting health care choices of geriatric patients. Communicating with older patients can be especially challenging, secondary to extensive medical histories, multiple medications, and physiologic barriers that may complicate the interaction.[9] Pharmacists should practice compassionate communication with geriatric patients and their care givers and should treat patients with dignity and respect, regardless of the cognitive or physical condition of the patient. Accommodations should be made for patients with hearing or visual impairments, such as speaking slowly and clearly, maintaining eye contact, and using visual aids written in a large type font and/or pictures and diagrams. A reassuring and supportive attitude while communicating can make the older patient feel comfortable in sharing their health care choices.

Informed Consent

Autonomy on the part of the geriatric patient and respect for autonomy on behalf of the pharmacist are manifest in the precept of **informed consent**. Informed consent has replaced paternalism in the decision-making processes of health care and allows the patient to make final decisions regarding health care choices only after receiving full disclosure regarding the risks and benefits of the available options. The five elements of informed consent that must be met for the patient to make a proper decision regarding health care choices are competence, disclosure, assurance of understanding, voluntariness, and signed authorization:

Competence refers to the ability of the patient to understand the decision at hand. Comatose patients and those with cognitive or psychological impairments lack competence and are unable to provide informed consent. This is especially an issue with mild cognitive impairment, dementia and delirium where a patient's ability to understand may wax and wane. Furthermore, medications may cloud a patient's mentation, creating further difficulties.

Disclosure of information must be appropriate based on contemporary professional standards or for what a reasonable person would expect to be told in a similar situation. Assurance of patient understanding must be determined by the health care provider. Understanding may be difficult to measure and the circumstances in which the information is disclosed may affect the patient's understanding. If a patient has poor health literacy, information must be disclosed in a manner they can understand. The clinician should have the patient explain what they understand about the choices to assess comprehension. Furthermore, in an emergency situation where time is of the essence, if the patient is emotionally distraught, or if medical terms are not clearly described, misunderstanding may occur. Voluntariness must be present and must not be affected by coercion or manipulation by health care professionals or relatives, or by medications or psychological disorders. Confusion can prevail when multiple family members disagree on the best choice for a patient, and the patient is unable or unwilling to oppose a choice which differs from her own perspective. Various cultures may involve family members or health care professionals to a greater or lesser degree in helping the patient make her own decision, and these differences must be evaluated to assure coercion is not present. Finally, authorization for any procedure must occur though a signature on a legally valid document. When all of the elements of informed consent are met, the patient has the right to make an autonomous decision and the decision should be respected by health care professionals.[10]

Informed consent is most frequently associated with participation in clinical research; however, written informed consent for nursing home residents with dementia treated with antipsychotic agents is mandated in some states and may become commonplace.[11,12] Nearly one third of elderly nursing home residents with dementia are receiving an antipsychotic medication, and those with impaired decision-making ability are 50% more likely to receive these medications. The combination of high utilization and patients with dementia makes the process of informed consent in this situation fraught with pitfalls.[13]

Privacy and Confidentiality

The Health Information Portability and Accountability Act of 1996, also known as the Privacy Rule or HIPAA, provides Federal protections for personal health information (PHI) held by covered entities (health care providers and health care institutions) and gives patients certain rights regarding the information.[14] A patient's understanding of his or her personal health record and how PHI is used allows the patient to assume responsibility for the accuracy and authorization of use of PHI. The basic rights under HIPAA are:

- Request a restriction on certain uses and disclosures of personal health information

- Upon request, obtain a paper copy of the notice of information practices

- Inspect and/or receive a copy of personal health record

- Request an amendment or correction to personal health record

- Obtain an accounting of disclosure of PHI

- Request for communication of PHI by alternative means or at alternative locations

- Revoke authorization to use or disclose PHI except to the extent that action has been taken

Application of HIPAA policies in the health care setting ensures that geriatric patients have the right to receive care in privacy (i.e., in the community pharmacy setting, medication counseling should be provided in a private area, away from other patients; in the nursing home, patients should receive their care, such as the administration of medications, in their room and not in the public areas of the facility). Pharmacy examples of HIPAA violations include the selling of prescription information to companies tracking prescribing patterns of physicians or the unauthorized speaking with family members regarding a geriatric patient's medications.

KEY POINT: Pharmacists have the obligation to ensure that PHI is only disclosed as patients permit.

Cultural Considerations

It is the professional responsibility of health care providers to become knowledgeable regarding the cultures of the patients they serve and understand the implications of these cultural beliefs on health behaviors. This understanding allows for the provision of culturally competent pharmacy care and avoids stereotyping and generalizations of people groups. There is data to show that lack of cultural competence can lead to disparities in health care access and provision;[15] information is available for pharmacists to determine and further develop their personal cultural competence.[16] Cultural considerations are important in understanding the health beliefs of patients from various generations, backgrounds, religions, and traditions.

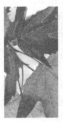

KEY POINT: Often patients have cultural beliefs that symptoms or side effects are just part of growing older and cannot be relieved. These beliefs may influence medication adherence.

Medication adherence in the elderly is affected by one's attitude toward self-efficacy (the belief that one can perform a specific behavior under differing conditions), medication-efficacy, confidence in the prescribers' knowledge, perceptions about natural products and home remedies, beliefs of control (over one's health), and illness perceptions.[17] Intergenerational relationships and the importance of traditional familial hierarchies influence health related behaviors and decision-making in the Southeast Asian, Japanese, and Hispanic cultures. Elders from Southeast Asian cultures base their beliefs on health care and medicine in the ancient practice of Chinese medicine. They characterize Western medicine as stronger, faster and curative compared to their folk medicines as weaker, slower, yet preventive. This belief system may explain why patients from Southeastern Asian cultures may be noncompliant with medications by taking lower doses.

Members of Native-American cultures believe in the interconnectedness of healing, spiritual beliefs, and community and look to modern medicine to alleviate modern ills such as hypertension and diabetes. They look to traditional Native-American remedies to cure common problems such as pain, or a "sick spirit" (defined as mental illness and/or alcoholism). Older Japanese-Americans respect healthcare practitioners as authoritarian figures, place a high level of trust in them and tend to allow healthcare practitioners to make treatment-related decisions for them.[18] Members of the African-American culture are more likely to express negative and suspicious beliefs about physicians' advice on medical treatments, including the prescribing of drugs, and report spiritual beliefs that God is ultimately responsible for health.[19] Patients with a faith-based lifestyle can perceive use of medications as a sign of disbelief or weakness. It is important for pharmacists to understand their patient's cultural beliefs so that medication counseling can be tailored, taking these beliefs into consideration.

What one thinks of illness and how it develops (i.e., the result of unhealthy habits, random occurrence, accidental, or punishment) and one's views on care for an illness (i.e., professional, self-care, do nothing), and treatments (i.e., holistic, scientific based, "natural" remedies) can all affect medication adherence. The "Greatest Generation" or "Traditionalists" may be noncompliant with pain medications as a result of stoicism; may delay in getting refills or may not complete a course of antibiotics as a result of hoarding (saving for a rainy day), or may be more dependent on home remedies as a result of self-reliance. The "Baby Boomer Generation," composed of an older (post World War II generation) cohort who expect a prescription to be written at every patient encounter and

a younger cohort (the Woodstock generation) at the other end of the spectrum, who rely on "natural products" for cures. Baby Boomers are interested in information related to their medications and generally accept patient counseling. The use of alternative medicine, including dietary supplements and herbal remedies, is increasing in all age groups and has doubled among geriatric patients since the year 2000.[20] Pharmacists should inquire about the use of alternative therapies when taking a medication history and when providing patient counseling regarding prescription medications. In counseling geriatric patients, pharmacists should be prepared to discuss alternative therapies and make recommendations when asked by their geriatric patient.

Shared Decision Making Capacity

Geriatric patients have the right to autonomy in decision making, but in reality, geriatric patients often participate in a shared decision making capacity that involves health care providers, family, and caregivers. As described above, various cultures approach health care decision-making as shared between the individual and one or more of these groups. However, ultimately the patient, if capable, must make his own informed choice. Pharmacists must be aware of cultures where strong extended family bonds or paternalism may overshadow an individual's right to make his or her own decisions. A patient has the best opportunity to maintain autonomy when working with an interprofessional team.

Surrogate Decision Making and Advanced Care Directives

A surrogate decision maker is an agent who acts on behalf of a patient who lacks the capacity to participate in a particular decision.[1] According to The Patient Self-Determination Act of 1991, health care organizations, including hospitals and nursing homes, that receive Medicaid and Medicare funds have the responsibility to explain to patients, staff, and families (through written information) that patients have a legal right to direct their medical and nursing care as it corresponds to existing state laws. This Federal regulation requires health care organization personnel to inquire of all adults admitted as inpatients as to whether they have an advance care directive (ACD) and to inform patients of their right to refuse treatment. The three primary purposes of the Patient Self-Determination Act are:

- to educate the public about state laws governing the refusal, withholding, and withdrawal of treatment at the end of life;

- to encourage wider use of ACDs to prevent the uncertainty among doctors and family members that often leads to prolonged treatment of the dying, and in some cases to lengthy court battles;

- to reduce the costs of treatment at the end of life by reducing unwanted and unnecessary intervention and the perceived need for defensive medicine.[21,22]

All states have regulations concerning ACDs, although their legal requirements may vary. Advance care directives are specific instructions, prepared beforehand, that are intended to direct a person's medical care, if (s)he becomes unable to do so in the future. ACDs allow patients to make their own decisions, and thus preserve some measure of control, regarding the medical care they would prefer to receive if they develop a terminal illness or a life-threatening injury (i.e., Alzheimer's disease, cerebrovascular accident, severe head injury). ACDs can also designate a surrogate to make decisions about medical care if the patient becomes unable to make or communicate those decisions. ACDs can avoid costly or specialized interventions that a patient may not desire, reduce personal worry and futile feelings of helplessness or guilt for family members, reduce overall health costs, and minimize legal concerns for those involved. Individuals are advised to keep a copy of the ACD with their personal papers and provide copies to their health care providers, family, and **proxy**.

The **living will** and the durable power of attorney for health care are ACDs important to the care of geriatric patients.[23] A living will may indicate specific care or treatments the individual consents to or refuses under certain conditions. Care or treatments may include CPR in the event

of cardiac or respiratory failure, "do not resuscitate" designations, artificial nutrition (intravenous or tube feedings), prolonged maintenance on a ventilator, antibiotic therapy, blood transfusions, spinal taps, blood cultures, initiation of dialysis, and organ donation. A durable power of attorney for health care is a legal document that allows an individual to appoint a proxy to make medical or health care decisions in the event the individual becomes unable to make or communicate such decisions personally. The durable power of attorney for health care does not allow the proxy to make legal or financial decisions for the individual. In an effort to simplify the health-related decision making processes at the end of life, states and organizations are combining ACDs into a single document described as an actionable medical order that can accompany the geriatric patient as they transition between and among levels of care. One such example is the MOLST document (Medical Orders for Life-Sustaining Treatment) utilized in the state of New York. Another popular form to document ACD is the Five Wishes™ form, which is recognized as a valid legal document in 40 states.[24]

Problems with Advanced Directives

Problems with ACDs include confronting a patient in distress with a list of possible procedures and requiring the individual to make decisions under duress. This can lead to unnecessary anxiety and poor decision making on the part of the patient. Other criticisms are that the language in ACDs can be vague or nonspecific and an individual's preferences may change with circumstances. Individuals should be counseled to discuss their health care issues with health care providers, family, and care givers and complete ACDs while they are in a state of good health. An alternative time to complete ACDs is during the preadmission process to a health care institution, prior to a planned medical procedure. A patient executing an ACD should have the ability to make decisions for oneself based on the information and choices presented, weighing the information to determine what the decision will mean for them on a personal level and then communicating that decision via the ACD. If a person is unable to follow this process, they are said to lack mental capacity.

A person may lack mental capacity due to a disability such as intellectual disability, dementia, brain injury, or mental illness, and this lack of mental capacity may be temporary. Legal capacity and the rights that go with it remain in effect until death unless a court of law determines that a person can no longer manage personal affairs in his or her own best interest and court intervention is necessary to protect the person. Health care practitioners, even if they think the person is incapable of making a decision, cannot overrule the person's expressed wishes unless a court declares the person legally incapacitated. Guardianship is a legal mechanism by which the court declares a person incompetent and appoints a guardian. The court transfers the responsibility for managing financial affairs, living arrangements, and medical care decisions to the guardian.[1]

Surveys of elderly African-Americans, whites, and Hispanics regarding attitudes towards completion of ACDs have revealed that African-Americans and Hispanics were less likely than white patients to have appointed a health care proxy, or completed an ACD. The differences in ACD prevalence were related to knowledge of health care proxies, availability of a potential health care agent, beliefs about the necessity of a formally appointed proxy in the presence of involved family, experience with life-prolonging technologies, age, and self-perceived health status. These findings highlight the need for healthcare providers to be sensitive to cultural differences while avoiding stereotyping patients and their beliefs around health care choices based on race and ethnicity.[25] Surrogate decision makers such as a health care proxy or guardian can benefit emotionally from the patient having ACDs in effect.

End-of-Life Decisions

ACDs provide a foundation for making end-of-life decisions when patients are unable to communicate their preferences for care. Many patients, however, are fully capable of making and communicating end-of-life decisions as they approach the end of their life. These patients are faced with choices that are based on their current experience, as opposed to the hypothetical situations covered by ACDs. For patients facing these dilemmas, end-of-life decisions are based on the expectation for their length of life weighed against their quality of life. Length of life decisions are based on the probability that death is highly likely and further efforts to postpone it are not likely to succeed. Quality of life decisions address the value or worth of life if the patient survives.

Life-Sustaining Treatments

Life-sustaining treatment is directed primarily at preserving life despite the disease, rather than at curing the disease. The use of ventilators, feeding tubes, dialysis, and cardiopulmonary resuscitation are considered life-sustaining treatments, while chemotherapy is a treatment often directed at curing disease. Artificial nutrition via gastric feeding tubes or intravenous feedings is considered a life-sustaining treatment, but is often likened to medical interventions instead of routine nursing care or comfort care.[26] After several court decisions regarding feeding tube issues, the American Medical Association changed its code of ethics on comas to allow physicians to ethically withhold food, water, and medical treatment from patients in irreversible comas or persistent vegetative states with no hope of recovery, even if death is not imminent.[27] Issues surrounding life-sustaining treatments are commonly in litigation and these laws will continue to be written.

Do-Not-Resuscitate Orders

When the decision is made to not revive a patient in the event of a cardiac or pulmonary arrest, a Do-Not-Resuscitate (**DNR**) order should be requested. A DNR may be written for a patient by the physician upon consultation with the patient (if possible), the family, or the proxy. The DNR order must be in writing and must be signed and dated by the physician. Patients and their families should be provided as much information regarding a DNR as it relates to the clinical situation so that an informed decision can be made. Often the cultural and spiritual beliefs of a patient and family guide the decision.

Assisted Suicide

Assisted suicide, also known as legal-assisted suicide or physician-assisted suicide, is the act of ending one's own life with the help of another person, i.e., a physician.[1] Most states have laws specifically prohibiting assisted suicide, but in the recent past, some few states have legalized assisted suicide which allows physicians to prescribe a fatal dose of medication to a patient whom the physician feels is likely to die within 6 months. Proponents of assisted suicide argue that persons should have the right to control their own destiny, including the right to control how and when they die. Opponents of assisted suicide point to the principle of nonmaleficence, arguing that taking a life is harmful by definition. Pharmacists may be involved in ethical dilemmas if requested to dispense prescriptions for medications to be used in assisted suicide.

Withholding and Withdrawing Treatments

Withholding treatment is a decision to forego initiation of treatment or medical interventions for a patient. When death is eminent and cannot be prevented by available means, it is morally permissible to withhold treatment that can yield only a precarious prolongation of a life that may involve a great burden for the patient or family.[1] Withdrawing (or discontinuing) treatment should be considered when the patient is in a terminal condition and there is a reasonable expectation of imminent death of the patient, or when the patient is in a non-cognitive state with no reasonable possibility of regaining cognitive function, and/or restoration of cardiac function will last for a brief period. Futility of treatment, as it relates to medical care, occurs when the healthcare practitioner recognizes that the effect of treatment will be of no benefit to the patient. Morally, the healthcare provider has a duty to inform the patient there is little likelihood of success. The determination as to the futility of a type of medical care is a scientific decision made by the physician.[1] Withdrawal of treatments may be selective such that treatments to provide comfort could be continued while therapeutic treatments are discontinued.

Although there is ample evidence to assist in the prescribing of safe and effective doses of medications, there is little evidence on when or how to stop or discontinue these same medications. Holmes et al. have proposed four criteria to consider when adding or removing medications from a geriatric patient's medication regimen:

- the patient's remaining life expectancy (based on actuarial charts and modified by the patient's current health status and history)
- the time required to obtain benefit from the medication (i.e., immediate for analgesics compared to years for antihyperlipidemic agents)
- the goals of care (a balance among prevention, treatment, and palliation)
- the treatment targets (relief of specific symptoms that agree with goals of care).[28]

Palliative Care

Palliative care is the active total care of a terminally ill patient whose disease is not responsive to curative treatment. Through the control of pain and other symptoms and by providing support for psychological, social, and spiritual issues allowing death to come naturally, palliative care should be encouraged in end-of-life situations. The goal of palliative care is to achieve the best possible quality of life for the dying patient and their family, while allowing the patient to organize the end of their life, participate in planning for their family's future, and help the family deal directly with their loved one's death.[3]

Hospice

Hospice is an interdisciplinary program of palliative care to give supportive care to the dying patient and his or her family, in the final phase of a terminal illness.[3] The focus of the care is on comfort and quality of life, rather than cure. The goal is to enable the patient to be comfortable and free of pain, so that they live each day as fully as possible and to this end, aggressive methods of pain control (including high doses of analgesics) may be used. The philosophy of hospice is to provide multidisciplinary support for the patient's emotional, social, and spiritual needs as well as medical symptoms as part of treating the whole person. Hospice is currently funded by Medicare for patients who are deemed to have a life expectancy of less than 6 months by their physician. A patient may choose to enroll in a hospice program if he or she meets this requirement. Hospice programs are available in the home or in freestanding facilities, nursing homes, or hospitals. Specific laws allow for dispensing opioid analgesics with fewer restrictions in hospice patients. Frequently, hospice patients require medications in specially compounded formulations to ease medication administration. Pharmacists may be involved in interprofessional discussions to optimize palliative therapies and to minimize treatments aimed at prolonging life in hospice patients.

Abuse, Neglect, and Safety Issues in the Elderly

Placement Issues

Aging creates losses of health, finances, loved ones, and independence. Assisting geriatric patients in compensating for losses may involve a change in the living situation to ensure safety and allow for access to the necessary health care. Alternatives for living situations for older patients include high rise independent living communities, assisted living communities, life care retirement communities, skilled nursing facilities, and nursing homes/long term care facilities. Each of these situations provides a specific type of care and planning in anticipation of a change in functional status can allow for the best environment to adequately meet the needs of the patient. Social issues that complicate illness in the geriatric patient include family and caregiver burnout, changes in family dynamics related to the illness, family guilt, patient reluctance or refusal to change the living situation, availability of the appropriate type of living situation, and financing for the health care. As in the case of ACDs, planning for potential living situations usually allows for more informed choices and smoother transitions.

Abuse and Neglect of the Elderly

If the social issues described above that complicate geriatric care are not adequately addressed, the geriatric patient can become vulnerable to the environment and experience poor outcomes. Elder abuse is classified as a type of domestic violence and is defined as any intentional, unintentional or negligent act or series of acts that cause harm or serious risk of harm to a vulnerable person, typically 69 years of age or older. The acts of abuse may be passive or active, and the abuser may not be aware of the consequences of his/her actions. Elder abuse may be classified as physical, emotional, financial, or sexual, involve neglect or abandonment, or any combination of these.[29] Elder abuse can occur in the home, in the community, or in health care institutions and screening tools are available for use by health care professionals to detect such abuse.[30] Misuse of medications, as to the point of oversedation or underuse of analgesic agents in a patient with chronic pain, is a form of physical abuse. In providing pharmaceutical care to geriatric patients, pharmacists should evaluate medication regimens, the frequency of refill requests, as well as the physical status of the patient to screen for possible abuse and medication misuse. Pharmacists, as well as all health care professionals, are responsible for reporting elder abuse to local or state authorities (i.e., Adult Protective Services, police, institutional administrators).

Decisions for People in Nursing Homes

Patients are often admitted to nursing homes because they are dependent on the services of others. Most nursing home residents suffer from some degree of physical impairment, many suffer from cognitive impairment and, in all, the ability to provide self-care is limited. Decision making for residents of nursing homes often involves ethical issues[31] and if residents of nursing facilities have ACDs in place or a named proxy, the decision making process related to health care issues is less problematic.

The Nursing Home Resident's Bill of Rights was incorporated into the 1987 Nursing Home Reform Law in order to assure residents maintained the same rights as individuals living in the community. An emphasis upon the resident's dignity and right to self-determination pervades the law, and facilities who receive Medicare or Medicaid funds are obligated to meet its requirements. The overall goal is to prevent a decline in health or quality of life as a consequence of care provided by a facility. A long term care ombudsman program is established to aid a resident or surrogate decision-maker if these rights are not honored. Common ethical issues encountered in the nursing home and their association to the Nursing Home Bill of Rights are summarized in Table 2-2.[32]

Socioeconomic Considerations

The economic and social conditions under which people live determine their health. Diseases are primarily determined by a network of interacting exposures that increase or decrease the risk for disease. The terms health disparities or healthcare inequality refer to the differences in the quality of health status, health outcomes, and the access to health care across groups of people.[33] Health disparities result from three primary factors:

- characteristics (personal, socioeconomic, and environmental) of people groups;

Table 2-2. **Nursing Home Resident's Bill of Rights**[32]

Nursing home residents have the right to:	Examples:
Be informed	Your rights as a nursing home resident Rules and regulations of the nursing home Address and phone number of ombudsman Available nursing home services Charges covered and not covered by Medicare/Medicaid Your medical condition and any changes Information must be provided in a language you understand
Participate in care	Care is adequate and appropriate Own assessment, care planning, treatment, and discharge Refusal of medication, treatments, physical restraints and chemical restraints Review of own medical record
Independent choices	What to wear Management of time, possessions, and personal finances Own physician and pharmacy
Privacy, dignity, and respect	Free from mental/physical abuse, involuntary seclusion, or corporal punishment Private and unrestricted communications Access to visitors and community organizations and the right to refuse visitors Self-determination Security of possessions Safety
Voice grievances without retaliation	Can be voiced to facility staff, outside representatives, visitors, or ombudsman
Be transferred or discharged only for medical reasons	Unless health/safety of others is at risk or lack of payment for services Requires 30 days notice Incorporates sufficient notice for preparation Includes right of appeal

- barriers encountered by people groups trying to enter the health care delivery system;

- quality of care received by people groups.

Geriatric patients can experience health care disparities as a result of the above factors. Specifically geriatric patients can experience problems accessing health care through:

- lack of insurance coverage (more likely to delay medical care and go without prescription medications, more likely be without health insurance or prescription insurance);

- lack of a regular source of care (more likely to avoid routine health care and receive fragmented care through emergency rooms or clinics);

- lack of financial resources to pay for health care;

- structural barriers (poor transportation, inability to schedule appointments quickly or conveniently, long wait times for care);

- health care financing system (likely to be enrolled in plans with limited coverage or with limited health care (physician and pharmacy) choices;

- health literacy (problems obtaining, processing, and understanding basic health information; this may lead to a poor understanding of when to seek care for symptoms);

- age (fixed incomes make paying for health care difficult, impaired mobility or lack of transportation makes accessing health care challenging, inability to use the internet as a source of information regarding health care and wellness).[34]

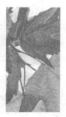

KEY POINT: From the pharmacy perspective, the ultimate health care disparity for geriatric patients is poor medication adherence, which can lead to poor health care outcomes.

Pharmacists have a professional obligation to assist geriatric patients in overcoming the socio-economic barriers that result in health care disparities by providing medication counseling and heath care information in a manner that is readily understandable by geriatric patients and assisting these same patients in obtaining the most affordable medications.

Financing Health Care

Health care in the United States is financed through a combination of health insurance programs and out-of-pocket expenses by patients. Many changes have occurred in health insurance plans since their introduction in the early 1900s and currently over 83% of health care expenditures are paid by private or public insurance programs.[35] Through the Centers for Medicare and Medicaid Services (CMS), the Federal government administers the publicly financed health insurance programs of Medicaid and Medicare. Medicaid is the tax based, jointly funded, Federal-State assistance program that provides coverage of health care costs to low-income people who meet eligibility requirements. Eligibility for, and services covered under Medicaid vary among states and some cases require recipients to provide a co-payment for services. Medicare is the federal health insurance program for persons 65 years or older, the disabled, and those with end-stage renal disease (ESRD). Medicare benefits are paid from an account that recipients have paid into during years of employment.[36] Prospective payment systems for health care services were instituted by the Federal government in 1999 in an effort to control costs for these programs.

In addition to the original Medicare fee-for-service program, Medicare offers beneficiaries the option to receive care through private insurance plans. These private insurance options are part of Medicare Part C and is now called Medicare Advantage. The most common type of Medicare Advantage plans are health maintenance organizations (HMOs). Medicare Advantage is a means of receiving health care and Medicare coverage. The beneficiary must specifically opt to receive Medicare coverage and care through an HMO, or other private plan insurance. Once the choice is made, the beneficiary must generally receive all of his or her care through the plan's providers in order to receive Medicare coverage. The main premise is that through preventive care and the use of a primary physician who acts as a gatekeeper to specialized care, health care costs can be reduced while beneficiary health can be maintained. Problems associated with Medicare Advantage plans are similar to those of patients receiving care from HMOs in that beneficiaries are limited to providers within the HMO, preapprovals are required for specialty care, and a complicated appeals process. Benefits to Medicare Advantage plans include reduced or absent deductibles and copays, and no claim forms to complete.[37]

With the passage of the Medicare Modernization Act of 2003 (MMA), Medicare Prescription Drug Coverage or Medicare Part D became available for Medicare beneficiaries, regardless of income, health status, or prescription drug usage (see Table 2-3). The Medicare Part D program provides beneficiaries with assistance paying for prescription drugs. Unlike coverage in Medicare Parts A and B, Part D coverage is not provided within the traditional Medicare program. Instead, beneficiaries must affirmatively enroll in one of many hundreds of Part D plans offered by private companies. The Medicare law establishes a standard Part D drug benefit. Plans must offer a benefit package that is at least as valuable as the standard benefit. The standard benefit is defined in terms of the benefit structure, not the particular drugs that must be covered.

The standard benefit includes an initial deductible amount and, after meeting the deductible the beneficiary pays 25% of the cost of covered Part D prescription drugs, up to an initial monetary coverage limit. Once the initial coverage limit is reached, the beneficiary is subject to another deductible, known as the "Doughnut Hole," or "Coverage Gap," in which they must pay the full costs of drugs. When total out-of-pocket expenses on formulary drugs reaches a second monetary coverage limit (including the costs of the deductible and coinsurance) the beneficiary reaches the "Catastrophic Coverage" benefit. A beneficiary entitled to Catastrophic Coverage

pays a modest copay for a generic or preferred drug and a slightly larger copay for other drugs, or a flat 5% coinsurance, whichever is greater. This out-of-pocket amount is calculated annually. A beneficiary who reaches the out-of-pocket threshold in one year has to begin to meet it again on January 1st of the next year. Because the deductible, initial coverage limit, and annual out-of-pocket threshold change each year according to the changes in expenditures for Part D drugs, beneficiary out-of-pocket expenses may increase annually. The Medicare law does not mandate a set premium amount. These costs as well as the list of covered drugs vary from plan to plan and from region to region. Beneficiaries should take time to review the various plans available to them in light of their current and anticipated needs and financial resources.

The MMA defines the drugs that are covered under Part D, and therefore the drugs for which payment will be made under Part D, in relationship to their coverage under Medicaid and under other parts of Medicare. A Part D drug is a drug that is approved by the Food and Drug Administration, for which a prescription is required, and for which payment is required under Medicaid. Biological products, including insulin and insulin supplies, and smoking cessation drugs are also covered under Part D. The MMA excludes from coverage those categories of drugs for which Medicaid payment is optional. Of particular significance to Medicare beneficiaries is the exclusion of drugs for weight gain (used in connection with treating weight loss), barbiturates (used to treat seizures in older people), benzodiazepines, and over the counter medications. Many of these excluded medications are used by geriatric patients. Part D plans are not required to pay for all covered Part D drugs. They may establish their own formularies, or list of covered drugs for which they will make payment, as long as the formulary and benefit structure are not found by CMS to discourage enrollment by certain Medicare beneficiaries. Each drug plan must develop its own exceptions process under which a plan enrollee may ask the drug plan to cover a non-formulary drug or to reduce cost sharing for a formulary

Table 2-3. Health Insurance Programs

Plan	Financing	Description	Covered Services
Private health insurance	Private business and patient cost sharing	Indemnity: beneficiary reimbursed upon claim submission; service benefit: health care provider reimbursed upon claim submission	Physician services, hospital services, optional prescription benefit
Medicaid	Public (federal and state governments)	Assistance for health care; co-pays may be required	Physician services and limited prescription benefit
Medicare Part A	Public (federal government)	Hospital insurance (HI)	Care for patients in hospitals, nursing facilities, hospice care, and home health services
Medicare Part B	Public (federal government)	Supplemental medical insurance (SMI)	Physician services, outpatient hospital care, durable medical equipment, and limited prescription benefit
Medicare Part C	Private insurance companies; patient premiums and copays	Medicare Advantage plans	Patients must have both Medicare Part A and Part B; provides Part A and Part B services and covers additional services
Medicare Part D	Public (federal government)	Prescription drug coverage	Outpatient prescription drugs, limited to formularies, and annual maximum; fee-for-service, preferred provider organizations (PPO)
Medicare Supplement	Private	MediGap	Portion of health care services for which the Medicare beneficiary has financial responsibility
Veterans benefits	Federal	Managed care provided within a closed system of veterans hospitals, clinics, and pharmacies	Hospitalization, home health, outpatient visits, prescription medications and skilled nursing according to veteran's eligibility

drug. Prescription drug coverage under Part D is voluntary. A beneficiary may purchase Part D coverage if she is entitled to Part A or enrolled under Part B. The beneficiary does not have to have both Part A and Part B coverage to choose prescription drug coverage. The beneficiary must enroll in a Part D plan that serves the geographic region in which she resides. The Part D benefit is premised on the notion that individual Medicare beneficiaries should have a choice of private drug plans in order to select a drug benefit that best meets their needs.[38]

Medicare Part D provides coverage for millions of American seniors who do not otherwise have prescription insurance, yet many seniors still lack prescription drug coverage. Its complex structure establishes barriers with enrollment selection of the prescription drug plan (formulary) with the best fit for the individual geriatric patient, and limits on annual benefit amounts with associated out-of-pocket expenditures.[39,40] Nursing home residents whose expenses are chiefly paid by Medicaid or private pay receive prescription drug coverage under Medicare Part D. Medicare Part D coverage in nursing homes is generally limited to plans that contract with long-term care pharmacies in order to assure that the drug packaging and dosage forms needed are easily available. In addition, immunosuppressants, oral antineoplastics, oral antiemetics, inhalant solutions, and insulin which are covered by Medicare Part B are also covered under Medicare Part D, creating a dilemma with appropriate billing for the long term care pharmacy.

Other Health Insurance Options

Two common options available to seniors when selecting private health insurance are fee-for service insurance and **managed care** plans (health maintenance organizations, HMOs, or preferred provider organizations, PPOs). Eligibility for private health insurance usually requires a medical examination to prove the patient is insurable and the insured patient pays out-of-pocket premiums and deductibles for health care services. Some employers provide health insurance which includes prescription drug coverage for vested retirees. Finally, the Department of Veterans Affairs provides health care to veterans, dependents and survivors according to eligibility; nearly 40% of veterans in the U.S. are over the age of 65 years and 7.84 million veterans are enrolled in the VA healthcare system.[41]

Challenges of Existing Models of Health Care Financing

The geriatric population, those 65 years of age and older, accounts for 36% of all hospital stays, 49% of all days of care in hospitals, and consumes almost one third of total U.S. health care expenditures.[42] Although this population composes about 12% of the U.S. population, it accounts for 34% of all prescription medication expenditures and 25% of OTC medication usage.[43] An estimated 91% of the U.S. population aged 65 and older has an annual prescription drug expense. Even with the availability of Medicare Part D, over one fourth of seniors (approximately 5 million) are reported to have no prescription medication coverage.[44]

The existing models of U.S. health care financing ultimately limit the individual patient's autonomy in making choices related to health care. The challenge is in achieving a balance between the access to health care and the provision of effective and affordable health care. Private health insurance plans commonly have a prescription drug benefit, but these may be rigid in requiring the patient to purchase maintenance prescriptions from specific pharmacies or from mail-order pharmacies, use formularies with associated tiered copayments for the prescribing of brand name drugs over generic drugs, and/or require prior authorization from the third-party payer for use of certain brand name drugs or drug classes.

When choosing between independent community pharmacies and chain community pharmacies for pharmacy services, ambulatory geriatric patients often price shop for prescriptions in a competitive market, made more widespread by the recently implemented inexpensive generic offerings at chain pharmacies. When seniors are admitted to long term care settings, either an assisted living facility or a skilled nursing facility, their choice of a provider of pharmacy services may be limited to those that can provide the medications in the packaging system used by the facility and/or those pharmacy providers who can provide the federally mandated consultant pharmacy services to the residents of the facility. Pharmacy services for residents of long term care settings are further complicated by the increasing use of formularies to manage prescriptions and control costs. Complications arise from the need to educate prescribers on the use of formularies and state pharmacy regulations regarding medication substitution issues

The emergence of managed care as a major health care force affecting older persons raises its own set of ethical issues. Whereas managed care offers older persons some attractive advantages, its propensity to reduce access to choice of care can be a major threat to health care for the more frail older patients. Geriatric patients are prime targets for efforts aimed at rationing health care because they consume disproportionately large amounts of medical care and because they are seen as having already lived their lives. Within the efforts to limit spending on older people, subtle approaches have been used and are cloaked in ethical concepts. Policy issues largely address questions of access and coverage, but these can be influenced by an individual clinician's beliefs about what elements of care are appropriate for older people. These beliefs, in turn, can reflect stereotypes and therefore, ethical issues arise at the bedside when decisions about initiating or continuing treatment are made.[31]

The geriatric patient is often in a state of dependency and there is disagreement on the value of a life lived with some level of dependency. If level of dependency is the primary outcome of health care, this implies that those who are dependent are no longer important to society. Much has been made about the money spent on health care in the last year of life. Costs related to health care increase when death approaches as the costs during the last month of life represent approximately 40% of the total costs for the last year of life.[45] Approximately 28% of the Medicare budget goes to the 5% of Medicare patients who die each year.[46]

In the provision of pharmaceutical care for geriatric patients, pharmacists have an obligation to work with patients, their caregivers, and third party payers to ensure that older patients receive the most appropriate medications to manage their health problems. Pharmacists should be prepared to discuss both the benefits and the limitations involved in obtaining affordable prescription medications, including the use of OTC medications in lieu of prescription medications, generic drugs, pill-splitting, tiered copayment benefit plans, prescription drug plans, mail order pharmacies, internet pharmacies, and prescription assistance programs from community coalitions, nonprofit organizations, and the Pharmaceutical Research and Manufacturers of America (PhRMA).

CASE 1: SKILLED NURSING FACILITY

SCENARIO ONE:

Subjective:
SS is a 90-year-old female resident of a skilled nursing facility for 8 years.

PMH:
Late-stage Alzheimer's disease; heart failure; receives nutrition via a nasogastric tube; confined to bed; occasional urinary incontinence. Within the past year, SS has been hospitalized four times due to the heart failure.

Medications:
Donepezil 10 mg at bedtime, aspirin 81 mg once daily, lisinopril 10 mg once daily, HCTZ 12.5 mg once daily, acetaminophen 650 mg every 6 hours as needed for pain (all medications are administered via the nasogastric tube).

Allergies:
NKDA (no known drug allergy).

SH:
BK (SS's daughter) is a court appointed guardian for SS and has had the physician sign a DNR order.

FH:
Non-contributory.

Objective:
BP 126/76, P 76, RR 24, oral T 97 F, Ht 5'1", Wt 118 lb

PE:

Chest examination revealed dyspnea, productive cough, rhonchi

Labs:

Sputum gram stain reported as: >25 WBC/hpf, <10 epithelial cells/hpf, many Gm (+) cocci in pairs. C&S reported as *Mycoplasma pneumonia*. Sensitive to erythromycin and azithromycin

Assessment:

SS is a 90-year-old female with community acquired pneumonia, cardiac risk factors, poor nutritional status, occasional urinary incontinence, and poor cognitive status. Signed DNR order is in the medical record.

Intervention:

Forty-eight hours after the above assessment was written, RT, the consultant pharmacist for the facility is completing the monthly drug regimen reviews. During the chart review for SS, RT noted the patient's diagnosis of community acquired pneumonia with no order for antibiotic therapy. When RT questioned the nurse regarding the lack of an order for an antibiotic, the nurse responded that because the patient is DNR, "No antimicrobial therapy is warranted in this situation."

Plan:

Contact physician for antibiotic order, as patient is not in cardiac or respiratory arrest.

Rationale:

1.   The court-appointed guardian for SS has had the physician sign a DNR (an order that states cardiopulmonary resuscitation [CPR] is not to be performed in the event of cardiac or respiratory arrest). At this point, the patient is not in cardiac or respiratory arrest, so an antibiotic should be ordered.

2.   The physician has a professional responsibility to SS to order an antibiotic to treat the pneumonia. The pharmacist has a professional responsibility to contact the physician and obtain an order for an antibiotic to treat the pneumonia.

3.   The ethical issues raised in this scenario include respect for patient autonomy (right to self determination) and surrogate decision making, beneficence (help others and promote patient welfare), and nonmaleficence (at least do no harm). If the pharmacist did not follow up with the physician to obtain an order for an antibiotic, the pharmacist would not respect the surrogate decision and would place SS in harm. Compare this ethical dilemma to the following scenario.

SCENARIO TWO:

Subjective:

SS is a 90-year-old female resident of a skilled nursing facility for 8 years.

PMH:

Late-stage Alzheimer's disease; heart failure; receives nutrition via a nasogastric tube; confined to bed; occasional urinary incontinence. Within the past year, SS has been hospitalized four times due to the heart failure. Within the past 3 months, SS has developed recurrent pneumonias with subsequent deterioration after each one (a total of four) pneumonias, each requiring hospitalization in addition to the four episodes with heart failure exacerbation.

Medications:

Donepezil 10 mg at bedtime, aspirin 81 mg once daily, lisinopril 10 mg once daily, HCTZ 12.5 mg once daily, acetaminophen 650 mg every 6 hours as needed for pain (all medications are administered via the nasogastric tube).

Allergies:

NKDA (no known drug allergy)

SH:

BK (SS's daughter) is a court-appointed guardian for SS and has had the physician sign a DNR order.

FH:

Non-contributory.

Objective:

BP 126/76, P 76, RR 24, oral T 97°F, Ht 5'1", Wt 118 lb.

PE:

Chest examination revealed dyspnea, productive cough, rhonchi

Labs:

Sputum gram stain reported as: >25 WBC/hpf, <10 epithelial cells/hpf, many Gm (+) cocci in pairs. C&S reported as *Mycoplasma pneumonia* Sensitive to erythromycin and azithromycin.

Assessment:

SS is a 90-year-old female with community acquired pneumonia (fourth pneumonia in 120 days with subsequent deterioration following each case), cardiac risk factors, poor nutritional status, occasional urinary incontinence, and poor cognitive status. Signed DNR order is in the medical record.

Intervention:

Forty-eight hours after the above assessment was written, RT, the consultant pharmacist for the facility is completing the monthly drug regimen reviews. During the chart review for SS, RT noted the patient's diagnosis of community acquired pneumonia with no order for antibiotic therapy. When RT questioned the nurse regarding the lack of an order for an antibiotic, the nurse responded that the physician stated, "No antimicrobial therapy is warranted in this situation." She further describes a consultation between the physician and the court appointed guardian for SS (the daughter) where the daughter stated that she understood her mother will not return to her previous level of functioning. Daughter stated that her mother would not wish to continue with multiple infections and poor quality of life. The surrogate decision is made to place SS in hospice.

Plan:

Withhold antibiotics. Assure pain and other symptom management is optimized.

Rationale:

1. Respect patient autonomy and withhold antibiotics. Assure beneficence by assuring patient is kept comfortable.

CASE 2: COMMUNITY PHARMACY

Subjective:

WW is a 78-year-old male retired from the telecommunications industry. He lives in his private residence with his wife of 56 years. He has no current health related complaints.

PMH:

Type 2 diabetes, hypertension, hyperlipidemia, depression, osteoarthritis, and macular degeneration.

Medications:

Pioglitazone 15 mg every morning, metformin 1000 mg twice daily, losartan 25 mg twice daily, furosemide 40 mg once daily, ezetimibe/simvastatin 10/40 once daily at bedtime, celecoxib 100 mg twice a daily, venlafaxine XR 75 mg every morning, aspirin 81 mg once daily, ocuvite once daily.

OTC Medications:

Multivitamin (senior formula) once daily, meclizine 25 mg as needed, calcium carbonate 500 mg as needed, docusate sodium 100 mg twice daily, fish oil 1000 mg twice daily, biotin 1000 mcg once daily, garlic 1000 mg once daily, purchases diabetic supplies to check blood glucose four times a day with a glucometer.

Allergies:

Penicillin, radioactive dyes.

SH:

Negative for tobacco and alcohol; receives Medicare Part D benefits.

FH:

Unknown.

Objective:

BP 166/78 (on self-check BP machine in the pharmacy), Ht 6'2", Wt 196 lb.

PE:

WDWNWM (well-developed, well-nourished white male) in no acute distress.

Labs:

Not available; WW stated that at his last physical (2 months ago), "Everything was A-OK!"

Assessment:

WW is 78-year-old male with elevated blood pressure who presents at the pharmacy counter and asks to speak with the pharmacist about the cost of his medications.

Plan:

1. Review WW's patient profile and complete a medication therapy management plan for WW.

2. Discuss with WW available alternatives for obtaining affordable prescription medications and reducing medication costs.

Rationale:

1. The older patient is frequently on a complicated medication regimen that often includes OTC products and dietary supplements. Pharmacists should develop medication therapy management plans especially for geriatric patients. Pharmacists should discuss these medication therapy plans with patients to insure the patients understand the indication and directions for use of each medication in their regimen.

2. Pharmacists should work with elderly patients to ensure that: those enrolled in Medicare Part D prescription drug plans are enrolled in one with a formulary most appropriate for their medication profile; generic alternatives are being dispensed when available; the most appropriate tiered copayment drugs are prescribed; patients are receiving medications from mail order pharmacies, if appropriate; patients are informed of the advantages and cautions of ordering prescription medications from internet sources; prescription assistance plans available from community coalitions, nonprofit organizations, and PhRMA are maximized for the patient's benefit.

Clinical Pearls

- *A geriatric patient who refuses aggressive (and expensive) chemotherapy for treatment of advanced stage breast cancer with the desire to preserve their children's inheritance is exerting personal autonomy in decision making.*

- *When considering the risk to benefit ratio of a medication with potential severe adverse effects (aspirin for myocardial infarction prophylaxis in a frail elderly patient) the pharmacist should take into consideration the patient's remaining life expectancy, the time required to obtain benefit from the medication, the goals of care, and the treatment targets.*

Chapter Summary

The tenets of biomedical ethics are important to the provision of health care and pharmaceutical care for the geriatric patient. Pharmacists respect patient autonomy by allowing patients to exercise their right of self-determination; display nonmaleficence when they act to prevent harm for the patient; display beneficence when they act for the good of the patient; and demonstrate justice when they allocate goods and services to their patients in an equitable manner.

Communication and decision making are important in providing health care for geriatric patients. Health care practitioners in general and pharmacists specifically should strive for effective communication with geriatric patients and assisting geriatric patients in having their personal choices regarding health care decisions made known and accomplished. Although a major benefit of managed care is that of shared risk, in reality the current health care system has the potential to limit access to choices of health care for geriatric patients.

Through the provision of accessible, convenient, confidential, and appropriate pharmaceutical care, the pharmacist can contribute to the resolution of health care disparities in the geriatric patient population. It is the professional responsibility of pharmacists to serve as patient advocates to ensure that these patients receive the pharmaceutical care to which they are entitled and that they desire.

Self-Assessment Questions

1. What is the difference between a living will and a durable power of attorney for health care?

2. How do informed consent, privacy, and confidentiality affect decision making in geriatric patient care settings?

3. What constitutes life-sustaining therapy?

4. What is the difference between palliative care and hospice care?

5. How do socioeconomic issues contribute to health care disparities geriatric patients, specifically in relation to medication adherence?

6. What are the differences between Medicaid and Medicare in terms of financing, eligibility, and benefits?

7. What options are available for geriatric patients to obtain affordable prescription medications?

References

1. Pozgar GD. *Legal and Ethical Issues for Health Professionals.* Sudbury, MA: Jones and Bartlett; 2005.

2. Lasser KE, Allen PD, Woolhandler SJ, et al. Timing of new black box warnings and withdrawals of prescription medications. *JAMA.* 2002;287(17):2215–2220.

3. Buerki RA, Vottero LD. *Foundations of Ethical Pharmacy Practice.* Madison, WI: American Institute of the History of Pharmacy; 2008.

4. Kidder RM. *How Good People Make Tough Choices.* New York: Quill; 2003.

5. Pence GE. *Classic Cases in Medical Ethics.* 4th ed. Boston: McGraw Hill; 2004.

6. Koch T. The challenge of Terri Schiavo: lessons for bioethics. *J Med Ethics.* 2005;31:376–378.

7. Steinbock B. The case for physician assisted suicide: not (yet) proven. *J Med Ethics.* 2005;31:235–241.

8. Van Den Haag E. A right to die? *National Review.* 1984;36(8):45–46.

9. Cappuzzo KA. Communicating with seniors and their caregivers. *The Consultant Pharmacist.* 2008;23(9):695–709.

10. Beauchamp TL, Childress JF. *Principles of Biomedical Ethics.* 5th ed. New York: Oxford University Press; 2001.

11. Texas Department of Human Services. Provider Letter #02-22 Informed Consent for Psychoactive Medication. June 2, 2002. Available at: http://www.dads.state.tx.us/providers/communications/2002/letters/PL02-22.html Accessed August 3, 2009.

12. Washington State Department of Social and Health Services. Policy 9.02. February 2009. Available at: http://www1.dshs.wa.gov/pdf/adsa/ddd/policies/policy9.02.pdf Accessed August 3, 2009.

13. Kamble P, Chen H, Sherer JT, Aparasu RR. Use of antipsychotics among elderly nursing home residents with dementia in the US. An analysis of national survey data. *Drugs Aging.* 2009;26(6):483–492.

14. Department of Health and Human Services. Understanding HIPAA. Available at: www.hhs.gov/ocr/privacy/hipaa/understanding/index.html Accessed January 17, 2009.

15. The National Academies Press. *Unequal Treatment-Confronting Racial and Ethnic Disparities in Health Care: 2002.* Washington, DC: Institute of Medicine; 2002.

16. Wells MI. Beyond cultural competence: a model for individual and institutional cultural development. *J Community Health Nurs.* 2000 Winter;17(4):189–199.

17. Chia L, Schlenk EA, Dunbar-Jacob J. Effect of personal and cultural beliefs on medication adherence in the elderly. *Drugs Aging.* 2006;23(3):191–202.

18. Stanford Geriatric Education Center at http://sgec.stanford.edu/ Accessed June 17, 2009.

19. Johnson KS. "You just do your part. God will do the rest": spirituality and culture in the medical encounter. *South Med J.* 2006;99(10):1163.

20. Sutherland JA, Poloma MM, Pendleton BF. Religion, spirituality, and alternative health practices: the baby boomer and cold war cohorts. *J Religion Health.* 2003;42(4):315–336.

21. Heitman E. The Patient Self-Determination Act and public assessment of end-of-life technology. Paper presented at International Society of Technology Assessment in Health Care Meeting; October 1992; Houston, TX.

22. Medline Plus Medical Encyclopedia. Advanced care directives. Available at: http://www.nlm.nih.gov/medlineplus/ency/article/001908.htm Accessed January 17, 2009.

23. Morrison RS, Zayas LH, Mulvihill M, et al. Barriers to completion of health care proxies. *Arch Intern Med.* 1998;158:2493–2497.

24. Aging with Dignity. 5 Wishes. Available at: http://www.agingwithdignity.org/5wishes.html. Accessed August 3, 2009.

25. Johnson KS, Kuchihhatla M, Tulsky JA. What explains racial differences in the use of advance directives and attitudes toward hospice care? *J Am Ger Soc.* 2008;56:1953–1958.

26. Steinbrook KE, Lo B. Artificial feeding-solid ground, not a slippery slope. *N Engl J Med.* 1988;318:286–290.

27. AMA Changes Code of Ethics on Comas. *Newsday.* April 24, 1986.

28. Holmes HH, Hayley DC, Alexander CG, et al. Reconsidering medication appropriateness for patients late in life. *Arch Intern Med.* 2006;166:605–609.

29. Conry M. Identifying, preventing, and reporting elder abuse. *Cons Pharm.* 2009;24(4):306–315.

30. Fulmer T. Screening for mistreatment of older adults. *Am J Nurs.* 2008;108(12):52–59.

31. Kane RL, Ouslander JG, Abrass IB. *Essentials of Clinical Geriatrics.* 5th ed. New York: McGraw Hill; 2004.

32. National Citizens' Coalition for Nursing Home Reform. Resident's Rights: An Overview. August 2003. Available at: http://www.nccnhr.org/uploads/Res-Rights03.pdf. Accessed August 3, 2009.

33. World Health Organization. Commission on the Social Determinants of Health. 2008. Available at: http://www.who.int/social_determinants/en/ Accessed June 17, 2009.

34. Goldberg J, Hayes W, Huntley J. Understanding health disparities. Health Policy Institute of Ohio. 2004. Available at: http://www.healthpolicyohio.org/pdf/healthdisparities.pdf Accessed June 17, 2009.

35. Larson LN. Financing health care in the United States. In: Smith MI, Wertheimer AI, Fincham JE, eds. Pharmacy and the U.S. Health Care System. 3rd ed. Binghamton, NY: Haworth Press; 2005:21–42.

36. HHS Frequent Questions. Available at: http://www.hhs.gov/faq/medicaremedicaid/85.html Accessed January 17, 2009.

37. Medicare Advantage. Available at: http://www.medicareadvocacy.org/FAQ_ManagedCare.htm Accessed June 28, 2009.

38. Center for Medicare Advocacy, Inc. Medicare Part D Prescription Drug Coverage. Available at: http://www.medicareadvocacy.org/FAQ_PartD.htm#whatIsD Accessed June 17, 2009.

39. Yin W, Basu A, Ahang JX, Rabbani A, et al. The effect of the Medicare Part D prescription drug benefit on drug utilization and expenditures. *Ann Intern Med.* 2008;148:169–177.

40. Lichtenberg FR, Sun SX. The impact of Medicare Part D on prescription drug use by the elderly. *Health Affairs.* 2007;26(6):1737–1744.

41. National Center for veterans analysis and statistics. VA benefits and healthcare utilization. April 17, 2009. Available at: www1.va.gov/vetdata/docs/4X6_spring09_sharepoint.pdf. Accessed August 3, 2009.

42. National Center for Chronic Disease Prevention and Health Promotion. *Healthy Aging: Preventing Disease and Improving Quality of Life Among Older Americans: At-a Glance 2000.* Atlanta, GA: Centers for Disease Control and Prevention; 2000.

43. Stuart B, Shea D, Briesacher B. Dynamics in drug coverage of Medicare beneficiaries: finders, losers, switchers. *Health Affairs.* 2001;20:86–89.

44. Henry J. Kaiser Foundation: Prescription Drug Trends, Fact Sheet. September 2008. Available at: http://www.kff.org/rxdrugs/upload/3057_07.pdf Accessed January 17, 2009.

45. Emanuel EJ. Cost savings at the end of life. *JAMA.* 1996;275:1907–1914.

46. Lubitz JD, Riley GF. Trends in Medicare payments in the last year of life. *N Engl J Med.* 1993;328:1092–1096.

General Biomedical and Pharmacotherapy Issues

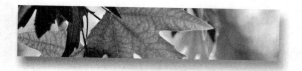

3

Biomedical Principles of Aging

LISA C. HUTCHISON

Learning Objectives

1. Compare the theories of biological aging.

2. Define successful aging.

3. Summarize the common physiologic changes associated with aging.

4. Outline the pharmacokinetic alterations which affect drug dosing in the elderly patient.

5. Identify age-related changes in pharmacodynamic sensitivity to medications.

6. Alter a standard drug regimen based upon pharmacokinetic and pharmacodynamic changes expected in an older adult.

Key Terms

GROWTH HORMONE: The peptide hormone, also called somatotrophin, which stimulates human cell growth and reproduction. The generic name of the recombinant DNA human growth hormone marketed in the United States is somatropin.

OXIDATIVE STRESS: Damage to a living cell as a result of normal oxidation reactions in the mitochondria that produce free oxygen radicals or free radical species generated by non-mitochondrial sources (e.g., the cytochrome P450 enzymes in the microsomes, or phagocytic cells during inflammation reactions).

SUCCESSFUL AGING: No single definition of successful aging has been agreed upon, but most believe it requires the achievement of old age with a few or no diseases or disabilities, high physical and cognitive functioning, and active engagement with life.

Introduction

The pharmaceutical care of older adults differs from that of younger adults for multiple reasons. Furthermore, considerations for the frail elderly are different from those of the healthy elderly patient. This chapter will focus upon the biologic changes that influence the use of medications in the elderly. After reviewing the most widely accepted theories of aging, the chapter will start with an overview of the physiologic changes which are normal or commonly seen with aging to provide the background needed to understand changes expected in the use of medications. When these factors are considered prior to treatment, drug-related problems can be minimized. While individually these factors appear straightforward, it is the need to integrate biologic changes seen in aging to design an optimal therapeutic regimen that increases the complexity of care in this population. Such are the challenges for the health care provider working with geriatric patients.

Physiology of Growing Older

There are commonly recognized physical characteristics that are associated with aging (e.g., hair graying, baldness and wrinkles) but no specific biomarkers predict morbidity or mortality due to aging. Because of this, one cannot make far-reaching assumptions regarding the magnitude of age-related biological changes for each individual at the last stages of adulthood. However, age remains the most significant risk factor for predicting death, so researchers continue to explore theories of aging in an effort to identify interventions which would reduce the significance of this risk factor.[1]

Theories of Aging

The multitude of differences seen in the aging adult contributes to a multitude of theories which attempt to explain the biology of aging. In the 1990s over 300 theories had been proposed.[2] These theories can be classified into three major categories: cellular, molecular or system decline.

Cellular Theories

Cellular theories of aging include the **oxidative stress** theory, wear-and-tear theory and the telomere theory. The oxidative stress theory proposes that aging occurs as a result of damage from free oxygen radical species that are normally produced within the cell, particularly by the mitochondria and the cytochrome P450 (CYP450) systems.[2,3] Once the cell's antioxidant defenses are unable to protect the cell from these free radical species, the oxidative damage accumulates and causes aging. This theory has support from many investigators who have used flies, worms, and rodents to show the impact of lower and higher oxidative stress.[4] The oxidative stress theory is also supported by epidemiologic studies in humans which indicate that people who consume a diet high in antioxidants found in fruits and vegetables live longer, healthier lives.[3,5] However, randomized, prospective studies which used vitamins E, A and C supplements in an attempt to reduce the morbidity or mortality of age-related diseases (cardiovascular, dementia) have not shown effectiveness.[6,7]

The wear-and-tear theory is related to the oxidative stress theory but is not grounded upon the generation of free oxygen radicals within the cell. Instead, it proposes that aging is the effect of the physiological work of cells, and this work is indirectly related to the organism's adverse living conditions.[2] Therefore, stressful living conditions would increase the work of cells and reduce lifespan.

Another cellular theory of aging centers upon the tendency for normal human cells to have a finite number of replications before the cell's telomeres shorten and are no longer able to support cell division. The telomeres provide "handles" for moving chromosomes and once they become too short, they are no longer functional and the cell cannot divide. This finite number is termed "Hayflick's limit" after the scientist who first described it and the theory is called the telomere theory. Cancerous cells do not experience the shortening of the telomeres and can divide an infinite number of times.[8]

Molecular Theories

Molecular theories of aging focus upon genetic regulation of cell function. The most accepted molecular theory is the genetic theory which suggests that aging occurs due to changes in gene expression that regulate the organism throughout all phases of life. Just as genes direct the body of an infant to grow and develop, they also direct the body of an octogenarian to decline and fail. Gene expression within a cell is thought to initiate cell death; this is termed *apoptosis*.[8] Other related theories such as the error catastrophe or somatic mutation theories, focus upon random molecular damage to DNA which accumulates over time until the genetic material can no longer be expressed or proteins produced are changed and are no longer effective.

System Decline Theories

System decline theories focus upon failures of the neuroendocrine system and the immune system to explain aging. Changes in the ability of the hypothalamic-pituitary-adrenal (HPA) axis are thought to signal each stage of life and in the final stage, the neuroendocrine system is unable to adapt to new stressors from the environment leading to decline and death.[9] Many individuals believe that every organism has its own "biological clock," which is programmed for the life expectancy of the species and the specific organism which fits into this line of thinking.

The immune system closely interacts with the neuroendocrine system to control and eliminate foreign organisms from the body without destroying the host. Failure of the immune system weakens the body's ability to fight infections or police for cancerous cells. This failure to recognize "self" triggers the failure of the body to survive. Mature T cells from healthy older adults as compared to frail elderly patients do not show a decline in function or adaptability, providing support for this theory.[8]

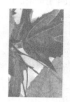

KEY POINT: No single theory of aging is likely to explain all of the changes which occur and lead to senescence of the individual.

Age-Related Biological Changes

Cardiovascular

A large body of literature is devoted to cardiovascular changes seen with aging but because cardiac disease is the leading cause of death in elderly patients, it is important in these studies to separate the changes seen with normal aging compared to those seen commonly with aging due to cardiovascular diseases. Morphologic changes that are thought to be due to aging alone include a decrease in myocytes within the myocardium, hypertrophy of the remaining myocytes, a stiffening of the ventricles, a reduced number of pacemaker cells in the sinoatrial node, valvular dilation and calcifications, and stiffening of the arterial wall.[10] These morphologic changes lead to a reduced ability to relax the heart (diastolic dysfunction) and a loss of the early filling from the atrial contraction. These changes are seen on echocardiogram which show an elevated left ventricular end-diastolic pressure and a reversal in the ratio of early to late filling velocity (E/A ratio).

The stiffening of the aorta and other large arteries predisposes the elderly patient to isolated systolic hypertension because the large vessels can no longer absorb the high pressures from systolic contraction of the heart. In turn, this predisposes the patient to orthostatic hypotension and syncope as the body is unable to compensate for the drop in pressure due to a diminished baroreceptor reflex tachycardia and peripheral vasoconstriction.[10]

Persistent elevation of catecholamines leads to a desensitization of beta-adrenergic receptors. The maximum predicted heart rate with exercise decreases with aging and has not shown to be reversible with athletic training. Endothelial dysfunction is also seen with aging possibly due to diseases such as hypertension, diabetes mellitus and dyslipidemias.[10]

Central Nervous System

Many older adults complain of memory loss, especially the very old, even when neuropsychological test results do not show cognitive impairment. Normal changes seen with aging include decrease in brain mass, cerebral blood flow and cerebral autoregulation. Dopaminergic, muscarinic and serotonin receptors tend to decrease although this decrease has not been directly associated with abnormal thinking. Crystallized cognitive abilities (i.e., vocabulary, accumulated knowledge and understanding proverbs) increase over the lifespan and remain intact throughout the normal aging process. However, fluid abilities (i.e., mental speed, novel problem solving), which rely more on short-term memory storage, peak in the mid-twenties and slowly taper until the mid-sixties.[11] At this point a steeper decline occurs. Fluid abilities are more affected by injury and disease, so their decline may not be solely due to normal aging and most elderly people readily compensate with this decline through crystallized intelligence.

The efficiency of sleep (amount of time spent in bed asleep) decreases with aging. Older persons tend to take the same amount of time to fall asleep as younger adults, but spend more time in Stage 1 and 2 non-REM (rapid eye movement) sleep and less time in Stage 3 and 4 and REM sleep. More awakenings contribute to the reduction in sleep efficiency and elderly persons frequently complain of non-restorative sleep problems. This leads to daytime napping and an earlier bedtime.[12]

Renal and Genitourinary

Kidney mass and weight decline by 10–43% over the lifespan. The number of glomeruli decreases and the glomerular basement membrane thickens.[13] Hence, glomerular function declines significantly with aging and the kidney has an increasingly difficult time maintaining fluid and electrolyte balance when presented with restrictions or overloads. The serum creatinine, a traditional indicator of renal function, may not increase in proportion to the decrease in kidney function due to the decrease in muscle mass seen in older adults. Tubular function is also impaired such that the kidney will not reabsorb sodium in concert with the body's needs.[14] When dietary sodium restrictions are imposed, the kidney does not respond rapidly and sodium losses continue in the tubules for a time. It is unwise to strictly limit sodium intake for most elderly patients.

The kidney's ability to dilute or concentrate the urine is also impaired with aging, most likely due to a loss of concentrating ability of the medullary tissue. Elderly patients have difficulty maintaining appropriate volume status if volume depletion or overload occurs.[10,13]

The urinary tract is also changed with aging. For women, the loss of estrogen with menopause may cause atrophic urethritis and diminished urethral resistance and the process of childbearing may cause weakening of the pelvic floor muscles. Although urinary incontinence is not considered a part of normal aging, these changes increase the risk for urinary incontinence due to stress or urge. Men may develop an enlarged prostate leading to urinary obstruction and an increased risk for overflow incontinence.[15]

Endocrine

Changes in the endocrine system have been associated with aging and aging theories. While some important hormones decrease with age, many others maintain secretion patterns and quantities that match those of young and middle-aged adults and still others are increased in the body's effort to maintain homeostasis (see Table 3-1). Several hormones secreted through the HPA axis do not deteriorate with aging. Concentrations of adrenocorticotropin, cortisol and antidiuretic hormone remain unchanged throughout the lifespan. Although levels of epinephrine and norepinephrine are higher in older adults than in younger adults, the response to stress is not blunted with hormones secreted through the HPA axis or the catecholamines. The thyroid decreases in size and fibrosis and lymphocytic infiltration increases within the gland. In spite of this, the serum concentrations of thyroxine and thyroid stimulating hormone (TSH) do not change significantly with aging unless disease is present. Insulin concentrations tend to increase with age, although this may be due to the increase in percentage of body fat which causes an increase in insulin resistance.[16]

Hormones which significantly decrease with normal aging include estrogen in women, testosterone in men, **growth hormone** and dehydroepiandrosterone (DHEA). The menopause occurs when cyclic estrogen production from the ovaries is replaced by a low continuous production at about 20% of pre-menopausal levels. This leads to uterine atrophy and a decrease in vaginal secretions which may further lead to dyspareunia and a decline in libido. In addition, hot flashes accompanied by perspiration, tachycardia, and vasodilation of the skin are reported in 50–75% of peri-menopausal women, frequently interrupting sleep. The mean age for menopause is 50 years, so most elderly women have had ample time to adjust to post-menopausal changes.[16] However, if a patient has been treated with estrogen therapy

Table 3-1. **Hormone Changes Seen with Aging**

Decreased Concentrations	Comments
Estradiol	Rapid increases and decreases seen during perimenopause with gradual reductions
Testosterone	Slow, subtle decrease after age 50
Dihydroepiandrosterone (DHEA)	Gradual decrease
Growth hormone	Pulse amplitude and duration decrease Pulse frequency is maintained
Calcitonin	Total decreased, but active levels intact
Renin	
Aldosterone	More difficult to maintain sodium and potassium balance
Erythropoietin	Relative to decrease in kidney size and function

No Change in Concentration	Comments
Adrenocorticotropic hormone (ACTH)	
Cortisol	Response to stress maintained
Antidiuretic hormone	Impairs ability to maintain fluid balance
Glucagon	
Prolactin	Nocturnal pulsatile secretion lost
Thyroxine	
Thyrotropin-stimulating hormone	

Elevated Concentrations	Comments
Epinephrine	Response to stress maintained
Norepinephrine	Response to stress maintained
Atrial natriuretic peptide	Increased due to renal resistance Leads to impaired salt wasting and difficulty in handling a decrease in salt intake leading to volume depletion with low sodium diet
Insulin	Increased due to increased peripheral tissue resistance
Parathyroid hormone	Increased to maintain serum calcium levels

through these years and subsequently has therapy discontinued, the patient is at risk for experiencing peri-menopausal symptoms.

The aging male does not experience the abrupt discontinuation of sex hormone production found in women. Testosterone production declines slowly over time, with many men never reaching a level where they would be considered androgen deficient. Sexual responses become slowed, decrease in intensity and exhibit an increase in refractory period. And, although the number of spermatozoa decrease, reproduction can take place even at the extremes of age for men.[15]

Growth hormone secretion by the pituitary diminishes with age regardless of continued secretion of growth hormone releasing factor in the hypothalamus. This hormone is responsible for maintenance of muscle mass and strength. DHEA concentrations in 85-year-old individuals are one fifth that of 30-year-olds. Although the exact actions of DHEA in humans are not clearly understood, animal studies indicate that it plays a role in prevention of obesity, diabetes mellitus, cancer and heart disease.[16]

Gastrointestinal

Gastrointestinal complaints are frequently expressed by older patients, however, many of these complaints are due to pathologic processes rather than a result of aging per se. For example, no important changes occur in the oral cavity that are strictly due to aging. Rather poor oral hygiene and lack of fluoridated water sources in childhood contribute to poor dental health in the older adult. Dry mouth is most often due to anticholinergic medications instead of aging. Esophageal function is preserved with aging except in patients with neurologic diseases such as neuropathy or stroke.[17]

The stomach, small intestine and large intestine are primarily unchanged with aging. Some researchers have noted atrophy of the stomach and of the villi in the small intestine that was believed to be associated with aging, while others have found no changes when disease was ruled out as a cause. Atrophic gastritis with a resultant achlorhydria, once thought to be universal with aging, is now known to be associated with perni-

cious anemia or infection by *Helicobacter pylori*.[17] Peristalsis may be slowed with aging resulting in an increased satiety from filling in the stomach and constipation from slowed emptying through the large intestine. Yet this commonly shared belief is not substantiated for all elderly.

The size and blood flow to the liver decrease as much as 1.5% per year after age 50. The number of hepatocytes is decreased and protein synthesis is diminished. The pancreas size may or may not be reduced with aging. Even with these changes, the normal function of the liver and pancreas is not appreciably altered as there is a tremendous reserve capacity in these two organs.[18]

Musculoskeletal and Connective Tissue

Muscles, skin and bones undergo many changes within the aging adult. Lean muscle mass changes dramatically with an average decrease of 30–40%. This change may be more due to increasing sedentary lifestyle than strictly due to aging itself. Nonetheless, elderly patients tend to replace lean body tissue with fat tissue over time unless they continue a rigorous exercise routine.

Skin changes are either intrinsic or extrinsic. Intrinsic changes include thinning of the skin and loss of elasticity. Extrinsic changes are related to the amount of time the skin has been exposed to the sun and are synonymous with photoaging. Sun exposure leads to fine and coarse wrinkling of the skin, leathery texture, telangiectasias, actinic keratoses, and a blotchy appearance. Generally, one can compare skin changes from the face or hands with the skin from the patient's buttocks to identify the differences between intrinsic and extrinsic aging. Body hair also may gray, thin and finally be lost altogether with aging except for hair on the face. Sebum secretion decreases with age, leading to dry, coarse skin and xerosis. Sweat glands also diminish with age and thermoregulation becomes more difficult as one grows older. These changes decrease the skin's ability to prevent infection.[19]

Bone remodeling occurs throughout the lifespan, but after age 30, there is a net bone loss of 0.7–1% per year. Bone loss is accelerated after menopause in women for approximately 5–10 years, after which it stabilizes.[20] The relative increase in bone resorption increases the risk of fracture in the elderly patient. Older individuals lose height at a rate of 0.6 cm per decade, mostly due to loss of height of the vertebrae and narrowing of the vertebral discs. This decrease is accelerated when compression fractures of the vertebra occur, leading to kyphosis. The long bones of the arms and legs do not shorten over time.

Respiratory

The lung tissue loses elasticity with age, but this is counterbalanced by changes in the chest wall and muscles so that total lung capacity is not changed. However, older individuals are unable to move air in and out of the lungs as quickly as younger individuals and all measures of air flow (i.e., forced expiratory volume in the first second [FEV1], forced vital capacity [FVC]) decrease with age. In addition there is an increase in residual lung volume and dead air space, partly related to more rapid closure of small alveoli upon expiration. This rapid closure, termed closing capacity, contributes to a reduction in arterial oxygen tension which falls linearly in association with age.[14]

Immunology/Hematology

Hemoglobin levels decrease with age, but this is more likely a phenomenon secondary to decreased erythropoietin synthesis due to decreased kidney size and function. In very old men, loss of testosterone may influence hemoglobin production. Other contributing factors could be presence of chronic inflammation, vitamin B12 deficiency or iron loss, none of which are directly due to aging per se. Therefore, anemia is not normal with aging, but is frequently encountered.[16]

Immunocompetence declines with age. This corresponds to one system-based theory of aging. The thymus decreases in size after puberty which affects T cells and cell-mediated immunity. Humoral immunity appears to be decreased as well with a lessened production of antibodies in response to antigen stimulation. In general, the older, frail patient is unable to mount the same immune response to an infectious insult, so we do not always see swelling, pain or erythema at the site of an infection and many elderly patients do not mount a fever or leukocytosis in response to systemic infections. This altered presentation makes diagnosis and monitoring of therapy difficult in the elderly patient.[9]

Sensory

Visual changes are universal with aging. By the age of 55, corrective lenses for reading and/or distance vision are needed by almost everyone. The loss of near vision associated with aging is called presbyopia. Accommodation to changes in lighting is more sluggish and glare becomes a problem. The ability to distinguish colors, particularly between greens and blues, is lost. Cataracts are likely to develop by the age of 70. Functional blindness increases with age to a prevalence of 17% in those age 90 and older.[20]

Hearing changes result from multifactorial changes seen with aging. First, cerumen in the ear canal is dryer and more likely to become impacted, which can contribute to hearing loss. Secondly, the inner ear may suffer degenerative changes, particularly from exposure to noise or atherosclerosis. This leads to loss of high frequency hearing referred to as presbycusis. Medications can contribute to hearing loss, specifically aminoglycosides, vancomycin and loop diuretics have been shown to cause irreversible hearing loss.[20,21]

Taste and smell perceptions also show decline in older adults. By the age of 80, the ability to perceive smells is reduced in half. Taste is less predictable, but some studies show that a higher threshold is required for sour, bitter and salty tastes, but not for sweet tastes. Medications such as metronidazole and captopril should be evaluated for their potential of causing dysgeusia before one assumes a change in taste is due to aging alone. These changes are important to address for patients with reduced appetite and malnutrition.[20]

Concepts of Successful Aging

With more individuals living into their eighties and nineties, there has developed a greater interest among the lay public, clinicians, and researchers about what constitutes **successful aging**. It is universally agreed that living longer is not enough to be successful if functional abilities are severely compromised. While the simplistic view that successful aging may be a product of an increased quantity of years plus an increased quality of years, more specific definitions and models to measure successful aging are needed.[22]

The biomedical model focuses upon longevity plus the absence of diagnosed chronic medical diseases, no psychiatric illness and little or no difficulty with the activities of daily living. Some researchers include participation in social activities as a part of this model. The social functioning model focuses upon the number of different social activities and the frequency of social contacts. Psychological models include measurement of self-efficacy, coping, self-worth, and goals. Socioeconomic models also exist. One of the strongest influences of self-perceived quality of life is an individual's feeling that they are in control of their lives and have a positive attitude toward their approach to problems.[23,24]

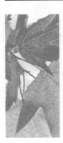

KEY POINT: The clinician must approach each patient individually to identify what areas constitute that person's definition of successful aging so pharmacotherapy decisions can be tailored to the patient's needs and desires.

Because the definitions of successful aging are still developing, it is difficult to classify every symptom and sign reported by an elderly patient as solely due to normal aging or due to common pathologies associated with aging. This classification is further clouded by the ageism in society. For example, loss of muscle mass is always noted as a consequence of aging, yet in one patient it may be due to lack of exercise and resistance training, in another due to lack of adequate vitamin D and protein intake and yet in another due to caregivers who tell the patient they should not be exercising at their age. Which of these causes is normal? Which one requires an intervention? Medical models tend to focus upon treating and preventing diseases which are commonly associated with aging. In some gerontological circles there is interest in identifying strategies to delay the overall effects of aging. This could aid in the ability to successfully treat all diseases because currently increased age is one of the most powerful risk factors for developing many disease states such as hypertension, diabetes and cancer.[22]

Anti-Aging Strategies

Many adults experiment with different strategies to reduce the effects of aging. Although no specific therapies are proven effective in reducing the overall effects of aging, several potential strategies may eventually show results. One such treatment is calorie restriction which focuses upon reducing caloric intake by 30–40% of the normal amount for the species while maintaining good nutritional balance. Animal models of yeast, worms, flies, rodents and dogs have proven this method to extend life, but only observational studies have been completed in humans as of yet.[25,26]

Antioxidant therapy using vitamin E, vitamin C or coenzyme Q10 is frequently used based upon the oxidative stress theory of aging. No studies have used these compounds to reduce aging or overall mortality, but several studies have attempted to reduce cardiovascular or central nervous system disease progression through supplementation of these antioxidants without success.[6,7]

Replacement of estrogen, testosterone, DHEA, and human growth hormone have been touted as compounds that may reverse aging processes. Estrogen therapy in post-menopausal women did not prove effective in reducing cardiovascular disease or Alzheimer's disease.[27-29] Testosterone therapy has been tried in older men with low normal serum concentrations over 6 months and found significant improvements in fat and lean body mass providing hope that this may prove to be a successful therapy in men.[30,31] Although the exact role of DHEA in the body is not yet clear, clinical trials evaluating the supplementation of DHEA in older individuals with low concentrations showed a slight increase in bone mineral density, increased lean body mass and an increase in perception of physical and psychological well-being.[30] Because these results were not consistent across all studies routine use of DHEA is not yet recommended.

Studies in adults with growth hormone deficiency show reversal of catabolism but studies with growth hormone as an anti-aging therapy did not add any benefit beyond that seen with resistance exercise training.[32] Access to growth hormone in the United States has been limited by Congress to conserve supplies for individuals with bonafide diagnoses known to respond to its administration, such as severe short stature syndrome in children and adult growth hormone deficiency. In spite of the lack of data, worldwide sales range from $1.5–2 billion with at least one third of this use for the off-label indication of prevention of aging.

Resveratrol is a compound found in red grape skins, blueberries, and lingonberries that is thought to activate genetically controlled enzyme production of sirtuins in the body. Sirtuins regulate cellular reaction to stress and may help to prevent cancer, reduce cardiovascular disease and extend life. Studies in yeast, fruit flies, nematodes and fish have shown that resveratrol, presumably through sirtuin activation, can effectively extend the lifespan.[33] It is thought that this compound may explain the French paradox in which a low risk of heart disease is seen in France although the population consumes a diet high in saturated fats. Prospective controlled studies in humans with resveratrol have not yet been performed.

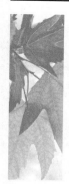

KEY POINT: Mankind has searched for the fountain of youth since the time of the Egyptian civilization. With the large variability in human genetic make-up coupled with environmental exposures, no one factor can be expected to halt the aging process.

Risk Factors for Functional Decline

Older adults report activity limitations more often than younger adults due to chronic medical conditions. Figure 3-1 shows how more medical conditions are reported as limiting activities in the youngest old, middle old, and oldest old. Of particular interest is the increase of senility and vision changes over these decades to the third and fourth most common reasons cited as limiting activity, behind arthritis/musculoskeletal and heart/circulatory conditions.[34] Activity is defined as work or everyday household chores.

Functional decline in older persons is commonly described as a loss of independence in their ability to take care of themselves. Initially, this is evaluated by observing a person's ability to perform activities like shopping, housekeeping, preparing meals, taking medications, handling finances and using public transportation (instrumental activities of daily living). As disability increases, functional decline may occur with personal care items such as bathing and dressing (activities of daily living). Functional decline generally results in a reduced quality of life and the elderly patient who experiences progressive disability will exhaust functional reserves and become more vulnerable to adverse outcomes, including adverse drug events. Functional decline can result from physical issues, medical problems, cognitive changes or a combination of these factors (see Table 3-2).[35,36] Hospitalization is frequently a time when the diminished reserve capacity of the elderly patient contributes to a rapid decline in functional abilities. The patient is frequently confined to bed in an unfamiliar environment and given multiple treatments and medications.

Medications can contribute to functional decline through multiple mechanisms. Mobility can be reduced with medications like metoclopramide and antipsychotic agents if a patient develops secondary parkinsonism symptoms from their administration. Steroids and statins can contribute to muscle weakness as can loop diuretics which may cause hypocalcemia. Drugs which alter mental status including benzodiazepines, opioids, and anticholinergics reduce an elderly person's ability to interact with others and the environment. Two

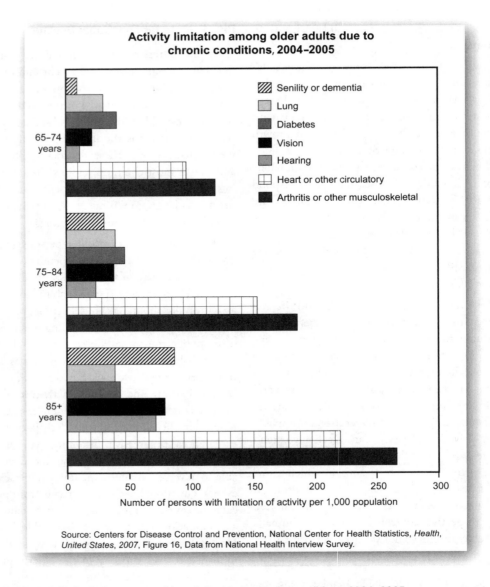

Figure 3-1. Activity limitation among older adults due to chronic conditions, 2004–2005.

of the most underappreciated drug side effects in older adults are anorexia and dysgeusia. Elderly patients, especially the frail elderly patient, frequently have weight loss, undernutrition, and a decrease in muscle mass. Use of medications such as digoxin, captopril, selective serotonin reuptake inhibitors and metronidazole may further increase the risk for anorexia and escalate functional decline.

Age-Related Changes in Medication Sensitivity

Over one third of prescription medications are taken by patients over the age of 65 even though this group makes up only 13% of the United States population. While most of this medication use results in improvements in morbidity and mortality, a significant proportion of elderly patients experience adverse drug events. One study in over 30,000 geriatric outpatients found that 27.6% of

Table 3-2. Risk Factors for Functional Decline

Physical
  Age
  Immobility
  Muscle Strength
  Exercise tolerance
  Decreased balance
  Undernutrition
  Weight loss
  Diminished lean body mass
Medical
  Hospitalization and length of stay
  Morbidity and disability from acute and chronic disease
Psychological
  Impaired cognition
  Depression

adverse drug events were preventable and 42.2% of preventable adverse events were serious, life-threatening, or fatal.[37] Another study identified that 28% of hospital admissions in the elderly were attributable to adverse drug events.[38] Use of medications in the elderly is one of the most challenging aspects of their health care. Important physiologic changes influence the pharmacokinetics and pharmacodynamics of medication use in older patients. A thorough understanding of these alterations will aid in optimizing pharmacotherapy and preventing adverse drug events in this vulnerable group of patients.

Age Related Changes in Pharmacokinetics

Absorption

Most medications are absorbed in the small intestine through passive diffusion.[39] Oral absorption of medications in the elderly patient can be delayed due to the slowing of transit time into the small intestine with no change in the overall absorption. Therefore, with chronic administration, this change makes little difference.[21] A medication administered for an acute illness or symptom, such as pain, will take longer to reach the time to maximal concentration, have a lower maximal

concentration and have a slowed onset of action. The assessment of medication effectiveness should be delayed appropriately in this situation.

A subset of elderly patients may have achlorhydria with decreased secretion of hydrochloric acid. This most often occurs in individuals with a history of peptic ulcer disease and/or gastric surgery. Treatment with high doses of proton pump inhibitors and histamine-2 blockers may also contribute. Patients with achlorhydria may have reduced absorption of vitamin B-12, iron and calcium.[40]

Little evidence is available to identify if significant changes occur with absorption of medications from transdermal patches. Changes in the skin associated with aging such as reduced blood flow and thinner skin should not be dismissed as possible enhancers or detractors of drug absorption through the skin. Studies with fentanyl transdermal patches in the elderly did not show statistically significant differences, however, great variability in absorption in all individuals may make such studies difficult to interpret. It is known that elevated body temperature will increase fentanyl absorption.[18] The cooler skin of the elderly may likewise inhibit absorption.

Distribution

The distribution of medication throughout the body occurs through the bloodstream. The relative decrease in total body water, lean muscle mass and the increase in percentage of body fat typically seen with older adults will alter the usual volume of distribution seen with medications.[41] Water-soluble medications will have a smaller volume of distribution; therefore smaller doses are required to attain the therapeutic response. If given the same dose as a younger adult, the older patient will have a higher serum concentration and be at risk for an increase in toxic effects. Aminoglycoside antibiotics are an example of a hydrophilic medication that exhibits a smaller volume of distribution in older patients with decreased total body water.[21] Similarly, drugs which distribute into lean muscle mass will also have a smaller volume of distribution and smaller doses should be used in the elderly. Digoxin has an average volume of distribution of 6–7 liters/kg in young adults but this average volume of distribution decreases to an average of 3–4 liters/kg in geriatric patients.

Lipophilic medications pose a unique problem in the older patient. With the increase in the percentage of body fat seen with most geriatric patients, one would anticipate that a larger dose of a fat soluble medication would be needed to fill up the larger volume of distribution.[40] However, because the clearance of a medication is directly related to its volume of distribution, the geriatric patient will not be able to clear fat soluble medications as quickly as a younger patient and these medications will accumulate, creating an increase for toxic effects. The equation which follows illustrates this relationship:

Elimination half-life (T½) =
(0.693 × volume of distribution)/clearance

As the volume of distribution increases with the elimination half-life held constant, it will take longer to clear the medication from the body. To avoid this problem, lipophilic medications should be used at reduced doses or increased dosing intervals. Benzodiazepines and antipsychotic medications are examples of medications that are lipophilic but have a high risk for accumulation in the elderly patient due to the larger volume of distribution.[42]

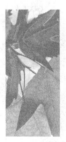

KEY POINT: The influence of the volume of distribution on the clearance of medications is overlooked in many package inserts, which report no difference in elimination between young adults and geriatric subjects.

Protein binding in the elderly patient may or may not be changed. Healthy older adults will have normal concentrations of albumin, alpha-1-acid glycoprotein and other proteins. However, malnutrition and frailty are associated with lower serum proteins, particularly of albumin. If a drug is highly protein bound, it will be unable to find sufficient binding sites in the serum and more un-

bound drug will be available to exert pharmacologic (and toxic) effects although its total serum concentration will still be within the therapeutic range. Phenytoin and warfarin are 99% protein bound, primarily to albumin. Their toxicity is increased in patients with hypoalbuminemia when the total serum concentration is within the therapeutic range because of the elevated free drug fraction in the serum.[43]

Metabolism

The smaller size and lower blood flow through the liver has one important effect on drug dosing in the elderly patient.[41] Because of these changes, drugs with high extraction during the first pass through the liver must be dosed cautiously. Less drug will be metabolized during the first pass through the liver and the drug will have a higher bioavailability in the elderly patient. Verapamil, propranolol and morphine are example medications that have a higher bioavailability in the older adult.

No researchers have studied metabolic capacity in young or middle-aged adults and then re-studied the same group of subjects once they had aged to over 65 years, so it is still not clear what the exact effect of aging alone may be on the various metabolic pathways.[44] Cross-sectional comparisons have shown a decrease in the function of CYP 2C19, no change in CYP 2D6 and a large variability in other isoenzymes. Because of the wide inter-individual variations in metabolism that exist for all age groups, we cannot be sure that all families of the cytochrome P450 system are diminished with aging. Esterase activity was reduced in one study of frail elderly subjects, but was not reduced in healthy elderly subjects.[18] Cautious clinicians anticipate decline in all Phase I reactions, oxidation, reduction and hydrolysis, for elderly patients when dosing medications which are metabolized through these pathways. Phase II reactions include glucuronidation, acetylation and sulfation have not shown significant decreases in older adults. Medications which are metabolized through these pathways do not require adjustment.

Drug metabolism also occurs in the small intestine, in renal cells and lymphocytic cells through CYP 3A4 enzymes or P-glycoprotein, however, studies show decreasing, increasing, or no change in activity. [45]

Elimination

While changes in liver metabolism are not completely understood, the reduced excretion of drugs through the kidneys is very well characterized for elderly patients. With age, renal mass and blood flow are reduced with a correlated drop in the functioning glomeruli. Although not every older patient has abnormal renal function, longitudinal studies indicate that the glomerular filtration rate drops on average by 1% for every year of age past 20 so that the oldest old who have survived six decades since their twentieth birthday will very likely have glomerular filtration rates (GFRs) of less than 59 mL/min. [41] Direct measurement of the GFR requires a 24-hour urine collection which is inconvenient and time-consuming for the patient, so most clinicians use an equation to estimate GFR or creatinine clearance, a closely related approximation of GFR, to evaluate a patient's renal function. The Cockcroft-Gault equation for estimating creatinine clearance is best validated for use in patients over the age of 75 years of age and has the most data for drug dosing adjustments. This equation is:

[(140-age in years) × (body weight in kg)]/[(72) × (serum creatinine in mg%)] × 0.85 for women[46]

For individuals more than 30% over their ideal body weight, it is appropriate to use their ideal body weight.

Controversy surrounds the application of this as well as other estimates of renal function in the dosing of medications. Individuals with low muscle mass generally have low serum creatinine concentrations. This gives rise to an over-estimate of kidney function when serum creatinine values below 0.8 mg% are used in the formula. Many clinicians advocate rounding extremely low serum creatinine values upward; however, studies have not supported this practice. [47,48]

The kidney also functions to secrete molecules in the tubules of the nephrons and to metabolize certain compounds. Both functions are re-duced with aging. Tubular secretion is reduced in proportion to the reduction in nephrons with a smaller kidney size. Approximately 10% of creatinine elimination is through tubular secretion rather than through filtration by the glomeruli, therefore, formulas for estimating creatinine clearance may not adequately account for this mode of elimination. [18] Certain medications can inhibit the secretion of creatinine or of other medications by the tubules. Trimethoprim and cimetidine are drugs that compete with creatinine for tubular secretion, so individuals receiving these agents may have an elevated serum creatinine that does not correctly reflect their level of renal dysfunction. Metabolism of insulin occurs in the renal cells, so with reduced numbers of functioning cells, a reduction in clearance will occur. Elderly patients with very poor renal function will experience an extended half-life of all insulin products such that regular insulin may exert effects lasting as long as a long-acting form of insulin would in a younger adult. Finally, activation of vitamin D occurs in the kidney with metabolism of 25-hydroxy-vitamin D3 to 1, 25-di-hydroxy-vitamin D3. But in the elderly patient with reduced kidney function, this activation does not occur at the rate necessary for calcium homeostasis. Many elderly patients are deficient in activated vitamin D with resulting hypocalcemia and subsequent hyperparathyroidism.

Although several important drugs are excreted through the biliary tree, no significant alterations in clearance associated with aging have been identified.

Age Related Changes in Pharmacodynamics

The cardiovascular system is frequently associated with pharmacodynamic changes in the elderly patient. This is partially because medications affecting the cardiovascular system are frequently used in the elderly patient. As the catecholamine level increases, down-regulation of cardiac beta-1-adrenergic receptors occurs which leads to a blunting of effect of antagonist agents such as metoprolol. [10] The risk for orthostatic hypotension due to antihypertensive agents is increased in older patients. [21] The diminished capacity of the baroreceptors to react to the drop in blood pressure with rising is one cause of this increased risk. In addition, the presence of isolated systolic hypertension accentuates the magnitude of the blood pressure drop. An increased sensitivity to medications that prolong the QT interval is seen, raising the risk for torsades de pointes.[49]

The second most common organ system with an altered sensitivity to the pharmacological effects of medications is the central nervous system. The brain of the elderly patient has a smaller reserve of neurotransmitters and cannot compensate for changes as easily as the younger brain.[49] The permeability of the blood brain barrier results in higher concentrations of psychoactive medications at the nerve endings. There is also an increased sensitivity to medications with anticholinergic properties. Even with medications thought to have minimal anticholinergic effects, such as second generation antihistamines and atypical antipsychotics, we frequently identify these side effects in elderly patients due to their increased sensitivity. Table 3-3 summarizes other

sometimes unexplained alterations in pharmacodynamic sensitivity to medications with specific recommendations are made to reduce the risk for adverse events.

Alterations at the End of Life

At the very end of life, additional pharmacokinetic and pharmacodynamic considerations must be addressed. Oral absorption may be impaired due to nasogastric suction and further slowing of the gastrointestinal tract may occur due to treatment with opiates. If the end of life period is particularly stressful (physical or psychologically) an increase in acid production may occur, increasing the risk for ulceration due to non-steroidal anti-inflammatory agents. Volume of distribution may be altered if the patient has edema or third space accumulation of fluid. Serum albumin concentrations may decrease if hepatic function is diminished or protein intake reduced. Fever and inflammation may decrease cytochrome P450 metabolism.

Table 3-3. **Pharmacodynamic Changes and Recommendations**

1. Start with very low doses of beta-adrenergic blockers and calcium channel blockers and titrate up slowly to avoid hypotension and bradycardia.

2. Avoid use of tricyclic antidepressants, antipsychotics, diuretics, angiotensin-converting enzyme inhibitors, alpha-adrenergic blockers, dopamine agonists, direct vasodilators, and opioids to minimize orthostatic hypotension.

3. Closely monitor use of diuretics and angiotensin converting enzyme inhibitors for fluid and electrolyte abnormalities and changes in oral intake of fluids, especially with emesis or diarrhea.

4. Avoid combination of medications that prolong the QT interval.

5. Start with very low doses of benzodiazepines and choose lorazepam or oxazepam due to their hydrophilic properties and Phase II metabolism.

6. Avoid drugs with anticholinergic properties. Even minor amounts of anticholinergic effect if present in multiple medications in the patient's regimen may be additive.

7. Begin with lower doses of warfarin to avoid the risk for overshooting the therapeutic INR range.

8. Anticipate a therapeutic response to anticonvulsants and immunosuppressants at the lower end of the therapeutic range.

9. Anticipate gastrointestinal hemorrhage from non-steroidal anti-inflammatory agents due to increased susceptibility.

10. Use a two-step tuberculosis skin test because of a decreased responsiveness in the elderly patients, particularly those residing in long term care facilities.

CASE 1: EMERGENCY ROOM

Setting:

Acute care hospital emergency room.

Subjective:

DH is a 79-year-old man who presents to the hospital with swelling and tenderness of his right lower extremity.

Past Medical History:

Atrial fibrillation, congestive heart failure, chronic kidney disease (baseline serum creatinine of 1.4 mg%), neuropathic pain.

Medications:

Furosemide 20 mg daily, fosinopril 40 mg twice daily, spironolactone 25 mg daily, metoprolol XL 25 mg daily, gabapentin 300 mg TID as needed for pain.

Allergies:

Penicillin caused "breathing problems."

Social History:

Retired engineer; lives with his wife.

Family History:

Non-contributory.

Objective:

Height 66 inches, weight 136.6 lb, blood pressure 132/80 mm Hg, heart rate 89 BPM, respiratory rate 15 per minute.

Physical examination:

Within normal limits except heart with irregularly irregular rhythm and right lower extremity with macular erythematous rash over right shin, pain to palpation and 4+ pitting edema.

Laboratory:

Complete blood count within normal limits except white blood count $16 \times 10^3 \times mm^3$ with 93.9% granulocytes, hemoglobin 10.2 g/dL, hematocrit 32.6%; electrolytes within normal limits. BUN 55 mg/dL, serum creatinine 1.7 mg/dL; PT 14.9 seconds, INR 1.2, PTT 26.9 seconds.

Assessment:

DH is a 79-year-old man with possible cellulitis.

Plan:

Admit to hospital, draw blood cultures and begin vancomycin 1 g every 24 hours for cellulitis. Check trough vancomycin level for further dosing adjustment and monitor BUN, serum creatinine, the white blood cell count and physical findings. Dosing adjustment for other renally eliminated medications. Evaluate patient for etiology of anemia and initiation of warfarin to prevent stroke.

Rationale:

Usual vancomycin dosage recommendations are 15-20 mg/kg/dose given every 12 hours in patients without renal insufficiency. The dose range for DH calculates as 930 mg to 1240 mg. Since 1000 mg is within this range and is a typical dose, it should be selected. DH weighs 62 kg, which is 1.8 kg below his calculated ideal body weight so his actual weight should be used to calculate his creatinine clearance and this calculation is 14 mL/min estimated by the Cockcroft-Gault equation. With this degree of renal insufficiency, vancomycin (a renally eliminated drug) will accumulate if dosed at the usual adult dosing range, so an extended interval is indicated. Drug information resources recommend every 24 hours or more.

Although the assessment does not mention that DH is dehydrated, the elevated BUN supports this possibility. A vancomycin trough level will guide further dosing more specifically regardless of the serum creatinine and hence the creatinine clearance calculation increases or decreases. The white cell count and physical findings will provide evidence of response to the antibiotic therapy.

The gabapentin dose for DH should be evaluated as it is renally eliminated. At a creatinine clearance of 14 mL/min, resources recommend a maximum dose of 300 mg daily. Furthermore, DH has a significant anemia, and his hemoglobin may decrease further with hydration. His anemia should be evaluated and appropriate therapy instituted. Finally, his records should be reviewed to identify why he is not anticoagulated to prevent embolism secondary to atrial fibrillation. If contraindications are not identified, warfarin should be added to his regimen.

Clinical Pearl

- *The most famous adage about pharmacotherapy for geriatric patients is "Start low, and go slow!" When we "start low," the changes in the volume of distribution, protein binding, and pharmacodynamics of an elderly patient are addressed. When we "go slow," the changes in metabolism and excretion are handled.*

Chapter Summary

Pharmacotherapy is one of the most challenging aspects of geriatric care because of age-related biologic changes. While many physiologic changes are common, few changes are due to aging itself. The impact that these changes have on the pharmacokinetics and pharmacodynamics of medications used to treat the older adult must be recognized in order to provide optimal pharmaceutical care. The pharmacist and other health care providers must apply these principles to avoid causing drug-related problems. As more is understood about the process of aging, more opportunities will arise to ensure that each patient has the tools needed to age successfully.

Self-Assessment Questions

1. What observational and interventional trials support or refute the most popular theories of aging such as the oxidative stress theory, genetic theory and system decline theories?

2. Which cardiovascular changes in older adults are a part of the normal aging process and which changes are more likely characterized as common in patients over the age of 65?

3. What are the expected changes seen in cognition as one grows older and how do they compare with changes seen in patients diagnosed with dementia?

4. What are the components of successful aging?

5. Which anti-aging therapies have been tested in humans and what are the results?

6. How do the changes associated with aging seen with lean body mass and body fat affect the volume of distribution of hydrophilic and lipophilic medications?

7. What would be the pharmacokinetic characteristics of the ideal drug for use with older patients?

8. What changes occur in Phase I metabolism as compared to Phase II metabolism in elderly patients?

9. Why are the changes in pharmacodynamics important to consider when choosing and dosing a medication for an elderly patient?

References

1. Hayflick L. Biological aging is no longer an unsolved problem. *Ann N Y Acad Sci.* 2007;1100:1–13.

2. Vina J, Borras C, Miquel J. Theories of aging. *Life.* 2007;59:249–254.

3. Harman D. Free radical theory of aging: an update Increasing the functional life span. *Ann N Y Acad Sci.* 2006;1067:10–21.

4. Muller FL, S LM, Youngmok J, Richardson A, Van Remmen H. Trends in oxidative aging theories. *Free Radical Biology & Medicine.* 2007;43:477–503.

5. Wright ME, Lawson KA, Weinstein SJ, et al. Higher baseline serum concentrations of vitamin E are associated with lower total and cause-specific mortality in the Alpha–Tocopherol, Beta–Carotene Cancer Prevention Study. *Am J Clin Nutr.* Nov 2006;84(5):1200–1207.

6. Peterson RC, Thomas RG, Grundman M, et al. Vitamin E and donepezil for the treatment of mild cognitive impairment. *N Engl J Med.* 2005;352(23):2379–2388.

7. vivekananthan D, Penn M, SK S, Hsu A, Topol E. Use of antioxidant vitamins for the prevention of cardiovascular disease: meta–analysis of randomised trials. *Lancet.* 2003;361:2017–2023.

8. Weinert BT, Timiras PS. Invited Review: Theories of aging. *J Appl Physiol.* 2003;95:1706–1716.

9. Vasto S, Candore G, Balistreri CR, et al. Inflammatory networks in ageing, age-related diseases and longevity. *Mech Aging Dev.* 2007;128(1):83–91.

10. Pugh KG, Wei JY. Clinical implications of physiological changes in the aging heart. *Drugs & Aging.* 2001;18(4):263–276.

11. Anstey KJ, Low L-F. Normal cognitive changes in aging. *Austr Fam Physician.* 2004;33(10):783–787.

12. Vaz Fragoso CA, Gill TM. Sleep complaints in community-living older persons: a multifactorial geriatric syndrome. *J Am Geriatr Soc.* 2007;55(11):1853–1866.

13. Epstein M. Aging and the kidney. *J Am Soc Nephrol.* 1996;7(8):1106–1122.

14. Oskvig RM. Special problems in the elderly. *Chest.* 1999;115(5 Supplement):158S–164S.

15. Meston CM. Aging and sexuality. *West J Med.* 1997;167(4):285–290.

16. Lamberts SWJ, van den Beld AW, van der Lely A-j. The endocrinology of aging. *Science.* 1997;278(5337):419–425.

17. D'Souza AL. Ageing and the gut. *Postgrad Med J.* 2007;83(975):44–53.

18. Cusack BJ. Pharmacokinetics in Older Persons. *Am J Geriatr Pharmacother.* 2004;2(4):274–302.

19. Fisher GJ, Kang S, Varani J, et al. Mechanisms of photoaging and chronological skin aging. *Arch Dermatol.* 2002;138(11):1462–1470.

20. Dharmarajan T, Ugalino J. The physiology of aging. In: Dharmarajan T, Norman R, eds. *Clinical Geriatrics.* New York: The Parthenon Publishing Group; 2003:9–22.

21. Hutchison LC, O'Brien CE. Changes in pharmacokinetics and pharmacodynamics in the elderly patient. *J Pharm Pract.* 2007;20(1):4–12.

22. Britton A, Shipley M, Singh-Manoux A, Marmot MG. Successful aging: The contribution of early-life and midlife risk factors. *J Am Geriatr Soc.* 2008;56(6):1098–1105.

23. Bowling A, Iliffe S. Which model of successful ageing should be used? Baseline findings from a British longitudinal survey of ageing. *Age Ageing.* 2006;35:607–614.

24. Bowling A, Seetai S, Morris R, Ebrahim S. Quality of life among older people with poor functioning: the influence of perceived control over life. *Age Ageing.* 2007;36:310–315.

25. The Calorie Restriction Society. Available at: http://www.crsociety.org/. Accessed December 3, 2009.

26. Walford RL, Mock D, Verdery R, McaccCallum T. Calorie restriction in Biosphere 2: alterations in physiologic, hematologic, hormonal, and biochemical parameters in humans restricted for a 2-year period. *J Gerontol A Biol Sci Med Sci.* 2002;57A:B211–224.

27. Resnick SM, Coker LH, Maki PM, et al. The Women's Health Initiative Study of Cognitive Aging (WHIS-CA): a randomized clinical trial of the effects of hormone therapy on age-associated cognitive decline. *Clin Trials.* 2004;1(5):440–450.

28. Shumaker SA, Legault C, Kuller L, et al. Conjugated equine estrogens and incidence of probable dementia and mild cognitive impairment in postmenopausal women: Women's Health Initiative Memory Study. *JAMA.* 2004;291(24):2947–2958.

29. Anderson GL, Limacher M, Assaf AR, et al. Effects of conjugated equine estrogen in postmenopausal women with hysterectomy: the Women's Health Initiative randomized controlled trial. *JAMA*. 2004;291(14):1701–1712.

30. Nair KS, Rizza RA, O'Brien P, et al. DHEA in elderly women and DHEA or testosterone in elderly men. *N Engl J Med*. 2006;355(16):1647–1659.

31. Emmelot-Vonk MH, Verhaar HJ, Nakhai Pour HR, et al. Effect of testosterone supplementation on functional mobility, cognition, and other parameters in older men: a randomized controlled trial. *JAMA*. 2008;299(1):39–52.

32. Liu H, Bravata DM, Olkin I, et al. Systematic review: the safety and efficacy of growth hormone in the healthy elderly. *Ann Intern Med*. 2007;146(2):104–115.

33. Baur JA, Sinclair DA. Therapeutic potential of resveratrol: the in vivo evidence. *Nat Rev Drug Discov*. 2006;5(6):493–506.

34. Prevention Centers for Disease Control. Health, United States. Figure 16. Available at: http://www.cdc.gov/nchs/hus.htm. Accessed December 3, 2009.

35. Hoogerduijn JG, Schuurmans MJ, Duijnstee MS, de Rooij SE, Grypdonck MF. A systematic review of predictors and screening instruments to identify older hospitalized patients at risk for functional decline. *J Clin Nurs*. Jan 2007;16(1):46–57.

36. Ferrucci L, Guralnik JM, Studenski S, Fried LP, Cutler GB, Jr., Walston JD. Designing randomized, controlled trials aimed at preventing or delaying functional decline and disability in frail, older persons: a consensus report. *J Am Geriatr Soc*. Apr 2004;52(4):625–634.

37. Gurwitz JH, Field TS, Harrold LR, et al. Incidence and preventability of adverse drug events among older persons in the ambulatory setting. *J Am Med Assoc*. 2003;189(9):1107–1116.

38. Bates DW, Leape LL, Petrycki S. Incidence and preventability of adverse drug events in hospitalized adults. *J Gen Intern Med*. 1993;8(6):289–294.

39. Hammerlein A, Derendorf H, Lowenthal DT. Pharmacokinetic and pharmacodynamic changes in the elderly. Clinical Implications. *Clinical Pharmacokinetics*. 1998;35(1):49–64.

40. McLean AJ, Le Couteur DG. Aging biology and geriatric clinical pharmacology. *Pharmacol Rev*. 2004;56(2):163–184.

41. Starner CI, Gray SL, Guay DR, Hajjar ER, Handler SM, Hanlon JT. Geriatrics. In: DiPiro JT, Talbert RL, Yee GC, Matzke GR, Wells BG, Posey LM, eds. *Pharmacotherapy: A Pathophysiologic Approach*. 7th ed. Available at: http://www.accesspharmacy.com/content.aspx?aID=3190958.

42. Greenblatt D, Harmatz J, Shader R. Clinical pharmacokinetics of anxiolytics and hypnotics in the elderly: therapeutic considerations: Pt 1. *Clinical Pharmacokinetics*. 1991;21(3):165–177.

43. Grandison M, Boudinot F. Age-related changes in protein binding of drugs: implications for therapy. *Clin Pharmacokinet*. 2000;38:271–290.

44. Belloto RJ. Altered pharmacokinetics in an aging population: a silent epidemic. In: Olsen CG, Tindall WN, Clasen ME, eds. *Geriatric Pharmacotherapy: A Guide for the Helping Professional*. Washington, DC: American Pharmacists Association; 2007:35–46.

45. Kinirons M, O'Mahony M. Drug metabolism and ageing. *Br J Clin Pharmacol*. 2004;57(5):540–544.

46. Cockroft D, Gault M. Prediction of creatinine-clearance from serum creatinine. *Nephron*. 1976;15:31–41.

47. Wolowich W, Raymo L, Rodriguez JC. Problems with the use of the Modified Diet in Renal Disease Formula to estimate renal function. *Pharmacotherapy*. 2005;25(9):1283–1285.

48. Bauer L. Creatinine clearance versus glomerular filtration rate for the use of renal drug dosing in patients with kidney dysfunction. *Pharmacotherapy*. 2005; 25(9):1286–1287.

49. Benoit S, Mendelsohn A, Nourjah P, Staffa J, Graham D. Risk factors for prolonged QTc among U.S. adults: Third national health and nutrition examination survey. *Eur J Cardiovasc Prev Rehabil*. 2005;12:363–368.

50. Blennow K, Fredman P, Wallin A, et al. Protein analysis in cerebrospinal fluid. II. Reference values derived from healthy individuals 18–88 years of age. *Eur Neurol*. 1993;33(2):129–133.

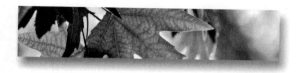

4

Geriatric Assessment

SUNNY A. LINNEBUR

Learning Objectives

1. Describe standard physical assessments necessary in geriatric patients.

2. Compare and contrast mood, behavioral, cognitive and functional assessments commonly utilized in clinical practice and research settings.

3. Describe important social assessments that should be performed in geriatric patients.

4. Explain changes that might be necessary for performing assessments in institutionalized patients and those with cognitive impairment.

Key Terms

ADL: Activities of daily living, such as bathing, dressing, and feeding.

ADVANCE DIRECTIVES: Legal documents that allow patients to have their medical decisions known and followed when receiving care.

GDS: Geriatric depression scale, a tool specifically for geriatrics patients to screen for depression.

IADL: Instrumental activities of daily living, such as shopping, paying bills, and managing medications.

MMSE: Mini-mental state examination, a tool commonly used for screening for cognitive impairment.

NPI-Q: Questionnaire that can be used in clinical practice to help with assessing neuropsychiatric symptoms of dementia.

TUG: Timed "up and go" test used to assess balance and fall risk in the elderly.

The author would like to thank Belynda Spooner, Pharm.D. candidate, Darla Eckley, Pharm.D. candidate, and Shannon Knutsen, Pharm.D. candidate, for their help in the preparation of this chapter.

Introduction

Due to the complexity of geriatric patients, assessment by health care providers typically requires more extensive investigation than for younger adults and may involve multiple health care practitioners. Furthermore, the frail elderly patient frequently presents with symptoms that are atypical for a specific disease. This makes diagnosis, treatment and monitoring a challenge. A full assessment should include the following: physical assessment and laboratory tests, a review of medical problems and medications, cognitive assessment, neuropsychiatric assessments, functional assessment, and social assessments. In addition to the evaluation of current medical problems, screening for diseases and plans for health promotion and disease prevention are also likely to be included when assessing relatively healthy elderly patients.

Caregivers, children, the medical power of attorney, and other individuals involved in the care for geriatrics patients should be included in visits if feasible to assist in reviewing medical information about the patient. Typically more than one visit is required in order to complete a comprehensive assessment of geriatric patients. It is also important to note that changes in the geriatric assessment may be required in those who are institutionalized or have dementia. Overall, the geriatric assessment should be tailored to the individual patient, based on their age, frailty, and living situation, and whenever possible, should include assessments from interdisciplinary team members and caregivers. Interdisciplinary team members who may be involved in assessing geriatric patients include physicians, nurse practitioners, physician assistants, nurses, pharmacists, social workers, physical therapists, occupational therapists, geropsychologists, dentists, and nursing aides and assistants. Although pharmacists can be involved in every step of the geriatric assessment, the most critical place for pharmacists to take an active role is in the assessment of medical problems and medications. Pharmacists are uniquely trained to identify drug-related problems and to make recommendations regarding drug therapy,

immunizations, and adherence. Capitalizing on the individual strengths of the geriatric interdisciplinary team members, including the pharmacist, allows for a more comprehensive assessment. The purpose of this chapter is to discuss in detail the steps involved in a comprehensive assessment of a geriatric patient and underscore its importance in the overall treatment plan for the patient.

KEY POINT: The geriatric assessment should be tailored to the individual patient, based on his or her age, frailty, and living situation.

Physical Assessment and Laboratory Evaluation

Physical assessment in the elderly requires typical elements performed in younger adults, with additions specifically based on the likelihood of chronic disease states, such as diabetes, chronic kidney disease, dementia, and depression being present. Physical assessment for a new patient should include reviews of all systems, vital signs, and examination of the eyes, skin, lungs, cardiovascular system, head and neck, musculoskeletal system, abdomen, and neurologic system. Many of the additional assessments necessary in elderly patients are to evaluate for the presence or consequences of chronic diseases. Of note, the physical assessments and laboratory evaluations described below are for "healthy" elderly patients, and may need to be altered or eliminated in more frail elderly patients depending upon the patient's goals.

Vital Signs

Typical vital signs (blood pressure, pulse, temperature, respiratory rate, and pain) are standard measurements necessary for a medical assessment in the elderly, and for the most part can easily be performed by a pharmacist. In the elderly, pain is especially important to evaluate due to the high incidence of osteoarthritis and chronic pain, and often needs investigation beyond a pain score. At a minimum, patients should also be evaluated for the location and type of pain they are experiencing. Blood pressure measurements in the elderly must be done with care. For example, it is important to select the correct size cuff (e.g., small, regular, or large), and it may be necessary to inflate the cuff to approximately 200 mmHg (or higher) prior to deflating the cuff, in order to make sure the correct systolic measurement is taken. An auscultatory gap is a common phenomenon among older patients with hypertension, so care must be taken to avoid a falsely low systolic reading. Orthostatic blood pressure measurements may also need to be evaluated due to aging, disease, and drug-related causes of orthostatic hypotension. When assessing the pulse it is important to note if the patient has a regular or irregular rhythm. As a standard vital sign, temperature should be checked at all visits. Any elevated temperature in the elderly is worrisome and should not be disregarded. Repeated temperature measurements greater than 99°F on two or more occasions, or an increase in temperature of more than 2°F above baseline usually indicate infection in an elderly patient.[1]

Patients with clinical signs or symptoms of infection, but with normal oral or tympanic temperatures, should have a rectal temperature measurement performed, as it can be more accurate in elderly patients.[2,3] Height and weight should be measured at the first visit, with weight being measured at all future visits. Weight and appetite should be evaluated to assess if the patient is under or overweight. Both obesity and malnutrition occur in the elderly, but in the very elderly malnutrition is more common. Multiple studies indicate that older adults who are undernourished have increased morbidity and mortality.[4] If the patient is obese, undernourished, or underweight, an intervention should be made. Referral to a dietician for nutrition counseling, a speech-language pathologist for a swallow study, or a dentist for an oral evaluation can be helpful in patients with malnutrition. Measured height can be compared with patient report to help identify if the patient may have vertebral fractures. If the patient is unable to get out of bed or has significant kyphosis, height can be estimated using knee height, forearm length, total arm length, or demi-span (the distance from the middle of the sternal notch to the tip of the middle finger).[5,6]

Ophthalmic, Otoscopic, and Oral Assessments

Eye examinations in the elderly should be performed by an optometrist at least annually. With increasing age, vision can deteriorate and there is an increased risk for ophthalmic disorders, such as glaucoma, macular degeneration, cataracts, and diabetic retinopathy. If driving, the patient should be assessed for the ability to see well enough to drive an automobile. Some states allow driver's licenses to last for many years (e.g., 10 years); during the time that the license is still active vision changes can occur and cause problems driving. To prevent accidents in the home or automobile, it is important to reassess vision periodically even if the patient is not complaining of vision changes. Also, the patient may need referral to an ophthalmologist if the optometrist cannot fully assess the patient or if they have complications of an ophthalmic disorder.

Ear examinations are also necessary in the elderly, as many may have hearing loss. Ears should be examined specifically for impacted cerumen, which is often due to dry cerumen and/or the use of hearing aids. The inability to hear can have negative consequences in the elderly, such as the appearance of cognitive impairment and preventing them from understanding their disease states and medications. In addition, impacted cerumen can make patients dizzy, predisposing them to falls. Hearing tests by an audiologist and further use of corrective hearing aids may improve quality of life. In patients with dementia, a finger rub or finger friction test can be utilized to assess hearing, and has been shown to have high sensitivity and specificity compared to audiometry.[7] Microphones with connected headsets (e.g., Pocket Talker) can also be used by health care practitioners to improve communication in patients with hearing impairment.

Oral problems often contribute to malnutrition in the elderly patient. Both medical providers and dentists can evaluate elderly patients for dryness, but dentists are better suited to evaluate for the number of teeth present, denture fit if applicable, the ability to chew food, and the presence of dental caries and oral cancers. If xerostomia is present, pharmacists can work with dentists and medical providers to reduce drug causes of xerostomia.

Skin Assessment

Skin examinations in the elderly should be particularly sensitive for dryness, cellulitis, edema, and cancer. Due to impaired sensation in the skin and impaired vision, elderly patients may not realize that their skin is dry, damaged, or infected. This is especially true for patients with diabetes who often suffer from neuropathies in their extremities as patient report may not be accurate. Edema is more prevalent in patients with congestive heart failure, but can occur in the elderly just due to poor circulation. Weight can also be used to help determine how much fluid overload is present. Skin cancer is more common in the elderly compared to younger adults[7] and the American Cancer Society (ACS) recommends that skin examinations should be done by a health care provider annually, with no age restriction.[9]

Pulmonary Assessment

Lung examinations in the elderly are similar to those in younger patients, taking into account that those with kyphosis may require a more meticulous assessment. Lung examinations for pulmonary edema that may accompany heart failure and chronic obstructive pulmonary disease including pulmonary function tests are useful to evaluate the severity of disease.

Cardiovascular Assessment

Cardiovascular examinations should evaluate the patient for murmurs and arrhythmias, such as atrial fibrillation. Blood pressure (both regular and orthostatic) as indicated above should be evaluated and assessed according to national blood pressure goals. For patients with hypertension, a fasting lipid panel should also be performed to evaluate if the patient has hyperlipidemia. If the patient has a sustained blood pressure of at least 135/80 mmHg, the United States Preven-tive Services Task Force (USPSTF) recommends screening the patient for type 2 diabetes, typically using a fasting plasma glucose concentration.[10] An electrocardiogram, carotid auscultation, and an echocardiogram may also be needed to further evaluate for arrhythmias, stroke risk, and heart failure, respectively. If the patient has a history of cardiovascular disease or cardiac risk factors, they should also be evaluated for peripheral vascular disease (PVD) with the ankle-brachial index. This simple calculation divides the systolic blood pressure in the ankle/foot by the systolic blood pressure in the arm to determine the index. A number below 0.8 is considered positive for PVD.

Musculoskeletal Assessment

The musculoskeletal examination in the elderly should evaluate range of motion in the joints, stability, strength, and the ability to rise from a sitting position, stand, bend forward, bend down, walk, and rotate the head around naturally. A proper amount of space is required to evaluate the patient. Some gait changes occur naturally with aging, such as narrowing or widening the stance. Gait and balance will also be discussed further under functional assessment.

Abdominal and Urologic Assessment

Palpation of the abdomen in the elderly is important to identify any masses and hernias. Abdominal examinations in the elderly often elicit a history of constipation. Chronic constipation is common in the elderly due to use of medications, decreased water and fiber intake, and lack of activity. A rectal examination may identify hemorrhoids and/or an enlarged prostate in men. Prostate cancer screening with a digital rectal examination and a prostate specific antigen (PSA) blood test should be offered to men annually, as long as life expectancy is at least 10 years.[9] An evaluation for colon cancer, such as a colonoscopy every 10 years, a flexible sigmoidoscopy every 5 years, or a double contrast barium enema every 5 years should also be offered.[9] Due to the invasiveness of colon cancer screening procedures, there is not an agreement on how long to continue testing. Typically if a patient is frail and would not choose to treat a detected cancer, there is no need to perform screening tests. Urologic examinations should focus on urinary retention, incontinence and benign prostatic hypertrophy. Many clinics now have ultrasound machines that can evaluate post-void residuals in patients with urinary retention, or it can be done with a urinary catheter. Pap smears in women can be stopped at age 70 if the last three are normal and all were normal in the last 10 years, or if the patient has had a total hysterectomy.[9] Elderly women should also be asked about vaginal dryness.

Neurologic Assessment

The thorough neurologic examination in the elderly can identify many subtle abnormalities including muscle strength, sensation, reflexes, sensory motor skills, coordination, tremor, muscle tone, and postural stability. In a study of older, community-dwelling adults without overt neurological disease, multiple subtle neurological abnormalities were associated with cognitive and functional decline and independently predicted mortality and cerebrovascular events.[11] In addition, cognition should be evaluated either with the neurologic examination, or separately. A discussion of cognitive assessment is found later in the chapter.

Other Assessments

Other evaluations that should be done in the elderly include an assessment of sleep, which is often abnormal and a foot examination to evaluate for pulses, dryness, nails, ulcers, and deformities. Patients with foot abnormalities or functional deficits can be referred to a podiatrist for further evaluation. In addition, a clinical breast examination and mammography is recommended annually in women if they are in good health,[9] and a dual-energy x-ray absorptiometry (DEXA) is recommended for all elderly women and high-risk men to evaluate their bone mineral density for osteoporosis. The DEXA should be performed on all eligible patients as long as they are able to lay down comfortably for the DEXA and are eligible for osteoporosis treatment. Medicare will cover one DEXA test every two years. Evaluating and assessing osteopenia or osteoporosis further can be facilitated by using the World Health Organization Fracture Risk Assessment Tool (FRAX) available online at http://www.shef.ac.uk/FRAX/.[12] The tool takes into account patient specific risk factors, such as age, race, country of origin, concomitant medications and disease state, and bone mineral density (if available) to estimate the 10-year probability of fracture. The tool can also be utilized to decide if drug treatment is warranted based on cost-effectiveness of treatment.

Laboratory Measurements

Typical baseline laboratory measurements that should be obtained in the elderly include: thyroid stimulating hormone (TSH); complete blood count (CBC); a basic metabolic panel to evaluate electrolytes and serum creatinine (SCr). In patients with a life expectancy of 3 years or more, a fasting lipid panel to screen for hypercholesterolemia is indicated. Utilizing the SCr, an estimation of creatinine clearance (CrCl) should be performed on all elderly patients at baseline and if the SCr increases significantly. Although it may underestimate the CrCl slightly, the Cockcroft-Gault equation is still the preferred equation to use in the elderly to estimate kidney function as discussed in Chapter 3.

Additional laboratory measurements are indicated in specific situations: a hemoglobin A_{1C} if the patient is diabetic; vitamin B12, if the patient is malnourished or has memory loss, anemia, depression, fatigue, or neuropathy; and, liver function tests (LFTs) if the patient is on medications that can raise these concentrations. After laboratory tests have been measured once, Medicare may not reimburse for them again for a certain time period. For example, unless the patient has an indication such as hyperlipidemia, hypertension, or coronary disease, Medicare may not reimburse for another screening fasting lipid panel for 5 years. Medicare also has restrictions on hemoglobin A_{1C}, which cannot be checked more often than once a month. Other laboratory measurements that are useful in the elderly include a serum 25-hydroxy vitamin D concentration, especially if the patient has osteoporosis, is obese, takes no vitamin D supplement, or is institutionalized; and a baseline creatinine kinase if the patient is going to be prescribed a statin.

KEY POINT: The type and frequency of laboratory examinations in the elderly are many times governed by Medicare reimbursement.

Assessments in Those Who Cannot Provide Self-Report

Physical examination and review of systems in patients who cannot provide self-report is often difficult and may rely on caregiver input. In patients who are institutionalized or who cannot provide self-report, some examinations and screenings may be eliminated, as the provider may be limited to bedside assessments, and certain screenings may not be necessary. Generally, the risks and benefits of the examination/screening can be reviewed by the provider, patient, family, or medical power of attorney to help determine how aggressive or limited to make the examination. Moreover, if the patient is bed-bound, certain exams may not be possible (e.g., DEXA). Vision and hearing assessment is typically only necessary for quality of life. However, if the patient is unable to respond, it is not possible to get accurate results. Studies of pain assessment in elderly patients with cognitive impairment indicate that self-report pain scales can still be used.[14,15] Based on several studies, it appears that elderly with cognitive impairment prefer the FACES rating scale, which utilizes facial expressions to rate their pain.[14,15]

Review of Medical Problems and Medications

The medical history of a geriatric patient can be extremely complex and time consuming to elicit. Many times the patient may not have previous medical records with them and may not fully remember their medical history, so care must be taken to order pertinent medical records from previous medical providers and hospitals. A complete medical history should include a family history, history of present illness, active medical problems, past medical problems, past hospitalizations, and past surgical procedures. It is especially helpful to identify dates of such past events, as dating of events can change current medical therapy. For example, if a patient had a coronary stent placed several years ago, it may be possible to reduce dual antiplatelet therapy as compared to a patient who had a coronary stent placed in the last several months. A functional health literacy assessment can also be performed to assess the patient's ability to obtain, process and understand basic health information and make appropriate health decisions.[16] Examples of formal assessments of health literacy include the Rapid Estimate of Adult Literacy in Medicine (REALM) and the Test of Functional Health Literacy in Adults (TOFHLA).[17,18]

A recent immunization history should be performed in every elderly patient, as multiple immunizations are indicated for older adults. All patients should be evaluated for a history of the 23-valent pneumococcal vaccination, yearly influenza vaccinations, herpes zoster vaccination, and a tetanus booster in the last 10 years. In most states, unvaccinated older adults can be referred to their local pharmacies for indicated immunizations.

A full medication assessment is also essential for geriatric patients. This should include current use of prescription drugs and over-the-counter vitamins, supplements, and herbal medications, in addition to the patient's pharmacy contact information. Past use of medications for chronic diseases, such as chronic pain, diabetes, hypertension, etc can also be useful in order to eliminate medication options for the future. A pharmacist can easily perform the medication assessment or provide valuable input to the medication assessment. Special insight from the pharmacist can help to identify drugs with no medical indications, drugs treating side effects of other drugs, duplications in therapy, drug-drug and drug-disease interactions, adverse effects, inappropriate or inadequate prescribing, non-adherence, and other such drug-related problems.

Pharmacists are integral in reducing drug-related costs for elderly patients. This can be accomplished in many ways, but typically includes increasing Medicare Part D formulary adherence to lower tier medications and recommendations for discontinuing medications. Pharmacists can also help patients to utilize pharmacy-specific drug discount programs (e.g., $4 generics), manufacturer patient assistance programs, and by ensuring the patient applies for extra assistance from state or federal programs (e.g., social security extra assistance, or Medicaid).

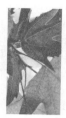

KEY POINT: Special insight from the pharmacist can help to identify drug-related problems, opportunities for reducing drug-related costs, and the need for patient education.

Along with a functional health literacy assessment, it is helpful to assess the older adults' understanding of their medications and disease states. An assessment of self-administration abilities for medications should also be included, and if the patient is found unable to perform these duties, plans for assistance should be made. Simple devices, such as pillboxes or calendars, can help many elderly patients remember to take their medications. For those with cognitive impairment or complex medication regimens, family members or caregivers may have to assist with medication adherence. Nonadherence in the elderly can be intentional (e.g., to save money or to prevent side effects) or nonintentional (e.g., too complex for patient to handle or forgetting to order refills). For institutionalized patients, medication adherence cannot be assumed because patients still have the ability to refuse their oral medications and unforeseen circumstances may prevent administration. Specific tools, such as the Morisky scale and the Drug Regimen Unassisted Grading Scale (DRUGS) and Medication Management Instrument for Deficiencies in the Elderly (MedMaIDE™) instruments, can assist the pharmacist in assessing the patient's capacity to manage medications, including adherence.[19,20] The Morisky scale consists of yes/no questions for the patient to ascertain if they forget to take medication, or if they purposefully choose to stop taking medication due to hassles or side effects. It has been adapted and validated for use in hypertension in seniors. The DRUGS evaluation involves asking the patient about each of his own medications against the prescribed directions, calculating a percentage correct of naming the drug, identifying the correct directions and time of day for administration. Poorer scores are associated with lower **mini-mental state examination (MMSE)** scores and increased risk of institutionalization. The MedMaIDE™ instrument is designed to identify if a patient understands what their medications are for, how to use medications, how to obtain medications and ability to administer medications.

Pharmacists providing medication therapy management (MTM) services will typically perform a thorough medical, medication, and adherence assessment. Pharmacists directly working with the primary care provider may have access to the medical records for the patient, but pharmacists providing services from a community pharmacy setting or through the Medicare Part D plan may only have access to the patient and medical and drug claims data. Pharmacists seeing patients in person for MTM can perform their own vital signs to evaluate the patient's drug therapy. Overall, pharmacists have the knowledge and ability to make many recommendations for patients to optimize their medications, improve adherence, reduce drug costs, and prevent adverse drug events.

Pharmacists providing MTM services or seeing geriatric patients in the community may refer patients to a geriatrician for a more thorough medical review. Moreover, interdisciplinary teams are important for quality care for complex geriatric patients. Depending on the state, pharmacists can directly refer patients to a physical therapist, occupational therapist, social worker, or dietician for additional assistance with their healthcare, functioning, or social issues although a physician's order may be necessary for Medicare to pay for the services.

Cognitive Assessment

Cognitive assessment in the elderly should be performed at one of the first visits and then yearly or as often as determined to be clinically relevant. There are multiple tools to assess cognition, but typically clinicians will utilize the MMSE, Mini-Cog, or the Seven-Minute Screen (7MS).[21-23] These tools are most utilized as they are quick to perform and are often reprinted for clinic use. They can be utilized in the outpatient or institutional settings. Pharmacists in many settings can easily initiate screening if they detect cognitive impairment, such as while performing MTM services or discussing adherence. In patients who may have complex cognitive impairment or for clinicians who are not comfortable with cognitive testing, referring patients to a geropsychologist, speech-language pathologist, or neurologist trained in cognitive testing can be useful.

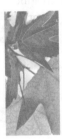

KEY POINT: There are multiple tools to assess cognition, but typically clinicians will utilize the Folstein Mini-Mental State Examination (MMSE), Mini-Cog, or the Seven-Minute Screen (7MS).

The MMSE is the most widely used clinical tool for assessing cognitive impairment associated with dementia, and is typically utilized to stage Alzheimer's Disease (AD) as mild, moderate or severe. It includes 11 questions assessing five different domains: short-term memory (recall), orientation, attention, language, and short-term memory (retention).[21] The maximum possible score for the test is 30 points. Typically a score of 24 to 30 indicates no cognitive impairment, 18 to 23 indicates mild impairment, 10 to 18 indicates moderate impairment, and less than 10 indicates severe cognitive impairment. The examination takes approximately 7–10 minutes to administer, but possibly longer if the patient has more severe cognitive impairment. Disadvantages

of the MMSE are that education level and language barriers can influence the results.

The Mini-Cog (Figure 4-1) is a combination three-item recall and a Clock Drawing Test (CDT). It is a simple, brief and valid screening tool designed to identify individuals at high-risk for dementia. Because the Mini-Cog takes approximately 3 minutes to administer, it is extremely simple for clinicians to remember and to utilize in their practice. Moreover, pharmacists can easily implement the Mini-Cog into their assessments when discussing adherence, ability to self-administer medications, or medication management services. The Mini-Cog assesses short-term and long-term memory, verbal comprehension, conceptualization, and executive functioning. The patient learns three unrelated words and is then asked to draw a clock with a time indicating ten minutes past eleven. Next, the patient is asked to recall the three items previously learned. The CDT acts as an assessment tool as well as a separation between the initial learning/recall of the three words. The Mini-Cog is scored based on points for each item recalled and a normal/abnormal clock. Although the Mini-Cog includes both the three-word recall and the CDT, some clinicians prefer to use only the CDT. The Mini-Cog has a sensitivity of 76–99% and a specificity of 89–93% at detecting cognitive impairment.[26] Multiple studies have compared the Mini-Cog to the MMSE and have found them to be equally effective.[26] Moreover, culture, education and language do not influence test results of the Mini-Cog.[26,27]

Additional screening tests for cognition include the 7MS and the St. Louis University Mental Status (SLUMS) The 7MS is another neurocognitive screening tool developed to provide improved sensitivity. The 7MS is composed of four brief tests: orientation, enhanced cued recall, clock drawing, and verbal fluency. The 7MS administration time ranges from 6–11 minutes and has performed better than the MMSE at evaluating very mild to mild AD, and it is not affected by gender, age or education level.[23,28] The SLUMS is similar in format to the MMSE, with a 30-point, 11-item scale. Patients are scored based on their level of education and classified as normal, having

DATE________ ID____________________AGE____GENDER M F LOCATION________________TESTED BY_______

MINI-COG ™

1) **GET THE PATIENT'S ATTENTION, THEN SAY: "I am going to say three words that I want you to remember now and later. The words are**
Banana Sunrise Chair.
Please say them for me now." (Give the patient 3 tries to repeat the words. If unable after 3 tries, go to next item.)
(Fold this page back at the TWO dotted lines BELOW to make a blank space and cover the memory words. Hand the patient a pencil/pen).

2) **SAY ALL THE FOLLOWING PHRASES IN THE ORDER INDICATED: "Please draw a clock in the space below. Start by drawing a large circle."** (When this is done, say) **"Put all the numbers in the circle."** (When done, say) **"Now set the hands to show 11:10 (10 past 11)."** If subject has not finished clock drawing in 3 minutes, discontinue and ask for recall items.

3) **SAY: "What were the three words I asked you to remember?"**

________ ________ ________ (Score 1 point for each) 3-Item Recall Score ☐

Score the clock (see other side for instructions): Normal clock 2 points; Abnormal clock 0 points — Clock Score ☐

Total Score = 3-item recall plus clock score ☐ ***0, 1, or 2 possible impairment; 3, 4, or 5 suggests no impairment***

Figure 4-1. The Mini-Cog™ tool is used to screen individuals at high risk for dementia.
Source: Reproduced with permission from S. Borson. Reprinted with permission of the author, solely for clinical and teaching use. All rights reserved.

mild neurocognitive disorder (MNCD), or having dementia. The SLUMS exam has been found to be comparable to the MMSE at detecting cognitive impairment, and appears to be possibly better at identifying mild neurocognitive disorder.[29]

Tools used in research must measure severity of disease and detect changes, and as such the tools are longer and take more time to administer. Clinical trials assessing cognition typically utilize the MMSE and Alzheimer's Disease Assessment Scale-cognitive subscale (ADAS-cog) for those with mild to moderate impairment and the MMSE and Severe Impairment Battery (SIB) for those with moderate to severe impairment.[24] The Clinician's Interview Based Impression of Change-Plus Caregiver Input (CIBIC-Plus) is complementary assessment of cognition and function utilized in clinical trials evaluating patients with cognitive impairment.[25] Pharmacists should be familiar with these instruments to provide adequate critique to study results.

The Alzheimer's Disease Assessment Scale was designed to measure severity of the most important symptoms of Alzheimer's disease.[30] The ADAS-Cog is a subscale that is considered the "gold standard" of cognitive tests used in clinical trials studying patients with mild to moderate cognitive impairment. Total scores range from zero to 70, with higher scores (greater than or equal to 18) indicating greater cognitive impairment. A four point change in 6 months is recognized as a clinically important difference.[31]

The SIB is a research tool designed to assess later stages of dementia.[24] Overall scores can range from 0–100 allowing for classification of degree of impairment with lower scores indicating greater cognitive impairment. The CIBIC-Plus differs from the ADAS-cog and SIB because it relies upon the caregiver interpretation of change in cognition and functioning from baseline to follow-up. The scoring ranges from one to seven points with four points indicating "no change." A score of one point is "very much improved" and a score of seven means "very much worse." The CIBIC-Plus is better at estimating decline rather than improvement.

Clinical interpretation of changes in the cognitive assessments described above is controversial. In general, as patients with dementia age, their scores on the assessments will decline. Clinical trials studying the effects of medications, such as cholinesterase inhibitors or memantine, and using some of the above measurements (e.g., MMSE, ADAS-cog, SIB) have found statistically significant improvements.[32] However, many experts question the clinical significance of these improvements.[33]

Neuropsychiatric Assessment

Because depression is common in the elderly, all geriatric patients presenting for the first time should be screened for depression. Screening after that can be done based on clinical suspicion for depression or periodically thereafter. Compared to younger adults, elderly patients with depression may not have typical signs and symptoms of depression. For this reason, the **Geriatric Depression Scale (GDS)** is a more specific screening tool for the geriatric population. The GDS is a self-report screening tool that relies on the patient to provide yes or no answers to questions about feelings/symptoms associated with depression.[34] It has been studied and validated in multiple geriatric populations and settings including outpatient settings, nursing home settings, inpatient settings, patients with normal cognition, patients with dementia, patients with visual impairment, patients who are non-English speaking, and when administered over the telephone.[35,36] The 15-item version is utilized more often when patients are fatigued or less time is available. In patients who are unwilling or unable to complete the GDS, both versions are also available in a validated informant version (GDS-I).[37,38]

Scoring and clinical application of the GDS is based on total points (e.g., 15 or 30), with some points awarded for positive responses and some points awarded for negative responses. A variety of scores have been utilized as cut-points to indicate depression; in general the higher the score the more severe the depression.

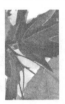 **KEY POINT:** The Geriatric Depression Scale (GDS) is a more specific screening tool for the geriatric population than other depression screening tools.

If the patient has dementia and needs to be assessed for depression, the GDS or GDS-I can be used as a screening tool. Additionally, the Dementia Mood Assessment Scale and the Cornell Scale for Depression in Dementia are screening tools that were developed specifically for this population. Both scales are completed by a caregiver or nursing staff.

In patients with dementia, psychotic and behavioral problems can also occur as the disease state progresses. Assessment of psychotic and behavioral problems in patients with dementia and the ability of the caregiver(s) to cope with the problems is important to evaluate the safety of the patient and the ability to stay in the same living situation. Several rating scales are available for assessment of behavior. The Neuropsychiatric Inventory (NPI), Behave-AD (Behavioral Pathology in Alzheimer's Disease Rating Scale), and **NPI-Q (Neuropsychiatric Inventory Questionnaire)** are commonly used assessments of behavioral problems.[39-41] The NPI, Behave-AD, and CIBIC-Plus are longer assessments, and as such are mainly utilized in research settings and clinical trials, while the NPI-Q was developed for clinical practice. The CIBIC-Plus, an assessment tool described above under Cognitive Assessment, includes components of behavioral assessment and is also utilized to evaluate these symptoms in clinical trials.

The NPI is a validated evaluation of neuropsychiatric symptoms based on a structured interview conducted by a provider with a caregiver and takes about 10 minutes to complete. The NPI includes 12 symptom domains rated for frequency and severity by the caregiver, for a total of 144 points. Higher scores indicate more severe neuropsychiatric illness. Clinical trials for drugs being studied for dementia often utilize the NPI as a secondary outcome. The NPI-NH can be completed by certified nurses' aides and licensed vocational nurses for use as a tracking agent for behavioral changes.[42] The Behave-AD is one of the earliest neuropsychiatric rating scales, and similar to the NPI, is often included in clinical trials of drug treatments in patients with Alzheimer's disease. The Behave-AD is a validated tool that evaluates 25 neuropsychiatric symptoms in seven categories, and includes a global rating of caregiver stress associated with the symptoms. The Behave-AD takes approximately 20 minutes to administer.

The NPI-Q is a validated questionnaire for clinical practice that can typically be completed in five minutes or less. The NPI-Q has the same symptom domains as the NPI; the caregiver-informant rates the severity of behavioral symptoms and the distress on the caregiver. Scores on the NPI-Q range from zero to 60, with higher numbers indicating increased severity of symptoms and increased stress on the caregiver.

Similar to the cognitive tests described previously, the definition of clinically significant changes in neuropsychiatric tests is debatable. Clinical trials studying drugs for Alzheimer's disease typically find statistically significant changes in these assessments, but it is very difficult to tell if these changes are clinically relevant as a whole. In patients who are complex, it may be useful to refer the patient to a neurologist or neuropsychologist for further evaluation and recommendation. Although pharmacists are likely to interact and recommend treatment for patients with neuropsychiatric symptoms, it is unlikely that they will be involved with neuropsychiatric screening other than utilizing the GDS screening tool for depression.

Functional Assessment

Functional assessments of geriatric patients should be performed at the initial visit and at regular intervals (e.g., annually) to assess for changes in function that might require changes in living situation. A comprehensive functional assessment should include assessing **activities of daily living (ADLs), instrumental activities of daily living (IADLs),** gait and balance, fall risk, and current level of physical activity. Geriatric nurses, social workers, occupational therapists, physical therapists, and caregivers are especially helpful in performing functional assessments of patients. Specifically, occupational therapists are typically trained in assessing and making recommendations to improve ADLs and IADLs. Physical therapists are helpful for assessing and intervening on gait and balance problems, fall risk, level of physical activity, and use of assistive devices for walking. Multiple tools are available to assist with assessing function. Utilizing these tools in clinical practice may help detect impairments that may not be adequately recognized by clinicians.[43]

Activities of daily living include self-care activities that are required to sustain existence and independence, such as bathing, dressing, toileting, transferring from bed or chair, continence, feeding, grooming, and walking. Patients should be evaluated to determine if they are capable of performing ADLs independently, with help, or if they are dependent on others to perform them. Based on the patient's ability to perform ADLs independently, they might require assistance that varies from needing to have a caregiver check on them several times a week, to living with a caregiver or in an assisted living facility, or living in a long term care center (e.g., nursing home). Physicians can also order home health care, including nursing, physical therapy, and occupational therapy, for patients who need assistance at home. Home health care agencies paid by Medicare are required to perform a formal assessment of the patient's need for care (Outcome and Assessment Information Set [OASIS]), including the ability of the patient to perform ADLs and IADLs.[44] These data are utilized by Medicare to monitor the quality of home health care, but can also be utilized by health care practitioners to monitor patient-specific quality of care.

Multiple tools are available to assist in documenting ADL assessments. The Katz ADL tool is one of the oldest tools utilized in clinical practice to assess ADLs, and takes about five minutes to administer.[45] The tool scores patients one point for being independent with six categories of ADLs and zero points for dependence with the activities. Higher points indicate more independence and functioning. The Alzheimer's Disease Cooperative Study Activities of Daily Living Inventory (ADCS-ADL) tool is a more detailed tool typically utilized in research settings and clinical trials and includes an assessment of ADLs and IADLs. The ADCS-ADL is a caregiver-rated questionnaire assessing 23 items; higher scores indicate better functioning.[46] This tool is capable of assessing function in a wider range of patients with cognitive impairment than the Katz ADL tool.

Instrumental activities of daily living consist of more complex activities that are necessary to have a higher level of functioning. The Lawton IADL tool is a commonly utilized tool in clinical practice and takes about 10 minutes to administer. It assesses the ability to complete the following eight tasks: ability to use a telephone, shop, prepare meals, maintain light housework, do laundry, travel independently, take medications, and handle finances.[47] Some IADLs are learned skills, and as such, the ability of the patient to carry out IADLs may be more a function of their environment and previous training than ADLs. A higher score on the Lawton IADL too indicates higher functioning. IADL tools can be completed by either the patient or a caregiver.

Falls, Gait, Balance, and Physical Activity

A patient's recent fall history (e.g., last 1–3 months) should be assessed at all medical visits and future fall risk should be assessed regularly (e.g., annually). Assessing fall risk requires assessment of many factors that can increase risk of falls, such as drugs (e.g., sedative/hypnotics), and disease states (e.g., heart disease, osteoarthritis, Parkinson's Disease), in addition to gait, balance and strength, and home safety (e.g., rugs, loose floor boards, stairs, cluttered areas).[48]

Both gait and balance can be assessed utilizing the Berg balance scale (BBS) and the **Timed Up and Go Test (TUG)**.[49,50] The BBS requires individuals to complete 14 balance-challenging tasks of varying difficulty without any assistive devices. For instance, the patient is asked to go from a sitting position to a standing position, the transfer between two chairs, to pick up an object from the floor, to stand in tandem stance, and to stand on one leg. Each item is scored on a five point scale with higher ratings associated with better performances. The highest number of points that patients can achieve is 56, with 45 points and up typically utilized as the cut-off for patients who are not likely to fall. This scale has good specificity (96%) for detecting non-fallers.[51] It takes approximately 10 to 15 minutes to administer and requires some equipment (e.g., chairs, stopwatch, yardstick, line on floor).

The TUG is easier and quicker than the BBS to assess fall risk. The patient must sit in a chair, safely rise from the chair, walk around a visibly colored marker (e.g., orange cone) three meters away, walk back, and then sit down in the chair. The patient must be instructed to do all of this as quickly and safely as they can. Patients can use their typical assistive devices while taking the test, but this typically slows them down. The test is timed; those who complete the test in less than 20 seconds have been shown to be independent in their transfers and mobility, and those requiring 30 seconds or longer have higher dependence and frailty. In another study of the TUG, investigators found that older adults who take longer than 14 seconds to complete the test are at a high risk of future falls.[52] Patients completing the test in a quicker fashion can still be counseled to consider exercise that is balance challenging, and those in the high-risk group should seek further assessment for falls and intervention.

Assessment of physical activity is also important in the ambulatory elderly, as increased physical activity has been shown to be an important predictor of functional status.[53] Surgeon general and American Heart Association (AHA) guidelines suggest 30 minutes or more of moderate physical activity on five or more days of the week.[53,54] The AHA guidelines also provide very detailed recommendations for strengthening and stability. Older sedentary adults can improve physical functioning by meeting these suggested physical activity levels; dropping below these levels has a negative effect on function.[53] Patients should be interviewed about the type of physical activity that they are involved with and the amount of time they are spending doing particular activities. Relatively brief counseling about walking and strength exercise has been shown to increase physical activity in elderly patients.[55]

Social Assessment

The social assessment in the elderly includes some aspects traditionally in a medical assessment of a new patient (e.g., smoking and alcohol status), but moves beyond that to include areas essential to caring for an older adult (e.g., independence, **advance directives**, insurance status, transportation/driving status, sexual activity, and life changes). Social workers can provide invaluable assistance and information for clinicians, patients, and caregivers when performing a complete social assessment.

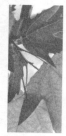 KEY POINT: The social assessment includes areas essential to caring for an older adult: independence, advance directives, insurance status, transportation/driving, sexual activity, and life changes.

Recent life changes should be assessed in order to fully appreciate goals that elderly patients may have for their healthcare. Many elderly will have faced new life changes, such as the death of a spouse, illness, moving from their home to an assisted living situation and/or dealing with the reality of their own eventual death. As such it is important to assess how patients deal with these changes and how they perceive themselves to determine their overall adaptability to life changes.

Social History: Tobacco and Alcohol Use

While most elderly do not start smoking in their advanced age it is important to assess their current smoking status, as those who do smoke probably have a significant smoking history. Similar to younger adults, patients should be asked about the length of their smoking history, how many packs or cigarettes per day they smoked, and any attempts to quit in the past. In addition, it is important to assess their willingness to quit. Many elderly may believe that they will not see a benefit from smoking cessation at this point in their lives. However, there is evidence to show that smoking cessation at any age, even after age $\geq$65 years old, is beneficial for reducing overall risk of death and disability.[56,57] If a patient is willing to quit smoking, assistance with a plan, whether non-pharmacologic or pharmacologic, should be offered.

In addition to tobacco use, alcohol consumption should be elicited from elderly patients. Occasional alcohol use may be permitted if it increases quality of life, but heavy alcohol use or even persistent use can cause complications in the elderly. For example, alcohol may increase a patients' risk for falls and fractures by impairing judgment and increasing balance problems. Secondly, chronic alcohol consumption may result in impaired hepatic function altering metabolism of medications. Since many elderly are on multiple medications there is a high likelihood they will be on at least one medication that is hepatically metabolized. Furthermore, it is important to assess alcohol consumption in elderly patients who become hospitalized to prevent delirium tremens, a potentially life threatening consequence of alcohol withdrawal. Older adults are likely to have a higher blood alcohol than younger people for a given dose of alcohol.[58] This can increase the risk of patients with chronic alcohol use developing delirium tremens when admitted to the hospital if proper assessment of alcohol use is not preformed.

Independence

Independence should be assessed as described above in the functional assessment. If the patient lives in an assisted living facility, the contact information for the facility should be recorded. A complete list of health care providers (e.g., specialists) should be recorded for future reference. Family and caregiver information should also be recorded at the initial visit and updated as needed. If the elderly patient has multiple family contacts, it is important to have a primary contact designated so health care providers are aware of whom to contact first. It is helpful to have this information available before a patient becomes severely ill.

Advance Directives

Assessment of advance directives is a vital, but sometimes neglected, part of the medical assessment of elderly patients. Advance directives are legal documents that allow patients to have their medical decisions known and followed when receiving care. These are so important to assess that in 1990 the Federal Patient Self Determination Act passed requiring that patients be asked at the time of admission to a healthcare service whether they have advance care plans.[59] Advanced directives must be documented when patients still have the capacity to make healthcare decisions. Once an initial assessment of advance directives is made, it is important to regularly reassess a patient's wishes since they can change as the patient ages or develops new health problems. Advance care plans can be revised up until the last moment of capacity to make decisions, so it is also important for healthcare providers to assess whether the most current decisions are on record.

Assessment to make sure elderly have advance directives in place or at least have thought about these issues is important for not only the patient but also the family. Having advance directives in place alleviates some of the stress and anxiety of family members when having to make decisions for loved ones.

Insurance Coverage

Another important assessment topic is insurance coverage, both government provided (Medicare, Medicaid, and military service) and private. Most elderly will have Medicare coverage and many will supplement coverage with an additional privately secured insurance plan. It is important to deter-

mine a person's eligibility for Medicare because Medicare coverage is associated with significant improvements in self-reported health trends for previously uninsured patients, especially for cardiovascular disease or diabetes.[61] Patients can enroll in Medicare Part A, B, and/or D. Medicare Part A covers hospitalizations; Part B covers outpatient medical visits, infusions, and medical supplies; and Part D covers prescriptions. However, Medicare coverage is not free of charge. Patients must pay deductibles and copays for products and services, unless they have supplemental coverage for these expenses. Medicare Part D covers prescription drugs for any person with Medicare. Some elderly may qualify for extra help if their individual savings and investments are worth less than 150% of the federal poverty levels. These dollar amounts fluctuate, so checking the Medicare and Social Security websites is important to fully investigate whether or not a patient may qualify for extra help. If the patient qualifies, then their Medicare copays may be reduced or eliminated.

For patients with Medicare Part D is it also advantageous to assess when and if they will be in the "doughnut-hole" coverage gap. Depending on the plan, during this time the patient may be responsible for all prescription drug costs until they spend up to a particular dollar amount designated by their selected Medicare Part D plan. Elderly patients with no prescription benefits while in this coverage gap may become nonadherent with their medications due to cost.

Transportation and Driving Assessment

Assessing transportation in the elderly is extremely important, as they may not have the ability to come to healthcare visits regularly, pick up their medications, shop for groceries, and have social outlets. Assessing an elderly individual's ability to appropriately operate a motor vehicle is an important balance between maintaining the individual's independence and personal and public safety. This assessment is particularly important for people with cognitive impairment or perception deficits such as decreased vision, arthritis, seizures, stroke, diabetes or Alzheimer's disease. Many elderly link driving with independence and rely on it for daily activities. Due to this, it may be difficult to convince them they are no longer safe to operate a mother vehicle. Social support from family and friends is essential to the decision for elderly patients to stop driving. Since many states do not require drivers to come into the Department of Motor Vehicles (DMV) each time they renew their licenses, caregivers, family members, clinicians and even the patient must play an important role in assessing driving ability. When a patient has been shown to be a likely unsafe driver, a referral should be made to the proper organization per each state's protocol; if a patient is no longer able to independently operate a motor vehicle, it becomes important to assess their ability to use other modes of transportation.

Patients who do not drive should be assessed for mode of transportation for outings. Depending on the living situation of the individual, transportation may be included with their housing. If not, those living in more rural areas may not have access to public transportation, while those in urban areas may have safety concerns with public transportation. In urban areas, non-profit programs such as Access-A-Ride can provide low-cost transportation for elderly patients with functional deficits. An assessment completed by a physician may be required to determine eligibility. Depending on the state, Medicaid may also provide some payment for transportation, including taxi fares. Pharmacists can help patients with transportation challenges by reviewing their local options for low-cost transportation and by referring patients to social workers who may have additional transportation resources.

Sexual Activity

An assessment of sexual activity may be overlooked in the elderly due to the perception that elderly patients are not sexually active. Sexual activity of elders is often underestimated and monogamy should not be assumed. Many elders are at risk of acquiring sexually transmitted diseases when sexually active with multiple partners or a single new untested partner. Of the total number of AIDS cases in the United States in 2005, more than 118,000 were in persons aged ≥ 50 years old.[62] As such, elderly patients should be assessed for sexual activity, and if active and not practicing safe sexual interactions, they should also be screened for and educated about sexually transmitted diseases.

On the other hand, many elderly suffer from the opposite problem, such as impotence, decreased libido or vaginal atrophy. Therefore, patients should also be questioned for their desire to remedy these problems and improve their sexual experience. In many instances these problems may be improved with medication or vaginal lubricants. Unfortunately, the biggest barrier to these improvements is often communication between the provider and patient.

CASE 1. COMPREHENSIVE INTERDISCIPLINARY GERIATRIC ASSESSMENT

Setting:
Ambulatory

Subjective:
Mrs. P is an 85-year-old woman who is new to the community. She recently moved to an assisted living facility in your area, as she was recently widowed. Previously, she lived with her husband in their own home. Her daughter requested she move into the assisted living facility, as it is close to her daughter's home. She relies on the assisted living to provide assistance for cooking, cleaning, and medication management. She is initiating care at a local Seniors Clinic for the first time. You provide clinical pharmacist services at the assisted living facility and at the Seniors Clinic where she is scheduled for a new patient appointment. Her daughter asks what to expect at the first visit.

Past Medical History:

Mild cognitive impairment, osteoporosis, hypertension, osteoarthritis, insomnia, and anemia.

Medications:

Acetaminophen, aspirin, alendronate, lisinopril, hydrochlorothiazide, zolpidem, ranitidine as needed, multivitamin, and calcium/vitamin D.

Social History:

No history of smoking; occasional alcohol socially.

Family History:

Sister died of a stroke 3 years ago, otherwise unknown.

Assessment:

Mrs. P and her daughter will undergo comprehensive geriatric assessment at the seniors clinic and want to know what to expect.

Plan:

Provide education to patient and caregiver on items involved in comprehensive geriatric assessment by an interdisciplinary team. Reassure that these assessments may take more than one visit.

1. Medical History: past medical records, immunization history (pneumococcal, influenza, herpes zoster, tetanus), history of falls and fall risk, gait and balance, physical activity and current diet, history of osteoporosis (past DEXA results).

2. Social History: and Functional Status: advance directives, assisted living contact information, transportation, driving ability, sexual activity, recent life changes, activities of daily living, instrumental activities of daily living, insurance status.

3. Review of Systems: pain assessment, sleep habits, bowel habits and bladder habits.

4. Physical Assessment: vital signs (including pain score), height and weight, hearing and eye tests, physical examinations, oral examination.

5. Laboratory: thyroid, vitamin B12, complete blood count, basic metabolic panel, fasting lipid panel, vitamin D.

6. Neuropsychiatric Assessment: screening for depression (GDS), cognition (MMSE, Mini-cog, SLUMS or 7MS), and possibly neuropsychiatric screening

7. Medication Review: review of her medications (including over-the-counter agents) for medication-related problems.

Rationale:

A comprehensive interdisciplinary geriatric assessment does not always occur in routine medical practice. Problems both simple and complex can be missed in assessment of the elderly patient due to atypical disease presentation and an attitude that many symptoms are normal in the aging adult. Establishing care at an interdisciplinary senior clinic will provide Mrs. P the best opportunity to attain optimal health and well-being.

The medical history will establish the baseline of disease states present and preventive services necessary for Mrs. P. Social and functional history will allow appropriate referrals for social services and support. The review of systems and physical assessment will identify what additional tests and evaluations may be needed and will discover if disease targets are being met (e.g., hypertension). Laboratory tests will evaluate Mrs. P's anemia, risk for osteoporosis and if there are reversible causes of possible cognitive impairment, such as hypothyroidism, low hemoglobin, or low vitamin B-12. The neuropsychiatric testing will establish the severity of the cognitive impairment and insomnia. Other causes of these problems such as depression may be established. Finally, a medication review will enable the assisted living facility and caregiver to know what medication management issues may be present. Establishing the pattern of use for prescription and over-the-counter medication use in this patient may uncover reversible causes of cognitive impairment (e.g., zolpidem) and insomnia.

CASE 2. REASSESSMENT BY A CONSULTANT PHARMACIST IN THE LONG TERM CARE SETTING

Setting:

Long-term care

Subjective:

Mrs. P is now 88 years old and is entering a long term care setting due to advancing dementia with hallucinations and delusions. The consultant pharmacist who serves the long-term care facility must identify needed evaluations for assessment of Mrs. P's medication regimen.

Past Medical History:

Alzheimer's disease, osteoporosis, hypertension, osteoarthritis, depression, hypothyroidism, constipation, hallucinations, delusions.

Medications:

Acetaminophen, low dose aspirin, ibandronate, lisinopril, levothyroxine, risperidone, rivastigmine, zolpidem, multivitamin, calcium/vitamin D, esomeprazole as needed, and milk of magnesia as needed.

Social History:

No history of smoking; no alcohol.

Family History:

Sister died of a stroke 6 years ago, otherwise unknown.

Assessment:

Additional information required for initial pharmacist consultation.

Plan:

Obtain the following information/tests:

Information from Mrs. P, her daughter or the nursing staff are needed including sleep habits, bowel habits, activities of daily living and insurance status (including formulary listings). Physical assessments should include her current vital signs, pain assessment using the FACES pain rating scale, height, and weight. Laboratory measurements for TSH, basic metabolic panel, and CBC requested. Neuropsychiatric evaluations to review include MMSE, NPI-NH and GDS-I. Frequency of administration of acetaminophen, risperidone, zolpidem, esomeprazole and milk of magnesia should be obtained from the medication administration record.

Rationale:

Both subjective and objective information will aid in evaluation of the effectiveness and risk/benefit of several of Mrs. P's medications. The continued need for risperidone, rivastigmine and zolpidem require special scrutiny of the objective neuropsychiatric assessments, as well as physical examination, laboratory findings and pain ratings. Inadequately treated pain, constipation or hypothyroidism in Mrs. P could manifest as agitation resulting in inappropriate use of psychotropic medications. New conditions such as hyponatremia or a urinary tract infection could also cloud the picture.

Whether Mrs. P has Medicare Part D or other insurance to cover prescription medications should be evaluated. Admission to a nursing home is an event which allows change to a different Medicare Part D insurer that includes a long-term care pharmacy provider, which may be advantageous to Mrs. P. Her medications should be reviewed to identify potential opportunity to convert to generic or preferred brand name prescriptions to reduce costs without reducing quality of care.

Chapter Summary

A comprehensive assessment of geriatric patients encompasses multiple types of assessments including medical, cognitive, neuropsychiatric, functional and social assessments. Elderly patients presenting to a primary care provider for the first time should attempt to bring previous medical records. If possible, family and caregivers for patients should also accompany them to the visits to provide supporting information. To complete all of the necessary assessments may take several visits with a primary care provider.

Self-Assessment Questions

1. How might the physical examination be different for ambulatory elderly compared to more frail, institutionalized elderly patients?

2. When screening for common disease states in the elderly, what laboratory parameters are commonly evaluated?

3. How is cancer screening for the geriatric patient different when the patient becomes older and frailer?

4. What specific areas should a pharmacist focus on when performing a medication assessment?

5. What are the major differences between the tools commonly utilized for cognitive assessment?

6. How might a clinician implement a tool into their clinical practice to evaluate geriatric patients for neuropsychiatric problems?

7. What are the tools available to help assess functional abilities and how can they be specifically utilized?

8. What are the important aspects of a complete social assessment for elderly patients?

9. Which interdisciplinary team members help contribute to a comprehensive assessment of a geriatric patient?

References

1. Bentley DW, Bradley S, High K, et al. Practice guideline for evaluation of fever and infection in long-term care facilities. *Clin Infect Dis.* 2000;31:640–653.

2. Darowski A, Najim Z, Weinberg J, et al. The febrile response to mild infections in elderly hospital inpatients. *Age Ageing.* 1991;20:193–198.

3. Varney SM, Manthey DE, Culpepper VE, et al. A comparison of oral, tympanic, and rectal temperature measurement in the elderly. *J Emerg Med.* 2002;22:153–157.

4. Reuben DB. Quality indicators for the care of undernutrition in vulnerable elders. *J Am Geriatr Soc.* 2007;55(suppl 2):S438–442.

5. Hickson M, Frost G. A comparison of three methods for estimating height in the acutely ill elderly population. *J Hum Nutr Diet.* 2003;16:13–20.

6. Haboubi NY, Hudson PR, Pathy MS. Measurement of height in the elderly. *J Am Geriatr Soc.* 1990;38:1008–1010.

7. Matteson MA, Linton A, Byers V. Vision and hearing screening in cognitively impaired older adults. *Geriatr Nurs.* 1993;14:294–297.

8. American Cancer Society. Cancer statistics 2008. Available at: http://www.cancer.org/docroot/PRO/content/PRO_1_1_Cancer_Statistics_2008_Presentation.asp?sitearea=PRO. Accessed October 16, 2008.

9. American Cancer Society. American Cancer Society guidelines for the early detection of cancer. Available at: http://www.cancer.org/docroot/PED/content/PED_2_3X_ACS_Cancer_Detection_Guidelines_36.asp?sitearea=PED. Accessed October 16, 2008.

10. U.S. Preventive Services Task Force. Screening for type 2 diabetes mellitus in adults: U.S. Preventive Services Task Force recommendation statement. *Ann Intern Med.* 2008;148:846–854.

11. Inzitari M, Pozzi C, Ferrucci L, et al. Subtle neurological abnormalities as risk factors for cognitive and functional decline, cerebrovascular events, and mortality in older community-dwelling adults. *Arch Intern Med.* 2008;168:1270–1276.

12. World Health Organization Collaborating Centre for Metabolic Bone Diseases. FRAX WHO fracture risk assessment tool. Available at: http://www.shef.ac.uk/FRAX/. Accessed October 16, 2008.

13. Stevens LA, Levey AS. National Kidney Foundation. Frequently asked questions about GFR estimates. Available at: http://www.kidney.org/professionals/kls/pdf/faq_gfr.pdf. Accessed October 16, 2008.

14. Taylor LJ, Herr K. Pain intensity assessment: a comparison of selected pain intensity scales for use in cognitively intact and cognitively impaired African American older adults. *Pain Manag Nurs.* 2003;4:87–95.

15. Manz BD, Mosier R, Nusser-Gerlach MA, et al. Pain assessment in the cognitively impaired and unimpaired elderly. *Pain Manag Nurs.* 2000;1:106–115.

16. Agness C, Murrell E, Nkansah N, et al. Poor health literacy as a barrier to patient care. *Consult Pharm.* 2008;23:378–382.

17. Davis TC, Long SW, Jackson RH, et al. Rapid estimate of adult literacy in medicine: a shortened screening instrument. *Fam Med.* 1993;25:391–395.

18. Parker RM, Baker DW, Williams MV, et al. The test of functional health literacy in adults: a new instrument for measuring patients' literacy skills. *J Gen Intern Med.* 1995;10:537–541.

19. Morisky DE, Green LW, Levine DM. Concurrent and predictive validity of a self-reported measure of medication adherence. *Med Care.* 1986;24:67–74.

20. Farris KB, Phillips BB. Instruments assessing capacity to manage medications. *Ann Pharmacother.* 2008;42:1026–1036.

21. Folstein MF, Folstein SE, McHugh PR. "Mini-mental state": A practical method for grading the cognitive state of patients for the clinician. *J Psychiatr Res.* 1975;12:189–198.

22. Borson S, Scanlan JM, Chen P, et al. The Mini-Cog as a screen for dementia: validation in a population-based sample. *J Am Geriatr Soc.* 2003;51:1451–1454.

23. Solomon PR, Hirschoff A, Kelly B, et al. A 7-minute neurocognitive screening battery highly sensitive to Alzheimer's disease. *Arch Neurol.* 1998;55:349–355.

24. Saxton J, Swihart AA, McGonigle-Gibson KL, et al. Assessment of the severely impaired patient: description and validation of a new neuropsychological test battery. *Psychol Assess.* 1990;2:298–303.

25. Knopman DS, Knapp MJ, Gracon SI, et al. The Clinician Interview-Based Impression (CIBI): a clinician's global change rating scale in Alzheimer's disease. *Neurology.* 1994;44:2315–2321.

26. Setter SM, Neumiller JJ, Johnson M, et al. The Mini-Cog: a rapid dementia screening tool suitable for pharmacists' use. *Consult Pharm.* 2007;22:855–861.

27. Borson S, Scanlan JM, Watanabe J, et al. Simplifying detection of cognitive impairment: comparison of the Mini-Cog and Mini-Mental State Examination in a multiethnic sample. *J Am Geriatr Soc.* 2005;53:871–874.

28. Solomon PR, Pendlebury WW. Recognition of Alzheimer's disease: the 7-Minute Screen. *Fam Med.* 1998;30:265–271.

29. Tariq SH, Tumosa N, Chibnall JT, et al. Comparison of the Saint Louis University mental status examination and the mini-mental state examination for detecting dementia and mild neurocognitive disorder—a pilot study. *Am J Geriatr Psychiatry.* 2006;14:900–910.

30. Zec RF, Landreth ES, Vicari SK, et al. Alzheimer disease assessment scale: useful for both early detection and staging of dementia of the Alzheimer type. *Alzheimer Dis Assoc Disord.* 1992;6:89–102.

31. Rockwood K, Fay S, Gorman M, et al. The clinical meaningfulness of ADAS-Cog changes in Alzheimer's disease patients treated with donepezil in an open-label trial. *BMC Neurol.* 2007;7:26.

32. Lanctot KL, Herrmann N, Yau KK, et al. Efficacy and safety of cholinesterase inhibitors in Alzheimer's disease: a meta-analysis. *CMAJ.* 2003;169:557–564.

33. Qaseem A, Snow V, Cross JT, Jr., et al. Current pharmacologic treatment of dementia: a clinical practice guideline from the American College of Physicians and the American Academy of Family Physicians. *Ann Intern Med.* 2008;148:370–378.

34. Yesavage JA, Brink TL. Development and validation of a geriatric depression screening scale: a preliminary report. *J Psychiatr Res.* 1983;17:37–49.

35. Wancata J, Alexandrowicz R, Marquart B, et al. The criterion validity of the Geriatric Depression Scale: a systematic review. *Acta Psychiatr Scand.* 2006;114:398–410.

36. Burke WJ, Roccaforte WH, Wengel SP, et al. The reliability and validity of the Geriatric Depression Rating

Scale administered by telephone. *J Am Geriatr Soc.* 1995;43:674–679.

37. Burke WJ, Rangwani S, Roccaforte WH, et al. The reliability and validity of the collateral source version of the Geriatric Depression Rating Scale administered by telephone. *Int J Geriatr Psychiatry.* 1997;12:288–294.

38. Brown LM, Schinka JA. Development and initial validation of a 15-item informant version of the Geriatric Depression Scale. *Int J Geriatr Psychiatry.* 2005;20:911–918.

39. Cummings JL, Mega M, Gray K, et al. The Neuropsychiatric Inventory: comprehensive assessment of psychopathology in dementia. *Neurology.* 1994;44:2308–2314.

40. Reisberg B, Borenstein J, Salob SP, et al. Behavioral symptoms in Alzheimer's disease: phenomenology and treatment. *J Clin Psychiatry.* 1987;48(suppl):9–15.

41. Kaufer DI, Cummings JL, Ketchel P, et al. Validation of the NPI-Q, a brief clinical form of the Neuropsychiatric Inventory. *J Neuropsychiatry Clin Neurosci.* 2000;12:233–239.

42. Wood S, Cummings JL, Hsu MA, et al. The use of the neuropsychiatric inventory in nursing home residents. Characterization and measurement. *Am J Geriatr Psychiatry.* 2000;8:75–83.

43. Pinholt EM, Kroenke K, Hanley JF, et al. Functional assessment of the elderly. A comparison of standard instruments with clinical judgment. *Arch Intern Med.* 1987;147:484–488.

44. Iezzoni LI. The demand for documentation for Medicare payment. *N Engl J Med.* 1999;341:365–367.

45. Katz S, Downs TD, Cash HR, et al. Progress in development of the index of ADL. *Gerontologist.* 1970;10:20–30.

46. Galasko D, Bennett D, Sano M, et al. An inventory to assess activities of daily living for clinical trials in Alzheimer's disease. The Alzheimer's Disease Cooperative Study. *Alzheimer Dis Assoc Disord.* 1997;11(suppl 2):S33–39.

47. Lawton MP, Brody EM. Assessment of older people: self-maintaining and instrumental activities of daily living. *Gerontologist.* 1969;9:179–186.

48. Tinetti ME, Speechley M, Ginter SF. Risk factors for falls among elderly persons living in the community. *N Engl J Med.* 1988;319:1701–1707.

49. Berg KO, Wood-Dauphinee SL, Williams JI, et al. Measuring balance in the elderly: validation of an instrument. *Can J Public Health.* 1992;83(suppl 2):S7–11.

50. Podsiadlo D, Richardson S. The timed "Up & Go": a test of basic functional mobility for frail elderly persons. *J Am Geriatr Soc.* 1991;39:142–148.

51. Bogle Thorbahn LD, Newton RA. Use of the Berg Balance Test to predict falls in elderly persons. *Phys Ther.* 1996;76:576–583.

52. Shumway-Cook A, Brauer S, Woollacott M. Predicting the probability for falls in community-dwelling older adults using the Timed Up & Go Test. *Phys Ther.* 2000;80:896–903.

53. Morey MC, Sloane R, Pieper CF, et al. Effect of physical activity guidelines on physical function in older adults. 2008;56:1873–1878.

54. Nelson ME, Rejeski WJ, Blair SN, et al. Physical activity and public health in older adults: recommendation from the American College of Sports Medicine and the American Heart Association. *Med Sci Sports Exerc.* 2007;39:1435–1445.

55. Dubbert PM, Morey MC, Kirchner KA, et al. Counseling for home-based walking and strength exercise in older primary care patients. *Arch Intern Med.* 2008;168:979–986.

56. Ossip-Klein DJ, Pearson TA, McIntosh S, et al. Smoking is a geriatric health issue. *Nicotine Tob Res.* 1999;1:299–300.

57. Schofield I. Supporting older people to quit smoking. *Nurs Older People.* 2006;18:29–33.

58. Penn ND, Corrado OJ, Pitchfork LJ, et al. Blood alcohol levels in acute elderly admissions to hospital. *Postgrad Med J.* 1989;65:20–21.

59. Emanuel LL. Advance directives and advancing age. *J Am Geriatr Soc.* 2004;52:641–642.

60. Aging with Dignity. 5 Wishes. Available at: http://www.agingwithdignity.org/5wishes.html. Accessed October 16, 2008.

61. McWilliams JM, Meara E, Zaslavsky AM, et al. Health of previously uninsured adults after acquiring Medicare coverage. *JAMA.* 2007;298:2886–2894.

62. Tangredi LA, Danvers K, Molony SL, et al. New CDC recommendations for HIV testing in older adults. *Nurse Pract.* 2008;33:37–44.

5

Adverse Drug Events in Elderly Patients

REBECCA B. SLEEPER

Learning Objectives

1. Define the terms adverse drug reaction, adverse drug event, adverse event, and adverse outcome.

2. Differentiate the concepts of error, near miss, therapeutic failure, and adverse drug withdrawal events.

3. Distinguish the most common sources of adverse drug events and identify scenarios in which elderly patients are most vulnerable.

4. Formulate strategies to prevent or react to common types of adverse events.

Key Terms

ADVERSE DRUG EVENT: Undesirable health outcomes associated with drug therapy.

ADVERSE DRUG WITHDRAWAL EVENTS: Adverse health events associated with discontinuation of drug therapy.

ERROR: In the context of drug therapy, error is a term used to describe inappropriate use of drug therapy (error of commission) or lack or drug therapy, its monitoring, or its documentation (omission).

NON-ADHERENCE: Failure to administer or continue drug therapy in the manner intended.

THERAPEUTIC FAILURE: Failure to achieve the therapeutic outcome for which a medication was prescribed.

Introduction

Adverse drug events are undesirable health outcomes in any patient population, but elderly populations are particularly vulnerable. Factors such as age related changes in drug sensitivity, the number or complexity of medications in a drug regimen or functional or cognitive barriers that affect access to care, administration of medications, or ability to self report problems may all influence the likelihood of an adverse health outcome. Although elderly individuals are vulnerable to errors of self-administration, vigilance on behalf of all members of the health care team is required to avoid problems originating at the level of the health professional or the health system. Given the proportion of adverse events deemed to be preventable, there is much that can be done to improve drug therapy outcomes. With the right strategies to evaluate medication appropriateness, pharmacists are in a position to identify medication related problems and make drug therapy interventions. This chapter will review the most common sources of adverse drug events among elderly populations, including preventable events.

Terms and Definitions

There are many different terms that are often used when discussing undesired health outcomes, however they are not all interchangeable. Table 5-1 lists the most common terminology, ranging from the most specific to the broadest. For the purposes of this chapter, the term **adverse drug event** (ADE) will be used as it is the broadest level definition that is still specific to drug therapy.

Not all ADEs are preventable. For instance, it will not always be possible to foresee the occurrence of an adverse effect that was not previously recognized as a common risk associated with a particular medication. On the other hand, ADEs include events that could have been prevented as a result of a variety of actions. These actions include careful reconciliation of drug selection or dose against past medical history, concomitant medications, allergy documentation, renal function and other clinical or laboratory parameters, evaluation of ability to afford or adhere to therapy, clear and accurate writing and transcribing of medication orders, appropriate product preparation, handling, and storage, timely monitoring, and where appropriate, documentation of care procedures.

Often, ADEs are characterized as unwanted effects of drug use or overuse, but health professionals should also remember that ADEs can occur as a result of lack of drug use, ineffective drug therapy, or withdrawal from a drug. The term **therapeutic failure** is used to describe unwanted outcomes associated with non-adherence, subtherapeutic dose, or failure to insure that the selected drug therapy has achieved the therapeutic goal for which it was prescribed. The term **adverse drug withdrawal event** describes adverse events that arise after drug discontinuation.

Table 5-1. Categories of Adverse Health Events

Term		Definition	Example
ADR	Adverse drug reaction	Implies a specific reaction usually related to the pharmacology of the drug	Nausea caused by codeine
ADE	Adverse drug event	Any injury due to drug therapy. Includes above, but not limited to side effects from typical use, can be any event related to medication use	Includes prescribing, dispensing, administration, adherence problems, and therapeutic failures
AE	Adverse event	Can be any adverse event, not just those related to medication	Deep vein thrombosis following hip replacement
AO	Adverse outcome	Any poor health outcome, may be related to medication, lifestyle, lack of medical intervention or lack of diagnosis	MI due to poor control of cholesterol

Other terms that are sometimes used in the literature include "**error**" and "near miss." Error is a term that implies some degree of negligence or malfeasance, however it does not necessarily connote that actual harm occurred as a result. Consider two examples of errors; in the first instance, a nurse in a long term care facility administers a medication to the wrong patient whereas in the second instance, the nurse administers the medication to the correct patient but documents the administration in the wrong resident's record. Both are examples of errors, but the consequences of each could be very different. When an error results in harm, it is often included under the ADE umbrella. However, when there is no harm, no "event" per se, an error may not be classified this way. "Near miss" is usually a retrospective definition, and implies a situation where there is no true "event." Examples of "near miss" situations are ambiguous medical orders that could potentially have resulted in error or harm but luckily did not due to clarification by a pharmacist, or an instance where a problem was identified and corrected before harm could result. The ADE literature may or may not include near misses in their evaluations, and if so, the distinction of "potential" ADE is often made. The term "medication misadventure" is sometimes used as an all-encompassing term that includes both actual errors and near misses. Routine evaluation of a health care institution's patterns of medication misadventures can help identify areas for improvement in patient safety.

Etiology and Epidemiology of ADEs in Elderly Populations
Prevalence of ADEs in Various Subgroups

It is a little difficult to pinpoint precise estimates of ADEs among elderly patients as the literature can vary in its use of errors, adverse drug reactions, or adverse drug events as the criteria for evaluating the prevalence of poor outcomes associated with drug therapy. In addition, not all studies have exclusively evaluated older populations, and prevalence rates differ by venue. For instance, various reports have estimated that 5.9% - 12.6% of emergency room visits for older patients are as-

sociated with ADEs.[1-3] A broader range of prevalence rates have been reported among elderly in the community setting, from 5.5% to 33% during 12-month observations.[4,5] In long term care, prevalence rates have been reported as ADEs per 100 resident months, and range from 1.89 to 9.8.[6,7] A meta-analysis of patients hospitalized for adverse drug related problems revealed that elderly patients, compared to younger populations, are more likely to be hospitalized as a result of drug related problems (16.6% vs. 4.1%).[8] What is more startling is the proportion of ADEs determined to be preventable, from 27.6% to 88%.[4-8] Worse, one study in the long term care setting determined 44% of preventable ADEs to be fatal, life threatening, or serious.[6]

 KEY POINT: ADEs are more common among elderly patients and serious, life-threatening, or fatal ADEs are often likely to be preventable.

In a recent Cochrane review of preventable adverse drug events in the ambulatory setting, cardiovascular drugs, analgesics and hypoglycemic medications accounted for a combined total of 86.5% of preventable ADEs, with 77.2% of preventable ADEs presenting with symptoms involving the Central Nervous System, renal or electrolyte status, or the GI tract.[9] Although many of the studies of ADEs in the ambulatory setting are not elderly specific, some of the highest rates of ADE incidence are reported from studies that enrolled cohorts of elderly patients.[9]

Drug therapy problems related to medications prescribed in the emergency room or during a hospital stay can affect a patient after discharge. Among a cohort of veterans aged 65 and older who were discharged from an emergency department, 31.8% were determined to have been prescribed suboptimal drug therapy. Among 421 patients discharged from the emergency department, 320 (34%) had an adverse outcome, defined as readmission or death, within 90 days of initial emergency department discharge, and a multi-variable analysis suggested a trend toward greater risk of adverse outcome among users of suboptimal therapy (HR 1.32, 95%CI 0.95–1.84).[10]

Adverse drug events are also costly, particularly among frail elderly, resulting in estimated health related expenditures of over $177 billion dollars per year.[11] Based on a current U.S. population of just over 3 billion,[12] the average expenditure per person per year could be estimated at roughly $60. By contrast the cost among long term care residents in one study was been estimated to be $4 billion per year.[13] Although this study was published in 1997, a comparison of U.S. census data for long term care demographics from both 1997 and more recently in 2004 indicate similar population sizes of 1.5–1.6 million. Therefore, while appearing to be a much smaller net cost, the average cost per person is actually significantly higher, at ≥$2,500 per year.[14,15]

Risk Factors and Categories of ADEs

Many risk factors for experiencing an ADE have been suggested, including increased age, female gender, history of prior ADR, prolonged hospital stay, fragmented medical care, and multiple disease states or poor health status, however, the only risk factor consistently reported in studies is polypharmacy.[16] Polypharmacy will be covered further in Chapter 6. In addition to identifying risk factors that increase vulnerability to an ADE, it is important to delineate categories of ADEs and describe the estimated prevalence ADEs within each category. The categories included in this chapter will include prescribing, dispensing, administration or adherence, and monitoring. Although the literature describing the prevalence of ADEs in each of these categories is not always elderly specific, it lends some perspective as to the source of many medication related problems.

Prescribing

Adverse drug events at this level occur as a result of inappropriate choice of drug, dose or regimen directions. There are several categories of medication related problems that can occur: medication without indication, indication without medication, duplicate medication, wrong drug, high dose, low dose, wrong route/formulation, wrong time/frequency, wrong duration, interaction (drug-drug, drug-supplement, drug-food or drug–disease interaction), and allergy or other contraindication.

Many studies report that the majority of ADEs can be traced back to the prescribing level. A Cochrane review in the ambulatory setting reported that the largest proportion of drug therapy problems occurred at this stage, with 64.7% of all preventable ADEs, and 56% of those causing hospitalization, being associated with prescribing.[9] Among a cohort of veterans over the age of 65 prescribed sub-optimal therapy upon emergency room discharge, the most common problems involved drug selection, drug-drug interaction, and drug-disease interaction.[9]

In general, prescribing problems can be related to lack of optimal drug therapy knowledge about either the medication being prescribed or the other medications already on the regimen. Dosing errors might occur as a result of failure to consider Geriatric dosage recommendations or adjustments based upon renal function. Failure to review or consider the pharmacology of the existing drug regimen can lead to drug interactions or selection of products that duplicate or compound the effects of one or more other medications, or drug-induced worsening of underlying conditions.

By contrast, the ultimate problem can sometimes lie not in whether the drug selected was appropriate for the indication, but whether the indication itself was appropriately assessed. For instance, consider an instance where a psychoactive medication is prescribed to calm agitated behavior without realizing that there is an underlying urinary tract infection with an atypical disease presentation. Another example is a patient who experiences tremor and tachycardia associated with excessive use of "as needed" albuterol prescribed for shortness of breath from COPD; what if an exacerbation of unrecognized or untreated co-morbid heart failure, as opposed to COPD, was actually the cause of the respiratory distress?

Perhaps the albuterol was not only excessive, but unnecessary. It is easy to imagine how such a scenario might lead to a prescribing cascade, where additional medication is added to treat problems associated with the initial prescribing choice. Atypical disease presentation and misinterpretation of presenting signs and symptoms can often be a source of sub-optimal drug selection. Although not all health professionals diagnose illness as part of their scope of practice, aspects of patient assessment and reporting of assessment data back to the team is a responsibility of all caregivers. Therefore, whether documenting in a chart, communicating over the phone, or interacting in a clinic or hospital setting, review of all pertinent patient data is important in order to take a deductive problem solving approach to illness presentation, and to avoid a "silo effect" where prescribing choices are made without evaluating all factors and drug therapy management is performed without assessment of the whole patient.

Sometimes, ADEs in this category can also be related to the documentation or record keeping associated with medication prescribing. Transcribing errors can occur in both the prescribing or dispensing categories due to illegible handwritten orders or the use of high-risk abbreviations (for example QD, QOD, or QID, if written illegibly could result a medication being taken at an interval ranging from every other day to up to four times a day). See Table 5-2 for a list of "Do not use" abbreviations.[17] However, transcribing errors are not the only source of documentation-related ADEs. For instance, failure to document or review allergies or previous adverse drug reactions could result in a choice of drug that inadvertently re-exposes the patient to the offending agent. Incomplete medical history documentation or failure to collect a current medication list can result in the selection of a drug that duplicates or interacts with other disease states or drugs. In addition, clinical record documentation is often the primary means of communicating the plan of care upon transfer between health care venues. For this reason, lack of clear or complete documentation could ultimately be the root cause of ADEs, not just in the prescribing category, but also in the following categories of dispensing, administration or monitoring. Upon a transfer between care venues, it could be difficult for the

Table 5-2. "Do Not Use" Abbreviations[17]

	Do Not Use	Use	Rationale
Official list	QD or QOD	"Daily" or "every other day"	Mistaken for each other and for "QID"
	U or IU	"Unit" or "International Unit"	Mistaken for "0," "4," "cc," "IV," or "10"
	Trailing zero/lack of leading zero	Xmg or 0.X mg	Missed decimal point resulting 10× error
	MS, MSO4, MgSO4	"Morphine sulfate" or "magnesium sulfate"	Confused with one another
Proposed list	> or <	"Greater than" or "less than"	Confused with "7," "L," or with one another
	Drug abbreviations	Spell out drug name	Multiple similarities between drug names
	Apothecary units	Metric units	Unfamiliar to many practitioners, confused with metric
	@	"At"	Mistaken for the number 2
	cc	mL	Mistaken for units
	μg	"mcg" or "microgram"	Mistaken for mg

patient or other health professionals in the new environment to correctly interpret the intent of the drug therapy prescribed in the previous venue. For instance, a medication that was intended to be continued for only a short time after hospital discharge may be continued indefinitely due to lack of documentation of the indication or desired duration of therapy.

Lastly, ADEs in this category can arise from the failure to consider how the drug is going to be administered or whether it will be feasible for the patient to adhere to the regimen. Will the patient self administer medications or will a caregiver assist with this process, and if so, to what extent? Does the individual performing this task understand the directions and are they capable of carrying them out? Can the patient afford to maintain the regimen through its desired duration? ADEs related to adherence are further discussed below, as even carefully selected drug therapy can go awry due to improper administration or poor adherence. However due consideration of whether medication administration, cost or adherence are practical for the patient is also part of the prescribing responsibility.

Dispensing

This category involves medication preparation, handling, pre-dispensing storage and security, dispensing, and related record keeping. The term "misfill" is often used to describe a situation where the product dispensed is not what was prescribed. It can also refer to situations where the correct drug is dispensed, but it is the wrong strength, route, formulation or directions. Labeling errors, such as wrong patient name, wrong prescriber or even wrong auxiliary stickers can also contribute to errors or at the very least contribute to confusion about medication use.

Misfill problems are only a part of the medication misadventures that can occur in this category. The pharmacist's responsibility to prepare and dispense pure and potent medicines rests on quality controls that insure proper aseptic technique during compounding, optimal equipment or clean room standards, stringent double check of calculations or titration/dilution volumes, maintenance

of inventory that is in-date and stored under the proper conditions, security against adulteration or diversion, and clear documentation of prescription records and dispensing activity.

Fortunately, this type of medication related problem is relatively infrequent. In the community pharmacy setting error rates are reported at 0.057%–1.7%, involving either drug product or drug labeling.[18,19] Most (67%) were classified as minor and these errors do not necessarily result in an ADE, however 22–60% of those classified as moderate were deemed to be preventable.[19] Problems classified as "med picking" errors in the hospital pharmacy setting are reported with a frequency of 0.04–2.9%, although error rates in floor-stock systems on nursing units are reported to have a higher incidence of 11.5%.[20-25] Despite this, given the enormous volume of prescription processing activity in many pharmacies, even a low percentage of error could potentially result in an unacceptably high absolute number of ADEs. In addition, the potential for these types of ADEs can be particularly frightening to patients because it can be difficult to completely defend one's self against them, especially when in an ill and vulnerable state.[26] These types of problems are often described as systems failures as there are often multiple breakdowns that must occur in order for the dispensing error to go from "near miss" to true ADE.[27] For instance, one study estimated that 30% of dispensing errors from a hospital pharmacy were not detected by the nurse administering the medication.[28]

When dispensing directly to the patient, medication counseling is an important defense against a dispensing error. Review of counseling points such as drug name, use, dose, route, time, directions, duration, storage/handling, what to expect, common adverse effects, self-monitoring techniques, and contact information in the event of questions or problems gives the patient an opportunity engage with the health professional and may trigger a realization that something is not right. This is optimally effective when patients also receive information from their prescriber about what is being prescribed so discrepancies can be identified. Although medication counseling is universally required with new prescriptions, it is a good idea at the time of refills too. Not only is this an opportunity to reinforce education and adherence, but a dispensing problem could be caught retrospectively by determining whether the patient has experienced an unexpected problem with their therapy.

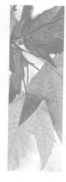

KEY POINT: For ambulatory patients, interaction with the pharmacist is the last opportunity for contact with a health professional before the patient starts a new medication. Careful medication counseling at this stage can be an important line of defense against adverse drug events.

When dispensing drugs within a hospital or to staff in a long term care facility, product changes hands without direct involvement of the patient. Although patients or their responsible parties should ask questions and be kept informed of prescribing choices and drug therapy outcomes, there are many other layers of safety procedures that must occur to prevent this type of problem. These include read-back verification when taking orders by phone, avoiding handwritten orders or high-risk abbreviations, verification of first-refills against the original order, the use of technology to support inventory management (whether bar code, inventory tag, or other system) and maintaining clear, traceable records of each health professional involved in medication transactions. Other quality assurance monitoring can identify areas of systemic weakness. These include spot inspections of check and double check procedures, periodic inspection/monitoring of equipment, temperature and other environmental parameters, and periodic records audits. Lastly, routine in-service education of personnel is vital to maintaining the most up to date standard of practice.

Administration and Adherence

Administration problems can be potentiated by patients themselves or by health professionals or caregivers who either assist with, or take over responsibility for, medication administration to the patient. Administration problems occur when, despite proper prescribing and dispensing, the patient receives or takes the wrong drug or dose, or the product is administered at the wrong time, frequency or with the wrong technique. **Nonadherence** is a failure to take or administer the medication as prescribed and can be a problem of either under-use or over-use. In some cases, problems similar to those discussed in the "dispensing" section can occur in the in the home or chronic care setting, as a result of the patient or caregiver improperly storing medication, keeping beyond the expiration date, or diverting the medication to someone other than the patient.

Medication related problems of this nature can be difficult to quantify, and statistics can vary depending on what variable is being evaluated. In chronic care settings the most frequent types of ADEs are associated with prescribing or monitoring, however, nursing home survey procedures generally do not consider these as part of the medication error review, where the accuracy of med pass procedures is the focus. One of the most common med pass errors is the failure to administer a medication within 1 hour before or one hour after the scheduled time. Due to the high number of medication doses typically administered during a given med pass interval, timely completion of the pass in under two hours is often difficult to achieve. Therefore high error rates based on this criterion are easily predicted but may not correlate to actual ADE rates. Excluding "wrong time" errors, a 2006 Institute of Medicine report estimated that the most common medication administration errors are administration of an unauthorized drug (44.8 %), omission of a prescribed drug (41.5 %), administration of the wrong dose (11%), via the wrong route (2%) or in the wrong form (0.4 %).[29] Another study of medication errors observed in 36 heath care facilities including both hospitals and skilled nursing facilities, a 19% error rate was observed with the most common problems being wrong time (43%), omitted dose (30%), wrong dose (17%), or unauthorized drug (4%). Seven percent of the events were characterized as potential adverse drug events.[30]

Unlike formal health care settings such as long term care, there is no formal "med pass audit" that is routinely performed in the home setting. The performance of medication evaluations in this setting are often not linked to a discrete health event such as a hospital or emergency department admission for ADE. In addition, there is usually no chart or clinical record against which to verify indications, transcribing of orders, or laboratory monitoring and no Medication Administration Record against which to verify administration of doses. Therefore, drug therapy reviews in this setting either evaluate non-adherence or identify potentially inappropriate medications based on list criteria, identification of interactions or therapeutic duplications, use of expired product, or continued use despite the presence of symptoms consistent with the side effect profile of one or more drugs on the regimen.

Non-adherence is a significant problem that contributes to both hospital and nursing facility admission.[31] It has been estimated that only 50% of filled prescriptions are correctly taken, and non-adherence rates among individuals over age 60 has been reported to occur at a frequency of 26–59%.[32] However it is not always possible to determine if the nature of such non-adherence is under-use, over-use, or incorrect use. In addition, non-adherence may be characterized as intentional or non-intentional. Intentional underuse occurs when the patient or caregiver determines a medication is ineffective, harmful or too costly without consulting a health care professional while intentional overuse may involve taking more of the medication than is prescribed to obtain more effect without consideration of the risks along with the prescriber. Health literacy studies shed some light on this problem by evaluating patient understanding of medication purpose, dose, use, and special instructions, but these studies do not consistently associate health literacy scores with observed ADEs.[33-35] In addition, it is not always clear if medication administration problems occur more commonly among individuals who self administer medications or who receive medication administration from a caregiver because outside of formal care settings it can be difficult to accurately identify the individual with pri-

mary control over this task. One Australian study comparing drug regimen reviews performed in a long term care setting to a home setting found that of 1,038 drug-related problems identified in 234 medication reviews, the number of problems among home-dwelling patients was higher than for long-term care residents (4.9 ± 2.0 vs. 3.9 ± 2.2; P < 0.001). In addition, the number of clinically-significant problems was higher among home dwelling patients (2.1 ± 1.1 vs. 1.5 ± 0.7; P < 0.001). However, the degree of self-administration among home dwelling patients was not known.[36]

Monitoring

Lack of monitoring is a significant contributor to preventable ADEs. One study among long term care residents determined 80% of ADEs occurred at the monitoring stage[7]. In a Cochrane review, inadequate monitoring was associated with 45.4% (22.2–69.8%) of adverse events in the ambulatory setting.[9] Although the number of monitoring-related ADEs was not as large as the number of prescribing related ADEs, the proportion of monitoring related ADEs that resulted in hospitalization was high, 61.2%, and as lack of monitoring was determined to be an "error of omission," the proportion of monitoring related ADEs deemed to be preventable was even higher, 72.2%.[9] Perhaps because of the preventable nature of monitoring-related ADEs, failure to supervise or monitor care was reported to be the third most common reason for a malpractice claim to be filed against a physician, after improper diagnosis and improper performance of a procedure.[37]

There are two primary areas of monitoring that are important for insuring optimal drug therapy outcomes: safety monitoring and efficacy monitoring. Lack of safety monitoring can be a source of preventable ADEs as a result of the failure to perform the recommended surveillance for known adverse effects of drug therapy or failure to interpret or react to clinical or laboratory data. Lack of efficacy monitoring is the failure to determine whether the drug therapy has achieved the therapeutic goal for which it was prescribed and can result in two problems, unnecessary exposure to adverse effects and cost of a medication that is not working, and exacerbation of the underlying undertreated condition.

Therapeutic failure is a term that is often used to describe this kind of ADE, and it can occur for many reasons, ranging from lack of adherence to sub-therapeutic dose or ineffective choice of drug for a particular patient. Therefore, therapeutic failures can occur as a result of prescribing, administration, or adherence problems. However, it is discussed within the context of monitoring because it is through drug therapy monitoring that the success of drug therapy is evaluated. When a therapeutic failure occurs, regardless of the reason why, efficacy monitoring should identify this problem, ideally before an adverse health outcome occurs. However, various studies have estimated that among patients admitted to the emergency room or hospital, 6.8–28% of drug related admissions were associated with a therapeutic failure[2,38,39]

Monitoring is a shared responsibility by multiple members of the health care team. Clinical and laboratory monitoring is usually ordered by the prescriber and carried out by other health professionals. Self-monitoring is performed by the patient or informal caregivers. In all cases, members of the team must be informed about the types of monitoring indicated, how and when monitoring should be performed, and how to report or react to the observed findings.

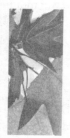 KEY POINT: Appropriate and timely monitoring is an important defense against preventable ADEs and various monitoring activities can be performed by the patient and all members of the health care team.

Adverse Drug Withdrawal Events

Defined as "clinical signs and symptoms that are related to the removal of a drug,"[40] **adverse drug withdrawal events** can occur when either a health professional or a patient decides to discontinue drug therapy or neglects to continue or adhere to drug therapy. Therefore, similar to therapeutic failures, adverse drug withdrawal events can be associated with the prescribing, administration, or adherence categories. There are two primary types of events that can occur, symptoms directly related to drug withdrawal, or symptoms of exacerbation of the untreated underlying disease state with the latter possibly being more common and occurring up to four months or longer after medication discontinuation.[41-44] Cardiovascular and central nervous system medications are most commonly associated with adverse drug withdrawal events and have been reported in both ambulatory and long term care populations.[43-45]

Although it has been suggested that receiving multiple medications, having multiple co-morbidities, having longer nursing facility stays, or hospitalization may be associated with increased risk of withdrawal events,[45] it is not clear which risk factors best explain an elderly patient's vulnerability to inappropriate removal of a medication. However, it does perhaps underscore the importance of accurate and current medical records documentation. Many different health professionals will interact with the patient or their record, often asynchronously, and be put in the position to attempt to assess the appropriateness of drug therapy. Without clear and complete documentation of the past medical history, current problem list, rationale for each drug on the regimen, goals of therapy, and desired duration of therapy, it could be very easy for the plan of care to be misinterpreted. Drugs may be improperly assessed as "inappropriate" due to lack of documentation of the clinical outcomes supporting use, prompting discontinuation. This action would be intended to be in the patient's best interest out of concern over unnecessary medication use, but there is a risk that this could ultimately result in an adverse drug withdrawal event. Likewise, without patient or caregiver counseling, verification of understanding, and reinforcement of adherence patients may be vulnerable to making choices to discontinue drug therapy without health professional supervision. In addition, risk of a withdrawal event increases as the duration of time since medication discontinuation increases, so the ability to review accurate history information, including past medication use, is important when evaluating new symptoms in elderly patients.[44]

Identifying ADEs

Due to the multiple sources of ADEs, there is need for a heightened level of vigilance to detect medication related problems. However, there is a lack of awareness of ADEs and a low potential for medication related problems to be considered as part of the differential diagnosis when an elderly patient presents to the hospital or emergency department.[46] For instance, in one study of 915 hospital admissions, a total of 102 adverse drug reactions were identified upon admission by the study team, and 45 of these were determined to have been directly related to the reason for admission. Among 38 of the admissions, 41 absolute contraindications were observed. Despite this, 56.9% of ADEs were not recognized by the attending physician upon admission. Among recognized ADEs drug withdrawal was the intervention taken 45% of the time, additional medication occurred in 45%, with the remainder addressed by dose adjustment. However, study authors determined that 27% of the drug interventions taken were not supported by scientific evidence.[46] In this study, patients with ADEs had longer hospital stays, than patients without ADEs, (14.6 days vs. 6.3 days).

Reduction of Adverse Drug Events

While there is a significant body of literature describing the prevalence and characteristics for ADEs, there is little literature that describes successful ADE reduction strategies. A 1996 randomized controlled trial of clinical pharmacist intervention to reduce inappropriate prescribing revealed that medication appropriateness (as measured by the Medication Appropriateness Index, discussed further in Chapter 6) improved and was sustained in the intervention group as compared to the control group at 3 and 12 months and that the rate of ADEs in the intervention group was 32.2% vs 40% (p = 0.19). Although this was not a statistically significant difference, this may have been due to lack of power.[47] An evaluation of inpatient geriatric units and outpatient geriatric clinics at 11 Veterans Affairs Hospitals compared usual care by attending physicians or house staff under their direction to team care, including a geriatrician, social worker, nurse and pharmacist. In the inpatient setting the team care was associated with reductions in inappropriate prescribing, unnecessary drug use, and drug underuse but not in serious adverse drug reactions. In the outpatient setting, team care was associated with fewer medical conditions with omitted medications, and a 35% reduction in the risk of serious adverse drug reactions.[48] By contrast, a trial evaluating the effectiveness of a computerized order-entry system with clinical decision support in two long term care facilities did not show a reduction in adverse drug events. This may seem surprising given the data suggesting that a high prevalence of ADEs occur within the prescribing category.[4,6] However, this model relied on information-technology based interventions and the clinical decision support mechanisms only addressed a small proportion of the adverse events identified. It was determined that more than half of the clinical alerts generated by the system were unnecessary or not clinically relevant. In addition, the alerts were directed at the prescriber only, and not the entire team.[49] Though a limited body of data, taken together these studies suggest that inter-professional intervention, including pharmacist participation, to improve medication appropriateness may be the most effective method to reduce ADE. However, more robust data is needed.

In order to do this on a wide scale, reliable tools for identifying inappropriate prescribing are needed. Although polypharmacy has been identified as a risk factor for ADE, reductions in drug number alone may not be enough. Due to the high prevalence of medication related problems associated with suboptimal prescribing choices, there have been many attempts to standardize definitions of inappropriate or suboptimal prescribing. The topic of suboptimal prescribing will be discussed further in Chapter 6. Within the context of this chapter, there is a great deal of interest in evaluating which of these measures of inappropriate prescribing is best to evaluate or predict ADEs. Theoretically, the ability to use validated screening tools to identify inappropriate prescribing should lead to a reduction on ADEs through improved drug therapy choices. However the data is mixed with respect to the best tool to achieve this. For instance, in a prospective cohort study, "inappropriate prescribing" was defined in one of four ways; contraindicated medications (based on the Beer's Criteria), drug-drug interactions, drug-disease interactions, or therapeutic duplications. Based on these definitions, over half the cohort was identified as having inappropriate prescribing. The 1-year ADE prevalence was 30.1% among individuals with inappropriate prescribing vs 13.5% among individuals with appropriate prescribing.[50] However, such criteria do not always consistently predict ADEs. For instance, many studies suggest list criteria such as the Beer's list does not predict, or is only associated with a small proportion of, ADEs among elderly patients.[51,52,53,54] By contrast, the STOPP and START criteria, validated in Europe, may identify a greater number of ADEs than the Beer's Criteria, but is still not established as a gold standard for identifying patients at risk for ADE.[55] Other criteria, such as the Medication Appropriateness Index, evaluate 10 criteria such as indication, effectiveness, dose, administration, drug-drug and drug-disease interactions, and cost.[56] However, it does not assess lack of medication and requires significant time and expertise to perform. Therefore, its use is not widespread in clinical practice. Further data is needed to determine the optimal tool to identify inappropriate prescribing, and it is anticipated that reductions in ADEs could be achieved with improvements in prescribing. However, even the best prescribing choices can be defeated by problems arising in the other domains of dispensing, administration, adherence or monitoring. Therefore there is perhaps no substitute for the vigilance of the health professional who continually evaluates drug therapy outcomes in the patients they serve.

Chapter Summary

Adverse medication events, as the broadest term for bad outcomes due to use of a medication, occur for a variety of reasons among older patients. Medication errors are important to study, but do not lead to adverse outcomes in most cases. Relative to younger populations, preventable ADEs in older populations tend to occur more frequently and are more likely to result in hospitalization. A high number of preventable ADEs are severe or life-threatening in nature. An ADE secondary to withdrawal of a medication, whether intentional or unintentional, can also be severe. While costs due to drug-related problems are reported to be over $177 billion per year in U.S. populations, costs in long-term care residents reach over $2500 per person per year.

The likelihood of experiencing an ADE in the areas of prescribing, dispensing, administering, non-adherence or monitoring increases as the drug regimen becomes more complex. Polypharmacy is the one risk factor for ADEs that is consistently identified by controlled studies. While prescribing ADEs are the most common type, health care professionals can help turn prescribing errors into near misses during dispensing, administration and monitoring stages. The ability of the pharmacist to recognize scenarios in which an elderly patient is vulnerable to an adverse drug event and taking action to correct potential problems is essential to professional practice.

CASE 1: ER PRESENTATION

Setting:
Emergency department

Subjective:
LM is an 86 year old female admitted to the emergency department with delirium. Her spouse presents to the emergency department with LM and verifies that LM adheres to her medication regimen but she does not self-monitor blood pressure or heart rate at home.

Past Medical History:
Atrial fibrillation (newly diagnosed one month ago), hypertension, chronic kidney disease, osteoarthritis, and GERD.

Medications:
Digoxin 0.25mg daily (added one month ago), metoprolol XL 25mg daily, warfarin 3 mg daily (added 1 month ago), acetaminophen 650 mg three times daily, omeprazole 20 mg daily, and multivitamin 1 tablet daily.

Allergies:
NKA

Social History:
Married to husband for 57 years; he reports no smoking, no alcohol, and limited daily exercise (short walk every morning).

Family History:
Not reported

Objective:
Weight: 113 pounds
Height: 64 inches
Blood pressure: 101/58 mmHg, Heart rate 52

Physical exam:
Elderly female with altered level of consciousness, no signs of bruising, bleeding, or other injury. The rest of examination is non-contributory.

Laboratory:
Sodium 138 mEq/L, potassium 4.0 mEq/L, chloride 99 mEq/L, CO2 27 mEq/L, BUN 33 mg/dL, creatinine: 1.2 mg/dL, glucose 109 mg/dL, INR 3.8 and digoxin level 2.4 ng/mL

Assessment:
Digoxin toxicity. Digoxin dose is excessive for LM's renal function (estimated CrCl 27 mL/min) and is a likely source of the clinical presentation.
Supratherapeutic INR

Plan:
1. Discontinue digoxin and monitor LM's level of consciousness, laboratory data, blood pressure, and heart rate. Adjust dose of beta blocker as needed to achieve rate control for atrial fibrillation.

2. Reduce warfarin dose from 3 mg daily to 2.5 mg daily, slightly more than a 15% decrease in weekly dose. Monitor for signs and symptoms of bruising, bleeding, TIA, PE or stroke. Reassess INR within 1 to 2 weeks.

Rationale:

1. LM is vulnerable to an adverse drug event associated with her digoxin therapy for several reasons. First, the dose prescribed is excessive for her estimated creatinine clearance. Second, this medication has not been appropriately monitored. Neither laboratory monitoring of serum digoxin concentration nor clinical monitoring of blood pressure or heart rate has been performed by the patient or her care providers. Lastly, the selection of digoxin may not be optimal for LM's Atrial Fibrillation and rate control achieved by her beta blocker therapy may be a better alternative. Digoxin toxicity is a potentially serious ADE that could have been prevented.

2. LM's supratherapeutic INR is also a result of failure to monitor drug therapy. This is an unwanted outcome, but thankfully LM has not experienced actual harm, and as such the laboratory assessment upon admission to the emergency department has resulted in the prevention of a serious ADE.

Case Summary:

This case illustrates adverse drug events that are associated with the prescribing and monitoring stages. The identification of ADEs in this case requires assessment of drug, dose, patient parameters such as creatinine clearance, and monitoring activity. Although explicit criteria such as the Beer's list would identify the dose of digoxin as potentially inappropriate, this criteria alone would not identify the problems associated with the lack of monitoring of the either the digoxin or the warfarin. Intervention at multiple levels could have prevented problems with both drugs. Selection of alternate drug therapy by the prescriber or the ordering of laboratory tests to evaluate the safety and efficacy of the prescribed dose are the primary actions that could have been taken. In addition, with education about home monitoring of blood pressure, heart rate, and clinical signs of adverse effects, LM could have performed her own assessment of medication safety and efficacy.

CASE 2: REFILL CLINIC

Setting:
Ambulatory care setting

Subjective:
JR is a 78-year-old male patient seen in the pharmacist's medication refill clinic due to running out of medication.

Past Medical History:
COPD, asthma, heart failure, hypertension, and h/o TIA 4 years ago.

Medications:
Fluticasone / salmeterol discus 1 puff twice daily, ipratropium metered dose inhaler, 2 puffs twice daily, albuterol metered dose inhaler, 1 puff as needed for shortness of breath, lisinopril 10 mg 1 tablet twice daily, metoprolol 25 mg 1 tablet twice daily, furosemide 80 mg 1 tablet every morning,

potassium chloride 20 mEq 1 tablet daily, omeprazole 20 mg 1 capsule daily, multivitamin 1 tablet daily, fluoxetine 20 mg 1 capsule daily, zolpidem 10 mg every night at bedtime, and naproxen (OTC) 220 mg twice daily.

Allergies:
PCN

Social History:
Lives alone, 44 pack-year history but currently does not smoke, reports occasional alcohol use. Does not exercise due to shortness of breath upon exertion.

Family History:
Not reported

Medication compliance:
JR displays some difficulty explaining what each drug on the regimen is for. He reports that the discus medication gave him sores in his mouth and he has not used it since. He is not sure how often he uses the ipratropium but states that he uses the albuterol "all the time." He reports he "tries to remember to take his medications" and that he takes them "most of the time." Pill counts checked against the refill dates on his prescription bottles indicate under use of all medications except furosemide and zolpidem. He reports he usually remembers these because they help him feel better. He reports that he uses the OTC naproxen twice a day but sometimes uses it three times if he is hurting a lot. He does not report any other over the counter medications.

Objective:
Weight: 177 pounds
Height: 69 inches
Blood pressure: 171/82 mmHg, heart rate 101 beats per minute, respiratory rate 18 per minute

Physical exam:
Afebrile, elderly male in mild respiratory distress. Physical examination is within normal limits except for dry mucous membranes and dry skin. Neurological examination reveals MMSE 23/30 (usual baseline 30/30).

Lab:
Sodium 133 mEq/l, potassium 3.4 mEq/L, chloride 98 meq/L, co2 31mEq/L, BUN 48 mg/dL, creatinine: 1.1 mg/dL, glucose 70 mg/dL. Complete blood count is within normal limits.

Assessment:
1. His electrolyte abnormalities may be associated with several factors, including dehydration (over use or excessive dose of furosemide), under-use of potassium, or over use of albuterol. His change in cognition could be associated with the electrolyte abnormalities or with over use or excessive dose of zolpidem. He also has several medications for which the indication is not clear.

Plan:
1. Reinforce compliance with medications for asthma, COPD, heart failure and hypertension. Include demonstration of administration techniques, and instructions to rinse his mouth after the use of the fluticasone/salmeterol. Education should be provided about the role of medications used for symptom management, including education about interactions between over the counter medications and prescription, recommendations for self-monitoring and when to report problems to the team.

2. Conduct a thorough medication history to determine the start dates and indications for the remaining medications on the regimen. Drug therapy should not be abruptly discontinued, but

in the absence of rationale for the use/continuation of the remaining medications, a slow taper can be pursued for one medication at a time. In particular evaluate need for zolpidem and implement a dose reduction to 5 mg to begin taper.

3. Clarify the continued need for medications identified as lacking indication (fluoxetine, omeprazole, and naproxen) and evaluate potential indications without medications (cardiovascular disease without aspirin). Do not discontinue medications until history has been investigated, as this patient may have ongoing symptoms related to mood, reflux or pain that are not well documented. However, consider that these medications may be potential targets for reduction or replacement.

Rationale:

It is not easy to distinguish the source of this patient's respiratory distress. It is possible that his asthma or COPD has been exacerbated by his non-adherence to fluticasone/salmeterol and ipratropium. An adverse drug event, oral thrush, may have been the reason for his self-discontinuation of the fluticasone/salmeterol. This may perhaps have been prevented by counseling about proper administration technique. It is also possible that his heart failure has been exacerbated by his non-adherence to lisinopril, metoprolol, and potassium, or because of a drug-drug or drug-disease interaction caused by the naproxen. With increasing symptoms of shortness of breath, JR has been relying on albuterol and furosemide, which may, in turn, be contributing to electrolyte abnormalities and dehydration. This, in combination with regular use of an excessive dose of zolpidem may further contribute to his change in MMSE score. The need for the zolpidem is not clear. He may have difficulty achieving restful sleep due to his shortness of breath or due to pain (as suggested by his regular need for naproxen). Alternatively, insomnia may be an adverse effect of his Prozac regimen, for which there is no clear indication. Finally, JR is also at risk of an unwanted health outcome due to untreated indication, as there currently no antiplatelet therapy on his regimen to prevent a second TIA.

Case Summary:

This case includes several examples of adverse drug events, polypharmacy and suboptimal drug therapy. JR's regimen is complex including multiple medications, some of which may be unnecessary. Adverse drug events associated with non-adherence have resulted in therapeutic failure. JR may also be experiencing ADEs associated with excessive dose. A multi-disciplinary approach to assess his disease state control and to assess the appropriateness of each medication is needed. List criteria alone will not be adequate to identify all of JR's medication related problems. In fact, the updated Beer's criteria would only identify fluoxetine 20 mg daily and naproxen use as potentially inappropriate. A pharmacist's assessment of medication appropriateness using considerations in the Medication Appropriateness Index will be crucial to identifying all the pertinent issues. Changes to his medication regimen should be made slowly, one at a time, so as not to precipitate an adverse drug withdrawal event.

Clinical Pearls

- There are multiple challenges to attaining optimal medication adherence among older patients. In addition to common barriers such as medication cost, access, or regimen complexity, health care beliefs are important. For instance, perceptions that symptoms are part of the aging process and therefore not likely to be alleviated by drug therapy can influence the patient's agreement with the plan of care. In addition, cognitive impairment can not only influence medication taking ability, but also the ability to accurately self-report adherence history.

- A Naranjo causality assessment is often used as method of determining the likelihood that an unwanted outcome was a result of an adverse drug effect. This is a validated tool that is very useful for evaluating adverse drug reactions, however other approaches are often needed when considering broader definitions of adverse drug events. This tool is less applicable for problems associated with non-adherence, adverse drug withdrawal events, or more complex problems due to drug-drug or drug disease interactions associated with polypharmacy.[57]

Self-Assessment Questions

1. What proportion of adverse drug events are considered to be preventable?

2. Why are elderly patients more or less vulnerable to hospitalization due to ADEs relative to younger patients?

3. What risk factor for ADEs is most consistently described in the literature?

4. In which category (prescribing, monitoring, dispensing, or administration) do the majority of adverse drug events occur?

5. What is the difference between an error and a near miss?

6. What are the two primary consequences of therapeutic failure?

7. For what period of time after medication discontinuation is an individual vulnerable to an adverse drug withdrawal event?

References

1. Budnitz DS, Pollock DA, Weidenbach KN, et al. National surveillance of emergency department visits for outpatient adverse drug events. *JAMA.* 2006;296:1858–66.

2. Yee JL, Hasson NK, Schreiber DH. Drug-related emergency department visits in an elderly veteran population. *Ann Pharmacother.* 2005;39:1990–5.

3. Pirmohamed M, James S, Meakin S, et al. Adverse drug reactions as cause of admission to hospital: Prospective analysis of 18,820 patients. *BMJ.* 2004;329(7456):15–9.

4. Gurwitz JH, Field TS, Harrold LR, et al. Incidence and preventability of adverse drug events among older persons in the ambulatory setting. *JAMA.* 2003;289:1107–16.

5. Hanlon JT, Pieper CF, Hajjar ER, et al. Incidence and predictors of all and preventable adverse drug reactions in frail elderly post hospital stay. *J Gerontol Med Sci.* 2006;61A:511–5.

6. Gurwitz JH, Field TS, Avorn J, et al: Incidence and preventability of adverse drug events in nursing homes. *Am J Med.* 2000;109:87–94.

7. Gurwitz JH, Field TS, Judge J, et al. The incidence of adverse drug events in two large academic long-term care facilities. *Am J Med.* 2005;118:251–8.

8. Beijer HJ, de Blaey CJ. Hospitalisations caused by adverse drug reactions (ADR): a meta-analysis of observational studies. *Pharm World Sci.* 2002 Apr;24(2):46–54.

9. Thomsen LA, Winterstein AG, Søndergaard B, Haugbølle LS, Melander A. Systematic review of the incidence and characteristics of preventable adverse drug events in ambulatory care. *Ann Pharmacother.* 2007 Sep;41(9):1411–26.

10. Hastings SN, Purser JL, Johnson KS, Sloane RJ, Whitson HE. Frailty predicts some but not all adverse outcomes in older adults discharged from the emergency department. *Am Geriatr Soc.* 2008 Sep;56(9):1651–7.

11. Ernst FR, Grizzle AJ. Drug-related morbidity and mortality: updating the cost-of-illness model. *J Am Pharm Assoc.* 2001;41:192–9.

12. U.S. Population Clock Projection, U.S. Census Bureau. Available at: http://www.census.gov/population/www/popclockus.html. Accessed 11/18/09.

13. Bootman JL, Harrison DL, Cox E. The health care cost of drug-related morbidity and mortality in nursing facilities. *Arch Intern Med.* 1997;157:2089–96.

14. Centers for Disease Control/National Center for Health Statistics. Vital and Health Statistics. Series 13 Number 147. The National Nursing home Survey:1997 Summary Available at: http://www.cdc.gov/nchs/data/series/sr_13/sr13_147.pdf. Accessed 11/18/09.

15. Centers for Disease Control 2004 National Nursing Home Survey. Available at: http://www.cdc.gov/nchs/fastats/nursingh.htm Accessed 11/18/09.

16. Hajjar E, Artz MB, Lindblad CI, Hanlon JT, Schmader K, Ruby C, Sloane R, Pieper C. Risk factors and prevalence for adverse drug reactions in an ambulatory elderly population. *Am J Geriatr Pharmacother.* 2003;1:82–89.

17. Official "Do Not Use" list. The Joint Commission. Updated 3/5/09.

18. Szeinbach S, Seoane-Vazquez E, Parekh A, Herderick M. Dispensing errors in community pharmacy: perceived influence of sociotechnical factors. *Int J Qual Health Care.* September 7, 2007.

19. Franklin, Dean B, O'Grady K. Dispensing errors in community pharmacy: frequency, clinical significance and potential impact of authentication at the point of dispensing. *Int J Pharm Pract.* 2007;15(4):273–81.

20. Woller TW, Stuart J, Vrabel R, et al. Checking of unit dose cassettes by pharmacy technicians at three Minnesota hospitals. *Am J Hosp Pharm.* 1991;48:1952–6.

21. Becker MD, Johnson MH, Longe RL. Errors remaining in unit dose carts after checking by pharmacists versus pharmacy technicians. *Am J Hosp Pharm.* 1978;35:432–34.

22. Mayo CE, Kitchens RG, Reese RL et al. Distribution accuracy of a decentralized unit dose system. *Am J Hosp Pharm.* 1975;32:1124–26.

23. Hassall TH, Daniels CE. Evaluation of three types of control chart methods in unit dose error monitoring. *Am J Hosp Pharm.* 1983;40:970–5.

24. Hoffman RP, Bartt KH, Berlin L et al. Multidisciplinary quality assessment of a unit dose drug distribution system. *Hosp Pharm.* 1984;19(Mar):167–169,173–174.

25. Hynniman CE, Hyde GC, Parker PF. How costly is medication safety? *Hospitals.* 1971;45(Sep 16):73–85.

26. Burroughs TE, Waterman AD, Gallagher TH, et al. Patients' concerns about medical errors during hospitalization. *Jt Comm J Qual Patient Saf.* 2007;33:5–14.

27. Leape LL, Bates DW, Cullen DJ, et al. Systems analysis of adverse drug events. ADE Prevention Study Group. *JAMA.*1995;274:35–43.

28. Cina JL, Gandhi TK, Churchill W, et al. How many hospital pharmacy medication dispensing errors go undetected? *Jt Comm J Qual Patient Saf.* 2006;32:73–80.

29. Aspden P, Wolcott J, Bootman JL, Cronenwett LR, eds. Institute of Medicine. Quality Chasm Series: Preventing Medication Errors 2006 Committee on Identifying and Preventing Medication Errors.

30. Barker, KN, Flynn EA, Pepper GA, Bates DW, Mikeal RL. Medication errors observed in 36 health care facilities. *Arch Intern Med.* 2002;162:1897–1903.

31. Peterson AM, Takiya L, Finley R. Meta-analysis of trials of interventions to improve medication adherence. *Am J Health Syst Pharm.* 2003;60:657–65.

32. van Eijken M, Tsang S, Wensing M, et al. Interventions to improve medication compliance in older patients living in the community: a systematic review of the literature. *Drugs Aging.* 2003;20:229–40.

33. Raehl CL, Bond CA, Woods TJ, Patry RA, Sleeper RB. Screening tests for intended medication adherence among the elderly. *Ann Pharmacother.* 2006 May;40(5):888–93.

34. MacLaughlin EJ, Raehl CL, Treadway AK, Sterling TL, Zoller DP, Bond CA. Assessing medication adherence in the elderly: which tools to use in clinical practice? *Drugs Aging.* 2005;22(3):231–55.

35. Hutchison LC, Jones SK, West DS, Wei JY. Assessment of medication management by community-living elderly persons with two standardized assessment tools: a cross-sectional study. *Am J Geriatr Pharmacother.* 2006 Jun;4(2):144–53.

36. Stafford AC, Tenni PC, Peterson GM, Jackson SL, Hejlesen A, Villesen C, Rasmussen M. Drug-related problems identified in medication reviews by Australian pharmacists. *Pharm World Sci.* 2009 Apr;31(2):216–23. Epub 2009 Feb 26.

37. Luce, JM. Medical malpractice and the chest physician. *Chest.* 2008;134:1044–50.

38. Kaiser RM, Schmader KE, Pieper CF, et al. Therapeutic failure related hospitalization in the frail elderly. *Drugs Aging.* 2006;23:579–86.

39. Franceschi A, Tuccori M, Bocci G, et al. Drug therapeutic failures in emergency department patients. A university hospital experience. *Pharmacol Res.* 2004;49:85–91.

40. Hanlon JT, Schmader KE, Gray S. Adverse drug reactions. In Delafuente JC, Stewart RB, eds. Therapeutics in the Elderly. 3rd ed. Cincinnati, OH: Harvey Whitney Books; 2000:289–314.

41. Woodward MC. Deprescribing: achieving better health outcomes for older people through reducing medications. *J Pharm Prac Res.* 2003;33:323–8.

42. Bain KT, Holmes HM, Beers MH, Maio V, Handler SM, Pauker SG. Discontinuing medications: a novel approach for revising the prescribing stage of the medication-use process. *J Am Geriatr Soc.* 2008;56(10):1946–52.

43. Graves T, Hanlon JT, Schmader KE, et al. Adverse events after discontinuing medications in elderly outpatients. *Arch Intern Med.* 1997;157:2205–10.

44. Kennedy JM, van Rij AM, Spears RA, et al. Polypharmacy in a general surgical unit and consequences of drug withdrawal. *Br J Clin Pharmacol.* 2000;49:353–62.

45. Gerety M, Cornell JE, Plichta D et al. Adverse events related to drugs and drug withdrawal in nursing home residents. *J Am Geriatr Soc.* 1993;41:1326–32.

46. Dormann H, Criegee–Rieck M, Neubert A, et al. Lack of awareness of community-acquired adverse drug reactions upon hospital admission: dimensions and consequences of a dilemma. *Drug Saf.* 2003;26(5):353–62.

47. Hanlon JT, Weinberger M, Samsa GP, Schmader KE, Utteck KM, Lewis IK, et al. A randomized, controlled trial of a clinical pharmacist intervention to improve inappropriate prescribing in elderly outpatients with polypharmacy. *Am J Med.* 1996;100:428–37.

48. Schmader KE, Hanlon JT, Pieper CF, et al. Effects of Geriatric evaluation and management on adverse drug reactions and suboptimal prescribing in the frail elderly. *Am J Med.* 2004;116:394–401.

49. Gurwitz JH, Field TS, Rochon P, et al. Effect of computerized provider order entry with clinical decision support on adverse drug events in the long term care setting. *J Am Geriatr Soc.* 2008;56:2225–33.

50. Chrischilles EA, vanGilder R, Wright K, Kelly M, Wallace RB. Inappropriate medication use as a risk factor for self-reported adverse drug effects in older adults. *J Am Geriatr Soc.* 2009;57:1000–6.

51. Rask KJ, Wells KJ, Teitel GS, Hawley JN, Richards C, Gazmararian JA. Can an algorithm for inappropriate prescribing predict adverse drug events? *Am J Manag Care.* 2005;11:145–51.

52. Page RL, Ruskin JM. The risk of adverse drug events and hospital-related morbidity and mortality among older adults with potentially inappropriate medication use. *Am J Geriatr Pharmacother.* 2006;4:297–305.

53. Laroche ML, Charmes JP, Nouaille Y, Picard B, Merle L. Is inappropriate medication use a major cause of adverse drug reactions in the elderly? *Br J Clin Pharmacol.* 2007;63:177–86.

54. Budnitz DS, Shehab N, Kegler SR, Richards CL. Medication use leading to emergency department visits for adverse drug events in older adults. *Ann Intern Med.* 2007;147:755–65.

55. Gallagher P, O'Mahony D: STOPP (Screening Tool of Older Persons' potentially inappropriate Prescriptions) application to acutely ill elderly patients and comparison with Beers' criteria. *Age Ageing.* 2008;37:673–9.

56. Hanlon JT, Schmader KE, Samsa GP, Weinberger M, Uttech KM, Lewis IK, Cohen HJ, Feussner JR. A method for assessing drug therapy appropriateness. *J Clin Epidemiol.* 1992, 45:1045–51.

57. Naranjo CA, Busto U, Sellers EM, et al. A method for estimating the probability of adverse drug reactions. *Clin Pharmacol Ther.* 1981;30:239–45.

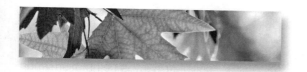

6

Polypharmacy and Other Forms of Suboptimal Drug Use in Older Patients

EMILY R. HAJJAR AND JOSEPH T. HANLON

Learning Objectives

1. Define the terms polypharmacy, and suboptimal drug use and discuss their prevalence and risks in the elderly.

2. Describe evidence based data that shows how polypharmacy and other forms of suboptimal drug use can be modified for elders in different settings.

3. Describe medication therapy management techniques that are used to improve polypharmacy and other forms of suboptimal drug use in the elderly.

Key Terms

BEER'S LIST OR CRITERIA: Common name for the 1997 and 2003 publication of potentially inappropriate medications for elderly patients.

MEDICATION APPROPRIATENESS INDEX: Tool for evaluating the appropriateness of drug therapy based on considerations of indications, dosage, concomitant drugs and disease states, and other factors.

POLYPHARMACY: The use of complex medication regimens, due either to multiple medications or to the use of unnecessary medications.

UNNECESSARY MEDICATION OR DRUG: Medication that is prescribed without a supporting indication, used for longer than intended, or continued despite adverse effects or lack of efficacy.

Introduction

Polypharmacy is commonly defined in one of two ways. The first definition is based on the use of multiple medications, purely classified by medication count.[1] Common cut-points of two, four, five, six, and nine medications have been used to categorize a patient as having polypharmacy.[2-10] Unfortunately, there is no consensus as to which number should be used to define polypharmacy, and studies aiming to quantify the prevalence of polypharmacy have arbitrarily chosen a number to operationalize their definition. Since most elderly patients often have multiple co-morbidities requiring multiple medications based on established medical guidelines, this definition is controversial because medication appropriateness is not considered. In fact, polypharmacy, measured by number of medication only, may be appropriate to treat a patient with a number of chronic medical conditions, such as heart failure, hypertension, and chronic kidney disease.

The second definition of polypharmacy is the administration of **unnecessary medications**.[11] This definition renders a clinical review necessary and takes medication appropriateness into consideration. Unnecessary drug use may be determined by application of three questions from the **Medication Appropriateness Index (MAI)** regarding a medication that lacks an indication or efficacy for a condition or a therapeutic duplication.[12] An example of unnecessary drug use would be a scenario where a patient with no history of gastrointestinal reflux or peptic ulcer disease receives an agent for stress-ulcer prophylaxis upon admittance to an intensive care unit and then has the drug continued when they are discharged from the hospital. In the outpatient setting, the gastrointestinal medication would be considered unnecessary as there is no longer an indication for the medication. Although this definition may be more clinically relevant, few studies have evaluated this definition of polypharmacy.

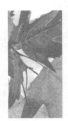

KEY POINT: It is important to understand which definition of polypharmacy is being used when interpreting clinical studies as the unnecessary drug use definition is more clinically relevant.

Prevalence of Medication Use

Elderly patients often have multiple co-morbidities requiring multiple prescription medications. A recent study found that 94% of men and women aged 65 and older took at least one medication in the previous week.[13] Moreover, over two thirds of both older men and women took five or more prescription medications.[13] Early evidence after the implementation of Medicare Part D suggests that prescription drug use may further increase in older adults who have increased access. One study using aggregate data from one large retail pharmacy chain estimated that Medicare Part D reduced out-of-pocket drug costs by 18% and increased use of prescription drugs by approximately 13%.[14] Using individual-level data from the same pharmacy chain, another study estimated a smaller effect for Part D: a 6% increase in monthly drug utilization and a 13% reduction in out-of-pocket costs.[15] This evidence demonstrates the fact that having to pay less for medications may actually increase the number of medications taken by elderly patients. Elders living in the community are also frequent users of non-prescription medications (over the counter [OTC] agents and dietary supplements).[16,17] Another study based on patient interviews reported that 13% of the elderly reported the use of a herbal product in previous 12 months.[18]

Medication use is even higher in older adults that are hospitalized or are long term care residents. In a study of hospitalized elders from Norway, almost half admitted taking 5 or more medications. A U.S. study using 1997 Medicare Current Beneficiary Survey data showed that 60% of older nursing home patients took 6 or more medications.[19] National U.S. data from the Centers for Medicare and Medicaid Services (CMS) reveal that 67.2% of older nursing home residents take 9+ medications daily.[20]

Most Common Drugs

When discussing polypharmacy, it is important to consider the specific prescription and non-prescription medications being used. Table 6-1 shows the most common prescription and over the counter medications used among non-institutionalized older adults.[13] It is important to realize that polypharmacy often entails the use of medications used to treat chronic conditions, and practitioners should be familiar with the commonly used medications. As shown a preponderance of this top ten list involved cardiovascular prescription medications. Uniquely, women more commonly reported the use of thyroid replacement therapy (i.e., levothyroxine) whereas men more commonly reported the use of an oral anticoagulant (i.e., warfarin). Both men and women commonly used two over the counter medications; aspirin and acetaminophen (Table 6-1). Regarding dietary supplements the top product,

a multivitamin, was the same for both older men and women (Table 6-2). Uniquely, men more commonly reported the use of an agent used for benign prostatic hyperplasia (i.e., saw palmetto). Table 6-3 shows the most common medication classes prescribed to older adults residing in U.S. nursing homes.[19] Of note, the use of anti-infectives (e.g., antibiotics), gastrointestinal (e.g., laxatives), and central nervous system medications (e.g., psychotropics) appears to be more common. For decades there has been concern that the use of CNS medication subclasses specifically psychotropic medications may be overused in nursing homes.[21] Specifically, national U.S. data from CMS reveal that almost half use an antidepressant, a quarter use an antipsychotic, 12% an anti-anxiety agent, and 4% use a hypnotic.[20]

Unnecessary Drugs

Few studies have quantified the prevalence of unnecessary drug use. A study of unnecessary drug use in a frail elderly Veterans Affairs (VA) population defined unnecessary drug use as a drug that lacks an indication, effectiveness, or is a therapeutic duplication. They found that 44% of veterans had at least one unnecessary medication at hospital discharge. The reasons for an unnecessary

Table 6-1. **Most Common Prescription and Over-the-Counter Drugs Used by Community Dwelling Elders**[13]

Men	Women
Aspirin	Aspirin
Lisinopril	Levothyroxine
Hydrochlorothiazide	Hydrochlorothiazide
Atorvastatin	Atorvastatin
Simvastatin	Metoprolol
Metoprolol	Lisinopril
Atenolol	Acetaminophen
Amlodipine	Atenolol
Furosemide	Alendronate
Levothyroxine	Simvastatin
Metformin	Amlodipine
Warfarin	Furosemide
Acetaminophen	Metformin
Ezetimibe	Conjugated estrogen

Table 6-2. **Most Common Dietary Supplements Used by Community Dwelling Elders**[13]

Men	Women
Mutlivitamin/minerals	Multivitamin/minerals
Vitamin E	Calcium
Vitamin B	Vitamin C
Vitamin C	Vitamin E
Calcium	Chondroitin/ glucosamine
Potassium	Potassium
Folic acid	Vitamin B
Chondroitin/ glucosamine	Vitamin D
Omega 3 fatty acids	Folic acid
Saw palmetto	Omega 3 fatty acids

Table 6-3. Top Medication Classes Used in Nursing Homes by Older Adults[19]

Medication Class	%
Analgesics/anti-pyretics	76.5
Gastrointestinal agents	74.5
Electrolytes, caloric supplements	71.0
Central nervous system agents	65.9
Anti-infectives agents	62.3
Cardiovascular agents	55.0
Topical or other agents	47.1
Renal/genitourinary tract agents	44.4
Hormones/synthetic substitutes	40.5
Respiratory agents	35.8
Anti-allergy agents	22.4
Blood formation/anticoagulants	17.7

 KEY POINT: Unnecessary drug use is a common problem in older adults.

Risk Factors for Unnecessary Drug Use

Risk factors for unnecessary drug use generally fall into sociodemographic, health status and access to health care categories. A study in a frail elderly veteran population at hospital discharge found that hypertension, having multiple prescribers, and the use of nine or more medications was associated with unnecessary drug use.[12] Another study in a veteran outpatient population found that an increased number of medications was associated with ineffective, not indicated or therapeutically duplicated medications.[22] White race, a low income as defined as less than $30,000 per year, an increased number of prescription medications, and lack of a belief in a "powerful other" for their health locus of control tended to be associated with unnecessary drug use in another veteran primary care population study.[23]

medication included lack of indication (33%), lack of efficacy (19%), and therapeutic duplication (8%). The most common unnecessary medications included gastrointestinal agents, central nervous system agents, and nutrients and minerals.[12] Another study in an outpatient VA population reported that approximately 60% of the patients had a medication that was ineffective, not indicated, or was a duplication of another drug. It was also noted that as the numbers of medication a patient was taking increased so did the average number of unnecessary drugs.[22] Evaluation of unnecessary drug use in another outpatient VA population and found that approximately 60% had at least one unnecessary medication. The most common reason for unnecessary drug use was lack of efficacy.[23]

In summary, it has been documented that older persons often take medications that are not necessary. Lack of indication and lack of effectiveness are the main reasons why most drugs were determined to be unnecessary. These medications are often used to treat chronic conditions and may actually be harmful to the patients.

Risks Associated with Polypharmacy

There is clear evidence that the use of multiple medications in older adults can lead to a variety of medication errors including those involving suboptimal prescribing, and drug non-adherence.[24,25] The use of multiple medications increases the risk of inappropriate prescribing regardless of the measure applied.[26-28] Another concern is the strong relationship between the number of medications and potential drug-drug interactions.[29] In addition medication adherence problems are much more common in older adults taking multiple medications.[30] These medication errors seen with multiple medications can also lead to medication related adverse patient events.[17] Specifically, the most consistent and important risk factor for one type of medication related adverse patient events (i.e., adverse drug reactions) is the use of multiple medications.[17] See Chapter 5 for further details.

The use of multiple medications also increases the risk of adverse health outcomes.[31,32] These adverse health outcomes include decline in functional status, increased health services use including nursing home admission, hospitalization and their associated increased costs.[31,32] Moreover, as the number of medications used increase the risk of the onset and exacerbation of specific geriatric syndromes including cognitive impairment, delirium, and falls also increases.[32,33]

In summary, polypharmacy negatively impacts a patient's health by increasing the risk of suboptimal prescribing, medication non-adherence, adverse drug reactions, cognitive impairment, delirium, and falls.

Other Forms of Suboptimal Drug Use

Another form of suboptimal drug use is underuse of medications.[24] This may involve an undiagnosed and untreated condition (e.g., depression) and diagnosed condition but omitted treatment (e.g., beta blocker post-MI) or the underuse of preventive treatment (e.g., calcium and vitamin D). Several groups from U.S. and Ireland have recently used explicit criteria to define underuse of medications. Additionally, one can apply the Assessment of Underutilization tool. A recent study using this instrument showed that nearly two thirds of community-dwelling veterans had evidence of underuse.[22]

The second form of suboptimal drug use is inappropriate medications[24] One set of explicit criteria developed via Delphi survey of geriatric experts is commonly referred to as the "Beers criteria."[24,26] They were originally developed as a way to measure the impact of a computerized feedback intervention on the prescribing of inappropriate medications in nursing home patients. They have been subsequently updated twice in this country and various U.S. and non-U.S. groups have adopted these for more specific use as quality indicator measure in various populations

of elders.[24] Table 6-4 shows a list of high-risk drugs developed by the Committee for Quality Assurance based in part on the Beers criteria.[28] Studies have shown that nearly one in five older patients are exposed to one or more of these high-risk medications.[24,26] Another approach to determining inappropriate drug use is after reviewing clinical chart information the Medication Appropriateness Index (Table 6-5). This instrument which consists of ten questions has been shown to detect inappropriate prescribing in up to 90% of patients with the most common problems seen with dosage, directions and medication cost.[27]

Interventions to Reduce Polypharmacy and Other Forms of Suboptimal Drug Use

There have been few intervention studies that have examined the impact on polypharmacy, defined as unnecessary medication use, and simultaneously other forms of suboptimal drug in older adults. One randomized, controlled trial evaluated the impact of a specialized inpatient Geriatric Evaluation and Management (GEM) team.[34] GEM is the systematic, interdisciplinary assessment of a frail older patient and the management of identified problems in physical, psychological, social and functional domains by a team of geriatric clinicians including pharmacists. This activity occurs in inpatient GEM units and outpatient GEM clinics. One important of component of GEM is the assessment, improvement and management of medications by geriatric-trained clinicians. They found that in frail elderly hospitalized veterans that GEM care reduced unnecessary medications by 0.5 per person more in comparison to the control group. This study also found significant improvements in underuse of medications measured by the Assessment for Underutilization of Medication and inappropriate medications use measured by the MAI.[34] A before-after study examined the impact of an interdisciplinary team on suboptimal drug use in 23 elderly veteran nursing home patients.[35] They found that this team approach significantly reduced 1.23 unnecessary drugs per patient from

Table 6-4. **National Committee for Quality Assurance Drugs to Avoid Criteria**[28]

Therapeutic Class/ Application	Drugs	
Antianxiety	Meprobamate (Equagesic, Equanil, Miltown)	
Antiemetic	Trimethobenzamide (Tigan)	
Analgesic	Ketorolac (Tordal)	
Antihistamine	Cyproheptadine (Periactin)	Hydroxyzine (Vistaril, Atarax)
	Dexchlorpheniramine (Polaramine)	Promethazine (Phenergan)
		Tripelennamine
	Diphenhydramine (Benadryl)	
Anti-infective	Nitrofurantoin	
Antipsychotic, typical	Thioridazine (Mellaril)	
Amphetamine	Amphetamine mixtures (Adderall)	Methamphetamine (Desoxyn)
	Benzphetamine (Didrex)	Methylphenidate (e.g., Ritalin, Methylin)
	Dextroamphetamine (Dexedrine)	Phendimetrazine (Prelu-2)
	Diethylpropion (Tenuate)	Phentermine (Ionamin, Adipex)
Barbiturate	Amobarbital-secobarbital (Tuinal)	Pentobarbital (Nembutal)
		Secobarbital (Seconal)
	Aprobarbital (Alurate)	
Benzodiazepine, long acting	Chlordiazepoxide (Librium)	Clidinium-chlordiazepoxide (Librax)
	Chlordiazepoxide-amitriptyline (Limbitrol)	Diazepam (Valium)
		Flurazepam (Dalmane)
Cardiovascular	Nifedipine (Procardia, Adalat)— short acting only	Guanadrel
		Guanethidine
Endocrine	Oral estrogen (e.g., Estinyl, Premarin)	Thyroid, desiccated
		Testosterone
Gastrointestinal antispasmodic	Atropine sulfate or Belladonna (in combination (Barbidonna, Bellergal-S, Butibel, Donnatal)	Hyoscyamine (Anaspaz, Cystospaz, Levsin, Levsinex)
		Propantheline (Pro-Banthine)
	Dicyclomine (Bentyl)	Scopolamine (Scopace, Transderm-Scope)
Hypoglycemic, oral	Chlorpropamide (Diabinese)	
Opioid analgesic	Meperidine	Propoxyphene combinations (Darvon CPD, Darvon N, Darvocet-N)
	Pentazocine (Talacen, Talwin, Talwin Cpd, Talwin NX)	
		Propoxyphene (Darvon)
Skeletal muscle relaxant	Carisoprodol (Soma)	Metaxalone (Skelaxin)
	Chlorzoxazone (Paraflex)	Methocarbamol (Robaxin)
	Cyclobenzaprine (Flexeril)	Orphenadrine (Norflex)
Vasodilator	Dipyridamole (Persantine) short acting only	Isoxsuprine (Vasodilan)
	Ergot mesyloids (Hydergine)	

Table 6-5. Medication Appropriateness Index

Questions to ask about each individual medication:

1. Is there an indication for the medication?
2. Is the medication effective for the condition?
3. Is the dosage correct?
4. Are the directions correct?
5. Are the directions practical?
6. Are there clinically significant drug-drug interactions?
7. Are there clinically significant drug–disease/condition interactions?
8. Is there unnecessary duplication with other medication(s)?
9. Is the duration of therapy acceptable?
10. Is this medication the least expensive alternative compared to others of equal utility?

admission to 2–3 months later. Moreover, significant improvements were also seen in the under and inappropriate prescribing as well.[35] Finally a randomized controlled trial of adding pharmaceutical care to the provision of acute GEM care resulted in significant improvements in inappropriate- and under-prescribing of medications.[36]

Medication Therapy Management Approach to Improving Polypharmacy and Other Forms of Suboptimal Drug Use

The first priority in managing polypharmacy and other forms of suboptimal drug use is to complete a thorough medication history. Asking the patient to bring in all prescription and nonprescription medications, including herbal and alternative therapies, to each healthcare visit will aid in this. Additional probing may be needed to fully ascertain the extent of over-the-counter products that a patient consumes. For example, products such as multivitamins, vitamin E, gingko biloba, ibuprofen, and calcium carbonate may be inadvertently left out since patients may not think to bring these items with them. Relating information such as side effects and drug inter-

actions with the patients can help to stress the importance of disclosing these products to all healthcare providers.

Once the healthcare provider has the complete medication list for a patient, they should then start to evaluate whether each medication is truly necessary for the patient. To start, each medication should correspond with a medical problem in the patient's past medical history or current problem list. Drugs that lack an indication should be evaluated to see if they are necessary for the patient. If there is no indication, discontinuation is reasonable for many medications, while others will need to be tapered to avoid any adverse drug withdrawal events. Drugs such as anticonvulsants, antidepressants, and corticosteroids may need to be tapered over a gradual period to minimize a resurgence of an undocumented underlying condition or withdrawal symptoms.[37] Medical conditions that have no associated medication should also be evaluated to see if additional therapy is warranted to fully treat the patient. It is also very important to evaluate any therapy that is prescribed to treat any adverse effects of another medication. An example of this would be the use of levodopa to treat Parkinson-like symptoms caused by metoclopramide. Sometimes this prescribing cascade cannot be avoided, but many times it unnecessarily contributes to the patient's medication regimen.[38] To help prevent a prescribing cascade, it is imperative to determine if any new symptoms that a patient experiences are the result of previous drug therapy or are the result of a medical condition.

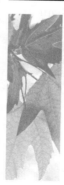

KEY POINT: The first step in identifying unnecessary drug use is to match each drug with an indication and every indication should be evaluated to assure appropriate medications per guideline recommendations, as befits the individual patient, is prescribed.

The healthcare provider must also decide whether the existing therapy is adequate or whether therapy modification or new drug therapy is necessary. Application of the Medication Appropriateness Index (Table 6-5) can help with this assessment. Many medical problems in the elderly do not require a medication to treat the condition or the risks associated with drug therapy outweigh potential benefits. Medications that are no longer effective or are a duplication of another medication should be discontinued. Once a medication is determined to be necessary, healthcare providers need to consider the drug's pharmacokinetics and side effect profile, and the patient's renal and hepatic function for proper dosing. Patient preference and prescription formulary information must also be considered when deciding what types of dosage forms are used. Most often starting doses in the elderly are reduced and many medications must be given in extended intervals to prevent toxicity from occurring compared to the dosing regimens prescribed for younger individuals. Healthcare providers should also become experts in prescribing a few select drugs to manage common problems in the elderly as they will become very familiar and comfortable know the dosing and predicted effects of those medications. Other co-morbid conditions and concomitant medications also need to be taken into account to avoid drug-disease or drug-drug interactions. Screening for drug-drug and drug-disease interactions before prescribing will help to reduce adverse outcomes. Limiting the use of "as needed" drugs and considering medications that can be dosed as few times per day as possible will help to enhance medication adherence. Patients and caregivers also need to be educated in both written and verbal means will also help to increase medication adherence. Considering generic options, utilizing compliance aids (e.g., pill boxes, medication calendars), and encouraging family support can help to improve medication adherence.[39-41] Establishment of clear and reasonable

therapeutic endpoints and monitoring plans and periodic review of medications are also important to screen for adverse drug reactions, therapeutic failures and adverse drug withdrawal events. See Chapter 5 for further details.

Medication reconciliation is another important process that helps to prevent polypharmacy and other forms of suboptimal drug use. Reconciliation should be done whenever a patient is transferred between levels of care such as hospital admission, hospital discharge, nursing home admission, or transfer to independent living. Constant reevaluation of a patient's medication regimen can prevent the addition medications that are only needed to treat acute problems along with ensuring that no medications are omitted. Medication reconciliation also helps transition a patient's medication regimen between various formulary restrictions. This is especially useful upon discharge of a patient back to independent living as it may be overwhelming for him to figure out formulary modification changes from an institution to his Medicare Part D plan on his own.

It is also very important to consider the necessity of medications as patients near the end of their life. Patients may be on many medications that are appropriate per disease state guidelines, but their usefulness is limited due to the fact that the goal of care has shifted from curative to palliative. Factors such as time until onset of medication benefit, goals of treatment, and remaining life expectancy need to be considered when considering starting or continuing medications as patients near the end of their life.[42] For example, adding a statin to the medication regimen of a cancer patient that has 3 months to live is not prudent as the time to benefit of that type of medication is beyond the patient's life expectancy. It is also not reasonable to add additional antihypertensive therapy to an end-stage Alzheimer's patient who is not experiencing any adverse effects from uncontrolled hypertension.

CASE: SUBOPTIMAL DRUG USE

Setting:
Inpatient ward

Subjective:
The patient is a 74-year-old black male who saw his primary care physician because he noticed when he woke up that his "heart wasn't beating right; it feels like it is going too slow." The patient denied chest pain, shortness of breath, nausea or vomiting. He did note feeling dizzy earlier in the day. Six weeks earlier the patient was started on diltiazem CD 180 mg daily by his primary care physician to further lower his blood pressure to goal. His physician also at that time decreased the dose of his metoprolol from 75 to 50 mg bid. Patient was sent to the hospital for admission.

Past Medical History:
Hypertension, type II diabetes, coronary artery disease s/p angioplasty 2 years ago, previous myocardial infarction, ejection fraction = 60%, peripheral vascular disease s/p left femoral to posterior bypass, and history of atrial fibrillation (4 years ago).

Medications on Admission:
Digoxin 0.25 mg daily, diltiazem CD 180 mg daily, metoprolol 50 mg bid, lisinopril 20 mg daily, imdur 30 mg daily, hydrochlorothiazide 12.5 mg daily, KCL 40 meq q am, EC ASA 325 mg qd, warfarin 5 mg daily, famotidine 20 mg at bedtime, vitamin C 500 mg daily, Lantus insulin 26 units at bedtime, Humalog insulin 8 units with meals, vitamin E 400 international units daily, ibuprofen 200 mg 2 tablets prn for headache, multivitamin daily, calcium/iitamin D 500 mg/200 international units bid.

Physical Examination:
Blood pressure 110/50 mmHg; pulse 38 BPM; respirations 14 per minute. The rest of the physical examination is unremarkable.

Pertinent Laboratory:
Potassium 6.9 mEq/L, serum creatinine 1.9 mg/dL, BUN 35 mg/dL, fasting glucose 102 mg/dL, WBC 5,800/mm^3, hematocrit 35%, digoxin level 2.78 ng/mL, INR 2.3, Electrocardiogram: bradycardia with normal sinus rhythm.

Hospital Course:
The patient was admitted to the coronary care unit and received Kayexalate® for increased potassium; digoxin, diltiazem, and metoprolol were held, but all other home medications were continued. Over the next few days, his heart rate and blood pressure increased to 82 BPM and 145/85 mmHg respectively. The patient was transferred to the geriatrics evaluation and management team and restarted on metoprolol. The pharmacist on the geriatrics team was asked to review the patient's home medications for appropriateness. After interviewing the patient and reviewing the records, the pharmacist provided the following medication assessment and plan.

Assessment:
1. Hospital admission secondary to medication-related adverse events: Use of multiple agents to treat hypertension without titration to maximum dose, use of digoxin and warfarin without current indication, and use of potassium chloride supplementation in the presence of an angiotensin converting enzyme inhibitor.

2. Home medications without a current indication for use in this patient: famotidine, warfarin, digoxin, and vitamin E.

3. Patient with significant cardiac history and diabetes mellitus without assessment or treatment for hyperlipidemia.

Plan:

1. Discontinue famotidine, diltiazem, digoxin, warfarin, and vitamin E due to lack of a current indication for use.

2. Reduce dose of ASA to 81 mg to reduce the risk for gastrointestinal bleeding.

3. Titrate metoprolol and lisinopril for a blood pressure goal of $\leq$ 130/80 mmHg.

4. Reevaluate need for hydrochlorothiazide in addition to two other antihypertensive agents.

5. Reevaluate need for KCl in light of increasing lisinopril dose and possible discontinuation of hydrochlorothiazide.

5. Reevaluate need for multivitamin and vitamin C. If the patient is eating a well balanced diet these supplements may be discontinued with little risk but with the benefit of a decreased pill burden.

6. Change from ibuprofen to acetaminophen for headaches as ibuprofen may worsen hypertension.

7. Order cholesterol panel and evaluate patient for statin therapy.

8. Refer to geriatric evaluation and management clinic pharmacist for medication therapy monitoring as an outpatient.

Rationale:

This patient is a classic example of polypharmacy evidenced by unnecessary drug use, as several of his prescribed and over-the-counter medications have no currently active medical indication. In addition, multiple drugs were prescribed at low doses for treatment of hypertension, increasing the pill burden and risk for drug-related problems. The digoxin dose is higher than recommended by the Beers' Criteria for an older adult, and the addition of diltiazem at the last office visit likely further elevated the digoxin serum concentration. Digoxin toxicity was further increased by the high serum potassium level which was a result of potassium supplementation along with use of an angiotensin converting enzyme inhibitor.

Furthermore, another form of suboptimal drug use may be present with underuse of a cholesterol-lowering medication, should his cholesterol panel reveal a low-density lipoprotein cholesterol over 100 mg/dL, which is likely in this patient with a long history of cardiovascular disease.

Clinical Pearl

- *OTC agents and herbal products are necessary pieces of information for a complete medication history. To obtain this information, asking questions as to what the patient uses to treat any complaint they have. For example: "what do you take when you get a headache?" This helps to prompt the patient to think about all of the OTC agents they use on a daily basis.*

Chapter Summary

Polypharmacy is a common phenomenon in older persons. While the use of multiple medications may be guideline adherent, particular attention needs to be focused on the use of unnecessary medications as negative patient health outcomes may avoided if unnecessary medications are removed from therapy. All healthcare professionals need to be aware of the use of unnecessary medications when managing the medication regimens of older patients and should adhere to the principles of geriatric pharmacotherapy when prescribing.

Self-Assessment Questions

1. What are the various definitions of polypharmacy and what are the pros and cons of each?

2. How can medication reconciliation help prevent adverse medication events?

3. What are the ten considerations that make up the Medication Appropriateness Index?

References

1. Stewart RB. Polypharmacy in the elderly: A fait accompli? *DICP.* 1990;24:321–323.

2. Bushardt RL, Massey EB, Simpson TW, Ariail JC, Simpson KN. Polypharmacy: misleading, but manageable. *Clin Interv Aging.* 2008;3(2):383–389.

3. Stewart RB, Cooper JW. Polypharmacy in the aged: Practical solutions. *Drugs Aging.* 1994;4:449–461.

4. Bjerrum L, Sogaard J, Hallas J, Kragstrup J. Polypharmacy: correlations with sex, age and drug regimen. A prescription database study. *Eur J Clin Pharmacol.* 1998;54:197–202.

5. Thomas HF, Sweetnam PM, Janchawee B, Luscombe DK. Polypharmacy among older men in South Wales. *Eur J Clin Pharmacol.* 1999;55:411–415.

6. Fialova, Topinkova E, Gambassi G, Finne-Soveri H, Jonsson PV, Carpenter I, et al. Potentially inappropriate medication use among elderly home care patients in Europe. *JAMA.* 2005;293:1348–1358.

7. Linjakumpu T, Hartikainen S, Klaukka T, Veijola J. Use of medications and polypharmacy are increasing among the elderly. *J Clin Epidemiol.* 2002;55:809–817.

8. Cannon KT, Choi MM, Zuniga MA. Potentially inappropriate medication use in elderly patients receiving home health care: a retrospective data analysis. *Am J Geriatri Pharmacother.* 2006;4:134–143.

9. Denneboom W, Dautzenberg MG, Grol R, De Smet PA. Analysis of polypharmacy in older patients in primary care using a multidisciplinary expert panel. *Br J Gen Pract.* 2006;56:504–510.

10. Roth MT, Ivey JL. Self-reported medication use in community-residing older adults: a pilot study. *Am J Geriatr Pharmacother.* 2005;3:196–204.

11. Montamat SC, Cusack B. Overcoming problems with polypharmacy and drug misuse in the elderly. *Clin Geriatr Med.* 1992;8:142–158.

12. Hajjar ER, Hanlon JT, Sloane RJ, Lindblad CI, Piper CF, Ruby CM, Branch LC, Schmader KE. Unnecessary drug use in frail older people at hospital discharge. *J Am Geriatr Soc.* 2005;53:1518–1523.

13. Qato DM, Alexander GC. Conti RM. Johnson M. Schumm P. Lindau ST. Use of prescription and over-the-counter medications and dietary supplements among older adults in the United States. *JAMA.* 2008;300:2867–2878.

14. Lichtenberg FR, et al. The impact of Medicare Part D on prescription drug use by the elderly. *Health Affairs.* 2007;26:1735–1744.

15. Yin W, et al. The effect of the Medicare Part D prescription benefit on drug utilization and expenditures. *Ann Intern Med.* 2008;148:69–177.

16. Hanlon JT, Fillenbaum GG, Ruby CM, Gray S, Bohannon A. Epidemiology of over-the-counter drug use in community dwelling elders. *Drugs Aging.* 2001;18:123–31.

17. Hanlon JT, Handler S, Maher R, Schmader KE. Geriatric pharmacotherapy and polypharmacy. In: Fillit H, Rockwood K, Woodhouse K, eds. *Brocklehurst's Textbook of Geriatric Medicine.* 7th Ed. London: Churchill Livingstone; 2008.

18. Bruno JJ, Ellis JJ. Herbal use among U.S. elderly: 2002 National Health Interview Survey. *Ann Pharmacother.* 2005;39:643–648.

19. Doshi JA, Shaffer T, Briesacher BA. National estimates of medication use in nursing homes: findings from the 1997 medicare current beneficiary survey and the 1996 medical expenditure survey. *J Am Geriatr Soc.* 2005;53(3):438–443.

20. Centers for Medicare and Medicaid Services. MDS quality measure/indicator report. January-March 2008. Available at: http://www.cms.hhs.gov/MDSPubQIandResRep/02_qmreport.asp?isSubmitted=qm3&group=03&qtr=13. Accessed September 8, 2008.

21. IOM. Committee on Nursing Home Regulations. Improving the quality of care in nursing homes. Washington, DC: National Academy Press; 2001.

22. Steinman MA, Landerfeld CS, Rosenthal GE, Berthenthal D, Sen S, Kaboli JK. Polypharmacy and prescribing quality in older people. *J Am Geriatr Soc.* 2006;54:1516–1523.

23. Rossi MI, Young A, Maher R, Rodriguez KL, Appelt CJ, Perera S, Hajjer ER, Hanlon JT. Polypharmacy

and health beliefs in older outpatients. *Am J Geriatr Pharmacother.* 2007;5:317–323.

24. Spinewine A, Schmader KE, Barber N, et al. Appropriate prescribing in elderly people: How can it be measured and optimized? *Lancet.* 2007;370:173–184.

25. Hughes CM. Medication non-adherence in the elderly. *Drugs Aging.* 2004;21:793–811.

26. Hanlon JT, Fillenbaum GG, Schmader KE, Kuchibhatla M, Horner RD. Inappropriate medication use among community dwelling elderly residents. *Pharmacotherapy.* 2000;20;575–82.

27. Hanlon JT, Artz MB, Pieper CF, Lindblad CI, Sloane R, Ruby CM, Schmader KE. Inappropriate medication use among frail elderly inpatients. *Ann Pharmacother.* 2004;38:9–14.

28. National Committee for Quality Assurance. Available at: http://www.ncqa.org/ Accessed 5/28/09.

29. Johnell K, Klarin I. The relationship between the number of medications and potential drug-drug interactions in the elderly. *Drug Safety.* 2007;30:911–918.

30. Gray SL, Mahoney JE, Blough DK. Medication adherence in elderly patients receiving home health services following hospital discharge. *Ann Pharmacother.* 2001;35:539–545.

31. Frazier SC. Health outcomes and polypharmacy in elderly individuals. *J Gerontol Nursing.* 2005;31 (9):4–11.

32. Hajjar E, Hanlon JT. Polypharmacy in the elderly. In: Calhoun K, Eibling DE, eds. *Geriatric Otolaryngology.* London: Informa Healthcare, 2006;667–673.

33. Inouye SK. Delirium in older persons. *N Engl J Med.* 2006;354:1157–1165.

34. Schmader KE, Hanlon JT, Pieper CF, Sloane R, Ruby CM, Twersky J, Dove- Francis S, Branch LG, Lindblad CI, Artz M, Weinberger M, Feussner JR, Cohen HJ. Effectiveness of geriatric evaluation and management on adverse drug reactions and suboptimal prescribing in the frail elderly. *Am J Med.* 2004;116:394–401.

35. Jeffery S, Ruby CM, Hanlon JT, Twersky J. The impact of an interdisciplinary team on suboptimal prescribing in a long-term care facility. *Consult Pharm.* 1999;14:1386–1389.

36. Spinewine A, Swine C, Dhillon S, Lambert P, Nachega JB, Wilmotte L, Tulkens PM. Effect of a collaborative approach on the quality of prescribing for geriatric inpatients: a randomized, controlled trial. *J Am Geriatr Soc.* 2007;55:658–665.

37. Iyer S, Naganathan V, McLachlan AJ, Le Couter DG. Medication withdrawal trials in people aged 65 years and older: a systematic review. *Drugs Aging.* 2008;25:1021–1031.

38. Rochon PA, Gurwitz JH. Optimising drug treatment for the elderly: the prescribing cascade. *BMJ.* 1997;315:1096–1099.

39. Murray MD, Birt JA, Manatunga AK, Darnell JC. Medication compliance in elderly outpatients using twice-daily dosing and unit-of-use packaging. *Ann Pharmacother.* 1993;27:616–621.

40. Murray MD, Darnell J, Weinberger M, Martz BL. Factors contributing to medication noncompliance in elderly public housing tenants. *Drug Intell Clin Pharm.* 1986;20:146–152.

41. Cramer JA. Enhancing patient compliance in the elderly: role of packaging aids and monitoring. *Drugs Aging.* 1998;12:7–15.

42. Holmes HM, Hayley DC, Alexander GC, Sachs GA. Reconsidering medication appropriateness for patients late in life. *Arch Intern Med.* 2006;166:605–609.

7

Cardiovascular

KRISTEN COOK AND JAMES E. TISDALE

Learning Objectives

1. Assess the significance of orthostatic hypotension and hypertension, appropriate goals for blood pressure, and first-line treatment recommendations in the geriatric population.

2. Discuss the benefits vs. risks of managing hyperlipidemias in elderly patients.

3. Recognize potential barriers in diagnosis and treatment of peripheral arterial disease in geriatrics and the considerations that must be taken when treating intermittent claudication.

4. Describe the benefits vs. risks of anticoagulation for stroke prevention in elderly patients with atrial fibrillation.

5. Discuss the evidence base for using β blockers, angiotensin-converting enzyme (ACE) inhibitors, diuretics, and digoxin in geriatric heart failure patients as well as appropriate considerations when administering these drugs to geriatric patients.

6. Describe the significance of stroke in geriatric patients and the different roles of primary and secondary stroke prevention.

7. Explain the appropriate and safe use of anticoagulants for prevention and management of venous thromboembolism in elderly patients.

Key Terms

ANTITHROMBOTIC: Prevents or interferes with the formation of a thrombus (clot).

DIGOXIN TOXICITY: Occurs when concentrations of digoxin increase above desired therapeutic levels. Arrhythmias are the most common manifestation and can be life threatening, especially in heart failure setting. Toxicity usually occurs in concentrations of >2 ng/mL but can occur at any level. The elderly are predisposed to toxicity.

FIBRINOLYTIC: A pharmacological intervention that dissolves an existing clot.

INTERMITTENT CLAUDICATION: A complication of peripheral arterial disease that presents as pain and fatigue caused by ischemia of muscles, usually in the lower extremities and typically brought on by walking.

ISCHEMIC STROKE: A type of stroke caused by a blood clot from a cardiac or noncardiac source that cuts blood flow off to a certain portion of the brain causing tissue cell death.

LEFT VENTRICULAR FUNCTION: Measure of how well the left ventricle is contracting and expelling blood to the aorta. Also known as systolic function and often measured by ejection fraction.

PULSE PRESSURE: The difference between the systolic and diastolic blood pressures.

RISK FACTOR: A condition which increases the potential for adverse outcomes in a patient, subgroup, or population. Risk factors can be modifiable (smoking, obesity) or not modifiable (age, sex).

THROMBOLYTIC: See *Fibrinolytic.*

Introduction

Cardiovascular diseases affect a large number of individuals in the United States each year. The prevalence and incidence of major cardiovascular diseases including coronary artery disease, hypertension, hyperlipidemias, stroke, heart failure, atrial fibrillation, and the others described in this chapter, increase with advancing age. In many instances, there are issues related to management of specific cardiovascular diseases, safety of medications used to manage cardiovascular conditions, adherence to therapy, and others that are particularly pertinent in the elderly population. In this chapter, the epidemiology, etiology, clinical presentation, standard treatment, and treatment/safety issues associated with major cardiovascular diseases in elderly patients will be discussed.

Orthostatic Hypotension
Etiology, Epidemiology, and Clinical Presentation in the Geriatric Population

Orthostatic hypotension is defined as a reduction in systolic blood pressure of $\geq$ 20 mmHg or a reduction in diastolic blood pressure of $\geq$ 10 mmHg within 3 minutes of standing.[1] Some evidence indicates that the prevalence of orthostatic hypotension increases with age, although the data are equivocal. The prevalence of orthos-

tatic hypotension in individuals > 65 years of age is approximately 20%, and is as high as 30% in individuals > 75 years of age.[2] The prevalence of orthostatic hypotension has been estimated to be as high as 50% in the frail elderly residing in nursing homes.[2]

Rather than having lower baseline blood pressures, elderly patients that develop orthostatic hypotension often have developed age-related increases in supine systolic blood pressure.[2] In the National Health and Nutrition Examination Survey II,[3] the relationship between postural changes on blood pressure and age and systolic blood pressure was evaluated in 8,574 Caucasian, nondiabetic individuals between the ages of 25–74 years. Logistic regression analysis revealed that age was not associated with postural changes in blood pressure (relative odds 1.07, 95% confidence intervals [CI] 0.89–1.19 for each 10-year increase in age). However, increases in supine systolic blood pressure were associated with postural changes in blood pressure (relative odds 1.59, 95% CI 1.49–1.70 for each 10 mmHg increase in systolic blood pressure). It has been suggested that the association between age-related increases in supine blood pressure and increased risk of orthostatic hypotension may be due to central autonomic degeneration resulting in baroreflex dysfunction in the presence of residual sympathetic outflow.[1,4]

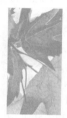

KEY POINT: Orthostatic hypotension that develops in association with advancing age is directly correlated with age-related increases in supine systolic blood pressure.

Orthostatic hypotension may be classified as acute or chronic. Acute orthostatic hypotension develops over a short period of time. Causes of acute orthostatic hypotension include dehydration, diarrhea, extreme heat, myocardial ischemia, adrenal insufficiency, vomiting, or, more rarely, sepsis. Importantly, acute orthostatic hypotension may be caused by medications, including antihypertensive agents. Antihypertensives that are more likely to cause orthostatic hypotension are those that are short acting, vasodilators, or volume depleting. These include centrally acting alpha receptor agonists, peripheral alpha receptor antagonists, nitrates and other vasodilators such as hydralazine or minoxidil, and loop diuretics. Other medications that can cause this include antipsychotic drugs, dopamine agonists, levodopa, marijuana, narcotics, sedatives, sildenafil, and tricyclic antidepressants.[2]

Chronic orthostatic hypotension develops gradually over a more prolonged period of time. Chronic orthostatic hypotension may develop as a result of pathophysiological changes including diminished baroreceptor sensitivity, diastolic dysfunction, or development of hypertension. In addition, chronic orthostatic hypotension may arise due to dysfunction of the autonomic nervous system, from causes such as brain stem lesions, Lewy Body dementia, multiple cerebral infarctions, myelopathies, Parkinson's disease, or multiple system atrophy.[2] Other etiologies of orthostatic hypotension may include alcoholism, amyloidosis, diabetes mellitus, and pernicious anemia.[2] Orthostatic hypotension may be more likely in patients with low body mass index.[5]

Most patients with orthostatic hypotension experience symptoms associated with postural change, including dizziness, lightheadedness, weakness, pre-syncope, syncope, blurred vision, nausea, dyspnea, neck pain, angina, and transient ischemic attacks.[1,2] Elderly patients are particularly susceptible to symptoms such as slurred speech, falls, confusion, and cognitive impairment. In some patients, symptoms may be worsened by prolonged standing, exertion, increased ambient temperature, or eating. Orthostatic hypotension is a common cause of hospitalization. In 2004, there were nearly 81,000 hospitalizations related to orthostatic hypotension.

Treatment Recommendations in the Geriatric Population

Since orthostatic hypotension most commonly occurs in elderly patients, standard adult treatment recommendations are the same for both groups. Recommendations for treatment of orthostatic hypotension are provided in Table 7-1. If the orthostatic hypotension is believed to be drug-induced, therapy with the causative agent should be discontinued. Patients should be advised to rise slowly from a sitting or supine to a standing position, particularly individuals that have undergone long periods of inactivity or bedrest. Patients should be counseled to avoid coughing, straining, or prolonged standing, especially in hot weather, as these activities reduce venous return to the heart.[2] Crossing the legs while standing and contracting muscles for 30 seconds may increase venous return. Raising the head of the bed by 20–30 degrees may minimize hypertension and overnight volume loss. Use of waist-high compression stockings and abdomen-binders may be helpful, as may increasing sodium and water intake.[2]

If nonpharmacological management is not sufficient to minimize or alleviate symptoms, drug therapy may be implemented. Drugs that are most often used for the management of orthostatic hypotension are fludrocortisone and midodrine. Fludrocortisone is a synthetic mineralocorticoid agent that promotes fluid and sodium retention.[1,2] The initial recommended dose of fludrocortisone is 0.1 mg orally daily. The dose may be titrated upward in weekly increments of 0.1 mg daily if necessary, until the maximum dose of 0.3 mg daily is attained, or pedal edema occurs.[1] Adverse effects of fludrocortisone include supine hypertension, ankle edema, headache, hypokalemia, and, rarely, heart failure in susceptible patients.[1,2] Elderly patients may be more susceptible to some of the adverse effects associated with fludrocortisone, particularly fluid overload and hypokalemia. Many elderly patients receiving this drug may require potassium supplementation, especially those taking higher doses.

In patients that continue to exhibit symptoms despite therapy with fludrocortisone, or in those patients in whom fludrocortisone is poorly tolerated, midodrine is a reasonable alternative. Midodrine is a peripheral selective α-receptor agonist.[1] The initial recommended midodrine dose is 2.5 mg orally three times daily during daytime hours; if necessary, the dose may be titrated upward in weekly increments of 2.5 mg per dose, until the maximum recommended dose of 10 mg three times daily is reached.[1,2] Adverse effects of midodrine include supine hypertension, pruritus, paresthesias, piloerection, bradycardia, and urinary retention.[1,2] Midodrine should not be administered to patients with a history of coronary artery disease, heart failure, urinary retention, acute kidney disease, or thyrotoxicosis. In addition, the risk of midodrine-associated bradycardia is increased when the drug is used concomitantly with other heart rate-lowering drugs, such as β-blockers, diltiazem, verapamil, amiodarone, or digoxin.

For patients with symptoms that do not respond to management with fludrocortisone or midodrine, other drug therapy options may be considered. Non-steroidal anti-inflammatory agents (NSAIDs) may increase blood pressure via prostaglandin inhibition.[1,2] Erythropoietin increases blood pressure by expanding blood volume. Caffeine, administered at a dose of 200 mg or taken as two cups of coffee every morning, may be effective. Other drugs that have been used to treat orthostatic hypotension include desmopressin acetate, pyridostigmine, yohimbine, and pseudoephedrine.

Barriers to Treatment in the Geriatric Population

There are few barriers to treatment in the geriatric population, once a diagnosis of orthostatic hypotension has been made. However, a barrier to treatment is the appropriate recognition and diagnosis of orthostatic hypotension. Blood pressure measurements are routinely performed with patients in the sitting position, limiting the ability to diagnose orthostatic hypotension. Clinicians should be aware of the potential for orthostatic hypotension in older patients, and should be alert to detect symptoms. The Joint National Committee on Prevention, Detection, Evaluation and Treatment of High Blood Pressure (JNC)-VII recommends that supine and standing blood pressure be measured periodically in all hypertensive patients > 50 years of age.[6]

Hypertension

Etiology, Epidemiology, and Clinical Presentation in the Geriatric Population

Cardiovascular disease (CVD) is the leading cause of mortality among individuals over the age of 65 years. Hypertension is one of the most prevalent and important **risk factors** contributing to CVD among adults. The prevalence of hypertension increases with advancing age, with elevated systolic blood pressure (SBP) of particular importance. Stratifying populations of elderly patients based on age reveals that 8% of the population over the age of 60 years have elevated SBP, while 25% of the population over the age of 80 years has elevated SBP.[7] Despite this increase in prevalence with age, it may not be accurate to assume that hypertension correlates with the increasing incidence of CVD events and mortality in all age subsets of elderly patients. A divergence in clinical outcomes has been observed among individuals with hypertension who are over 65 years of age as compared with those over 85 years.

In patients between the ages of 65 and 84 years, survival rates are lowest in those individuals with SBP greater than 180 mmHg. However, in patients over the age of 85 years, differences in survival rates in those with SBP less than 130 mmHg compared to those with SBP greater than 180 mmHg are less clear. One study evaluated the relationship between blood pressure and survival in patients over the age of 85 years, found that the risk of death was actually highest among individuals with SBP less than 140/90 mmHg, who would have been defined as "at goal" per JNC-VII guidelines.[6,8]

The relationship between diastolic blood pressure (DBP) and risk may also change with age. A negative relationship has been demonstrated between lower DBP and total mortality.[9] In a population of 7557 patients over the age of 60 (average age of 70 years), lower DBP was associated with increased mortality rates across all strata of SBP.[9] This suggests that a high **pulse pressure** may be a better predictive factor of CVD events in this population. Elderly patients may also have more variation in their blood pressure readings than younger patients. This is referred to as labile hypertension, and may be due to loss of elasticity of arterial walls, changing the manner in which baroreceptors respond.[10] Labile hypertension has not been proven to be an independent risk factor for cardiovascular disease.[11] However, in patients with labile hypertension, these blood pressure variations emphasize the need for several blood pressure measurements to be taken, including home readings, prior to treatment decisions.

Based on these data, the association between hypertension and CVD outcomes among individuals over the age of 60 is well-established. However, it appears that the association between hypertension and CVD outcomes is not as clear among the strata of elderly patients who are of extremely advanced age, in whom high pulse pressures may actually be associated with increased mortality. Therefore, the optimal blood pressure goal across all strata of older individuals remains unclear.

Standard Adult Treatment Recommendations

The standard of care for the treatment of hypertension in the adult population is well-established by the JNC-VII guidelines.[6] Normal blood pressure in the adult is defined as 120/80 mmHg, with hypertension defined at blood pressure > 140/90 mmHg for the general population. Medication therapy to achieve goal blood pressure is recommended for adult patients, and these recommendations are extended to older adults, defined using the age criteria of greater than or equal to 50 years. General recommendations can be found in Table 7-1. Goal blood pressure can be achieved with monotherapy or combination drug therapy, although the guidelines recommend that medication therapy should be initiated at low doses and titrated slowly to avoid orthostatic hypotension, to which elderly patients are more susceptible.

Treatment Recommendations in the Geriatric Population

The JNC-VII guidelines are well-supported and well-respected, but it is reasonable to examine whether these recommendations apply to all subgroups in the elderly population. To determine this and to select specific medications that are the best choices for treatment, one must consider the

Table 7-1. **Standard Treatment Recommendations**

Disease State	Treatment
Orthostatic hypotension	Non pharmacological: • Rise slowly from a sitting or supine to a standing position • Avoid coughing, straining, or prolonged standing, especially in hot weather • Cross the legs while standing and contract muscles for 30 seconds • Raise the head of the bed by 20–30 degrees • Use waist-high compression stockings and abdomen-binders • Increasing sodium and water intake Pharmacological: If drug-induced: discontinue causative agent Fludrocortisone 0.1 mg po daily (maximum dose 0.3 mg po daily) Unresponsive to or intolerant of fludrocortisone: midodrine 2.5 mg po three times daily, maximum dose 10 mg po three times daily

Table 7-1. **Standard Treatment Recommendations (cont'd)**

Disease State	Treatment

Hypertension	Goals:
	    General population: <140/90 mmHg
	    Diabetes or chronic kidney disease: <130/80 mmHg
	
	Initial treatment (no compelling indications):
	    140–159/ or 90–99 mmHg: thiazide diuretic
	    ≥160/ or ≥100 mmHg: two drug combo of thiazide diuretic + ACEI/ARB/ β-blocker/calcium channel blocker
	
	Treatment with compelling indications:
	    Heart failure: diuretic, β-blocker, ACEI, ARB, aldosterone antagonist
	    Post myocardial infarction: β-blocker, ACEI, aldosterone antagonist
	    High coronary disease risk: diuretic, β-blocker, ACEI, calcium channel blocker
	    Diabetes: diuretic, β-blocker, ACEI, ARB, calcium channel blocker
	    Chronic kidney disease: ACEI, ARB
	    Recurrent stroke: diuretic, ACEI

Hyperlipidemias	Goals (see Table 6-2): Nonpharmacological: • Therapeutic lifestyle changes: dietary modifications (<7% of total calories from saturated fat; dietary cholesterol <200 mg daily; ≤10% of total calories from polyunsaturated fat; ≤20% of total calories from monounsaturated fat; total fat intake should not exceed 25–30% of total calories; carbohydrates and protein should comprise 50–60% and 15%, respectively, of total calories. • Weight reduction • Increase physical activity Pharmacological: • Initiate therapy with a statin drug; other options include a bile acid sequestrant or nicotinic acid, but a statin is preferred • Evaluate LDL at 6 weeks; if not at goal, increase dose of statin, or add ezetimibe, bile acid sequestrant, or nicotinic acid

(continued)

Table 7-1. **Standard Treatment Recommendations (cont'd)**

Disease State	Treatment
Acute coronary syndromes/coronary artery disease	**ST segment elevation myocardial infarction:** • oxygen (if the oxygen saturation is <90%) • sublingual nitroglycerin • aspirin 162–325 mg orally • intravenous nitroglycerin • morphine should also be administered for relief of pain and anxiety. • reperfusion therapy with primary percutaneous intervention (PCI) or fibrinolysis (alteplase, reteplase, tenecteplase, or streptokinase) with concomitant administration of intravenous unfractionated heparin or subcutaneous low-molecular weight heparin should be administered as appropriate. In patients that undergo primary PCI, adjunctive therapy with unfractionated heparin and abciximab should be administered. *Non-ST segment elevation myocardial infarction/unstable angina:* • oxygen (if the oxygen saturation is <90%) • sublingual nitroglycerin • aspirin 162–325 mg orally • intravenous nitroglycerin • morphine should also be administered for relief of pain and anxiety. • intravenous unfractionated heparin or subcutaneous enoxaparin, fondaparinux, or bivalirudin • clopidogrel should be administered to patients for whom a noninvasive strategy is planned • in patients for whom an early invasive strategy (i.e., early PCI) is planned, intravenous abciximab or eptifibatide should be administered, starting at the time of PCI, and continued for 12 hours (eptifibatide) or 18–24 hours (abciximab). *Secondary prevention of coronary events:* • To reduce the risk of subsequent coronary events, patients with documented coronary artery disease should receive aspirin 75–162 mg daily indefinitely. • For patients that undergo PCI with placement of a bare metal stent, the aspirin dose should be 162–325 mg daily for a minimum of 30 days; for a sirolimus-eluting stent, 162–325 mg daily for 3 months; for a paclitaxel-eluting stent, 162–325 mg daily for 6 months; in all cases, the aspirin dose should be 75–162 mg daily thereafter indefinitely. • Patients with non-ST segment elevation myocardial infarction who are managed medically should receive clopidogrel 75 mg orally daily for a minimum of 9 months. For patients that underwent PCI with placement of a stent, clopidogrel should be administered for a minimum of 12 months. • All patients should receive long-term therapy with an oral β-blocker, ACE inhibitor or angiotensin receptor blocker (ARB), and lipid-lowering therapy.

(continued)

Table 7-1. **Standard Treatment Recommendations (cont'd)**

Disease State	Treatment

Peripheral arterial disease	**Nonpharmacological:**
	• Exercise rehabilitation programs (first line for symptomatic IC)
	  ■ Supervised program with 30–45 minutes at least 3×/week
	• Surgical (failure to other therapy, severe symptoms, risk vs. benefit analysis prior)
	• PTA (percutaneous transluminal angioplasty), Stent placement, vascular bypass, endarterectomy
	
	Pharmacological:
	• Risk factor reduction
	  ■ Smoking cessation, hyperlipidemia, hypertension, diabetes (see other chapters)
	• **Antithrombotic** therapy (indicated for asymptomatic and symptomatic)
	  ■ First line: aspirin 75–325 mg daily
	  ■ Alternative: clopidogrel 75 mg daily
	• **Intermittent claudication** symptoms (first line: exercise rehab program)
	  ■ Cilostazol 100 mg twice daily
	  ■ Alternative: Pentoxifylline 400 mg TID

Venousthromboembolism	**Prevention of VTE:**
	• Low risk (minor surgery in mobile patients; mobile medical patients):
	  ■ Early ambulation
	• Moderate risk (most general, open gynecologic, urologic; medical patient on bed rest/sick):
	  ■ LMWH, LDUH, or fondaparinux
	• High risk (hip or knee arthroplasty; hip fracture surgery; major trauma):
	  ■ LMWH, fondaparinux, or warfarin
	   *If moderate or high risk with high risk of bleeding: mechanical prophylaxis with graduated compression stocking or intermittent pneumatic compression
	Treatment of VTE:
	• Acute treatment
	  ■ UFH IV or subcutaneous, LMWH, or fondaparinux (must overlap for ≥5 days and can stop after INR >2.0) + warfarin
	  ■ Massive PE with hemodynamic compromise: consider **thrombolytics**
	  ■ Cancer + VTE: LMWH at least 3 months
	  ■ LMWH first line if can treat on outpatient basis
	• Chronic treatment:
	  ■ Warfarin (INR goal 2–3); LMWH if warfarin contraindicated
	  ■ Treatment duration: 3 months to lifelong depending on risk and etiology
	  ■ Compression stockings: proximal DVT at least 2 years

(continued)

Table 7-1. **Standard Treatment Recommendations (cont'd)**

Disease State	Treatment

Stroke	Hemorrhagic stroke: no pharmacological treatment
	• Ischemic stroke:
	  ■ Acute:
	    — IV tissue plasminogen activator 0.9 mg/kg (max. 90 mg) if able to give within 3 hours of onset
	    — Aspirin 160–325 mg daily within first 48 hours of onset (if received tPA do not start for 24 hours)
	    — tPA intra-arterially within 6 hours onset in select patients
	
	• Secondary prevention:
	  ■ Cardioembolic:
	    — Warfarin (INR goal 2–3)
	  ■ Noncardioembolic:
	    — Acceptable first line choices: aspirin 25 mg/ER-dipyridamole 200 mg twice daily, clopidogrel 75 mg daily, aspirin 50–325 mg daily
	    — AHA/ ASA Council 2008 guidelines update has changed recommendation to preference of aspirin/ER-dipyridamole combination over aspirin alone. Although cost must be factored in and above all remain acceptable options.
	    — Alternative: ticlopidine 250 mg twice daily
	  ■ Risk factor modification:
	    — Statin therapy with intensive lipid lowering (goal LDL <100, optional <70)
	    — Hypertension management
	    — Smoking cessation, glycemic control, limited alcohol intake, weight management
	  ■ Primary prevention:
	    — Aspirin 75–160 mg daily for high risk patients (10 year event risk of ≥10%)
	    — Risk factor modification
	  ■ Transient ischemic attack (TIA)
	    — Implement appropriate secondary prevention and risk factor modification

(continued)

Table 7-1. **Standard Treatment Recommendations (cont'd)**

Disease State	Treatment

Heart failure	Chronic management:
	• Stage A: (High risk for developing heart failure)
	   ■ Control concomitant disease states and risk factors: hypertension, atherosclerotic disease, diabetes, arrhythmias, thyroid disorders, tobacco abuse, excessive alcohol, illicit drug use, inactivity
	   ■ ACE I for high risk patients (hx of atherosclerosis, HTN, or diabetes with other cardiovascular risk factors)
	   ■ ARBs can be used in all cases for those intolerant to ACE Is
	• Stage B: (Structural heart disease, no symptoms HF)
	   ■ All Stage A recommendations
	   ■ β blockers (metoprolol succinate, bisoprolol, carvedilol) and ACE I in all with hx of MI, reduced LVEF
	• Stage C: (Prior of current symptoms of HF with reduced LVEF)
	   ■ All recommendations for Stage A, B
	   ■ Dietary salt <2 grams
	   ■ All patients on ACE I and β blocker (metoprolol succinate, bisoprolol, carvedilol)
	   ■ Diuretics as needed for fluid retention
	   ■ Aldosterone antagonists (spironolactone or eplerenone), digoxin, hydralazine/nitrate combo in select patients
	• Stage D: (Refractory HF)
	   ■ All recommendation for Stage A, B, C
	   ■ End of life/palliative care decisions
	   ■ Consider palliative continuous positive inotrope (dobutamine, milrinone) infusions
	   ■ Referral for LV assist device, cardiac transplantation in appropriate patients
	
	Heart failure with preserved LVEF (diastolic):
	• Control hypertension (use of ACE I should be considered)
	• Diuretics for fluid retention
	• Low sodium diet
	• β blockers and calcium channel blocker for rate control in atrial fibrillation

Atrial fibrillation	*Ventricular rate control:* Normal **left ventricular function**: diltiazem, verapamil or β-blocker Left ventricular dysfunction: digoxin combined with β-blocker or amiodarone *Conversion to sinus rhythm:* Direct current cardioversion, or Normal left ventricular function: amiodarone, dofetilide, flecainide, ibutilide, propafenone Left ventricular dysfunction: amiodarone, dofetilide, ibutilide *Maintenance of sinus rhythm:* Normal left ventricular function: propafenone or flecainide Left ventricular dysfunction: amiodarone, dofetilide, sotalol *Stroke prevention:* Warfarin titrated to INR 2–3, unless <75 years of age and no other risk factors for ischemic stroke, then aspirin can be used

ACEI, angiotensin-converting enzyme inhibitor; ARB, angiotensin receptor blocker; INR, international normalized ratio.

literature upon which the JNC-VII recommendations for older patients are based.[6] Specifically, the clinical trials that included at least some elderly patients that also met criteria for inclusion in the JNC-VII guidelines include the Systolic Hypertension in the Elderly Program (SHEP), the Swedish Trial in Old Patients with Hypertension (STOP), the Systolic Hypertension in Europe (Syst-Eur), and the Medical Research Council (MRC) trial.[12-15] Collectively, these trials enrolled patients with an average age of 74 years. Study populations were large, ranging from 1,627 to 4,736 subjects. All of the trials lasted at least two years and showed a reduction in the risk of endpoints such as stroke or cardiovascular death. Three of the four trials used a thiazide diuretic and β-blocker as the antihypertensive agent and one used an ACE inhibitor and calcium channel blocker. Based on evidence from these trials, it would seem that the data support antihypertensive treatment in older patients and that thiazide diuretics, β-blockers, ACE inhibitors, or calcium channel blockers could all be recommended. For patients in the age ranges represented in these clinical trials, these are likely valid conclusions.

Blood pressure goals established for the adult population are appropriate for patients over the age of 65, and remain valid endpoints throughout the seventh decade of life. Current treatment recommendations are appropriate among this population. However, not all of the trials were designed to evaluate high blood pressure in older populations, with only the SHEP trial exclusively for patients with isolated systolic hypertension over the age of 65 years. The MRC trial enrolled no patients over 80 years of age, and only a small number of patients in this age group were represented in the other three studies, including fewer than 1,500 of a total 15,000 subjects. Minimum baseline blood pressure values were 170/77 mmHg; therefore, patients with blood pressure above the JNC-VII goal of 140/90 mmHg but below 170 mmHg systolic were not adequately represented, and none of the trials achieved the JNC goal of 140/90 mmHg. These points raise concerns regarding the reliability with which blood pressure goals and treatment recommendations for patients over the age of 50 years can be extrapolated to all subgroups of elderly patients, particularly individuals of very advanced age.[12-15]

A few studies have focused on individuals over the age of 80 years.[12-19] The results of a meta-analysis of these studies showed a significant reduction in the incidence of non-fatal stroke events among patients over the age of 80 years, but there was no significant reduction in the risk of myocardial infarction, cardiovascular mortality or mortality from any cause.[16] Instead, there was a troubling trend towards an increased risk of mortality, although this was not statistically significant.

Other subgroup analyses of these trials suggest that the hypertension treatment benefit persists and even increases for patients over the age of 70 years. The benefit is particularly evident in men, in patients with other cardiovascular risk factors, and in those patients with the widest pulse pressures. These data suggest that treatment is particularly justified among individuals with systolic pressures greater than 160mmHg. However, these data do not determine whether the benefit persists for those over age 80 years.

The Hypertension in the Very Elderly Trial (HYVET) enrolled 3845 subjects over the age of 80 years, with an average follow-up period of 21 months.[20] The baseline systolic blood pressure was 173/90 mmHg in the treatment and control groups, and the treatment blood pressure goal was less than150/80 mmHg. The treatment intervention was a diuretic or placebo, with the possible addition of an ACE inhibitor in the treatment group. The results showed a significant decrease in rate of fatal/ nonfatal stroke (30%), incidence of death from stroke (39%), rate of death from any cause (21%), and incidence of heart failure (64%) associated with antihypertensive therapy.[20] The benefits began to appear in the treatment group at one year. Limitations of the trial included the fact that, based on demographic characteristics of patients enrolled, the elderly population enrolled in this study was likely healthier than the typical elderly population. Therefore, the results may not be applicable to the frail elderly population. Exact causes of death were difficult to validate in some cases; evidence was required to classify as a death from stroke. Rapid, unexpected deaths were classified as cardiac causes. Nonetheless, the incidence of death from all causes was significantly reduced in the antihypertensive treatment group. This study also demonstrated that thiazide diuretics, with or without the addition of an ACE inhibitor, have been associated with the most favorable outcomes among patients of advanced age.

Based on this review of the data, the importance of treatment to JNC-VII recommended blood pressure goals appears well-supported for patients between the ages of 60–80 years. While the benefits have been less clearly demonstrated among patients of more advanced age, the results of the HYVET trial suggest that treatment with thiazide diuretics as preferred agents to a goal blood pressure of 150/80 mmHg is justified. It is recognized that decisions about antihypertensive medication are often guided by the presence of other cardiovascular risk factors and non-cardiovascular co-morbidities.

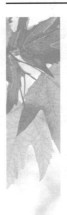

KEY POINT: Standard JNC blood pressure goals are appropriate for patients over the age of 65 years and continue to be beneficial in patients between the ages of 70 and 80 years. These treatment goals need to re-evaluated in patients 80 years of age and over, and may need to be relaxed from the JNC-VII guidelines.[6]

Barriers in Treatment of the Geriatric Population

Adverse outcomes can be associated with failure to initiate an appropriate dose and titrate on an appropriate schedule. Therapeutic goals, frailty, patient prognosis, and age-related decline in kidney function must be considered when initiating and titrating therapy, although once a maintenance dose has been achieved reduction of antihypertensive medication based upon age or creatinine

clearance is inappropriate without assessment as to whether the patient has been tolerating the regimen and has achieved the desired therapeutic goal. Instead, increasing the frequency of monitoring may be a prudent precaution. For example, elderly patients with reduced creatinine clearance are particularly vulnerable to hyperkalemia associated with ACE inhibitors, requiring increased frequency of serum chemistry monitoring. Due to age-related changes in pharmacokinetics and pharmacodynamics, some classes of antihypertensive medication, including β-blockers, centrally acting α-agonists, peripheral α-antagonists, nitrates, and other vasodilators present special concerns for older patients,[21] as noted in Chapter 3.

Hyperlipidemias

Etiology, Epidemiology, and Clinical Presentation in the Geriatric Population

Approximately 25% of adults have elevated plasma low-density lipoprotein (LDL) concentrations.[22] Roughly 63% of patients with elevated plasma LDL concentrations are aware of the condition, and about 41% of those with elevated LDL are taking lipid-lowering medications.[22] Serum concentrations of total cholesterol and LDL increase throughout life, and hyperlipidemia is a common condition in elderly patients.

Published data indicate that the risk associated with elevated plasma cholesterol concentrations observed in younger patients persists in the elderly population. In a multicenter, longitudinal study of 4066 men and women 65 years of age or older (average age 79.2 years at initiation of study), there was a significant correlation between increasing plasma cholesterol concentrations and the increased adjusted relative risk of death due to coronary heart disease over a 4-year period.[23] In addition, in a prospective cohort study of patients 80 years and older, higher plasma high-density lipoprotein (HDL) concentrations were shown to be associated with survival during a 2-year period.[24] Men who survived during this period had mean plasma HDL concentration of 43.4 ± 10.3 mg/dL, compared with 36.7 ± 7.6 mg/dL in those who died (p = 0.001). Similarly, women who survived had higher plasma LDL concentrations than those who did not (49.3 ± 14.9 mg/dL vs. 42.2 ± 11.5 mg/dL, p = 0.001).

A meta-analysis of 61 prospective observational studies that enrolled almost 900,000 adults was performed to determine the relevance of blood pressure and total cholesterol on vascular mortality.[25] The investigators reported that a prolonged reduction in total cholesterol concentration of 1 mmol/L (38.6 mg/dL) from mean "usual" concentrations was associated with the following age-related reductions in the hazard ratio (HR) for death due to ischemic heart diseases: age 40–49 years, HR 0.44 (95% CI 0.42–0.48); age 50–59 years, HR 0.58 (0.56–0.61); age 60–69 years, HR 0.72 (0.69–0.74); age 70–79 years, HR 0.82 (0.80–0.85); 80–89 years, HR 0.85 (0.82–0.89). Therefore, while the magnitude of reduction in HR for death due to ischemic heart disease diminished in patients between 70–79 years and 80–89 years, the reduction in hazard remained statistically significant in both age groups. In addition, there was a strong and significant inverse relationship between plasma HDL concentration and hazard of death due to ischemic heart disease in every age group. However, paradoxically, the hazard ratio for ischemic stroke associated with a 1 mmol/L (38.6 mg/dL) lowering of plasma cholesterol concentration compared to "usual" values was reduced only in patients between the ages of 40–59 years, and was increased in patients between the ages of 80–89 years (HR 1.06, 95% CI 1.00–1.13). The investigators were unable to explain the absence of an independent positive association of cholesterol with stroke mortality at older ages.

Standard Adult Treatment Recommendations

Treatment recommendations for hyperlipidemias are based on the guidelines of the Third Report of the National Cholesterol Education Program (NCEP) Expert Panel on Detection, Evaluation and Treatment of High Blood Cholesterol in Adults (Adult Treatment Panel III).[26] Treatment goals as recommended by the ATP III guidelines are presented in Table 7-2. In 2006, the American Heart Association (AHA)/American College of Cardiology (ACC) updated their guidelines for secondary prevention of patients with coronary and other vascular disease.[27] These guidelines recommend that the LDL goal for patients with coronary heart disease be < 100 mg/dL, but also indicate that it is reasonable to treat to a lower target of < 70 mg/dL. The ATP III guidelines do not recommend altering treatment decisions based on age.

Standard treatment includes therapeutic lifestyle changes to reduce the dietary intake of saturated fats, weight reduction and increasing physical activity.[26] For patients for whom therapeutic lifestyle changes are insufficient to achieve target serum LDL concentrations or for patients with serum LDL concentrations that are sufficiently high to warrant initiation of drug therapy

Table 7-2. Serum LDL Cholesterol Concentration Treatment Goals and Cutpoints for Therapeutic Lifestyle Modifications (TLC) and Drug Therapy[19]

Risk Category	LDL Goal (mg/dL)	LDL at Which to Initiate TLC	LDL at Which to Initiate Drug Therapy
CHD or CHD risk equivalents (10-year risk > 20%)	<100	≥100	≥130 (100–129 drug optional)
2+ risk factors (10-year risk 10–20%)	<130	≥130	≥130
2+ risk factors (10-year risk < 10%)	<130	≥130	≥160
0–1 risk factor	<160	≥160	≥190 (160–189 drug optional)

CHD, coronary heart disease; LDL, low density lipoprotein.

simultaneously with therapeutic lifestyle changes (Table 7-2), drug therapy is initiated.

Treatment Recommendations in the Geriatric Population

Relatively few studies have been conducted to determine the benefits associated with management of hyperlipidemias in the elderly population. Observational studies suggest that benefits of treatment of hyperlipidemias are evident in the very old population. Aronow et al.[29] conducted a prospective, observational study in 1410 male and female nursing home residents (mean age 81 ± 9 years) with a history of prior myocardial infarction and serum LDL concentration ≥ 125 mg/dL; 48% of these patients were taking statins. At 3 years of follow-up, statin use was associated with significant relative reductions in the risk of death due to coronary heart disease or non-fatal myocardial infarction, stroke, and heart failure. In addition, statins were associated with a significant reduction in the risk of new coronary heart disease in patients older than 90 years of age. Statin therapy significantly reduced the risk of new stroke in patients ≤ 90 years of age, but not in those older than 90 years. In a study with a similar design,[30] the same authors evaluated 529 elderly patients with diabetes (mean age 79 ± 9 years) with prior myocardial infarction and mean serum LDL concentration ≥ 125 mg/dL; 53% of these patients were taking statins. Therapy with statin drugs was associated with significant reductions in the incidence of new coronary events and stroke at 2 ½ years of follow-up.

The pravastatin in elderly individuals at risk of vascular disease (PROSPER) trial[31] randomized 5,804 patients between the ages of 70–82 years with a history of or risk factors for vascular disease to receive therapy with pravastatin 40 mg daily or placebo. The mean serum LDL concentration in randomized patients was 147 ± 31 mg/dL. In patients randomized to receive pravastatin, serum LDL concentrations were relatively reduced 34%, and the incidence of primary endpoint events (composite endpoint of death from coronary heart disease, nonfatal myocardial infarction, and fatal or nonfatal stroke) was significantly reduced

by 15% in pravastatin-treated patients. Pravastatin therapy was not associated with a significantly greater deterioration of cognitive function than placebo, and there was no significant difference between the groups in the incidence of myalgias. However, there was significantly higher incidence of new cancers in the pravastatin group compared with that in the placebo group; these findings require further study and corroboration. Overall, however, the results of the PROSPER trial indicate that elderly patients appear to benefit from lipid-lowering therapy.

The relative reduction in the primary endpoint associated with pravastatin in the PROSPER trial was smaller than expected, for reasons that are not entirely clear. Subgroup analyses revealed that the benefits associated with pravastatin therapy appeared to more pronounced in men; there was not a significant reduction in the incidence of the primary endpoint in women. In addition, the hazard ratio for the study endpoints was more favorable in patients with a history of vascular disease compared with those who had no prior history of vascular disease. Overall, however, despite the smaller than expected magnitude of risk reduction associated with pravastatin in this study, the results of PROSPER indicate that lipid-lowering therapy with pravastatin reduces the risk of coronary death, nonfatal myocardial infarction, and fatal or nonfatal stroke in elderly patients.

Sub-group analyses of other large randomized trials provide support for the benefits of lipid-lowering therapy in elderly patients.[28,32] The Cholesterol Treatment Trialists[28] performed a meta-analysis of 14 randomized studies of statin drugs for management of hyperlipidemias, which included 90,056 patients. The results of this analysis suggest that elderly patients achieve significantly benefit associated with lipid-lowering therapy. The relative risk for a major coronary event in patients > 65 years of age was 0.81 (95% CI 0.76–0.88), compared to 0.74 (95% CI 0.69–0.79, p = 0.01) in patients ≤ 65 years of age. Although there appeared to be greater benefit in patients ≤ 65 years old, statin therapy was associated with a significant reduction in the risk of major coronary events in patients > 65 years of age.[28] This study also found a significant reduction in the risk of major coronary events in patients 75 years of age or older (RR 0.82 [99% CI 0.70–0.96], p = 0.002), suggesting that "older" elderly patients benefit from lipid-lowering therapy as well.

Barriers to Treatment in the Geriatric Population

Elderly patients may be at increased risk of developing statin-induced myopathy.[33] In addition to age, risk increases with polypharmacy, reduced renal function and female sex, all common characteristics of many elderly patients. Consequently, elderly patients must be counseled regarding the symptoms of statin-induced myopathy, and must be advised to seek medical attention should the symptoms develop and should be diligently questioned regarding potential symptoms of statin-induced myopathy during routine follow-up visits.

Factors such as frailty, advanced dementia, or patient preferences for palliative-only interventions are often a reason to defer or discontinue drug therapy. In such instances, strict diets and other lifestyle restrictions are also often relaxed or abandoned.

Acute Coronary Syndromes/ Coronary Artery Disease
Etiology, Epidemiology, and Clinical Presentation in the Geriatric Population

Coronary artery disease is the leading cause of death in the U.S. and throughout the world, particularly in the elderly population.[34] The average age at which individuals experience a first myocardial infarction is 66 years for men and 70 years for women. Acute coronary syndromes (ACS) account for roughly 35% of all deaths among individuals ≥ 65 years of age.[35] Eighty-three percent of all individuals that die from ischemic heart disease are > 65 years of age. Although only 6% of the population of the U.S. is > 75 years of age, 60% of all deaths related to myocardial infarction occur in that population.[35] In addition, elderly patients are at higher risk for adverse outcomes associated with ACS. For each 10-year increase in age, the odds of in-hospital mortality associated with ACS increase by 70%.[36] Greater than 50% of patients ≥ 75 years of age develop heart failure due to systolic or diastolic dysfunction following a myocardial infarction.

Patients with an ACS typically present with crushing, squeezing substernal chest discomfort that may be accompanied by pain/discomfort in the arm, back, or jaw. Additional symptoms may include nausea, vomiting, or shortness of breath. Elderly patients are more likely to present with atypical symptoms than younger patients. A higher proportion of elderly patients experiencing a myocardial infarction complain of dyspnea, diaphoresis, nausea and vomiting, and syncope as primary complaints compared with younger patients, while a substantially lower proportion of elderly patients complain of chest discomfort. Some elderly patients experiencing a myocardial infarction may be completely asymptomatic. This renders the diagnosis of myocardial infarction more difficult in the elderly. Serum troponin I and/or creatine kinase concentrations are elevated in patients experiencing a myocardial infarction. Some patients demonstrate elevated ST segments on the electrocardiogram (ST-segment elevation myocardial infarction [STEMI]), while others do not (non-ST segment elevation myocardial infarction [NSTEMI]). Elderly patients with ACS are more likely than younger patients to present with nondiagnostic ECGs.

Standard Adult Treatment Recommendations

(a) *STEMI:* Standard treatment recommendations are presented in Table 7-1. Initial therapy includes oxygen (if the oxygen saturation is < 90%) sublingual nitroglycerin, aspirin 162–325 mg orally, and intravenous nitroglycerin. Morphine should also be administered for relief of pain and anxiety. Reperfusion therapy with primary percutaneous intervention (PCI) or fibrinolysis (alteplase, reteplase, tenecteplase, or streptokinase) with concomitant administration of intravenous unfractionated heparin or subcutaneous low-molecular weight heparin should be administered as appropriate. In patients that undergo primary PCI, adjunctive therapy with unfractionated heparin and abciximab should be administered.[37]

(b) *NSTEMI:* Initial therapy includes oxygen (if the oxygen saturation is < 90%) sublingual nitroglycerin, aspirin 162–325 mg orally, and intravenous nitroglycerin (Table 7-1). Morphine should also be administered for relief of pain and anxiety. Patients should receive intravenous unfractionated heparin or subcutaneous enoxaparin, fondaparinux, or bivalirudin. Clopidogrel should be administered to patients for whom a noninvasive strategy is planned. In patients for whom an early invasive strategy (i.e., early PCI) is planned, intravenous abciximab or eptifibatide should be administered, starting at the time of PCI, and continued for 12 hours (eptifibatide) or 18–24 hours (abciximab).[38]

(c) *Secondary prevention of coronary events:* To reduce the risk of subsequent coronary events, patients with documented coronary artery disease should receive aspirin 75-162 mg daily indefinitely (Table 7-1). For patients that undergo PCI with placement of a bare metal stent, the aspirin dose should be 162–325 mg daily for a minimum of 30 days; for a sirolimus-eluting stent, 162–325 mg daily for 3 months; for a paclitaxel-eluting stent, 162–325 mg daily for 6 months; in all cases, the aspirin dose should be 75–162 mg daily thereafter indefinitely. Patients with NSTEMI who are managed medically should receive clopidogrel 75 mg orally daily for a minimum of 9 months. For patients that undergo PCI with placement of a stent, clopidogrel should be administered for a minimum of 12 months. All patients should receive long-term therapy with an oral β-blocker, ACE inhibitor or angiotensin receptor blocker (ARB), and lipid-lowering therapy.[39]

Treatment Recommendations in the Geriatric Population

Although some studies have been conducted regarding the efficacy of specific treatment strategies in the elderly, many trials of pharmacological interventions for ACS and secondary prevention have included relatively small populations of elderly patients. This has resulted in some cases in a lack of data regarding the safety and efficacy of specific pharmacological therapy in the elderly. Much more research regarding the efficacy of management strategies for ACS and secondary prevention of ACS in elderly patients is needed.

(a) *STEMI:* Relatively few studies have described the efficacy of treatment strategies in elderly patients with STEMI. Data from small randomized studies suggests that PCI is more effective than **fibrinolytic** therapy for reducing the incidence of reinfarction and need for target vessel revascularization in elderly patients. The efficacy of PCI and fibrinolytic therapy appear similar within the first 3 hours following symptom onset, but PCI is more effective in elderly patients that present > 6–12 hours following symptom onset.[40]

In view of the fact that a large proportion of hospitals do not have cardiac catheterization laboratories, fibrinolytic therapy remains a viable option in patients with STEMI. Some data indicate that elderly population may derive a larger degree of mortality reduction associated with fibrinolytic therapy than younger populations.[40] Advanced age is not a contraindication to receive fibrinolytic therapy, as mortality benefit has been demonstrated in patients up to 85 years of age, despite the fact that age and age-related comorbidities are associated with an increased risk of fibrinolytic-associated intracranial hemorrhage. Therefore, fibrinolytic therapy should be administered to elderly patients up to the age of 85 years who do not have contraindications to therapy. Due to the increased risk of intracranial bleeding and the relative lack of data regarding the efficacy of fibrinolytic agents in patients ≥ 85 years, therapy with these drugs is not generally recommended in this population, but further research is necessary.[40] Either unfractionated heparin or low molecular weight heparin can be administered with fibrinolytic agents as adjunctive therapy in the elderly population. In patients ≥ 75 years of age, higher rates of intracranial hemorrhage have been reported in association with enoxaparin compared with those due to unfractionated heparin when used as adjunctive therapy with tenecteplase. However, when enoxaparin doses are adjusted appropriately for declining kidney function in the elderly, data suggest that enoxaparin may be more effective than unfractionated heparin as adjunctive therapy with fibrinolytics for improving outcomes.

Some evidence suggests that elderly patients with STEMI may derive greater benefit associated with the administration of intravenous β-blockers than younger patients.[40] However, these data apply to patients within the range of 65–75 years of age; the study did not include patients > 75 years old. Other data suggest that patients with STEMI who are 70 years of age or older are particularly susceptible to the hypotensive and bradycardic effects of intravenous β-blockers, and may be at greater risk of developing cardiogenic shock associated with these drugs. Therefore, administration of intravenous β-blockers to elderly patients experiencing STEMI with hemodynamic compromise is not recommended.[40]

(b) *NSTEMI:* Data regarding the magnitude of benefit associated with glycoprotein IIb/IIIa receptor inhibitors in elderly patients with NSTEMI are variable and equivocal. Some studies suggest that elderly patients with NSTEMI derive similar benefits associated with this class of drugs as younger patients, while one study reported worse outcomes associated with eptifibatide compared with placebo in patients ≥ 80 years of age.[35] Older age has been identified as a risk factor for bleeding associated with glycoprotein IIb/IIIa receptor inhibitors. In addition, eptifibatide and tirofiban undergo renal elimination, and therefore the risk of bleeding associated with these drugs increases with worsening kidney function. In elderly patients, glycoprotein IIb/IIIa receptor inhibitors are associated with the greatest benefits when administered at the time of a PCI, and when the drugs are not administered to patients with kidney disease.[35] Additional research regarding the benefits vs. the risks of glycoprotein IIb/IIIa receptor inhibitors in patients with NSTEMI who are not undergoing PCI is needed.

(c) *Secondary prevention of coronary events:* Subgroup analyses of elderly patient populations in randomized trials indicate that older patients may derive greater benefit from specific adjunctive therapies for secondary prevention. For example, oral β-blocker therapy is associated with a greater degree of reduction in the relative risk of reinfarction and mortality in elderly patients with a prior myocardial infarction than in younger patients.[40] Similarly, elderly patients derive greater reduction in risk of subsequent coronary events associated with aspirin therapy than younger patients.[35] Secondary prevention with ACE inhibitors or ARBs is equally beneficial in elderly patients compared with younger patients.

Barriers to Treatment in Geriatric Population

As discussed, many elderly patients with ACS present with atypical symptoms and/or nondiagnostic ECGs, rendering the diagnosis of ACS more difficult. In addition, ACS are more likely to occur in elderly patients with a larger number of comorbid conditions, sometimes confusing the diagnosis. These factors often result in misdiagnosis or delays in diagnosis, which in turn delays appropriate treatment. Further, prehospital delays in seeking appropriate treatment for ACS are more likely in elderly patients, as a result of atypical or absent symptoms and socioeconomic or cognitive factors.[40]

The proportion of elderly patients with STEMI who are eligible for reperfusion therapy, either with fibrinolytic agents or PCI, is substantially lower than in younger populations, due to a higher prevalence of exclusion criteria. Overall, elderly patients are at higher risk for adverse effects associated with many agents used for the management of ACS or for secondary prevention, in part due to diminished kidney function. Many studies of pharmacological therapy for acute management of ACS and for secondary prevention have included only small numbers of elderly patients. Therefore, there is a relative lack of data regarding efficacy and safety of specific therapies, and this has led to under-use of life-prolonging drugs in the elderly, including fibrinolytic agents, β-blockers, ACE inhibitors, and others. Adherence to treatment guidelines in elderly patients should be strongly encouraged.

An extension of this issue includes use of dual antiplatelet therapy which has also shown an increased risk is for bleeding complications in older patients. Clinicians may hesitate to treat older patients with dual antiplatelet therapy. However, when applied for the appropriate indication for the recommended duration of therapy, and with proper adjustments for renal function, drug-drug interactions and fall risk reduction allow this therapy to be given safely. Patient education on bleeding risks and proper follow-up are essential.

Peripheral Arterial Disease

Etiology, Epidemiology, and Clinical Presentation in the Geriatric Population

Peripheral arterial disease (PAD) is a common form of atherosclerotic disease. PAD is often not diagnosed because it is frequently asymptomatic, especially in the elderly population. PAD is associated with increased cardiovascular morbidity and mortality, and is often thought to be an indicator of systemic atherosclerosis. The annual incidence of major cardiovascular events in patients with PAD is estimated to be 5–7% in patients.[41]

The prevalence of PAD increases with age. The Rotterdam Study evaluated the incidence of PAD and intermittent claudication (IC) in 10,275 patients in the Netherlands in the very elderly and the normal adult population. The incidences of PAD and IC in men between the ages of 55–59 years were 6.6% and 1%, respectively. For women between the ages of 55–59, the incidences of PAD and IC were 9.5% and 0.7%, respectively. In patients >85 years of age, the incidences of PAD and IC in men were 52% and 6.0%, respectively, and in women the incidences of PAD and IC were 59.6% and 2.5%.[42]

In 2001, the cost to Medicare of treating PAD was estimated at $4.37 billion dollars.[43] This cost estimate did not include medications, durable medical equipment, or rehabilitation programs. In the Medicare population, 6.8% of patients received treatment for PAD in 2001. The proportion of the Medicare population undergoing treatment for PAD increased with age: 4.5% (65–74 years), 7.5% (75–84 years), and 11.8% (>85 years). Approximately 88% of costs were inpatient-related.[43] These reported incidences are lower than those in other studies, and suggest that earlier detection and prevention may help with inpatient costs associated with PAD in this population.

Patients between the ages of 50–69 years with a history of smoking or diabetes and those older than 70 years should undergo a review of vascular symptoms, including walking impairment and claudication symptoms.[44] Exercise treadmill tests are sometimes used to evaluate functional limitation and response to therapy, but may not be feasible in the elderly population. Walking ability may be limited as a result of functional decline or co-morbid conditions such as arthritis or pulmonary disease. The 6-minute walk test is an alternative in the elderly.[44]

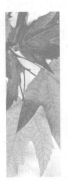

KEY POINT: Appropriate evaluation of lower extremity fatigue and walking limitations should be performed in the elderly, as it is common to attribute these symptoms to deconditioning due to advancing age, when the patient may in fact have PAD.

Standard Adult Treatment Recommendations

The ACC/AHA Practice Guideline for Management of Peripheral Arterial Disease and the American College of Chest Physicians (ACCP) Guidelines on Antithrombotic Therapy for Peripheral Artery Occlusive Disease outline general treatment recommendations (Table 7-1).[44-45] Pharmacological treatment can be divided into two categories: antithrombotic therapy to prevent occlusion/reduce cardiovascular event rates and drug therapy for intermittent claudication symptoms. PAD is a form of atherosclerotic disease, and risk reduction in the form of smoking cessation, glycemic control, hyperlipidemia management, and hypertension therapy should be emphasized.

The treatment guidelines do not generally make distinctions between the elderly and general adult population. Emphasis is placed on screening patients > 70 years of age for PAD.[44] Surgical interventions can also be helpful in patients with PAD who do not respond to pharmacotherapy and continue to experience significant impairment in daily life.

Treatment Recommendations in the Geriatric Population

Since the incidence of PAD is significantly higher in the older population, many of the studies included in the ACC/AHA and ACCP guidelines include patients older than 65 years. However, few studies include patients over the age of 80 years.

Treatment of PAD focuses on risk factor reduction (Table 7-1). Risk reduction should continue to be a goal of treatment in the geriatric population. PAD should be considered a clinical form of atherosclerotic disease and goals for risk factor management treated accordingly.

Antithrombotic therapy has been assessed in several trials that included patients with PAD. The Antithrombotic Trialists' Collaboration was a large meta-analysis that helped form recommendations for PAD. However data in elderly patients were not specifically available.[46] The CAPRIE trial compared the efficacy of clopidogrel 75 mg versus aspirin 325 mg in 19,185 patients with vascular disease. In the subgroup of patients with symptomatic PAD, the average age was 64.3 years. No patient exclusions were made based on age. *Posthoc* subgroup analyses of patients with PAD revealed a significant reduction in the relative risk of vascular events of 23.8% in favor of the clopidogrel group.[47] As no studies exclusively evaluate antithrombotic therapy in the geriatric population, treatment decisions are based upon the assumption that the available data can be extrapolated to this population. As seen in other disease states, caution is required when making this assumption.

Exercise rehabilitation programs are recommended for all patients with symptoms of claudication. These programs should include 30–45 minutes of treadmill or track walking three times per week for at least 12 weeks initially.[44] Many of the studies evaluating such programs are small. The findings of a Cochrane database review that included 10 trials, 8 of which included patients > 65 years, support the efficacy of exercise programs in patients with intermittent claudication.[48] Another exercise trial that focused on the geriatric population (n = 61, mean age 70.5 years) reported a 134% increase in treadmill distance walked until the onset of claudication symptoms.[49] The benefits of such programs have not been tested extensively in the older population, but most studies have been positive, and, given the other health benefits of exercise, should be considered an option for all older patients.

Cilostazol is currently the only recommended pharmacotherapy for symptoms of intermittent claudication. The evidence in support of the efficacy of pentoxifylline is inconclusive, but this agent may be used as an alternative in patients that are intolerant of cilostazol. Most trials used to establish the efficacy of cilostazol did not exclude elderly patients, but the average age of participants was in the mid-60s.[50-52]

Barriers and Issues in Treatment in the Geriatric Population

Bleeding risk must be considered in any patient receiving aspirin or clopidogrel therapy, but this is particularly important in elderly patients because of the higher risk of bleeding events in this population. In the Clopidogrel in Unstable Angina to prevent Recurrent Events (CURE) trial, the incidence of bleeding complications in the aspirin/placebo group increased with advancing age: 2.1% (< 65 years), 3.1% (65–74 years), 3.6% (>75 years). The bleeding incidence was higher in patients in the aspirin & clopidogrel group: 2.5% (<65 years), 4.1% (65–74 years), 5.9% (>75 years).[53] This antiplatelet combination is not currently recommended for the management of PAD. The geriatric population may experience a higher incidence of complications associated with gastrointestinal bleeding than the younger population. Aspirin or clopidogrel should be used at the lowest dose proven effective, which is 81 mg and 75 mg, respectively, for the management of PAD. Symptoms of bleeding and complete blood counts should be monitored closely in the geriatric population to detect occult bleeding.

Declining kidney function also must be considered in pharmacotherapy for PAD. Kidney function must be monitored in patients on cilostazol therapy. If the serum creatinine is > 2.5 mg/dL, concentrations of cilostazol and its active metabolites can be significantly increased and the drug should be used with caution.[54] Pentoxifylline doses must be adjusted to 400 mg twice daily in patients with estimated creatinine clearance 10–50 mL/min and to 400 mg once daily in patients with estimated creatinine clearance < 10 mL/min.

Heart failure is common in the geriatric population. Cilostazol should not be administered to patients with heart failure of any New York Heart Association classification, as other phosphodiesterase III inhibitors have been shown to decrease survival rates in patients with heart failure. Cilostazol undergoes a significant degree of metabolism by cytochrome p-450 3A4 enzymes. Elderly patients take a larger number of medications than younger patients, and the greater potential for drug interactions requires consideration. Cilostazol is an arterial vasodilator and can exacerbate hypotension and cause dizziness. Geriatric patients needs to be screened for orthostasis and hypotension prior to initiating therapy with cilostazol, as these conditions are often more common in this population.

Heart Failure
Etiology, Epidemiology, and Clinical Presentation in the Geriatric Population

The incidence of heart failure increases with age. According to national statistics from the AHA/American Stroke Association, the incidence of heart failure is 9.3% in men and 4.8% in women between the ages of 60–79 years. In patients ≥ 80 years of age, the incidence increases to 13.8% in men and 12.2% in women.[22] In 2009, heart failure is estimated to cost the U.S. $37.2 billion.[22] The incidence of mortality associated with heart failure is also higher in the geriatric population. Concomitant disease states that contribute to development of heart failure or precipitate heart failure, including hypertension, atrial fibrillation, coronary artery disease, and diabetes mellitus are also more common in the elderly.

Changes in anatomy and physiology of the cardiovascular system contribute to the incidence of heart failure in older patients, including increased vascular stiffness and decreased endothelial function, which increases ventricular afterload.[49] In older adults, diminished response to β-adrenergic stimulation occurs due to decreased receptor density and sensitivity. Elderly patients have higher plasma concentrations of catecholamines, but are less responsive to circulating catecholamines.[54] Left ventricular (systolic) function is often preserved and normal in older patients, but diastolic function is often impaired. This type of heart failure is sometimes referred to as "diastolic dysfunction," but this is not an official term. The incidence of heart failure with preserved left ventricular function is high in the geriatric population, especially in women. The Cardiovascular Health Study evaluated heart failure in community dwelling older adults (average age 79 years), and found that 55% of these patients with heart failure had preserved left ventricular function.[56] Management strategies are different for patients with heart failure and preserved left ventricular function, and distinguishing the presence of this type of heart failure is of great importance in the elderly.

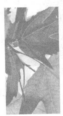

KEY POINT: Diagnosis and clinical presentation of heart failure can be more complicated in older patients. Chronic deconditioning can mimic heart failure symptoms.

Chronic lung disease can mimic shortness of breath and rales heard on auscultation. Peripheral edema can be caused by venous insufficiency and medications such as calcium channel blockers and NSAIDs. Atypical presentation of heart failure also occurs in the elderly, with such symptoms as anorexia, confusion, generalized weakness, and fatigue. Subjective complaints can render diagnosis of heart failure difficult in the elderly, and echocardiography should be used as an objective measure to determine left ventricular function. The use of B-type natriuretic peptide (BNP) for diagnosis and monitoring of treatment in elderly patients can be complicated, as plasma BNP concentrations tend to be higher in the elderly and interpretation of normal concentrations with the different assays can be difficult.[55-58] More trials are needed to determine the role of BNP monitoring in the elderly.

Standard Adult Treatment Recommendations

Heart failure management for adults is described in the 2009 update of the 2005 ACC/AHA guidelines and the Heart Failure Society of America (HFSA) 2006 guidelines (Table 7-1).[59-60] In the AHA/ACC guidelines, patients are categorized into Stages A-D based on the progression of heart failure. One of the aims of this classification is to identify those at risk for preventative measures. The New York Heart Association (NYHA) classification system categorizes patients who have already developed heart failure into class I-IV based on symptoms and functional status. Appropriate pharmacological treatment depends on the staging of heart failure.

Treatment Recommendations in the Geriatric Population

Several of the trials used in the national guidelines included patients over the age of 65 years. However, many of these trials only included a small percentage of patients over 80 years of age, and some included no patients older than 80 years. The HFSA guidelines include a small subsection regarding treatment of elderly patients. The primary specification in regards to pharmacotherapy in elderly patients is to use ACE inhibitors and β-blockers in the absence of contraindication in those over age 80 years. The strength of this recommendation in the older population is based on cohort and case control studies, while in the very old (over age 80) it is based simply on expert opinion.[60]

A review of the literature reveals some studies of the pharmacotherapy of heart failure in patients over the age of 80 years. Many of these studies are *post hoc* analyses of major trials or meta-analyses of several smaller studies. The evidence in major drug classes is discussed below. Efficacy of diuretic therapy in heart failure is not specifically addressed, but these agents are typically effective in older patients. There are also limited data re-

garding the efficacy of hydralazine/nitrate and aldosterone antagonist therapy in the elderly.

β-blockers: The Study of the Effects of Nebivolol Intervention on Outcomes and Rehospitalisation in Seniors with Heart Failure (SENIORS)[61] was a randomized, placebo controlled trial that evaluated a β-1 selective blocker, nebivolol, in patients ≥70 years with heart failure, regardless of left ventricular ejection fraction. The mean age of participants was 76 years in both groups. The primary outcome was all-cause mortality or cardiovascular hospital admission (time to first event). Significantly fewer patients in the nebivolol group reached the primary outcome (p = 0.039); differences in efficacy between the groups became apparent at 6 months of therapy. No difference was found in cardiovascular hospital admissions, and, based on subgroup analyses in the age groups 75–85 years versus those > 85 years, age was found not be a significant influence on primary outcome. This study did not allow patients with significant kidney disease or hepatic dysfunction to enroll, which may limit the generalizability of the study's results to the entire elderly population.[61]

A subgroup analysis of the Metoprolol CR/XL Randomized Intervention in Heart Failure (MERIT-HF) study evaluated the efficacy and tolerability of metoprolol-XL in patients ≥ 65 years (average age 72 years).[62] The analysis found that there were significant reductions in all-cause mortality (37%), sudden death (43%), and hospitalization (36%) associated with metoprolol XL compared with placebo in this elderly population. The analysis also showed significant benefit specifically for patients over the age of 75 years. However, in patients 65 years of age or older, there was a significantly larger proportion of patients that discontinued therapy with metoprolol XL. In addition, older patients achieved a lower dose than younger patients (146 mg vs. 168 mg). Further, there were significantly fewer older patients taking ACE inhibitors, and a larger proportion of older patients with atrial fibrillation or past myocardial infarction. This analysis is limited in that it was performed *post hoc*, and that the trial was not originally designed to determine differences in efficacy in elderly patients.[62] The Carvedilol Open Label Assessment (COLA) II study[63] evaluated the tolerability of carvedilol in patients ≥ 70 years, and demonstrated that 80% of patients achieved a specified carvedilol dose and maintained therapy for at least 3 months. As evidenced by these two larger studies, β-blockers appear to provide benefit with respect to decreased mortality and hospitalization and are as well-tolerated in elderly patients as in the younger population. β-blockers should be recommended for use in elderly patients with heart failure.

ACE Inhibitors: No large placebo controlled trials have analyzed the efficacy of ACE inhibitor therapy specifically in the elderly population with heart failure. Several landmark trials included patients over the age of 65 years. However, there is not as much evidence in the very old population. In one study, patients in nursing homes who were on ACE inhibitors or digoxin were evaluated retrospectively. The average age of patients in the ACE inhibitor group was 84 years, while the average age in patients in the digoxin group was 85 years. Outcomes assessed were overall mortality, hospital admissions, and rate of functional decline. Compared with the digoxin group, there was a significant reduction in the relative risk of mortality (0.89, 95% CI 0.83–0.95) in the ACE inhibitor group. There was only a non-significant trend toward a reduced incidence in hospitalization, but there was a significant reduction in the rate of physical decline in patients taking ACE inhibitors. This evaluation did not distinguish between heart failure with or without preserved left ventricular function, and no consideration was given to doses or previous therapies.[64]

A systematic overview of the efficacy of ACE inhibitors in five large trials was conducted, and included 12,763 patients.[65] The analysis found that the incidence of mortality was lower (23% vs. 26.8%) in patients taking ACE inhibitors compared with those not receiving ACE inhibitor therapy. In addition, the incidence of readmission for heart failure was lower in the ACE inhibitor group (13.7% vs. 18.9%). The mean age of patients in this analysis was 61 years. In a subgroup analysis of specific age groups, there was a smaller

mortality benefit in patients older than 75 years. Three of the major trials included only patients that were post-myocardial infarction.[65] Despite the lack of an overwhelming amount of evidence specifically in elderly patients, ACE inhibitors should be used in the elderly population with heart failure, if tolerated. The benefits of ARBs have been demonstrated to be comparable to that of ACE inhibitors in younger patients with heart failure. ARBs may be tried in elderly patients that do not tolerate ACE inhibitors.

Digoxin: In the Digoxin Investigation Group (DIG) study,[66] patients with heart failure were randomized in double-blind fashion to receive therapy with digoxin or placebo. Patients were stratified by age, and the outcomes assessed were mortality, hospitalizations for heart failure, hospitalization for **digoxin toxicity**, and withdrawal of digoxin therapy. The study included 2,092 patients between the ages of 70–79 and 425 patients 80 years of age and older. The analysis found that the benefit of digoxin with respect to reducing the incidence of hospitalizations due to heart failure was independent of age. However, age was found to be a significant predictor of hospitalization for digoxin toxicity and withdrawal of digoxin therapy.[66] Digoxin did not reduce the incidence of mortality. Digoxin therapy should only be used in elderly patients with left ventricular systolic dysfunction who remain symptomatic despite maximally tolerated doses of a β-blocker, ACE inhibitor, and diuretic. Some studies have demonstrated a lower target range for serum digoxin concentrations of 0.5–0.8 ng/mL that provides as much benefit for heart failure management as higher serum concentrations.[67-68] This lower therapeutic serum concentration range is acceptable in older patients, especially in view of their increased risk of digoxin toxicity.

Combination Therapy: The Trial of Intensified versus standard Medical therapy in Elderly patients with Congestive Heart Failure (TIME-CHF) was conducted to determine whether intensive management is more effective than standard medical therapy. The study enrolled 499 patients with a mean age of 82 years in the very old age group and 69 years in the younger group.[69]

The study compared therapy guided by plasma BNP concentrations with symptom-guided therapy. The primary outcomes were hospitalization-free survival and quality of life measures at 18 months. There was no significant difference in the primary outcomes between the BNP-guided and symptom-guided groups. The BNP-guided group achieved higher doses of ACE inhibitors and β-blockers, and was regarded as the more aggressive treatment group. When the patients were stratified into age groups of 60–74 years and ≥ 75 years, it was found that the younger group may benefit more from the BNP-guided therapy. In the group that was ≥ 75 years of age, benefit from BNP-guided therapy was not apparent, and in fact this treatment strategy was potentially harmful.[69] This trial suggests that increasing drug doses aggressively may not benefit patients with heart failure that are 75 years of age or older. These findings warrant further investigation.

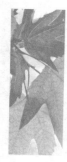

KEY POINT: Therapy with β-blockers and ACE inhibitors should be attempted in elderly patients with heart failure unless there are contraindications. Lower starting doses and slower dose titration may be necessary to maximize safety and tolerability.

Barriers and Issues in Treatment of the Geriatric Population

Proper diagnosis of heart failure can be a barrier to proper treatment, because the symptoms can mimic other common disease in the elderly. In addition, hesitation to attempt titration of heart failure medications due to risk for adverse effects can also be a barrier to proper treatment. Titration of doses of medications for heart failure management can be more difficult in elderly patients. For each class of medications, there are specific issues of which to be aware in the elderly. When initiating therapy with β-blockers, the lowest dose should be used. Starting doses for the three

β-blockers with proven efficacy in heart failure are: metoprolol XL 12.5–25mg once daily, bisoprolol 1.25 mg twice daily; carvedilol 3.125mg twice daily.[70] Heart failure symptoms should be stable before initiation of therapy, and doses should be increased every 2–4 weeks to target doses or the maximally tolerated dose. Therapy with ACE inhibitors/ARBs should also be initiated at lowest dose possible and titrated every 1–2 weeks. Hypotension and bradycardia can limit the ability to titrate the dose in the elderly. Carvedilol may be associated with a slightly higher risk of hypotension than other β-blockers, due to its α-blocking properties. Staggering the time of administration of doses of medications that can lower blood pressure and eliminating other anti-hypertensive agents are strategies that can be used to reduce risk and increase tolerability.

Hyperkalemia is a concern with the use of ACE inhibitors/ARBs and aldosterone antagonists. Chronic kidney disease in elderly patients further increases the risk. Careful monitoring of serum creatinine and potassium concentrations, particularly in elderly patients, is necessary with each dose increase.

Elderly patients may be more sensitive to volume depletion associated with diuretics, and kidney disease may reduce diuretic efficacy in some patients. Thiazide diuretics are not useful for patients with estimated creatinine clearance < 30 mL/min therefore loop diuretics are needed. Hypotension and kidney function should be monitored carefully in these patients. Potassium loss can be a concern with loop diuretics, especially in patients taking digoxin. Hypokalemia can increase the sensitivity of cardiac tissue to effects of digoxin and increase the risk of digoxin toxicity. Monitoring of serum potassium concentrations should be performed on a regular basis.

The half-life of digoxin is increased significantly in patients with kidney disease. The usual half-life of digoxin is 30–40 hours, but in patients with kidney disease the half-life can be as long as 4–6 days.[70] Dose adjustment can be performed by altering the dosing interval or decreasing the maintenance dose. Suggested adjustments based on dosing interval or total daily dose include: for patients with estimated creatinine clearance >50 mL/min, administer every 24 hours; creatinine clearance 10–50 mL/min, administer every 36 hours give or 25–75% of the usual dose; creatinine clearance < 10 mL/min, administer every 48 hours or give 10–25% of the usual dose.[70] Decreased skeletal muscle mass or volume depletion in the elderly reduces the volume of distribution of digoxin and increase the risk of toxicity.

Polypharmacy increases the risk of drug interactions and can contribute to higher toxicity risk. All patients with heart failure should also be counseled regarding avoidance of non-prescription NSAIDs. Elderly patients may be more likely to use these medications as a result of comorbid disease states such as osteoarthritis. Acetaminophen should be recommended in lieu of NSAIDs.

A few recent studies have demonstrated a possible link between heart failure and cognitive impairment or dementia. Proposed mechanisms include decreased cerebral blood flow leading to further ischemia and possibly degeneration of neurons.[71-73] Further analyses are needed in this area, but it is reasonable to make sure that cognitive screening is performed in elderly patients with heart failure.

Atrial Fibrillation
Etiology, Epidemiology, and Clinical Presentation in Geriatric Population

The prevalence of atrial fibrillation increases with aging. Atrial fibrillation is present in approximately 0.5% of patients between the ages of 50–59 years; in individuals >65 years, the prevalence is roughly 5%, and rises to 8–10% in patients > 80 years.[74-75] The incidence of atrial fibrillation is less than 0.1% per year in individuals under the age of 40 years, but increases to 1.5% and 2.0% per year in women and men, respectively, over the age of 80 years.[76]

Atrial fibrillation is associated with a two-fold increase in the incidence of cardiovascular mortality. In addition, atrial fibrillation increases the risk for ischemic stroke 5-fold, and is responsible for approximately 15% of all strokes in the U.S.[77]

Atrial fibrillation may be responsible for as many as 24% of all strokes in individuals between the ages of 80–89 years.[78]

Risk factors for atrial fibrillation include hypertension, coronary artery disease, heart failure, valvular heart disease, and rheumatic heart disease. The common feature of these conditions is the development of left atrial hypertrophy, which leads to derangements in atrial impulse conduction and refractoriness. Hyperthyroidism is a potentially correctable cause of atrial fibrillation. This arrhythmia may occur following thoracic surgery, including coronary artery bypass graft surgery, pulmonary resection, or esophagectomy. In these situations, the arrhythmia is usually transient, lasting only a few days. Drug-induced atrial fibrillation appears to be uncommon, but has been reported in association with binge-drinking of alcohol (the so-called "holiday heart" syndrome). In addition, bisphosphonate drugs have recently been associated with inducing new cases of serious atrial fibrillation; this is particularly pertinent to the elderly population, as many elderly patients with osteoporosis take these drugs for prevention of fractures. The association between bisphosphonate drugs and new-onset serious atrial fibrillation is not certain, and requires further study.

Atrial fibrillation appears on the electrocardiogram (ECG) as an irregularly irregular rhythm with no visible p waves, but rather an "undulating baseline," representing chaotic atrial electrical activity. Ventricular rates during atrial fibrillation generally range from 100–180 beats per minute. Symptoms associated with atrial fibrillation are typically dependent on the ventricular rate, and include palpitations, dizziness, lightheadedness, near-syncope, syncope, shortness of breath, and, in patients with underlying coronary artery disease, angina. Elderly patients have atypical presentations or may be asymptomatic. An evaluation of pulse may reveal irregular hear rate in an otherwise asymptomatic individual. In some patients, the first symptom of atrial fibrillation is a stroke. Depending on the degree to which cardiac output is compromised, patients may become hypotensive and hemodynamically unstable.

Standard Adult Treatment Recommendations

Treatment recommendations are provided in the AHA/ACC/European Society of Cardiology (ESC) guidelines for management of patients with atrial fibrillation.[76] The primary goals of therapy include: (a) ventricular rate control, (b) conversion to sinus rhythm, (c) reduction in the frequency of episodes (for patients with paroxysmal atrial fibrillation), and (d) stroke prevention.

(a) *Ventricular rate control:* Diltiazem, verapamil, or a β-blocker are first line agents for controlling ventricular rate. If contraindicated, digoxin or amiodarone is recommended. The goal of therapy is reduction in ventricular rate to < 100 bpm or, if that cannot be achieved, reduction in ventricular rate > 20% from the pretreatment value with alleviation of patient symptoms.[76]

(b) *Conversion to sinus rhythm:* Conversion of atrial fibrillation to sinus rhythm is safe in patients in whom the episode of atrial fibrillation has persisted for < 48 hours. However, if the patient's episode of atrial fibrillation has persisted for ≥ 48 hours or if the duration is unknown, conversion to sinus rhythm with DCC or drugs may be dangerous, because, after 48 hours, the possibility exists that a clot may have formed in the left atrium. The process of converting atrial fibrillation to sinus rhythm may dislodge the clot and cause a stroke. Therefore, in many institutions, a transesophageal echocardiogram (TEE) is performed in patients with atrial fibrillation of ≥ 48 hours or of unknown duration. If a left atrial clot is detected by TEE, conversion to sinus rhythm is deferred, and anticoagulation is initiated for at least 4 weeks. However, if no left atrial clot is detected by TEE, sinus rhythm may be restored.[76]

Although there are no comparative trials of DCC vs. drug therapy, DCC is generally believed to be more effective. Pharmacological conversion of atrial fibrillation to sinus rhythm may be achieved with dofetilide, ibutilide, amiodarone, propafenone or flecainide and the exact agent is selected according to presence of contraindications.

(c) *Reduction in the frequency of episodes of atrial fibrillation:* This goal of therapy is commonly referred to as "maintenance of sinus rhythm." Several randomized studies have compared rate-control and rhythm control strategies finding no advantage of rhythm control therapy over rate control therapy with respect to incidence of mortality or stroke. However, some data generated in these studies suggested that there may be trends towards worse outcomes, including mortality, associated with rhythm control strategies, presumably as a result of proarrhythmic effects of the drugs. Therefore, drug therapy for reduction of frequency of episodes should be reserved for patients with paroxysmal atrial fibrillation who continue to experience symptoms despite optimal doses of drugs for ventricular rate control.[76]

Propafenone, flecainide, amiodarone, sotalol, or dofetilide are potential choices for maintenance of sinus rhythm, however propafenone and flecainide are contraindicated in patients with left ventricular dysfunction. Amiodarone has been shown to be more effective than sotalol, is rarely associated with the proarrhythmia known as torsades de pointes, and therefore is a preferred drug by many clinicians; however, amiodarone is associated with a long list of noncardiovascular adverse effects, including pulmonary fibrosis, thyroid dysfunction, hepatotoxicity, photosensitivity, blue-grey skin discoloration, corneal microdeposits, and others.

(d) *Stroke prevention:* A summary of the most recommendations of the American College of Chest Physicians (ACCP) for stroke prevention in atrial fibrillation is provided in Table 7-3.[79] The majority of patients require warfarin therapy; however, patients under the age of 75 years with no other risk factors for ischemic stroke may take aspirin. An alternative, but similar approach to stroke prevention in atrial fibrillation is based on the CHADS2 score (Table 7-4).[80]

Treatment Recommendations in Geriatric Population

Treatment recommendations for ventricular rate control, conversion of atrial fibrillation to sinus rhythm, and reduction of the frequency of episodes for patients with paroxysmal atrial fibrillation are the same in elderly patients as in younger patients. With respect to stroke prevention, there are two accepted approaches, both based on the presence of additional risk factors for stroke.[79-80]

Table 7-3. Stroke Prevention in Atrial Fibrillation–American College of Chest Physicians Recommendations[78]

Patient Category (Risk Factors)	Recommended Drug	Dose/Target
Prior ischemic stroke, TIA, or systemic embolism	Warfarin	INR 2.5 (range 2.0–3.0)
$\geq$ 2 of the following: • Age > 75 years • Hypertension • Diabetes mellitus • Heart failure	Warfarin	INR 2.5 (range 2.0–3.0)
One of the following: • Age > 75 years • Hypertension • Diabetes mellitus • Heart failure	Warfarin or Aspirin However, guidelines strongly recommend warfarin in this population	INR 2.5 (range 2.0–3.0) 75–325 mg po qd
< 75 years of age and no other risk factors for ischemic stroke	Aspirin	75–325 mg po qd

INR, international normalized ratio; TIA, transient ischemic attack.

Table 7-4. Stroke Prevention in Atrial Fibrillation–CHADS$_2$ Risk Stratification[79]

CHADS$_2$ Score	Degree of Risk	Recommended Stroke Prevention Strategy
0	Low	Aspirin 325 mg po daily
1	Moderate	Aspirin 325 mg po daily or warfarin (INR 2.0–3.0)
$\geq$ 2	High	Warfarin (INR 2.0–3.0)

CHADS$_2$ score calculated as follows:

Congestive heart failure	1 point
Hypertension	1 point
Age $\geq$ 75 years	1 point
Diabetes mellitus	1 point
Stroke or TIA history	2 points

INR, international normalized ratio; po, orally; TIA, transient ischemic attack.

Based on the ACCP guidelines,[79] patients over the age of 75 years who have one or more additional risk factors for stroke, such as hypertension, diabetes, and/or heart failure should receive warfarin therapy, unless a compelling contraindication to anticoagulation exists, such as a pre-warfarin International Normalized Ratio (INR) > 2.0, a history of alcoholism, anticipated poor adherence, or a current bleeding diathesis. Patients over the age of 75 years who have no additional risk factors for stroke may be treated with warfarin or aspirin; the majority of these patients are treated with warfarin. Elderly patients under the age of 75 who do not have other risk factors for stroke, such as hypertension, diabetes, and/or heart failure, may be treated with aspirin. However, the majority of elderly patients have at least one additional risk factor for stroke, and therefore the majority of elderly patients with atrial fibrillation should be treated with warfarin titrated to an (INR) of 2.0–3.0 (target 2.5) (Table 7-3).[72] An alternate, but similar approach is the calculation of the CHADS2 score, which incorporates age > 75 years as one risk factor, and calculates a risk factor score based on the presence of specific risk factors, including advanced age (Table 7-4).[80]

Barriers to Treatment in the Geriatric Population

Elderly patients are at greater risk for adverse effects associated with some of the antiarrhythmic agents used for the management of atrial fibrillation. For example, elderly patients are more likely to experience constipation associated with verapamil or diltiazem. In addition, drugs such as sotalol, ibutilide, and dofetilide are associated with the risk of the potentially life-threatening ventricular arrhythmia known as torsades de pointes; elderly patients are at greater risk of experiencing this drug-induced proarrhythmia. Further, as a result of declining kidney function, elderly patients may be at higher risk of experiencing elevated serum digoxin concentrations and associated digoxin toxicity. A number of the adverse effects associated with amiodarone occur with increased frequency in elderly patients, including sinus bradycardia, hypothyroidism, pulmonary fibrosis, and neurologic adverse effects, such as ataxia, tremor, peripheral neuropathy, insomnia, and impaired memory. As a result of these considerations, digoxin (at doses greater than 0.25 mg daily) and amiodarone are included in the Beers criteria for potentially inappropriate drug use in older adults.[81]

There are numerous considerations for the use of warfarin in elderly patients which are discussed here, and in the VTE section of this chapter. Conflicting data exist regarding whether elderly patients are at increased risk of bleeding complications associated with warfarin therapy. However, it is well-established that the risk of warfarin-induced bleeding complications is increased in the very old population (patients > 80 years of age). Warfarin therapy is not contraindicated in this population, but careful monitoring of INR and signs and symptoms of bleeding is warranted. In addition, many elderly patients are at risk of falls; in patients with a history of falls, or who appear to be at risk of falling, careful assessment of the risks and benefits of warfarin therapy is often performed. Conventional thinking has been that if a therapeutically anticoagulated patient falls and hits his/her head, an intracranial hemorrhage may result, which may be as catastrophic as a thromboembolic stroke. In the frail elderly population who are at risk of falling, aspirin therapy is often substituted for warfarin therapy, because of the risk of intracranial hemorrhage. However, evidence suggests that the risk of a patient falling and experiencing a significant cerebral bleed during warfarin therapy is low. Man-Song-Hing et al.[82] utilized a Markov decision model incorporating previously published literature regarding the risk of accidental fall and cerebral bleeding during warfarin therapy in patients who were 65 years of age or older. The authors concluded that warfarin therapy was associated with a larger number of quality-adjusted life-years than aspirin therapy or no antithrombotic therapy (12.90 vs. 11.17 vs. 10.15, respectively). In addition, the authors concluded that, based on sensitivity analysis, risk of falling was not an important determinant of optimal antithrombotic therapy. Therefore, perceived risk of falling may not be a sufficiently important factor to discourage warfarin administration for stroke prevention in elderly patients with atrial fibrillation.

Since elderly patients are usually taking a substantially larger number of medications than younger patients, there is a greater potential for drug interactions associated with warfarin that could increase the risk of supratherapeutic INR and bleeding. Careful assessment of concomitant drug therapy, particularly drugs that inhibit the function of cytochrome P-450 2C9, and appropriate adjustment of warfarin dose, where appropriate, is important in the elderly population. This is often especially problematic with antibiotic drugs, as these are usually prescribed on an acute, short term basis. Routine warfarin monitoring schedules can not always capture INR excursions caused by interaction as antibiotic prescribing will not often coincide with a predictable schedule, so the ability to identify a drug interaction is dependent upon prospective drug regimen review by the prescriber and pharmacist at the time of antibiotic initiation.

Stroke

Etiology, Epidemiology, and Clinical Presentation in the Geriatric Population

Stroke is a significant cause of morbidity, and is the third leading cause of death in the U.S. The risk of stroke doubles every 10 years after the age of 55.[22,83] The cost of stroke care is high as many patients have residual effects, and was estimated to be $68.9 billion in 2009.[22]

The incidence of mortality associated with stroke rises with age, demonstrating a need for prevention and education in the geriatric population. Median survival after a first stroke in patients age 60–69 years is 6.8 years for men and 7.4 years in women. In patients age ≥ 80 years, median survival is 1.8 years for men and 3.1 years for women.[22] As many as 26% of patients receive institutionalized care after stroke.[22] Risk factors for stroke, such as hypertension and atrial fibrillation, also are more prevalent in the geriatric population.

Ischemic stroke accounts for approximately 87% of cases, while hemorrhagic stroke accounts for the remaining 13%.[22] This ratio takes into account all age groups and is representative of the older population. Clinical presentation does not differ greatly in the geriatric population. Comorbid disease states, such as dementia, may make recognition of stroke symptoms more difficult. Patients and caregivers require significant education with respect to stroke recognition, as time of treatment from onset is an important factor in determining outcome.

Standard Adult Treatment Recommendations

The standard of care is based on national guidelines (Table 7-1), which are to be applied to the general adult population, and do not make specific recommendations for the elderly population.

The source of stroke (hemorrhagic, noncardioembolic, cardioembolic) and time of onset of stroke symptoms are important factors in the treatment of stroke. Thrombolytic therapy should only be used if the presentation is within 3 hours of onset and the etiology of the stroke is ischemic. The only FDA approved thrombolytic drug for management of stroke in the U.S. is tissue plasminogen activator (t-PA), and patients must be evaluated for inclusion and exclusion criteria for its use (Table 7-1). The source of the stroke affects whether antiplatelet or anticoagulant treatment is administered.

The optimal antiplatelet medication for secondary prevention of stroke is not completely clear. Aspirin, extended release (ER) dipyridamole with aspirin, and clopidogrel all are acceptable choices per guidelines. The AHA/ASA guidelines have suggested that ER dipyridamole with aspirin may be a better choice based on the European/Australian Stroke Prevention in Reversible Ischaemia Trial (ESPRIT) and other previous trials.[84] Since publication of the AHA/ASA guidelines, the Prevention Regimen For Effectively Avoiding Second Strokes (PRoFESS) trial has been published,[85] in which the efficacy of clopidogrel was compared with that of ER dipyridamole combined with aspirin for secondary prevention of strokes. In this study, the efficacy of both treatment strategies on stroke recurrence was similar. All of these therapies remain first-line options, although cost is a significant factor, as aspirin therapy costs much less than the other two therapeutic strategies. Future studies are required to determine whether there is a clear benefit associated with specific treatment strategies. Ticlopidine is an alternative agent for patients who cannot tolerate other antiplatlets. Use of ticlopidine is very limited due to adverse effects including bone marrow suppression, diarrhea, and aplastic anemia. Transient ischemic attack (TIA) should be considered reason for secondary prevention.

The Management of Atherosclerosis with Clopidogrel in High-Risk Patients (MATCH) trial[86] evaluated the efficacy of the addition of aspirin therapy to clopidogrel for reducing the incidence of vascular events, including stroke. This trial included patients with a history of stroke within the previous 3 months plus additional risk factors for vascular events. All patients received clopidogrel 75 mg daily, and were randomized to receive either aspirin 75 mg daily or placebo. This study found no significant decrease in vascular events with the combination of aspirin and clopidogrel compared with clopidogrel alone. However, there was a significantly higher incidence of life-threatening bleeding in patients treated with the combination of clopidogrel and aspirin.[86] Therefore, combination therapy with clopidogrel and aspirin is not recommended for secondary prevention of stroke.

Treatment Recommendations in the Geriatric Population

The majority of the trials used in development of the national guidelines for stroke included patients over age 65 years, most with a mean age in the 60s. The guidelines are applicable to most geriatric patients with special considerations discussed in this section. However, the subgroup of patients over the age of 80 years was not as well-represented in this evidence base.

The National Institute of Neurological Disorders and Stroke (NINDS) study of the efficacy of tissue plasminogen activator for ischemic stroke enrolled patients with mean age of 67 ± 10 years.[87] There have been several follow-up studies specifically in patients over the age of 80 years. Overall, these studies have shown that thrombolytic therapy should not be withheld in patients with stroke who are ≥ 80 years, if other criteria for receiving the medication are met. Although some trials showed that a higher proportion of younger patients achieved a favorable outcome associated with thrombolytic therapy than in patients ≥ 80 years of age, there was still benefit reported in the very elderly population.[88-90] A lower proportion of patients ≥ 80 years of age experiencing benefit from thrombolytic agents may be partially explained by a larger number of comorbid conditions in the very old population, and the fact that the very elderly population experience more severe strokes in some trials. Several of the studies were retrospective reviews or *post hoc* analyses of data and must be interpreted in that context. However, there is a substantial amount of evidence that age should not be an automatic exclusion to thrombolytic therapy.[88-91] The Chinese Acute Stroke Trial (CAST)[92] and the International Stroke Trial (IST)[93] were major studies that established the benefit of early aspirin therapy in patients with ischemic stroke, and their data are applicable to the geriatric population who cannot receive thrombolytic therapy. In the CAST trial, 28% of patients were over the age of 70 years, while 26% of patients enrolled in the IST trial were ≥ 80 years of age.[92-93]

Several of the landmark trials of secondary prevention of stroke included patients over the age of 65 years, and secondary prevention recommendations should be applied to all age groups. The Antithrombotic Trialists' Collaboration investigated the efficacy of antiplatelet therapy in patients over age 65 years of age, and reported that this group derives similar benefits as younger patients.[94] Some studies have shown lower rates of appropriate anticoagulation or antiplatelet therapy after stroke in the geriatric population, and it should be emphasized that the use of these agents for secondary prevention should be advocated in elderly patients, as this is often the highest risk group. The role of primary prevention in the geriatric population, especially the very old, is not as clear, as there are few data. If a patient's 10-year risk for coronary heart disease is >10%, primary prevention should be considered. Future trials should provide more guidance for primary prevention of stroke in the elderly.

Hormone replacement therapy for older women has been found to increase the risk of stroke and should be avoided or used for the shortest duration possible. Post-stroke depression, dementia and the development of seizures are common, as is dysphagia (discussed in Chapter 10), functional decline associated with loss of mobility or contractures, and somnolence. Drug therapy such as antidepressants, cholinesterase inhibitors, memantine, antiepileptics, nutritional supplements, appetite stimulants, muscle relaxants and psychomotor stimulants may often get added to a patient's regimen as interventions for these various problems. In such instances critical evaluation of patient outcomes is necessary as this is often a source of polypharmacy related problems.

Barriers and Issues in Treatment in the Geriatric Population

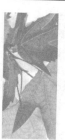

KEY POINT: Patients and caregivers should be educated regarding symptoms of stroke so that symptoms can be recognized, facilitating early presentation to the emergency room for treatment.

A potential barrier to early presentation in the geriatric population is transportation to the emergency room. It should be stressed that patients must call 911 immediately if stroke symptoms occur.

There is a risk of bleeding in association with any of the above medications used for acute treatment or prevention. Some evidence shows small increases in bleeding risk associated with these agents as age increases, but there is also evidence to the contrary. The risks and benefits of therapy in each patient must be weighed. Factors such as frailty, falls, previous gastrointestinal bleed, peptic ulcer disease, polypharmacy, life expectancy, and patient preference should be weighed. Specific concerns with warfarin in the geriatric population are discussed in the venous thromboembolism section and are pertinent to consider in the setting of stroke. The lowest possible drug doses should be used in the elderly, including aspirin 81 mg.

Dose adjustment for patients with kidney and/or hepatic disease is always a consideration in the geriatric population, as there is age-related decline in kidney and hepatic function. Extended-release dipyridamole with aspirin and aspirin monotherapy should be avoided in patients with estimated creatinine clearance < 10 mL/min, and clopidogrel therapy should be avoided in patients with severe kidney disease. Dipyridamole should also be used with caution in patients with severe hepatic impairment. Caution should also be exercised in older patients with syncope or orthostatic hypotension, as dipyridamole can exacerbate these conditions due to its vasodilatory properties.

Venous Thromboembolism

Etiology, Epidemiology, and Clinical Presentation in the Geriatric Population

The incidence of venous thromboembolism (VTE) is higher in the geriatric population compared with that in younger patients. Age should be considered when assessing a patient's risk of VTE. In a large study of 342,000 patients in France, the overall rate of VTE in the population was 1.83/1000 patients, but was 10/1000 patients in those ≥ 75 years of age.[95] In addition to this higher risk, mortality associated with VTE is also higher in the geriatric population.

Risk factors for VTE, including malignancy, hormone replacement therapy, heart failure, severe lung disease, major surgery, and use of erythropoiesis-stimulating agents are more common in the geriatric population. Immobility also plays a large role in determining risk. Paralysis from stroke can cause significant immobility, and recovery after surgery or procedures may put geriatric patients at higher risk. Older adults tend to have several of these risk factors, which are cumulative with respect to conferring risk.

Orthopedic procedures such as total hip replacement, total knee replacement, and hip fracture surgeries are more common in the geriatric population. Immobility after these procedures carries a higher risk in older patients. Incidences of DVT from 7–14 days after these procedures in patients not undergoing VTE prophylaxis are as high as 40–60%.[96] The administration of VTE prophylaxis reduces these incidences to 1–10% in the 3 months following surgery.[96] Geriatric patients need aggressive monitoring and appropriate prophylaxis to prevent higher morbidity and mortality after these procedures and during their rehabilitation.

The clinical presentation of VTE is similar in the geriatric population to that in younger populations. Diseases such as heart failure and chronic obstructive pulmonary disease that occur more frequently in the older population can complicate the diagnosis of pulmonary embolism. Changes in the frequency or quality of shortness of breath and chest pain can be more difficult to detect in patients with those diseases, and symptoms related to those diseases can fluctuate. In addition, heart failure can cause significant lower extremity edema which can complicate the diagnosis of deep vein thrombosis (DVT), although edema associated with DVT is typically unilateral. Advanced diabetic neuropathy and paralysis from stroke can also cause difficulty in recognizing changes in pain and temperature in lower extremities.

Standard Adult Treatment Recommendations

New guidelines for prevention and treatment of venous thromboembolism were released in 2008 by ACCP.[96-97] A summary of standard treatment can be found in Table 7-1. Risk assessment should be performed for each hospitalized patient and written policies and protocols should be in place to specify appropriate prophylaxis measures. Both mechanical and pharmacological methods are described in the guidelines. Treatment of VTE should be performed in an outpatient setting if possible, using low molecular weight heparin.[97] Duration of treatment depends on risk factors and identification of cause of VTE. No distinctions are made regarding the geriatric population in the guidelines, with the exception of recommending extra attention to dose adjustments of anticoagulants in the elderly population with kidney disease. Specific recommendations regarding VTE prevention in patients undergoing total hip and knee replacement or hip fracture surgeries are in the guidelines, as these procedures are commonly performed in the geriatric population. Bleeding, kidney function, and development of postthrombotic syndromes should be monitored. Graduated compression stockings are recommended for prevention of postthrombotic syndrome for proximal DVT.

Treatment Recommendations in the Geriatric Population

The ACCP guidelines provide a strong basis for treatment recommendations in the geriatric population, and the majority of the analyses that form the basis for the guidelines include many patients above the age of 65 years, and some above 80 years.[96-97] Treatment recommendations for prevention of VTE should be advocated for the geriatric population. There is some evidence that physicians are less likely to use anticoagulation therapy in the older population. The risk vs. benefit ratio for VTE management is clearer than with indications such as atrial fibrillation, for which there may be more treatment alternatives. However, with respect to prophylaxis of VTE, physicians' attitudes regarding risks associated with anticoagulation in elderly patients may be more of a factor. Mechanical methods should not be used as the sole method of prophylaxis, unless the patient is high risk for bleeding. Low molecular weight heparin (LMWH), fondaparinux, or warfarin should be used for VTE prophylaxis patients undergoing total knee and total hip replacement. For patients undergoing hip fracture surgery, an additional option is low-dose unfractionated heparin (LDUH).[96] Considerations for dose adjustment of these agents for kidney disease in the geriatric population are discussed below. The duration of prophylaxis should be at least 10 days and up to 35 days after orthopedic surgery. Immobility and speed of recovery must be considered in the geriatric population, and the duration of prophylaxis may need to be extended, depending on course of recovery. Evidence for routine prophylaxis in nursing home patients and homebound geriatrics is not established and no recommendations can be made.[98]

Evidence for treatment of VTE in geriatric patients is very similar to that in the normal adult population. The majority of the studies that form the basis for the ACCP guidelines include older adults. LMWH and fondaparinux administration facilitates outpatient treatment of DVT, which should be a goal for older patients as well. It is recommended that unfractionated heparin (UFH) be used for initial treatment in patients with severe kidney disease, which could encompass some of the geriatric population. The duration of anticoagulation treatment of VTE depends in part on the number of VTE events experienced and whether risk factors can be eliminated. If immobility was a suspected cause of VTE, and is not expected to change, an older patient may continue anticoagulation treatment for longer than the recommended 3 months, even after a first event. Intensity of anticoagulation with warfarin for long term treatment of VTE in the geriatric population should be an INR of 2.0–3.0.

The use of thrombolytic agents for management of pulmonary embolism should be reserved for patients with hemodynamic compromise.[99] Contraindications for use of thrombolytics for pulmonary embolism include history of cerebrovascular accident, which may prohibit their use in the geriatric population.[99] Precautions also include age > 75 years, due to increased bleeding risk.[99]

Several issues pertaining to elderly patients must be considered regarding therapy with warfarin, which is used for long term treatment of VTE and also for VTE prophylaxis. The initial recommended warfarin dose in elderly patients is ≤ 5 mg daily, according to the ACCP guidelines.[100] In a large cohort study that included 2,359 patients ≥ 80 years of age, average weekly doses of warfarin were analyzed, stratified by age.[101] The investigators reported that the average weekly warfarin dose decreased by 0.4mg for every year of age. The average daily dose for men and women ≥ 80 years of age was 4.0 mg and 2.0–3.6 mg, respectively. The recommended initial daily dose of 5mg would have been too high for 82% of women and 65% of men > 70 years of age in this study.[101]

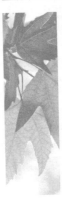

KEY POINT: In the geriatric population, therapy with warfarin should be initiated at 4–5 mg daily with frequent early INR monitoring. If other factors such as heart failure, malnourishment (decline in total protein and albumin), or debilitation are present, an even lower dose should be considered.

The ACCP guidelines also suggest that for patients that desire less frequent INR monitoring, the intensity of anticoagulation can be lowered to a goal INR of 1.5–1.9 after the first 3 months of conventional therapy (INR 2.0–3.0).[97] This lower target may sometimes be suggested for geriatric patients, as they are perceived to be at higher risk for bleeding. However, the Extended Low-intensity Anticoagulation for Thrombo-embolism Investigators (ELATE) trial compared the lower intensity warfarin regimen (INR 1.5–1.9) to the more conventional regimen (2.0–3.0) for prevention of VTE, and found the conventional regimen to be more effective than lower intensity warfarin, with incidences of recurrent VTE of 0.6% per patient-year and 1.9% per patient-year, respectively. The lower intensity recurrence

rate does provide benefit when compared with placebo rates in other studies.[97-102] Further, the lower intensity regimen was not associated with a lower incidence of bleeding compared with the conventional regimen.

Barriers and Issues in Treatment in the Geriatric Population

Numerous considerations are pertinent with respect to anticoagulation for VTE in older adults. Dose adjustments of LMWH and fondaparinux for patients with kidney disease must be considered. For patients requiring VTE prophylaxis with estimated creatinine clearance < 30 mL/min, the dose of enoxaparin should be 30 mg subcutaneously once daily. For patients requiring VTE treatment who have an estimated creatinine clearance < 30 mL/min, the enoxaparin dose should be 1 mg/kg once daily. The manufacturers of dalteparin and tinzaparin suggest caution with use of these drugs in patients with severe kidney disease and mention the potential need to monitor anti factor Xa activity. Fondaparinux should be used with caution in patients with estimated creatinine clearance 30–50 mL/min, and the drug is contraindicated in patients with estimated creatinine clearance < 30 mL/min.[103] These medications are administered subcutaneously, and the ability of the geriatric patient to perform self-injections or the ability of a caregiver to consistently administer injections should be evaluated before the patient is placed on outpatient treatment.

Several concerns related to warfarin therapy are particularly important in elderly patients. Geriatric patients may have less access to transportation and may have difficulty meeting the monitoring requirements for warfarin therapy. Alternatives in this case may include continued treatment with LMWH/ fondaparinux or the possible use of point-of-care INR monitoring. Medicare now has expanded coverage for point-of-care testing for patients undergoing chronic warfarin therapy for VTE. Point-of-care testing is only approved after the patient has been on anticoagulation therapy for 3 months, has undergone face-to-face education, and is not monitoring more than once weekly.[104] The patient's dexterity should also be assessed to determine whether the patient has the capacity to perform this monitoring.

Older adults may be more sensitive to the effects of warfarin. As discussed above, elderly patients generally require lower warfarin doses, and higher initiation doses in the past may have contributed to some of the data indicating a higher risk of bleeding in the geriatric population. Lower body weight and volume of distribution may also be factors. Hypoalbuminemia, malnourishment, or decreased dietary vitamin K intake may also contribute to higher sensitivity. A few studies have suggested that receptor sensitivity may be altered or greater inhibition of vitamin K dependent clotting factors may occur in the elderly,[105] but currently there are few data to support this. Management of warfarin therapy is also complicated by the potential for numerous drug interactions, as polypharmacy tends to be more common in the geriatric population.

Bleeding is a major concern for any patient on anticoagulation therapy, and even more so in the geriatric population. The risk of falls must be assessed and considered in the risk versus benefit analysis as discussed in the atrial fibrillation section.

CASE 1: DEEP VEIN THROMBOSIS

Setting:
Ambulatory anticoagulation clinic

Subjective:
JT is an 80-year-old male referred to your anticoagulation clinic for initiation of therapy with enoxaparin and warfarin after his deep vein thrombosis diagnosis today. The patient presents using walker and appears very unsteady with movement.

Past Medical History:
Hypertension
Osteoarthritis
Heart failure (left ventricular ejection fraction 30%)
Hyperlipidemia
Chronic kidney disease
Coronary artery disease, coronary artery bypass graft (CABG) x 3 in 2001

Medications:
Hydrochlorothiazide 25 mg daily
Lisinopril 10 mg daily
Metoprolol XL 100 mg daily
Furosemide 20 mg daily as needed
Aspirin 81 mg daily
Simvastatin 40 mg bedtime
Ibuprofen 600 mg three times daily prn

Allergies:
NKA

Social History:
Married to wife x 60 years. She sets up a medication organizer weekly for the patient and reports that he is adherent to regimen. Non-smoker. Drinks 1 beer nightly and 1 cup of regular coffee each morning.

Family History:
Mother: diabetes and Alzheimer's disease
Brother: Parkinson's disease

Objective:
Weight: 168 pounds
Height: 70 inches
Blood pressure: 125/72 mmHg
AST: 27 IU/L(15–46)
ALT: 48 IU/L (11–66)
Creatinine: 2.2 mg/dL

Assessment:
Deep vein thrombosis requiring anticoagulation with warfarin and enoxaparin complicated by kidney disease, heart failure, and potential falls risk.
Heart failure well-controlled on diuretic, β blocker, and ACE inhibitor. Ibuprofen should not be used in this patient as it is an NSAID.
Hypertension well-controlled. Hydrochlorothiazide not beneficial in patients with creatinine clearance < 30 mL/min.

Plan:
1. Given patient's significantly impaired renal function estimated creatinine clearance 28 mL/min), enoxaparin should be administered at a dose of 1 mg/kg once daily, based on the patient's weight of 76 kilograms (= 80 mg once daily). Assess ability to perform injections or educate caregiver on technique for injections. Assess the risk of falls with questions regarding frequency of falls, daily activities, orthostatic symptoms, etc. Warfarin therapy should be initiated at a dose less than 5 mg daily in this patient given his age, concomitant medications, mobility problems, and heart failure. Recommend warfarin 3 mg daily. Recheck INR in 5–7 days. Patient likely requires more frequent monitoring as he is at high risk for complications for the above reasons.

2. Continue current heart failure therapy. Discontinue ibuprofen and recommend scheduled acetaminophen for osteoarthritis pain.

3. Discontinue hydrochlorothiazide. Recommend home blood pressure monitoring and, if needed, increase lisinopril dose.

Rationale:
1. Enoxaparin dose must be reduced due to diminished kidney function. Warfarin therapy is initiated at lower dose because of age, medications, falls risk, and heart failure. Osteoarthritis can interfere with ability to perform injections. Potential for falls needs special attention, as falls may lead to more severe complications for patients on warfarin.

2. Diuretics, ACE inhibitors, and β blockers are all therapies indicated for heart failure patients and should be used in the geriatric population. Ibuprofen is an NSAID that can exacerbate fluid retention in heart failure, complicate kidney disease, and lead to higher risk of gastrointestinal bleeds in patients taking warfarin.

3. Hydrochlorothiazide provides little blood pressure benefit for patients with creatinine clearance < 30 mL/min. Home blood pressures can be used to assess control off medication. Lisinopril is not at target dose for heart failure and the dose could be increased to benefit both heart failure and hypertension.

Case Summary:
The geriatric patient needs a thorough assessment when anticoagulation therapy is initiated. Elderly patients are typically taking a larger number of medications and have more disease states and social issues that need to be addressed compared with younger patients.

CASE 2: ORTHOSTATIC HYPOTENSION

Setting:
Long-term care setting

Subjective:
LM is an 89-year-old female resident of a long term care facility who has been experiencing multiple falls, some resulting in injuries such as bruising and skin tears. Over the last 6 months, her ambulation status has declined from independent to wheelchair level. She complains of pain in her legs when walking more than short distances across the nursing unit.

Past Medical History:
Hypertension
Alzheimer's disease
Hypothyroidism
Osteoarthritis

Medications:
Amlodipine 10 mg daily
Donepezil 10 mg at bedtime
Levothyroxine 0.88 mg every morning
Celecoxib 200 mg daily
Furosemide 40 mg every morning

Allergies:
NKA

Social History:
Widowed with 2 adult children living in town, retired photographer and owner of an art supply store

Family History:
Unknown

Objective:

Vitals:
Weight: 129 pounds
Height: 64 inches
Blood pressure: supine 177/82 mmHg, standing 105/60mmHg
Heart rate: 78 bpm

Physical Exam:
HEENT: Normocephalic, no evidence of trauma, PERRLA, EOMI. Dry mucous membranes
CV: Regular rate and rhythm
Respiratory: Clear to auscultation bilaterally
Abdomen: Soft, non-tender, no masses or guarding
G/U: Skin intact, assisted with toileting and personal hygiene by staff
Extremities: Bilateral 2+ edema to lower extremities; skin dry, dark bruising and skin tear to right elbow and forearm
Neuro: Alert and oriented to person only. MMSE 18/30, stable over last 12 months

Lab:
TSH 2.45, Free T4 0.98

Serum chemistry: Na 135, K 3.8, Cl 99, CO2 25, Glucose 101, SCr 0.9, BUN 42
CBC: WBC 7.0, RBC 4.5, Hgb 11.9, Hct 34.1, Platelet 255
UA: clear

Pain assessment:

Using the faces pain scale, no pain is occurring at rest. Upon walking LM complains of moderate-severe pain.

Assessment:

Orthostatic hypotension resulting in falls, possibly associated with medications. While each of her medications could relate to falls by some mechanism, the drug of primary concern is furosemide. Medication without clear indication: furosemide. This is being used to treat edema, but the etiology of the edema is not clear, and could be induced or exacerbated by her current drug therapy. Decrease in ambulation status associated with increased pain upon walking and recent falls

Plan:

Recommend discontinuation of amlodipine, Celebrex, and furosemide, and replacement with hydrochlorothiazide 25 mg daily and acetaminophen 500 mg four times daily. Recommend physician evaluation for peripheral vascular disease and intermittent claudication, and to rule out heart failure or other causes of edema. Monitor vitals (including orthostatic hypotension assessments), edema, and pain daily, and follow-up serum chemistry within 30 days.

Rationale:

LM may be experiencing falls due to orthostatic hypotension associated with uncontrolled supine hypertension and an unnecessary loop diuretic. Her sodium and potassium, though in the normal range, are lower than optimal and continued use of a diuretic without potassium supplementation can further exacerbate electrolyte status. Her SCr:BUN ratio and dry mucous membranes suggest she is a little dehydrated. Although she is currently experiencing bilateral edema, she does not have a diagnosis that explains the cause of the edema. She current takes two medications that could be causing, or at least exacerbating, the edema. These are amlodipine and celecoxib and if edema were to improve or resolve upon discontinuation, the furosemide would not be necessary. The amlodipine is not currently controlling her hypertension. Hydrochlorothiazide alone may not either, but is a reasonable initial choice and combination therapy can be considered if necessary. It is difficult to assess the efficacy of celecoxib for osteoarthritis. There is no pain at rest, and she may achieve similar pain control scheduled acetaminophen while avoiding NSAID side effects. The pain upon walking could suggest peripheral vascular disease with intermittent claudication and she should be evaluated for this. Ruling out heart failure as a cause of her edema is important because the choice of drug therapy for PVD depends upon her comorbidities. LM does have other risk factors for dizziness and falls, including dementia, cholinesterase inhibitor use, and a thyroid disorder. However, these conditions have been stable on the current drug therapy, and any considerations for adjustments should be deferred until after the effects of the above changes are observed.

Case Summary:

This case illustrates several examples of drug therapy problems in a frail elderly patient. These include (1) the use of medication to treat a symptoms without investigating the underlying cause, (2) a prescribing cascade where new medications are prescribed to treat side effects of existing medications, (3) failure to assess efficacy of the drug regimen, and (4) a potential unrecognized and untreated medical condition.
Furosemide has been prescribed to treat edema, but it is not clear if the edema was caused by medication side effects, PVD, or heart failure. Failure to assess the root cause has not only resulted in the lack of intervention for a potential underlying problem, but the new medication prescribed to treat the edema is now causing new problems such as orthostatic hypotension and dehydration, and LM continues to experience supine hypertension and pain interfering with ambulation despite amlodipine and celecoxib use. The underlying problem is cardiovascular, but has implications for functional status and quality of life.

Clinical Pearls

- *Elderly patients can have atypical presentations of heart failure with symptoms such as anorexia, confusion, generalized weakness, and fatigue. Echocardiography should be used to identify heart failure and determine left ventricular function to guide therapy.*

- *An auscultatory gap is a common phenomenon among older patients with hypertension. This is a phenomenon of particular importance to the elderly patient. If palpation of the radial pulse is not performed to insure adequate inflation of the cuff in an elderly patient, the re-emergence of Korotkoff sounds at the bottom of the gap can be mistaken as the systolic pressure. This can result in a falsely low reading.*

Chapter Summary

The prevalence and incidence of vascular diseases increases with advancing age, and are highest in the elderly population. Treatment guidelines exist for many cardiovascular diseases, but in many instances specific recommendations for elderly patients are lacking. For some treatments, elderly patients derive greater benefit than younger patients. However, in many cases, elderly patients are more susceptible to the adverse effects associated with drugs used to treat cardiovascular diseases, and close monitoring in this population is particularly warranted.

Self-Assessment Questions

1. How does the presence or absence of hypertension in elderly patients in different subgroups affect their expected survival and how do blood pressure goals differ in the subgroups?

2. What are some potential barriers in diagnosing peripheral arterial disease and the risks associated with not overcoming them?

3. What criteria are used to determine whether an elderly patient with atrial fibrillation should receive warfarin or aspirin for stroke prevention?

4. What are the documented benefits of treating elevated serum LDL cholesterol in elderly patients?

5. What are the risks and benefits of using β blocker, ACE inhibitors, and digoxin in elderly patients with heart failure?

6. How does the risk of stroke change with every decade over age 55?

7. What are some co-morbidities in elderly patients that complicated anticoagulation for venous thromboembolism?

References

1. Freeman R. Neurogenic orthostatic hypotension. *N Engl J Med.* 2008;358:615–624.

2. Gupta V, Lipsitz LA. Orthostatic hypotension in the elderly: diagnosis and management. *Am J Med.* 2007;120:841–847.

3. Harris T, Lipsitz LA, Kleinman JC, et al. Postural change in blood pressure associated with age and systolic blood pressure. The National Health and Nutrition Examination Survey II. *J Gerontol.* 1991;46:M159–M163.

4. Shannon JR, Jordan J, Diedrich A, et al. Sympathetically mediated hypertension in autonomic failure. *Circulation.* 2000;101:2710–2715.

5. Luukinen H, Koski K, Laippala P, et al. Prognosis of diastolic and systolic orthostatic hypotension in older persons. *Arch Intern Med.* 1999;159:273–280.

6. Chobanian AV, Bakris GL, Black HR, et al. Seventh Report of the Joint National Committee on prevention,

detection, evaluation and treatment of high blood pressure. *Hypertension.* 2003;42:1206–1252.

7. Staessen J, Amery A, Fagard R. Isolated systolic hypertension in the elderly. *J Hypertens.* 1990;8:393–405.9

8. Rastas S, Pirttila T, Viramo P et al. Association between blood pressure and survival over 9 years in a general population aged 85 and older. *J Am Geriatr Soc.* 2006;54:912–918.

9. Protogerou AD, Safar ME, Iaria P, et al. Diastolic blood pressure and mortality in the elderly with cardiovascular disease. *Hypertension.* 2007;50:172–180.

10. Freis E. Use and abuse of antihypertensive drugs in the aged. *Bull NY Acad Med.* 1980;56:697–702.

11. Maddens M, Imam K, Ashkar A. Hypertension in the elderly. *Prim Care.* 2005;32:723–753.

12. Prevention of stroke by antihypertensive drug treatment in older persons with isolated systolic hypertension. Final results of the Systolic Hypertension in the Elderly program (SHEP). SHEP Cooperative research group. *JAMA.* 1991;265:3255–3264.

13. Dalhof B, Hansson L, Lindholm LH, et al. Morbidity and mortality in the Swedish trial in old patients with hypertension (STOP–hypertension). *Lancet.* 1991;338:1281–1285.

14. Staessen JA, Fagard R, Thijs L, et al. Randomized double blind comparison of placebo and active treatment for older patients with isolated systolic hypertension. The Systolic Hypertension in Europe (Syst–Eur) trial. *Lancet.* 1997;350:757–764.

15. Medical Research Council working party. MRC trial of treatment of hypertension in older adults; principle results. *BMJ.* 1992;304:405–412.

16. Gueyffier F, Bulpitt C, Boissel J, et al. Antihypertensive drugs in very old people: a subgroup meta–analysis of randomized controlled trials. *Lancet.* 1999;353:793–796.

17. Amery A, Birkenhager W, Brixko R, et al. Efficacy of antihypertensive drug treatment according to age, sex, blood pressure, and previous cardiovascular disease in patients over the age of 60. *Lancet.* 1986;2:589–592.

18. Coope J, Warrender TS. Randomized trial of treatment of hypertension in elderly patients in primary care. *BMJ.* 1986;293:1145–1151.

19. Casigla E. Spolaore P, Mazza A, et al. Effect of two different therapeutic approaches on total and cardiovascular mortality in a cardiovascular study in the elderly. *Jpn Heart J.* 1994;35:589–600.

20. Beckett NS, Peters R, Fletcher AE, et al. Treatment of hypertension in patients 80 years of age or older. *N Engl J Med.* 2008;358:1887–1898.

21. Hämmerlein A, Derendorf H, Lowenthal DT. Pharmacokinetic and pharmacodynamic changes in the elderly. Clinical implications. *Clin Pharmacokinet.* 1998;35:49–64.

22. American Heart Association. Heart disease and stroke statistics: 2009 update. Dallas, Texas. American Heart Association. 2009.

23. Corti MC, Guralnik JM, Salive ME, et al. Clarifying the direct relation between total cholesterol levels and death from coronary heart disease in older persons. *Ann Intern Med.* 1997;126:753–760.

24. Landi F, Russo A, Pahor M, et al. Serum high-density lipoprotein cholesterol levels and mortality in frail, community-living elderly. *Gerontology.* 2008;54:71–78.

25. Prospective Studies Collaboration. Blood cholesterol and vascular mortality by age, sex, and blood pressure: a meta-analysis of individual data from 61 prospective studies with 55,000 vascular deaths. *Lancet.* 2007;370:1829–1839.

26. Expert Panel on Detection, Evaluation, and Treatment of High Blood Cholesterol in Adults. Executive Summary of the third report of the National Cholesterol Education Program (NCEP) Expert Panel on Detection, Evaluation and Treatment of High Blood Cholesterol in Adults (Adult Treatment Panel III). *JAMA.* 2001;285:2486–2497.

27. Smith SC, Allen J, Blair SN, et al. AHA/ACC guidelines for secondary prevention for patients with coronary and other atherosclerotic vascular disease: 2006 update. *Circulation.* 2006;113:2363–2372.

28. Cholesterol Treatment Trialists' (CTT) Collaborators. Efficacy and safety of cholesterol–lowering treatment: prospective meta–analysis of data from 90 056 participants in 14 randomised trials of statins. *Lancet.* 2005;366:1267–1278.

29. Aronow WS, Ahn C, Gutstein H. Incidence of new atherothrombotic brain infarction in older persons with prior myocardial infarction and serum low-density lipoprotein cholesterol >or=125 mg/dl treated with statins versus no lipid-lowering drug. *J Gerontol A Biol Sci Med Sci.* 2002;57:M333–M335.

30. Aronow WS, Ahn C, Gutstein H. Reduction of new coronary events and new atherothrombotic brain infarction in older persons with diabetes mellitus, prior myocardial infarction, and serum low-density lipoprotein cholesterol >/=125 mg/dl treated with statins. *J Gerontol A Biol Sci Med Sci.* 2002;57:M747–M750.

31. Sheperd J, Blauw GJ, Murphy MB, et al. The pravastatin in elderly individuals at risk of vascular disease (PROSPER): a randomized, controlled trial. *Lancet.* 2002;360:1623–1630.

32. Aronow WS. Treatment of high-risk older persons with lipid-lowering drug therapy. *Am J Ther.* 2008;15:102–107.

33. Rosenson RS. Current overview of statin-induced myopathy. *Am J Med.* 2004;116:408–416.

34. Murray CJ, Lopez AD. Mortality by cause for eight regions of the world: Global Burden of Disease Study. *Lancet.* 1997;349:1269–1276.

35. Alexander KP, Newby K, Cannon CP, et al. Acute coronary care in the elderly, part I: non-ST-segment elevation acute coronary syndromes. A scientific statement for healthcare professionals from the American Heart Association Council on Clinical Cardiology; in collaboration with the Society of Geriatric Cardiology. *Circulation.* 2007;115:2549–2569.

36. Granger CB, Goldberg RJ, Dabbous O, et al. Predictors of hospital mortality in the Global Registry of Acute Coronary Events. *Arch Intern Med.* 2003;163:2345–2353.

37. Antman EM, Hand M, Armstrong PW, et al. 2007 focused update of the ACC/AHA 2004 Guidelines for the Management of Patients With ST-Elevation Myocardial Infarction: a report of the American College of Cardiology/American Heart Association Task Force on Practice Guidelines (Writing Group to Review New Evidence and Update the ACC/AHA 2004 Guidelines for the Management of Patients With ST-Elevation Myocardial Infarction). *J Am Col Cardiol.* 2008;51:210–47

38. Anderson JL, Adams CD, Antman EM, et al. ACC/AHA 2007 guidelines for the management of patients with unstable angina/non-ST-elevation myocardial infarction: a report of the American College of Cardiology/American Heart Association Task Force on Practice Guidelines (Writing Committee to Revise the 2002 Guidelines for the Management of Patients With Unstable Angina/Non-ST-Elevation Myocardial Infarction): developed in collaboration with the American College of Emergency Physicians, American College of Physicians, Society for Academic Emergency Medicine, Society for Cardiovascular Angiography and Interventions, and Society of Thoracic Surgeons. *J Am Col Cardiol.* 2007;50:e1–157.

39. Grines CL, Bonow RO, Casey DE Jr., Gardner TJ, Lockhart PB, Moliterno DJ, et al. Prevention of premature discontinuation of dual antiplatelet therapy in patients with coronary artery stents. A Science Advisory from the American Heart Association, American College of Cardiology, Society for Cardiovascular Angiography and Interventions, American College of Surgeons, and American Dental Association, with representation from the American College of Physicians. *Circulation.* 2007;115:813–818.

40. Alexander KP, Newby LK, Armstrong PW, et al. Acute coronary care in the elderly, part II: ST-segment elevation myocardial infarction: A scientific statement for healthcare professionals from the American Heart Association Council on Clinical Cardiology: in collaboration with the Society of Geriatric Cardiology. *Circulation.* 2007;115:2570–2589.

41. Norgren L, Hiatt W, Dormandy M et al. Inter-Society Consensus for the Management of Peripheral Arterial Disease (TASC II). *J Vasc Surg.* 2007;45 (Suppl 8): S5A–S67A.

42. Meijer W, Hoes A, Rutgers D, et al. Peripheral arterial disease in the elderly: The Rotterdam Study. *Arterioscler Thromb Vasc Biol.* 1998;18:185–192.

43. Hirsch A, Hartman L, Town R, et al. National health care costs of peripheral arterial disease in the Medicare Population. *Vasc Med.* 2008;13:209–215.

44. Hirsch A, Haskal Z, Hertzer N, et al. ACC/AHA 2005 Practice Guidelines for the Management of Patients with Peripheral Arterial Disease (Lower Extremity, Renal, Mesenteric and Abdominal Aortic): A Collaborative Report from the American Association for Vascular Surgery/Society for Vascular Surgery, Society for Cardiovascular Angiography and Interventions, Society for Vascular Medicine and Biology, Society of Interventional Radiology, and the ACC/AHA Task Force on Practice Guidelines. *Circulation.* 2006;113:e463–e654.

45. Sobel M, Verhaeghe R. Antithrombotic therapy for peripheral artery occlusive disease: American College of Chest Physicians Evidence-Based Clinical Practice Guideline 8th Edition. *Chest.* 2008;133:815–843.

46. Antithrombotic Trialists Collaboration. Collaborative meta-analysis of randomized trials of antiplatelet therapy for prevention of death, myocardial infarction, and stroke in high risk patients. *BMJ.* 2002;324:71–86

47. CAPRIE Steering Committee. A randomized, blinded, trial of clopidogrel versus aspirin in patients at risk of ischaemic events (CAPRIE). *Lancet.* 1996;348:1329–1339.

48. Leng GC, Fowler B, Ernst E. Exercise for intermittent claudication. Cochrane Database of Systematic Reviews. 2000; Art. No. CD000990.

49. Gardner A, Katzel L, Sorkin J, et al. Exercise rehabilitation improves functional outcomes and peripheral circulation in patients with intermittent claudication: a randomized controlled trial. *J Am Geriatr Soc.* 2001;49:755–762.

50. Robless P, Mikhailidis D, Stansby G. Cilostazol for peripheral arterial disease. Cochrane Database Syst Rev 2008; (1): CD003748.

51. Hiatt W, Money S, Brass E. Long term safety of cilostazol in patient with peripheral artery disease: The CASTLE study (Cilostazol: A Study in Long term effects). *J Vasc Surg.* 2008;47:330–336.

52. Beebe H, Dawson D, Cutler B, et al. A New Pharmacological treatment for intermittent claudication: results of a randomized, multicenter trial. *Arch Intern Med.* 1999;159:2041–2050.

53. Plavix package insert. Bristol Myers Squibb/Sanofi U.S. Rev. 11/97, Rec 2/98.

54. Clinical Pharmacology Online database. Tampa, FL: Gold Standard, Inc.; 2008. Available at: http://www.clinicalpharmacology–ip.com. Updated August 2008.

55. Alexander KP, O'Connor C. The elderly and aging. In: Topol E, ed. *Textbook of Cardiovascular Medicine.* 3rd ed. Philadelphia: Lippincott Williams & Wilkins; 2007:561–586.

56. Kitzman D, Gardin J, Gottdiener J, et al. Importance of heart failure with preserved systolic function in patients ≥65 years of age. *Am J Cardiol.* 2001;87: 413–419.

57. Redfield MM, Rodeheffer RJ, Jacobsen SJ, et al. Plasma natriuretic peptide concentration: impact of age and gender. *J Am Coll Cardiol.* 2002;40:976–982.

58. Maisel AS, Clopton P, Krishnaswamy P, et al. Impact of age, race, and sex on the ability of B-type natriuretic peptide to aid in the emergency diagnosis of heart failure: results from the Breathing Not Properly (BNP) multinational Study. *Am Heart J.* 2004;147:1078–1084.

59. Hunt SA, Abraham WT, Chin MH, et al. 2009 focused update incorporated into ACC/AHA 2005 guide-

lines for diagnosis and management of heart failure in adults: a report of the American College of Cardiology Foundation/American Heart Association Task Force on Practice Guidelines. *J Am Coll Cardiol.* 2009;53:el–90.

60. Adams K, Lindenfeld J, Arnold J, et al. Executive summary: HFSA 2006 comprehensive heart failure practice guideline. *J Cardiac Fail.* 2006;12:10–38.

61. Flather MD, Shibata MC, Coats AJ, et al. Randomized trial to determine the effect of nebivolol on mortality and cardiovascular hospital admission in elderly patients with heart failure (SENIORS). *Eur Heart J.* 2005;26:215–225.

62. Deedwania PK, Gottlieb S, Ghali J, et al. Efficacy. Safety and tolerability of beta adrenergic blockage with metoprolol CR/XL in elderly patients with heart failure. *Eur Heart J.* 2004;25:1300–1309.

63. Krum K, Hill J, Fruhwald F, et al. Tolerability of beta blockers in elderly patients with chronic heart failure: The COLA II study. *Eur J Heart Fail.* 2006;8:302–307.

64. Gambassi G, Lapane KL, Sgadari A, et al. Effects of angiotensin converting enzyme inhibitors and digoxin on health outcomes of very old patients with heart failure. *Arch Intern Med.* 2000;160:53–60.

65. Flather MD, Yusuf S, Keber L, et al. Long term ACE inhibitor therapy in patients with heart failure or left ventricular dysfunction: a systematic overview of data from individual patients. *Lancet.* 2000;355:1575–1581.

66. Rich MW, McSherry F, Williford WO, et al. Effect of age on mortality, hospitalizations and response to digoxin in patients with heart failure: The DIG Study. *J Am Coll Cardiol.* 2001;38:806–813.

67. Rathore SS, Curtis S, Wang Y, et al. Association of serum digoxin concentration and outcomes in patients with heart failure. *JAMA.* 2003;289:871–878.

68. Adams KF, Gheorghiade M, Urtesky B, et al. Clinical benefits of low serum digoxin concentrations in heart failure. *J Am Coll Cardiol.* 2002;39:946–953.

69. Pfisterer M, Buser P, Rickli H, et al. BNP-guided vs. symptom-guided heart failure therapy: the trial of intensified vs. standard medical therapy in elderly patients with congestive heart failure (TIME–CHF) randomized trial. *JAMA.* 2009;301:383–392.

70. Clinical Pharmacology Online database. Tampa, FL: Gold Standard, Inc.; 2008. http://www.clinicalpharmacology-ip.com. Updated August 2008.

71. Chengxuan Q, Winblad B, Marengoni A, et al. Heart failure and risk of dementia and Alzheimer's disease. *Arch Intern Med.* 2006;166:1003–1008.

72. Vogels R, Oostermann J, Harten B, et al. Profile of cognitive impairment in chronic heart failure. *J Am Geriatr Soc.* 2007;55:1764–1770.

73. Vogels R, Scheltens P, Schroder-Tanka J, et al. Cognitive impairment in heart failure: A systematic review of the literature. *Eur J Heart Fail.* 2007;9:440–449.

74. Go AS, Hylek EM, Phillips KA, et al. Prevalence of diagnosed atrial fibrillation in adults: national implications for rhythm management and stroke prevention: the Anticoagulation and Risk Factors in Atrial Fibrilla-tion (ATRIA) study. *JAMA.* 2001;285:2370–2375.

75. Wolf PA, Abbott RD, Kannel WB. Atrial fibrillation as an independent risk factor for stroke: the Framingham study. *Stroke.* 1991;22:983–988.

76. Fuster V, Rydén LE, Cannom DS, et al. ACC/AHA/ESC 2006 guidelines for the management of patients with atrial fibrillation-executive summary: a report of the American College of Cardiology/American Heart Association Task Force on Practice Guidelines and the European Society of Cardiology Committee for Practice Guidelines (Writing Committee to Revise the 2001 Guidelines for the Management of Patients With Atrial Fibrillation). *Circulation.* 2006;114:700–752.

77. Fang MC, Chen J, Rich MW. Atrial fibrillation in the elderly. *Am J Med.* 2007;120:481–487.

78. Lakshminaryan K, Solid CA, Collins AJ, et al. Atrial fibrillation and stroke in the general Medicare population; a 10-year perspective (1992–2002). *Stroke.* 2006;36:1969–1974.

79. Singer DE, Albers GW, Dalen JE, et al. Antithrombotic therapy in atrial fibrillation: American College of Chest Physicians evidence-based practice guidelines (8th ed). *Chest.* 2008;133:546–592

80. Gage BF, Waterman AD, Shannon W, et al. Validation of clinical classification schemes for predicting stroke: results from the National Registry of Atrial Fibrillation. *JAMA.* 2001;285:2864–2870.

81. Fick DM, Cooper JW, Wade WE, et al. Updating the Beers criteria for potentially inappropriate medication use in older adults. Results of a U.S. consensus panel of experts. *Arch Intern Med.* 2003;163:2716–2724.

82. Man-Son-Hing M, Nichol G, Lau A, et al. Choosing antithrombotic therapy for elderly patients with atrial fibrillation who are at risk for falls. *Arch Intern Med.* 1999;159:677–685.

83. Goldstein L, Adams R, Alberts M, et al. American Heart Association/ American Stroke Association Guidelines Primary Prevention of Ischemic Stroke. *Stroke.* 2006;37:1583–1633.

84. Adams R, Albers G, Alberts M, et al. Update to the AHA/ASA Recommendations for the prevention of stroke in patients with stroke and transient ischemic attack. *Stroke.* 2008;39:1647–1652.

85. Sacco R, Diener H, Yusuf S, et al. Aspirin and extended release dipyridamole versus clopidogrel for recurrent stroke. *New Engl J Med.* 2008;359:1238–1251.

86. Diener H, Bogousslavsky J, Brass L, et al. Aspirin and clopidogrel compared with clopidogrel alone after recent ischaemic stroke or transient ischaemic attack in high risk patients (MATCH): randomized, double-blind, placebo-controlled trial. *Lancet.* 2004;364:331–337.

87. National Institute of Neurological Disorders and Stroke rt–PA Stroke Study Group. Tissue plasminogen activator for acute ischemic stroke. *N Engl J Med.* 1995;333:1581–1587.

88. Sylaja P, Cote R, Buchan A, et al. Thrombolysis in patients older than 80 years with acute ischemic stroke:

Canadian Alteplase for Stroke Effectiveness Study. *J Neurol Neurosurg Psychiatr.* 2006;77:826–829.

89. Berrouschot J, Rother J, Glahn J, et al. Outcome and severe hemorrhagic complications of intravenous thrombolysis with tissue plasminogen activator in very old (≥80 years) stroke patients. *Stroke.* 2005;36:2421–2425.

90. Tanne D, Gorman M, Bates V, et al. Intravenous tissue plasminogen activator for acute ischemic stroke in patients aged 80 years and older. *Stroke.* 2000;31:370–375.

91. Engelter S, Bonati L, Lyrer P. Intravenous thrombolysis in stroke patients of ≥80 versus <80 years of age: a systematic review across cohort studies. *Age Ageing.* 2006;35:572–580.

92. Chinese Acute Stroke Trial Collaborative Group. CAST: randomized placebo controlled trial of early aspirin use in 20,000 patients with acute ischemic stroke. *Lancet.* 1997;349:1641–1649.

93. International Stroke Trial Collaborative Group. IST: a randomized trial of aspirin, subcutaneous heparin, both, or neither among 19,435 patient with ischemic stroke. *Lancet.* 1997;349:1569–1581.

94. Albers G, Amarenco P, Easton D, et al. Antithrombotic and thrombolytic therapy for ischemic stroke. *Chest.* 2008;133:630–669.

95. Oger. E. Incidence of venous thromboembolism: A community based study in western France. *Thromb Haemost.* 2000;83:657–660.

96. Geerts W, Bergquist D, Pineo G, et al. Prevention of venous thromboembolism: American College of Chest Physicians Evidence-Based Clinical Practice Guideline (8th edition). *Chest.* 2008;133:381S–453S.

97. Kearon C, Kahn S, Agnelli G, et al. Antithrombotic therapy for venous thromboembolic disease: American College of Chest Physicians evidence-based clinical practice guideline (8th edition). *Chest.* 2008;133:454S–545S.

98. Jacobs. L. The use of oral anticoagulants (warfarin) in older people. *J Am Geriatr Soc.* 2002;50:1439–1445.

99. Activase package insert. Genentech. U.S. Rev. 5/02, Rec 12/05.

100. Ansell J, Hirsh J, Hylek E, et al. Pharmacology and management of vitamin K antagonists: American College of Chest Physicians evidence based clinical practice guidelines (8th edition). *Chest.* 2008;133:160S–198S.

101. Garcia D, Regan S, Crowther M, et al. Warfarin maintenance dosing patterns in clinical practice: implications for safer anticoagulation in the elderly population. *Chest.* 2005;127:2049–2056.

102. Kearon C, Ginsberg JS, Kovacs MJ, et al. Comparison of low-intensity warfarin therapy with conventional-intensity warfarin therapy for long-term prevention of recurrent venous thromboembolism. *N Engl J Med.* 2003;349:631–639.

103. Clinical Pharmacology Online database. Tampa, FL: Gold Standard, Inc.; 2008. Available at: http://www.clinicalpharmacology-ip.com. Updated August 2008.

104. CMS. Decision memo for prothrombin time (INR) monitor for home anticoagulation management (CAG-00087R). March 19, 2008.

105. Shepherd A, Hewick D, Moreland T, et al. Age as a determinant of sensitivity to warfarin. *Br J Clin Pharmacol.* 1977;4:315–320.

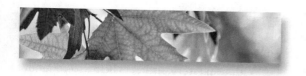

8

Respiratory Issues of Aging

MICHAEL R. BRODEUR AND SEAN M. MIRK

Learning Objectives

1. Assess the applicability of general adult treatment guidelines for COPD, asthma, pneumonia, influenza, and tuberculosis to all older adults.

2. Recommend appropriate drug therapy and treatment goals for various respiratory disorders in older adults.

3. Critically review the medical literature representing treatment of COPD, asthma, pneumonia, influenza, and tuberculosis in older adults.

4. Describe common problems encountered by older adults associated with therapies for respiratory disorders and recommend solutions to these problems.

Key Terms

DRUG-RESISTANT STREPTOCOCCUS PNEUMONIAE (DRSP): Although usually sensitive to penicillin, S. pneumonia resistance to beta lactam, macrolide, fluoroquinolone and tetracycline antibiotics is becoming more widespread. Acquisition of antibiotic resistant pneumococcal strains is associated with previous antibiotic use, time spent in institutional settings (nursing homes or hospitals) and recent respiratory infections.

HERD IMMUNITY: Resistance to spread of an infection in a community based upon a high proportion of individual members having resistance to the infection.

IMMUNOSENESCENCE: The waning of the immune system that occurs with age.

REACTIVATION: TB reactivation occurs from a previously dormant focus seeded at the time of primary infection. Symptoms of cough, weight loss and fatigue develop insidiously over weeks to months before diagnosis.

TRIVALENT INACTIVATED INFLUENZA VACCINE: Inactivated preparations of subvirion influenza virus components are prepared for intramuscular administration. Three viral types are identified each year for inclusion in the product.

Introduction

A host of age-related changes occur in the respiratory system. While some of these changes are normal in aging, most are secondary to environmental effects or from complications due to specific disease states. When pulmonary insults occur in the elderly patient, such as chronic obstructive pulmonary disease (COPD), asthma, and infection, the loss of reserve capacity in the lung prevents adequate response to the stressors imposed. Pulmonary decompensation can be rapid and difficult to reverse. This is readily apparent in the frailest of patients.

This chapter covers respiratory-related illnesses common in the older population. COPD and asthma are reviewed first as many drug therapies for these disease states are problematic in the elderly patient. This is followed by infectious respiratory illnesses including influenza, community- and hospital-acquired pneumonias and tuberculosis. Institutionalized patients have important differences from patients in the community. However, in any setting, adequate use of preventive measures and rapid response when exacerbations occur can reduce the morbidity and mortality associated with these illnesses. Pharmacists must take a leading role in assuring patients, caregivers and other health care professionals are educated to recognize and implement optimal pharmacotherapy to prevent and/or treat respiratory illnesses in the older patient.

COPD/Asthma

Etiology, Epidemiology and Clinical Presentation Specific to Geriatrics

Respiratory diseases are common disorders in older adults and account for significant morbidity and mortality. Chronic obstructive pulmonary disease (COPD) is the fourth leading cause of death in the United States and affects 20% of adults.[1,2] The prevalence of asthma in older adults is difficult to assess due to underdiagnosis, misdiagnosis and undertreatment; however, most studies indicate a prevalence of approximately 7%. Differentiating the two conditions can be prob-

lematic for the experienced clinician, especially because asthma and COPD may co-exist in the same patient.

With respiratory disorders being so common, special attention should focus on the issues that are unique in the elderly: potential for medication adverse effects especially in those patients with multiple medical comorbidities; drug interactions in patients receiving polypharmacy, particularly medications that may worsen asthma and COPD; and issues of effective medication delivery, specifically with reference to inhaled medications. In addition there are many age-related changes that occur within the respiratory system which can affect the course of both asthma and COPD.

Age-related changes affecting the respiratory system include:

- Loss of height secondary to osteoporosis leading to a decrease in lung volume

- Neurologic conditions may affect the swallowing mechanism, leading to aspiration

- Non-asthmatic older patients have less perception of bronchoconstriction despite similar levels of decreases in forced expiratory volume over 1 second (FEV 1) after a methacholine challenge test.

- Bronchodilator response to inhaled beta agonists declines with age. No data to support any age-related difference in response to inhaled anticholinergic medications[3]

The misconception that asthma is a childhood disease leads to symptoms being overlooked by both patients and physicians. Patients are fearful of having a chronic illness with the associated burdens and the potential of dying. A majority of elderly patients who develop asthma after the age of 65 have their first asthmatic symptoms proceeded immediately or concomitantly with an upper respiratory tract infection. This may delay the diagnosis of asthma because patients attribute their respiratory symptoms to lingering effects from the upper respiratory tract infection. Other conditions and diseases may present with respiratory symptoms such as heart failure and gastroesophageal reflux in which cough is a common complaint. Treatment of asthma is more complicated in older patients compared to younger patients. While younger patients may be managed with medications as needed, older patients most often require continuous therapy complicated by frequent dosing with multiple medications.

Summary of Standard Treatment in General Adult Population

The management of COPD has been summarized in national and international guidelines that stress similar treatment modalities. The Global Initiative for Chronic Obstructive Lung Disease was designed to increase awareness of COPD and improve prevention and management with the ultimate goal of reducing disease-related morbidity and mortality. The goals of treatment for COPD are to improve the quality of life, exercise tolerance, sleep quality, and survival; and to reduce dyspnea, nocturnal symptoms, exacerbations, use of rescue medications, and hospitalizations. The diagnosis of COPD should be considered in any patient who has dyspnea, chronic cough or sputum production, and/or a history of exposure to risk factors for the disease. The diagnosis should be confirmed by spirometry.[2] A post-bronchodilator FEV1/forced vital capacity (FVC) ratio < 0.70 confirms the presence of airflow limitation that is not fully reversible. The FEV1/FVC ratio is used to stratify the severity of disease and guide management. (Figure 8-1) Treatment regimens include medications with different mechanisms of actions (Table 8-1). However, only smoking cessation and supplemental oxygen therapy have been proven to improve the course of COPD. Smoking cessation is most effective in early disease, but all patients who smoke should be encouraged to quit.

Similar to COPD, a stepwise approach to the treatment of asthma is recommended. Step 1 utilizes short acting beta agonists on an as needed basis; steps 2 to 6 emphasize inhaled corticosteroids (ICS) as the preferred regimen with the daily dose of ICS increasing as the steps progress. Alternative treatment options include leukotriene receptor modifiers, cromolyn, and theophylline. Omalizumab should be considered in patients who have allergies although there is limited data

in its efficacy in older adults. These treatment steps have been designed for the general adult population and maybe applied to older adults with some modifications.

For both COPD and asthma, proper inhaler technique is critical to successful therapy. The following strategies should be employed when counseling patients using inhalers:

- Be familiar with various inhaler devices and how to use them. Placebo devices are a valuable training aid
- Demonstrate the technique to the patient
- Encourage patients to demonstrate the use of their inhaler
- Re-check inhaler technique at each visit until the patient has mastered the technique. Consider re-checking this every 2 to 3 months thereafter
- Spacer devices are an essential tool
- Minimize the number and types of inhaler devices

Review of Evidence Base Supporting Treatment Recommendations for Elderly Patients

A systematic search of the medical literature evaluated the inclusion of older adults in clinical trials in COPD.[4] After reviewing two decades worth of information, the authors concluded that while older adults were not specifically excluded from the trials, they are underrepresented. The average age of the subjects recruited was 58–69 years and very few subjects over the age of 80 years participated in the trials. In addition subjects with comorbidities such as asthma, other respiratory disorders and cardiovascular diseases were excluded from these trials. Approximately 40% of clinical trials excluded subjects with ECG abnormalities and cardiovascular disease such as recent myocardial infarction, unstable angina, arrhythmias and heart failure. This is concerning given the potential for cardiovascular side effects associated with therapy for COPD which include QT interval prolongation, tachycardia and other arrhythmias, worsening of myocardial ischemia and congestive heart failure, and electrolyte disturbances.

Another systematic search of the medical lit-

Table 8-1. Commonly Used Drugs in the Management of COPD and Asthma

Class: Medication Examples	Indications for Use	General Adult Treatment Principles	Geriatric Considerations
Short-Acting β 2 Agonists (SABA) Inhaled and oral bronchodilators Albuterol Pirbuterol Terbutaline sulfate (oral tablets only). Levalbuterol hydrochloride Levalbuterol tartrate	Asthma: Treatment of choice for relief of acute symptoms and prevention of exercise-induced bronchospasm; generally used as needed. COPD: For relief of acute symptoms.	Asthma: Use of SABA > 2 days a week for symptom relief (not prevention of EIB) generally indicates inadequate asthma control and the need for initiating or intensifying anti-inflammatory therapy. Chronic use of SABA not recommended. COPD: Improves breathlessness but not other patient-oriented outcomes. In stable COPD, there is an associated improvement in FEV1.	Combinations of bronchodilators improve efficacy and reduce risk of AEs versus increasing the dose of a single agent. This sound strategy supports combination therapy using ipratropium and albuterol, for example, rather than quadrupling the dose of either one of those agents alone. Possible SE: tachycardia, palpitations, tremor, feeling nervous, insomnia, HA, N/V. Geriatric pts may be more susceptible to these effects.
Anticholinergics, Inhaled bronchodilator Ipratropium bromide Tiotropium	Asthma: Ipratropium may be used as an alternative bronchodilator for patients intolerant of SABA COPD: May be more effective than long-acting β 2 agonist in relieving the symptoms of COPD.	Asthma: Effective as bronchodilator but not as potent as β 2 agonists. Ipratropium provides additive benefit to SABA in moderate or severe exacerbations not responding to β 2 agonists alone. COPD: Improves symptoms and quality of life and decreases exacerbations, hospitalizations, and deaths; improves sleep. Decreases rescue inhaler use and office visits.	Inhaled ipratropium has an excellent safety profile in the elderly, and it should be considered for use when additional bronchodilator therapy is necessary. Ipratropium has a slow onset of action; it requires 30–60 min for maximal effect. Possible SE: dry mouth, abnormal taste in mouth, bitter, nasal congestion, dry nasal mucosa, tachycardia. Tiotropium: Ensure that the patient has the dexterity to be able to place the capsule in the HandiHaler, do not swallow the capsule; for inhalation use only.

(continued)

Table 8-1. Commonly Used Drugs in the Management of COPD and Asthma (cont'd)

Class: Medication Examples	Indications for Use	General Adult Treatment Principles	Geriatric Considerations
Inhaled Corticosteroids: Inhaled anti-inflammatory Beclomethasone dipropionate Budesonide Flunisolide Fluticasone propionate Mometasone furoate Triamcinolone	Asthma: The most effective long-term control therapy for persistent asthma regardless of severity.	Pt should be started on higher and more frequent doses and then tapered down once control has been achieved. Response is delayed with symptom improvement occurring within the first 1–2 wk in most pts and full therapeutic benefits in 4–8 wk Risk of systemic toxicity minimal with low to moderate doses and increases with high doses (greater than 1000 mcg/day). Local AEs (e.g., oropharyngeal candidiasis, hoarseness, cough and dysphonia) can be reduced by use of a spacer device and rinsing mouth after use Use the lowest dose that maintains the asthma control. Assess pt's inhaler technique, adherence & environmental measures before increasing dose. Adding a LABA to a low or medium dose of inhaled corticosteroids may be more effective than doubling the dose of steroids to maintain asthma control. COPD: Decreases exacerbations in patients with moderate to severe disease. No effect on mortality.	Long-term use of inhaled corticosteroids at recommended doses has been associated with a good safety profile. Adverse effects are dose related. Local effects of the mouth and pharynx include candidiasis and dysphonia. Systemic absorption of inhaled corticosteroids has been associated with skin bruising, cataracts, and reduced bone mineral density. An increase risk of pneumonia has been associated with high doses (1000 mcg/day) of fluticasone.

(continued)

Table 8-1. **Commonly Used Drugs in the Management of COPD and Asthma (cont'd)**

Class: Medication Examples	Indications for Use	General Adult Treatment Principles	Geriatric Considerations
Long-Acting β 2 Agonists (LABA) Inhaled bronchodilator Formoterol Salmeterol	Asthma: Used as adjunctive long-term therapy with inhaled corticosteroids, which is more effective than increasing the dose of corticosteroids alone. Can be used for nocturnal asthma.	NOT used as monotherapy due to absence of anti-inflammatory properties. NOT effective for acute severe asthma due to slow onset (20–30 min). Formoterol has faster onset than salmeterol Need to continue short acting β agonist for acute exacerbations while on long-acting β 2 agonists.	Use in the elderly should be closely monitored. Geriatric pts may be more susceptible to SEs of beta agonists e.g., tachycardia, palpitations and tremor. This risk is higher in pts with pre-existing coronary artery disease. Other SEs also include nervousness, insomnia, HA, N/V. May cause dose-dependent drop in serum potassium and QT interval prolongation; use cautiously in pts with arrhythmia and pre-existing coronary artery disease. Although not clearly established, airway responsiveness to β-agonist medications may also decrease with age.
Methylxanthine: Oral bronchodilators Theophylline	Asthma: sustained-release theophylline may be used as alternative, not preferred, therapy for step 2 (mild persistent asthma). It may be also used as an adjunctive with inhaled corticosteroids	Rarely used in practice. Monitoring of theophylline concentration is essential. Severe cardiac arrhythmia, seizures and death can occur at serum concentration only twofold greater than optimal therapeutic concentration.	Use not recommended due to safety concern. Patients over age 75 have a 16-fold greater risk of life-threatening events or death than pt under age 25 at comparable serum theophylline level. Dose should be reduced. Elderly patients should be started with a 25% reduction of the adult dose.
Combined Medication: Inhaled bronchodilator and steroid Budesonide and formoterol Fluticasone and salmeterol	Asthma: Use is recommended for step 3 moderate persistent asthma.	The combination gives the advantage of providing bronchodilation while reducing airway inflammation. LABA also allows reduction in corticosteroid dosage (by 50%). Onset is rapid (within 1 wk). Compliance can be also improved with the combination.	Refer to each component.

(continued)

Table 8-1. Commonly Used Drugs in the Management of COPD and Asthma (cont'd)

Class: Medication Examples	Indications for Use	General Adult Treatment Principles	Geriatric Considerations
Corticosteroids: Oral anti-inflammatory Methylprednisolone Prednisone Dexamethasone	Asthma: Indicated in patients with acute severe asthma not responding completely to aggressive inhaled β 2 agonists. Also used long term to treat pts with severe persistent asthma. COPD: Long-term treatment with oral corticosteroids is not recommended in COPD. Can be used for short periods for management of COPD exacerbations.	May take 6–8 hours for pulmonary function improvement. Most patients achieve 70% predicted FEV1 within 48 hours and 80% by day 6. Full dose should be continued until patient's peak flow reaches 80% of predicted normal or personal best. Tapering the steroid dosage after short course is unnecessary. Following attempts should be made 1) optimize therapy with inhaled corticosteroids, 2) keep oral steroids to the minimum dose possible, 3) use relatively short acting agents e.g., prednisone and methylprednisolone, 4) attempt to control symptoms with alternate-day dosing.	Long-term use of corticosteroids may lead to or exacerbate osteoarthritis, diabetes, hypertension, cataracts and (rarely) depression of the immune system and susceptibility to infections. This can be troublesome in the elderly because many of these complications occur in the elderly even without steroid use. Myopathy, increased skin fragility, loss of attention span and memory, and mood swings may also occur in geriatric patients with long term steroid use. Monitor closely with long-term steroid use.
Leukotriene Modifiers: Oral anti-inflammatory Montelukast Zafirlukast Zileuton	Asthma: Effective in prevention of allergen-induced asthma, exercise induced asthma and aspirin-induced asthma.	Can be also used as adjunctive therapy with inhaled corticosteroids. Can be used as daily medication for mild persistent asthma, but is less preferred than low-dose inhaled corticosteroids. Liver function monitoring is essential. Possible adverse effects: headache, nausea, diarrhea, infection.	Geriatric patients may be more susceptible to some of the adverse effects, e.g. headache and mild infection. Females >65 years of age appear to be at an increased risk for ALT elevations. QT interval prolongation is possible with Zileuton. Montelukast appears to be the safest one among the three.
Mast Cell Stabilizers: Inhaled anti-inflammatory Cromolyn sodium Nedocromil sodium	Asthma: Indicated for prophylaxis of mild persistent asthma (step 2).	May be particularly effective for allergic asthmatics on a seasonal basis. May also be used as preventive therapy before exercise or unavoidable exposure to known allergens. Coughing and wheezing are possible after inhalation of each agent; bad taste and headache are possible after nedocromil use.	Well tolerated.

(continued)

Table 8-1. Commonly Used Drugs in the Management of COPD and Asthma (cont'd)

Class: Medication Examples	Indications for Use	General Adult Treatment Principles	Geriatric Considerations
Monoclonal Antibody: Anti-allergen Omalizumab	Asthma: Indicated for treatment of moderate to severe persistent allergic asthma not well controlled by high doses of inhaled corticosteroids.	Dose is based on IgE serum levels prior to treatment and body weight. Dosing adjustment during treatment should be based on significant changes in body wt, NOT IgE levels during or <1 year following discontinuation of therapy. Possible SE: Injection site reactions, anaphylaxis, viral infection, upper respiratory tract infection, sinusitis, headache, sore throat.	Specific geriatric considerations have not been established. Elderly patients might be more susceptible to adverse effects.

erature evaluated the inclusion of older adults in clinical trials in asthma.[5] The average age of the subjects in these clinical trials ranged from 25 to 49 years with some trials excluding older adults. Of the articles reviewed, approximately 17% had no specific exclusions or contained information on exclusions. Existing clinical trials need to be interpreted with caution because exclusion of patients of advanced age and multiple medical comorbidities was common. The asthma treatment algorithms emphasize long-term pharmacologic treatment with careful attention placed on self-management.

Inhaled beta agonists can cause both pulmonary and extrapulmonary adverse effects. In a meta-analysis of randomized placebo-controlled trials of beta agonists in 6,623 patients (mean age 52.2 years) with obstructive airway disease cardiac adverse events were classified as mild such as minor changes in heart rate and clinically unimportant changes in the level of serum potassium. There was an increase in the risk for adverse cardiovascular events (relative risk [RR], 2.5), largely caused by an increase in the risk of sinus tachycardia. The likelihood of major cardiovascular events did not reach statistical significance.[6] In absolute terms, approximately one additional event occurred in the beta-agonist group for every 200 patients treated over a 6-month period.[7] The Salmeterol and fluticasone propionate and survival in chronic obstructive pulmonary disease trial, commonly referred to as the TORCH trial (n = 6184, 1542 patients in the salmeterol arm, mean age 65 years), found cardiovascular causes contributed to mortality in 3% of patients, with no significant difference between the salmeterol and placebo groups.[8] The Salmeterol Multi-Center Research Trial (SMART), designed to test the safety of salmeterol, had about 26,000 participants, was stopped early because of safety concerns. As a result of the study, the Food and Drug Administration (FDA) issued a public health advisory for long-acting beta-2 agonists (LABA) in 2005. It warned that these medications can cause a "small but significant risk in asthma-related deaths." The FDA also required the addition of "black box" safety labels to LABAs. There has been considerable debate over the use of beta

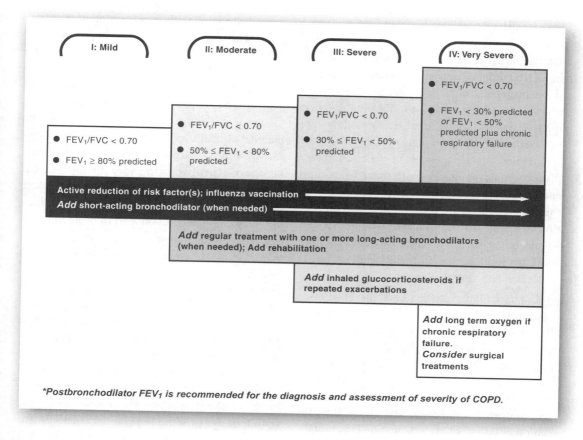

Figure 8-1. Therapy at each state of COPD. *Source:* Reprinted with permission from reference 2.

agonists in the management of moderate and severe COPD. Supporters of beta-agonists believe that clinical trials clearly show short- and LABAs improve dyspnea, quality of life and reduce respiratory exacerbations in patients with COPD.[9] While proponents argue that anticholinergics have equal or superior efficacy to beta-agonists in improving lung function parameters without creating tolerance over time as seen with regular use of beta-agonists.[9] In elderly asthmatic patients, LABA should be used only in combination with ICS due to these safety concerns and the potential for cardiac comorbidities. It would be prudent to carefully assess the cardiac risk factors before instituting a LABA in a patient with COPD.

In patients with moderate to severe COPD, ICS should be used to reduce exacerbations. A meta-analysis of 12 randomized controlled trials assessing ICS demonstrated one fewer exacer-bation for every 12 patients with moderate-to-severe disease who were treated for 18 months.[10] ICS are associated with a variety of adverse effects; the most common are the local effects in the upper airways such as thrush and dysphonia. These complications can be minimized through the use of spacers and rinsing the mouth after inhalation of the drug. Due to the increase risk of osteoporosis and osteopenia in older adults, treatment with ICS has been evaluated to examine if these agents pose any increased risk of reduced bone mineral density. In the TORCH trial patients treated with fluticasone alone or in combination with salmeterol reported a non-significant increase in the incidence of fractures compared with placebo (5.4%, 6.3% and 5.1% respectively).[8] In a subset of TORCH participants were (n = 658) specifically assessed for changes in bone mineral density, the prevalence of osteoporosis was significant. Specifically, about 70% of all patients had osteopenia or osteoporosis indicating that abnormal bone health is a common problem in COPD. Higher doses of ICS like that used in the management of asthma have been associated with increased bone turnover, but data on bone mineral density and fracture at these doses are not available.[11] Those patients requiring oral corticosteroids for management of their respiratory disease should be on adequate doses of calcium and vitamin D at minimum. Bisphosphonates are the drugs of choice for the treatment and prevention of glucocorticoid induced osteoporosis and should be considered if the patient will require continuous glucocorticoid therapy unless there is a documented contraindication.

Cataracts and glaucoma have also been associated with ICS. The TORCH study performed slit lamp examinations in a safety subset of 658 subjects using high-dose ICS (fluticasone, 500 mcg, twice daily). Only 29% of patients did not have cataracts at baseline examination. There were no differences in the development of new cataracts compared with the placebo group. Thus, the relation of ICS to cataract formation is not totally clear.[12] In a systematic review of the literature an expert panel found grade C evidence that ICS are associated with cataracts in young asthma patients, however the risk may be elevated in older patients.[13] This same expert panel found that the risk of glaucoma with ICS use to be small, probably dose dependent and found insufficient evidence to conclude if any specific ICS formulation had an increased risk.[13]

Common Problems Encountered When Treating Elderly Patients with COPD

Elderly patients may be more vulnerable to problems using inhaler devices properly due to poor eyesight, poor hand strength, arthritis, and coordination difficulties. Older adults are underrepresented in studies evaluating different inhaler types and results are often extrapolated from younger adults predominately with asthma and not COPD. However, most patients regardless of their age, should be able to acquire and maintain adequate technique when given appropriate instruction with the exception of those patients with significant cognitive impairment.[14,15] Spacer devices may be used with metered dose inhalers (MDIs) when patients have difficulty with hand-breath coordination. Spacers improve drug delivery and reduce systemic absorption. Common problems encountered by older adults include difficulty connecting the MDI to the spacer, difficulty activating the device, and unnecessary repetitive firing into the spacer. Up to 85% of patients who were prescribed spacer devices did not use them.[16,17] Dry powder inhalers (DPI) have been developed to overcome difficulties encountered with MDIs and have been viewed as more "patient friendly" by patients and health care providers. However, in general, DPIs require a higher peak inspiratory flow (PIF) than MDIs for effective drug delivery since a minimum inspiratory flow is required to disaggregate and disperse the drug powder in the inhaled airstream.[18] In a study specifically designed to assess the use of DPIs in elderly patients with mild and moderate COPD, a large percentage of participants were unable to generate adequate PIFs for optimum use of some popular DPI devices. An analysis showed that both age and COPD disease severity were independent variables influencing PIF.[19]

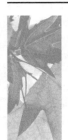

KEY POINT: DPIs require a higher PIF than MDIs for effective drug delivery. Many elderly patients with mild and moderate COPD are unable to generate adequate PIFs for optimum use of some popular DPI devices.

Another common issue encountered in the elderly is cognitive impairment and the ability to use inhalers correctly. Not surprisingly elderly people with significant cognitive impairment were unable to learn to use a standard MDI. Patients with mild-to-moderate dementia may be able to use either an inhaler with a spacer device or an inspiration-triggered inhaler. However, only those patients that had no cognitive impairment were able to demonstrate perfect inhaler technique.[15] Subsequent studies have shown that patients with a Mini-Mental State Examination (MMSE) test score of less than 23 out of 30 or the inability to copy intersecting pentagons are unlikely to master MDI technique. Executive domains are important determinants of an adequate inhaler self-administration technique with or without overt cognitive impairment on the MMSE.[19,20] A majority of this research has been conducted in a frail elderly population during hospitalizations for rehabilitation and additional research has been called for in a community-based sample. In addition to cognitive impairment, patients having difficulties with exhalation, hand-breath coordination and breath-holding are likely to have difficulty with any inhaler, therefore, frailty may be a central issue.[21] It would be appropriate to assess a patient's cognitive function prior to initiating therapy with an inhaler to establish a baseline and aide in the selection of an inhaler device. It is not known whether patients with mild-to-moderate dementia can retain inhaler skills as their cognitive function declines. Therefore, planned regular review of technique should take place to test competence and changes made to therapy as necessary.[15] Furthermore, supervision of inhaler use is recommended for patients with cognitive impairment.

It is a myth that nebulizers are more effective than correctly administered inhalers. An evidence based review of effectiveness reported that nebulizers, DPIs, and MDIs have comparable effectiveness when used properly.[22] The appropriate use of nebulizers does contain some complexities such as the need to disassemble, wash, dry, and reassemble the nebulizer between treatments. Nebulizer compressors require periodic maintenance, such as filter replacement.[23] Subjectively, older adults often seem to prefer nebulizers; perhaps this is due to the sensation that is given by the taste and sight of the mist, however no objective evidence has been published to support this notion and patient compliance with home nebulizer therapy in COPD patients was on average 57% in one study.[24] Appropriate candidates for nebulizer therapy are those patients with very poor hand-breath coordination such as those with Parkinson's disease or severe osteoarthritis of the hands.

Older adults are more likely to develop complications while receiving asthma therapy which manifest as adverse reactions to pharmacotherapy (Table 8-1), therefore, it is prudent to provide more intense monitoring.[25] Most elderly patients will require continuous treatment programs to control their disease. In part, this may be because bronchodilator response to inhaled beta agonists declines with age.[26] Even in mild disease older adults should receive regular preventive treatment with ICS, given the poor perception of bronchoconstriction by older asthmatic patients.[27] If symptoms persist despite ICS, the addition of a LABA should be considered. Due to concerns about the safety of beta-2 agonists in older adults, LABA should be only used concomitantly with ICS and these patients should have regular cardiac assessments including periodic electrolyte monitoring to rule out hypokalemia.

A critical component of self-management is the provision of a written asthma plan that instructs patients on how to deal with changes in asthma symptoms. In a study that investigated the risk factors associated with hospitalization for asthma, 40% of elderly people with asthma reported that they did not know everything they needed to know to manage flare-ups, adjust their medications or avoid asthma triggers.[5] Most did not have a peak flow meter, and of those who did, 29% did not know what to do in case of an abnormal reading. It is imperative that written asthma plans and adequate peak flow counseling are provided to older adults with asthma. If cognitive impairment is present, caregivers should be educated on the steps needed to adjust therapy and when to seek help.

Adverse effects from beta agonists may occur more frequently in elderly patients, especially in those with pre-existing cardiac disease. Levalbuterol, the R-isomer of albuterol, has been touted as producing fewer adverse effects and superior bronchodilation when compared to albuterol. Studies in asthma and COPD have shown mixed results. If an elderly patient has minimal response to albuterol or significant adverse effects, levalbuterol may be considered as an alternative. However, current evidence does not support routine use of levalbuterol as the beta agonist of choice in the elderly.

Inhaled anticholinergic medications may increase intraocular pressure and have other ocular adverse effects. This is important in the elderly population because of the high prevalence of glaucoma, macular degeneration, and other ophthalmologic problems. Several case reports have correlated the use of a loose-fitting mask while administering ipratropium bromide to anisocoria due to unilateral mydriasis.[28] Prolonged pupillary dilation can occur if the drug is sprayed directly into the eye and this is especially concerning regarding tiotropium, because of the prolonged duration of action of the agent. Avoiding contact with the eyes seems to be the best management strategy; studies of ipratropium given at four times the recommended dose in patients with normal angle glaucoma had no effect on intraocular pressure, pupil dilation, and accommodation.[29]

Inhaled anticholinergic medication is poorly absorbed making systemic side effects unlikely. The most common adverse effect with inhaled anticholinergic medications is dry mouth but this rarely leads to discontinuation. Inhaled anticholinergic agents have a relatively low incidence of cardiovascular or respiratory adverse effects although supraventricular tachycardias, increased cardiovascular risk, and paradoxical bronchoconstriction have been reported.[6] This notion was challenged recently in a systematic review and meta-analysis of patients using ipratropium or tiotropium which showed an increased risk for cardiovascular events.[30] The analysis included 17 trials that lasted from 6 weeks to 5 years with nearly 15,000 patients. Patients treated with inhaled anticholinergics were more likely to reach the primary endpoint of cardiovascular death, myocardial infarction, and stroke (1.8% vs 1.2%). When the studies were analyzed based on length, the risk remained elevated in the long-term studies and short-term studies did not reach statistical significance. These findings remind the clinician to carefully monitor COPD patient receiving long-term inhaled anticholinergic therapy.

Theophylline is generally avoided in the elderly due to its narrow therapeutic index and potential to cause major systemic side effects and drug interactions (see Table 8-1). If theophylline must be used, serum concentrations should be monitored and a lower therapeutic range of 8–12 mg/L be targeted in elderly patients.[31]

Pneumonia
Etiology, Epidemiology, and Clinical Presentation Specific to Geriatrics

Pneumonia, in combination with influenza, is the sixth leading cause of death from all causes and the number one cause of death from infection in the elderly population in the United States.[32] The cost of care to treat pneumonia is more in the elderly compared to a younger population, in part due to a greater percentage of elderly patients requiring hospitalization, which is often due to a higher prevalence of comorbid conditions.[33] Along with an increase in hospitalization rates for pneumonia, the elderly also require longer lengths of stay compared to younger patients. These factors translate into greater cost, with nearly half of the dollars spent on pneumonia used to treat elderly patients.[33]

The predisposition to pneumonia in the elderly population remains unclear. Higher rates of comorbid conditions amongst the elderly, rather than aging itself, may be responsible for a higher incidence of pneumonia. Risk factors that may contribute to a higher incidence of pneumonia in the elderly are listed in Table 8-2.[33,34]

Listed in Table 8-3 are common causes of pneumonia in the elderly population. In all care settings the most commonly identifiable agent in elderly patients with pneumonia is *Streptococcus pneumoniae*, however, 50% of all cases are caused by unknown organisms. Good sputum specimens are hard to obtain from elderly patients limiting the ability to identify an infectious agent. **Drug-resistant S. pneumoniae (DRSP)** is on the rise in elderly patients, especially patients with a history of prior antibiotic therapy, alcoholism, immune suppression (including corticosteroid therapy) and multiple comorbidities.[35-7] *Pseudomonas aerugino-*

Table 8-2. Risk Factors for Pneumonia in Elderly Patients

Comorbidities	Chronic obstructive pulmonary disease Diabetes mellitus Heart failure Liver disease Malignancy Neurologic disorders
Age-related changes	Decreased cough reflex Rigid chest wall Decreased FEV1 Poor mucociliary clearance of microorganisms Impairment in immune system[a] Increases in oropharyngeal gram-negative and S. aureus colonization
Oral hygiene	Xerostomia[b] Poor dentition/dental plaque
Functional status	Reduced mobility Incontinence Impairment in daily living activities Reduced quality of life
Risk for aspiration	Stroke Dementia Impaired swallowing
Others	Cigarette smoking Malnutrition Prior antibiotic therapy Use of corticosteroids

[a] May be age-related and/or due to medications that effect the immune function.
[b] May be related to dehydration or medications that effect oral secretions.
Source: Adapted from references 33, 34, and 70.

sa and gram-negative enteric bacilli are uncommon causes of community-acquired pneumonia, however nursing home residents and patients with exposure to the healthcare environment (i.e., hemodialysis clinic, recent hospitalization) have a higher incidence of these pathogens.[37] If *P. aeruginosa* or gram-negative enteric bacilli is the identifiable cause of pneumonia, it may be attributed to the presence of risk factors such as aspiration, prior antibiotic therapy, and pulmonary comorbidities.[36-8] Atypical pathogens have been found to cause a higher frequency of infection in patients age 65–79 than in patients 18–39 years.[34] These pathogens (especially *Chlamydia pneumoniae*) may spread epidemically among nursing home patients.[39] Due to the clinical complexities in elderly patients and frequent transitions of care between hospitals, nursing homes, and the com-munity, a detailed history is needed to determine the most likely causative infectious agent and ensure an appropriate empiric therapy is selected.

Elderly patients may not present with classical symptoms of pneumonia which may lead to a delay in treatment and adverse outcomes. Older patients may present with atypical or nonspecific manifestations such as confusion, weakness, lethargy, failure to thrive, worsening of a chronic illness, change in mental status, episodes of falling and general deterioration.[33,34] Chronic illnesses (i.e., COPD, heart failure, diabetes mellitus) can mask the presence of an infection and the decompensation of these chronic illnesses may be the first sign of pneumonia.[33,34]

Upon examination, fever and chest consolidation may not be present in the elderly. The onset of

Table 8-3. Common Identifiable Etiologic Pathogens for Pneumonia in Elderly Patients[a]

Outpatient/non-ICU treated	ICU treated
Pneumococcus (including DRSP)[b]	Pneumococcus (including DRSP)[b]
H. influenzae, M. catarrhalis[c]	Atypical pathogens: M. pneumoniae, pneumoniae and Legionella spp.[d]
Atypical pathogens: M. pneumoniae, pneumoniae and Legionella spp.[d]	Enteric gram-negative organisms[e]
Enteric gram-negative organisms[e]	H. influenzae, M. catarrhalis
S. aureus (including MRSA)[f]	S. aureus (including MRSA)[f]
Anaerobes[g]	Respiratory viruses[h]

[a] Listed in decreasing order of occurrence
[b] Increased incidence of DRSP in elderly patients with a history of prior antibiotic therapy, alcoholism, immune suppression and multiple comorbidities
[c] Especially in cigarette smokers
[d] Increased incidence in patients with bronchiectasis, COPD with recent antibiotics, and/or on corticosteroid therapy
[e] Including P. aeruginosa
[f] Increased incidence after influenza infection or in patients with diabetes or CKD
[g] Increased incidence in patients with neurological illness or impaired swallowing due to aspiration
[h] Includes: influenza A & B, adenovirus, respiratory syncytial virus and parainfluenza.
Source: Adapted from references 35–37.

fever in response to pneumonia is less frequent in the elderly, in part due to a lower baseline temperature and a blunted thermoregulatory process.[33,34,40] Also, elderly patients may not mount a white blood cell response. The presence of tachypnea, as defined by a respiratory rate of 25–30, in the elderly is an important physical finding, indicating the possibility of a lower respiratory tract infection.[33,34,40] Oxygen saturation less than 90% and an elevated white blood cell count are also supportive findings. These atypical presentations may delay diagnosis and increase the time taken to administer antibiotic therapy. Timely administration of antibiotic therapy is critical in reducing mortality.[40]

A chest radiograph (CXR) is recommended in all patients in whom infection is suspected to define the presence and severity of pneumonia.[35] In the elderly population this approach is important since typical clinical features of pneumonia may be reduced. It is recommended to obtain blood cultures only in severely ill patients with no history of antibiotic use prior to admission. Sputum gram stain and culture (before antibiotic therapy) may also be a reasonable diagnostic test to acquire but only in patients that can produce a quality specimen.

Summary of Standard Treatment in General Adult Population

The Infectious Disease Society of America/ American Thoracic Society (IDSA/ATS) has developed consensus guidelines for the treatment of pneumonia.[35,41] Treatment will vary depending on clinical setting, comorbidities and length and route of therapy. Empiric therapy regimens provide coverage for the overwhelming majority of pneumonia-causing pathogens (see Table 8-4). Utilizing the IDSA/ATS recommendations and taking into account important elements for local resistance patterns to develop guideline-based protocols has been shown to reduce mortality in several studies.[42] Along with implementation of institutional guidelines, administration of antibiotic therapy within 4 to 8 hours of arrival to the hospital for pneumonia has been shown to lower mortality rates in two large retrospective studies.[43,44] Once the diagnosis of pneumonia has been made, timely administration of antibiotic is crucial in decreasing mortality.

A respiratory fluoroquinolone or a macrolide plus a β-lactam antibiotic is recommended as empiric therapy.[35,42] Both cover the majority of expected pathogens (including DRSP). Mono-

Table 8-4. **Commonly Used Antibiotics for the Treatment of Pneumonia in the Elderly**

Class and Medication Examples	Spectrum of Activity	General Adult Treatment Principles	Geriatric Considerations
Macrolide: Azithromycin Clarithromycin	Covers: *S. pneumonia, H. influenza*, atypical pathogens	Used as monotherapy if no recent antibiotic exposure or comorbidities exist.	Monitor for potential drug-drug interaction.
β-lactam: Amoxicillin Cefpodoxime Cefuroxime Cefprozil Ceftriaxone Cefotaxime	Covers: *S. pneumonia, H. influenza* (amoxicillin only if non-ß-lactamase producing), atypical pathogens, gram-negative bacilli	Used in combination with a macrolide.	Dose or frequency may need to be adjusted in patients with renal impairment.
Respiratory Fluoroquinolone: Levofloxacin Moxifloxacin Gemifloxacin	Covers: *S. pneumonia, H. influenza*	Used as monotherapy for outpatient or general ward treatment or in combination in ICU.	Dose adjustment may be required in patients with renal impairment. Monitor for potential drug-drug interaction. Most notable drug interactions include: antacids/calcium products, iron salts and zinc salts (administer 2–4 hours before or after fluoroquinolone); and warfarin. Monitor for QT prolongation. Risk for tendonitis and tendon rupture increase with age > 60 years, concomitant steroid therapy and lung, kidney or heart transplant; therapy should be discontinue with first signs of tendon pain, swelling, or inflammation.
Clindamycin: Clindamycin	Covers: *S. pneumonia*, anaerobic pathogens	Used in combination with fluoroquinolones for aspiration pneumonia	Monitor for *C. difficile* mediated diarrhea
Antipneumococcal, antipseudomonal β-lactam: Piperacillin-tazobactam Cefepime Imipenem Meropenem	Covers: *P. aeruginosa*, gram-negative bacilli	Used in combination when *Pseudomonas* infection is an issue.	Dose adjustment may be required in patients with renal impairment. Imipenem and meropenem may exacerbate seizures, especially in patients with CNS disorders.

(continued)

Table 8-4. Commonly Used Antibiotics for the Treatment of Pneumonia in the Elderly (cont'd)

Class and Medication Examples	Spectrum of Activity	General Adult Treatment Principles	Geriatric Considerations
Aminoglycosides: Gentamicin Tobramycin Amikacin	Covers: *P. aeruginosa*	Used in combination for patients admitted to the ICU for CAP, or for aspiration pneumonia and nosocomial pneumonia.	Dose adjust for renal impairment. Monitor for neurotoxicity, nephrotoxicity and ototoxicity.
Miscellaneous: Vancomycin Linezolid	Covers: DRSP, MRSA	Used for the treatment of MRSA.	Monitor for nephrotoxicity or ototoxicity and dose adjust for renal impairment with vancomycin. Monitor for serotonin syndrome if concomitant use of SSRI or TCA and instruct to avoid high tyramine content with linezolid.

therapy with a macrolide is not recommended for elderly patients with comorbidities (liver or renal disease, heart failure, diabetes, malignancy, asplenia, immunosuppressant condition or on immunosuppressant drugs) or at significant risk for DRSP, especially in areas with known macrolide-resistant *S. pneumoniae*.[35,42] The other common modification to empiric therapy is when *P. aeruginosa*, MRSA or anaerobic aspiration pneumonia is suspected. Risk factors for *P. aeruginosa* include severe COPD, chronic/frequent use of oral corticosteroids, alcoholism and prior antibiotic therapy. If *P. aeruginosa* is suspected, an antipneumococcal, antipseudomonal β-lactam should be considered; for anaerobic aspiration pneumonia clindamycin plus a fluoroquinolone is preferred (alternately, beta-lactam/beta-lactamase).[35,41] Once the causative pathogen is determined, therapy should be tailored.

Appropriate supportive care of severe sepsis and septic shock, respiratory failure and decompensated comorbidities are crucial to improving outcomes.[34,42] Noninvasive ventilation may be appropriate in patients with underlying COPD or who are in respiratory distress. Treatment of severe sepsis and septic shock in elderly patients with pneumonia does not significantly differ from that of other infections. Prophylactic therapy for

deep venous thrombosis should be considered for patients at high-risk for thrombosis.

Finally, all individuals over the age of 50 should be vaccinated yearly for influenza. Elderly patients ≥ 65 years should also have the 23-valent polysaccharide pneumococcal vaccine (PPSV).

 KEY POINT: Administration of the pneumococcal and influenza vaccine in appropriate patients is associated with reduced morbidity and mortality.

Review of Evidence Base Supporting Treatment Recommendations for Elderly Patients

To determine if all-cause mortality, length of hospital stay, and readmission rate were associated with implementation of pneumonia guidelines in elderly patients, a study utilizing data from Medicaid and Medicare for Utah was conducted.[45] Patients ≥ 66 years old with a diagnosis of pneumonia were enrolled in the study. The mean age of the 17,728 patients analyzed was 72 years (SD ± 12 years). An increase in guideline compliance was associated with a significant decrease in

30-day readmission rate (OR 0.86) and mortality (OR 0.92).[45]

The efficacy of the PPSV has been established in the elderly population in several large studies.[46-49] These studies have not shown PPSV to significantly decrease the risk of pneumonia. However, adults immunized with PPSV were less likely to die if admitted to the hospital for pneumonia and had decreased occurrences of complications like bacteremia and meningitis secondary to *S. pneumoniae*. Of particular interest is a prospective study conducted in Swedish patients ≥ 65 years old.[49] The study aimed to determine the effectiveness of PPSV and influenza vaccine at reducing hospital needed treatment and death caused by influenza, pneumonia and invasive pneumococcal disease.[49] Of the 258,754 patients enrolled in the study 48% were vaccinated (72,107 had both vaccines; 29,346 only influenza; and 23,249 only PPSV). The PPSV and influenza vaccine together produced an additive effect at decreasing hospitalization (OR 0.63) and length of hospital treatment for influenza and pneumonia significantly (5.2 versus 7.5 days; 9.9 versus 11.3 days, respectively).[49] Also, the two vaccines demonstrated an additive effect at reducing mortality due to pneumonia (OR 0.65).[49]

Common Problems Encountered When Treating Elderly Patients with Pneumonia

Although the need to perform severity assessment is considered critical in stratifying therapy and achieving desirable outcomes, tools such as the Pneumonia Severity Index (PSI) and the British Thoracic Society (CURB-65) lack validation in the elderly population.[34,42] Therefore, caution is warranted when these tools are used to determine hospital admission in the elderly patient with pneumonia. The PSI may oversimplify the decision to admit an elderly patient by relying heavily on age and comorbidities. Most elderly patients with fever would reach class III with the PSI, regardless of function status.[42] In contrast, CURB-65 lacks direct assessment of comorbidities. The IDSA/ATS recommends that subjective factors that are not detected in clinical decision support tools be taken into account when determining site-of-care in the elderly.[44] Such subjective factors include:

- Ability to reliably take oral medications
- Outpatient resources (i.e., caregivers for dependent patients)
- Decompensation of comorbidities (i.e., COPD, heart failure, diabetes mellitus, or renal insufficiency)
- Psychosocial needs or other medical conditions requiring hospitalization (e.g., psychiatric illness, homelessness, poor functional status, or vomiting)
- Treatment failure or lack of response to previous empiric therapy
- Access to IV therapy

 KEY POINT: Appropriate risk stratification and timely administration of antibiotics is important in reducing mortality due to pneumonia.

In general, elderly patients may not improve as quickly as younger patients due in large part to an altered immune system. It is common for elderly patients that have severe illness, bacteremia, alcoholism, COPD and multiple comorbidities to have a delay in resolution.[34,42] The duration of hospitalization, drug therapy and intravenous to oral switch (IV to PO switch) depends on clinical response of the patient. Patients with improvement in cough, sputum production, dyspnea, fever (afebrile on two separate occasions 8 hours apart), white blood cell count, and who are able to tolerate oral medications may be considered clinically stable.[34,42] IV to PO switch of antibiotic therapy is possible once a patient becomes clinically stable; due to excellent bioavailability and board spectrum bactericidal activity of the fluoroquinolones in patients without gastrointestinal issues. Guidelines recommend a minimum of 5 days of therapy and patients should be afebrile for at least 48 to 72 hours before stopping therapy.[35]

Smoking cessation, improvement of malnutrition and attention to aspiration risk should be addressed in elderly patients. Vaccinating the appropriate patients with both the PPSV and influenza vaccine is also recommended.[35,41] The influenza vaccine and influenza treatment are discussed more fully in the next section All patients 65 and older should receive the PPSV. If a patient younger than 65 receives the vaccine, they should be re-vaccinated at age 65. Re-vaccination should also occur if elderly patients have an anatomic or functional asplenia or have an immunocompromising condition; an additional dose should be given at least 5 years after the previous dose.

Influenza

Etiology, Epidemiology, and Clinical Presentation Specific to Geriatrics

Influenza season in the United States typically occurs between late fall and early spring. Each year nearly 226,000 hospitalizations and 36,000 deaths occur in patients 50 and older.[50-2] About 90% of all deaths contributed to influenza occur in individuals ≥ 65 years.[50-2] Furthermore, individuals with underlying medical conditions, such as cardiopulmonary diseases, are at the greatest risk for serious complications and death.[50,51]

Clinical manifestation of influenza include abrupt onset of fever, headache, chills, nonproductive cough, myalgias, malaise, sore throat, rhinitis and conjunctive inflammation.[50] It is difficult to distinguish symptoms of influenza from symptoms of the common cold or other viral respiratory infections. Typically acute symptoms of uncomplicated influenza last for 3–7 days. However, it is common for patients to have a nonproductive cough, respiratory compromise and severe malaise for much longer periods of time (10–21 days).[50]

In the elderly, secondary bacterial infection of the lower respiratory tract are common. Symptoms may progress with severe respiratory compromise or the patient may experience a delayed worsening of symptoms.[50,53] Agents involved in bacterial superinfections include *Hemophillus influenzae*, *Staphylococcus aureus*, and *S. pneumoniae*.[53] Older patients with comorbidities such as heart failure and COPD are at high risk for complications due to secondary bacterial pneumonia.[53]

Summary of Standard Treatment in General Adult Population

Updated recommendations by the CDC's Advisory Committee on Immunization Practices occur annually. The recommendations include the use of influenzae vaccine and antiviral agents against influenza A and B. All patients ≥ 50 years old should receive the **trivalent inactivated influenza vaccine** (TIV) annually; at this time the safety and effectiveness of the live attenuated influenza vaccine has not been established in the elderly.[50] In times of vaccine shortage, the age cut-off is raised to ≥ 65 years old. In addition, those at high risk for complications (i.e., with chronic pulmonary disorders, chronic cardiovascular disorders or immunocompromised) and individuals that can transmit influenza to patients at high risk (i.e., healthcare workers, LTCF and home care employees, family members) should also be immunized. Avoidance and good hygiene are also vital in preventing the spread of influenza. Antiviral therapy with neuraminidase inhibitors should not serve as an alternative to vaccination for the prevention of influenza but may be used during periods of widespread influenza outbreaks in individuals who have not received the influenza vaccine.

Review of Evidence Base Supporting Treatment Recommendations for Elderly Patients

Studies have attempted to characterize the rate of effectiveness of the influenza vaccine across age groups and those with impaired immunological status. In elderly populations, effectiveness may be decreased due to **immunosenescence** or increased due to **herd immunity** to various strains of influenza that different generations were exposed to in previous decades. Furthermore, the main outcomes measured in studies influence the rate of effectiveness that is reported. As noted above, only the TIV vaccine is recommended for use in the elderly, and studies of safety and effectiveness described below are limited to this product.

The effectiveness of influenza vaccine was evaluated in a large, placebo-controlled, randomized trial in community-dwelling individuals in the Netherlands. Without regard to age, the effectiveness of the influenza vaccine at reducing influenza respiratory illnesses (IRI) was 50%.[54] After stratification for age, the vaccine effectiveness dropped significantly in individuals ≥ 70 years (23% compared to 57% in individuals ≥ 60 years).[54]

The effectiveness of influenza vaccine at reducing IRI has also been studied in nursing homes. In a retrospective analysis IRI rate was significantly lower in vaccinated nursing home residents compared to unvaccinated residents (OR = 0.58, imputed vaccine effectiveness estimate of 42%).[55] Like the Netherlands study, when effectiveness was stratified for age, the vaccine was more effective in younger residents (65–84 years) than older residents (≥ 85 years). Overall, it is estimated that the effectiveness of influenza vaccination in the elderly ranges from 30% to 40%.

Although the influenza vaccine may not be as effective against IRI in the elderly population, vaccination against influenza may help prevent serious complications. A systematic review published in 2005 reviewed the effectiveness (reduction in symptomatic cases) of influenza vaccination in individuals ≥ 65 years. In all, 64 studies were reviewed (5 randomized, 49 cohort, and 10 case-control). The analysis of the studies demonstrated that the vaccines effectiveness against IRI was 23% for residents living in nursing homes (or equivalent setting) but was not significantly effective against IRI in community-dwelling individuals.[56] Vaccination of nursing home and community-dwelling individuals showed effectiveness at preventing hospital admission for influenza and pneumonia (45% and 26%, respectively) and all-cause mortality (60% and 42%, respectively).[56] Also, individuals in nursing homes that were vaccinated were significantly less likely to have pneumonia or die from influenza or pneumonia.[56]

Adequate data supporting clinical effectiveness for the treatment and prevention of influenza using neuraminidase inhibitors in older patients is lacking. A meta-analysis published in 2003 found the reduction in median time to alleviation of symptoms, for zanamivir and oseltamivir compared to placebo, in the intent-to-treat population for high risk individuals (≥ 65 years or chronic medical conditions) was not statistically different from controls.[57] Furthermore, the use

of oseltamivir versus placebo showed no difference in preventing influenza. No trials on zanamivir given to high risk patients, as defined by this study, were included.[57] The lack of significant difference in the treatment and prevention of influenza in high risk patients may be due to a lack of power to detect a difference.

Common Problems Encountered with Influenza in Elderly Patients

Despite clear benefits of preventing complications with vaccination against influenza, the estimated coverage in the United States is low. For the 2005–2006 and 2006–2007 seasons, the National Health Interview Survey estimated national influenza vaccine coverage for individuals ≥ 65 years was 65% and 66%, respectively.[50] This rate of coverage is low compared to the goal of 90% coverage for individuals ≥ 65 years set by the Healthy People 2010 objectives.[58]

 KEY POINT: Improving influenza vaccine coverage amongst the elderly population will greatly diminish adverse outcomes related to influenza.

Neuraminidase inhibitors may be used for the treatment of severe or complicated influenza. These agents have been shown to decrease the severity and duration of illness in the general population. Although evidence is less convincing in elderly people oseltamivir and zanamivir can be used for prophylaxis against influenza during an outbreak. Renal dose adjustment is required for oseltamivir if creatinine clearance is less than 30 mL/min. Zanamivir is an inhaled agent and may cause severe bronchospasms. This agent should be avoided in patients with pulmonary disorders or acute airway reactivity to influenza. Furthermore, elderly patients with arthritis, poor dexterity, vision problems, weakness and impaired cognition, may have difficulty with the inhaler device.

It is not recommended to use amantadine or rimantadine for the treatment or prevention of influenza in the United States due to their CNS side effects such as confusion, anxiety and seizures. Both require dose adjustment in the geriatric population.[50]

Tuberculosis

Etiology, Epidemiology, and Clinical Presentation Specific to Geriatrics

Tuberculosis (TB), caused by *Mycobacterium tuberculosis*, has been declining in recent years in the United States due to increased awareness and selective prevention therapy including treatment of latent infection. The elderly have the highest case reports among all age groups.[59] Disease in the elderly mostly occurs in community-dwelling individuals; however, patients that reside in nursing homes and long-term care facilities (LTCF) are at a 2–3 times higher risk for TB disease.[60,61] Furthermore, the rate of tuberculin reactivity is associated with the length of stay in a nursing home and in nursing homes with known recent infectious cases.[60,61]

Elderly patients are at higher risk for TB infection due to higher rates of exposure and infection that occurred early in the twentieth century. The increasing likelihood of latent infection combined with immunosenescence increases the likelihood of **reactivation**. Reactivation of a primary infection in the elderly accounts for 90% of TB disease.[60,61] Despite improvements, prevention and control of TB in the elderly population remains a challenge.

The tuberculin skin test (TST) is used to diagnose *M. tuberculosis* infection. It contains a 5-tuberculin unit dose of purified protein derivatives (PPD) injected intradermally to form a wheal. Interpretation of TST results 48–72 hours after administration should be stratified occurring to risk groups. Patients that do not have signs or symptoms of TB disease, but have a positive TST may have latent TB infection (LTBI). Elderly patients may not be able to mount an immune response to provide a positive result to the TST. Therefore, a two-step TST is recommended. If the patient's first TST is negative, a second TST should be given 1–3 weeks later. A positive TST regardless if it was the first or two step TST warrants a chest radiograph and further investigation to determine treatment modality.

Although relatively uncommon, a false-positive TST can occur, especially in patients that have recently received the bacilli Calmette-Guérin (BCG) vaccine or those infected with atypical mycobacteria. BCG is not used in the United States. However, foreign-born individuals may have received the BCG vaccine. Cell-mediated immunity to PPD declines over time in individuals who have received the BCG vaccine.[60,61] Older patients with a positive TST result should be treated for LTBI or *M. tuberculosis* infection, regardless if a history of BCG vaccine is noted in the patient's chart, especially in individuals that came from endemic areas of TB or have been exposed to TB.[60,61]

LTBI may not be detected in the elderly population because of an inability to mount an immune response to the PPD. A false-negative TST occurs in patients with febrile illness, HIV and other viral disease and in patients taking corticosteroids or other immunosuppressive drugs.[60,61] The rate of false-negative in the elderly is more common than in the general population.[59] In the elderly, lack of a reaction to TST cannot conclusively rule out TB disease or infection.

Summary of Standard Treatment in General Adult Population

The American Thoracic Society, CDC, and Infectious Disease Society of America have developed treatment recommendations for TB.[62] Control of TB is focused on breaking the chain of transmission. This can be achieved in the United States by: (1) rapid detection of TB (2) screening high-risk groups, (3) effective treatment of LTBI and active TB and (4) preventing TB transmission into the community.[62] The preferred treatment for LTBI is isoniazid (INH) with daily rifampin as an alternative. For the treatment of active TB, all appropriate specimens should be obtained before empiric therapy is started. Direct observational therapy and therapy that covers multidrug resistant TB based on local resistance patterns is recommended.[62] Baseline and monthly monitoring of liver function tests (LFT) are recommended for individuals with HIV and chronic liver disease.

Review of Evidence Base Supporting Treatment Recommendations for Elderly Patients

Recommendations for tuberculosis treatment do not differ between adults and the elderly population according to guidelines. Studies have not focused upon the elderly specifically; however, co-morbidities and social issues may require adjustments to be made in standard treatment plans. The majority of TB cases in elderly patients in Western societies are probably treatment-sensitive; most infections in the elderly are due to reactivation of disease that was acquired prior to availability of antituberculous therapy early in the 20th century.[60,61] The most challenging component in treating elderly patients is selecting the highest effective treatment regimen while diminishing the probability of major adverse reactions. Table 8-5 reviews the common agents used in TB.

Common Problems Encountered When Treating Elderly Patients with This Condition

Despite elderly individuals having the highest rate of infection, some view TB as a problem of younger individuals. This, in part, is due to the emergence and focus on HIV-associated TB that predominately occurs in younger individuals.[63] Also, healthcare professionals may not always identify a possible TB infection since symptoms may be less pronounced, non-specific or confused with other pulmonary, heart or malignant disease; radiological findings may be "atypical"; and the frequency of false-negative TST occurs more frequent in the elderly population. These factors contribute to a possible delay in diagnosis which can result in a higher rate of mortality and spread of TB.[63]

Anti-tumor necrosis factor (TNF)-α treatment was recently identified as a risk factor for

Table 8-5. First-line Agents Used for the Treatment of LTBI or Active TB

Class: Medication Examples	General Adult Treatment Principles	Geriatric Considerations
Isonicotinic acids: Isoniazid	First-line treatment as monotherapy for LTBI or in combination for active TB	Monitor liver function and counsel patient on alcohol consumption. Supplement with pyridoxine 25 to 50 mg/day to prevent peripheral neuropathy. Monitor for drug interactions. May increase concentration of phenytoin, carbamazepine, warfarin, diazepam; corticosteroids may decrease levels of INH.[a]
Rifamycins: Rifampin Rifabutin Rifapentine	First-line treatment as monotherapy for LTBI or in combination for active TB.	May turn urine reddish/orange. Monitor liver function and counsel patient on alcohol consumption. Monitor for drug interactions. Rifampin may decrease concentrations of methadone, digitalis glycosides, cyclosporine, warfarin, oral hypoglycemic drugs, corticosteroids, theophylline, phenytoin, ketoconazole, protease inhibitors, non-nucleoside reverse transcriptase inhibitors.
Miscellaneous: Pyrazinamide Ethambutol	Used in combination for active TB.	Monitor liver function and counsel patient on alcohol consumption. Monitor uric acid levels. Counsel patient to report any visual disturbances if taking ethambutol. Adjust dose for renal impairment.

[a]Not a complete list of drug interactions; it is important to screen all medications for drug interactions carefully.

reactivation of TB in older adults. Studies have been published using an active-surveillance database and the FDA's Adverse Event Reporting System which indicate that treatment with infliximab or etanercept is associated with a five-fold overall increased risk of TB.[64-68] Based on these findings it is recommended to screen all patients for LTBI or active disease before starting anti-TNF-α treatment.

Some LTCF are reluctant to admit residents with a diagnosis of TB due to the difficulty in treating elderly patients successfully and for fear of increasing the risk of transmission to others currently in the facility. For elderly patients newly admitted to a LTCF or nursing home, screening with two-step TST and treatment for LTBI per established guidelines is recommended.[60,61]

Hepatic toxicity with INH has a higher incidence in individuals over 35 years of age, and this was a main reason for restricting treatment for LTBI in the elderly.[69] Intolerance to INH has been documented in older individuals and the risk for INH-hepatitis is the highest in individuals ≥ 50 years (2.3% risk). In patients at high risk for hepatotoxicity, those with HIV and chronic liver disease, it is recommended to perform baseline and monthly LFT. Symptomatic monitoring of INH-induced hepatitis may not be optimal in elderly individuals with impaired communication or cognition skills or chronic comorbidities.[60,61] Therefore, it may be appropriate to also monitor LFT in these individuals.

All agents used in treatment of TB have significant toxicities and drug interactions of importance in older adults. Elderly patients, in particular those with diabetes, uremia, malnutrition or history of alcohol abuse are at higher risk for peripheral neuropathy from INH. To prevent peripheral neuropathy, pyridoxine 25 to 50 mg/day may be given. INH has also been shown to increase serum concentrations of some benzodiazepines and anticonvulsants. See Table 8-5.

Use of rifampin with pyrazinamide for the treatment of LTBI is strongly discouraged due to the potential for severe hepatotoxicity.[62] See Table 8-5. A complete medication review for potential drug interactions should be completed prior to initiating therapy and concomitant use of known hepatotoxic agents should be avoided.

CASE 1: ASTHMA

Setting:
Skilled nursing facility

Subjective:
MD is an 82-year-old woman who has been a long time resident of the skilled nursing facility. Recently the nursing staff has noted that she is having increasing shortness of breath and nighttime awakenings, which they attribute to a worsening of her asthma.

Past Medical History:
Late onset asthma, osteoarthritis, hypertension, recently diagnosed with glaucoma, and depression.

Medications:
Fluticasone 250 mcg/salmeterol 50 mcg inhaler 1 inhalation BID, albuterol 0.083% solution 3 mL via nebulizer four times a day PRN, acetaminophen 500 mg four times a day, furosemide 20 mg daily, metoprolol 50 mg BID, and sertraline 50 mg daily and sertraline 50 mg daily. There is an order for timolol 0.5% ophthalmic solution 1 gtt BID initiated 2 weeks ago.

Allergies:

No known drug allergies

Social History:

Negative for tobacco and alcohol use

Family History:

Mother died of old age, father died of a MI at age 81

Objective:

Height 5'2", Weight 101 pounds, blood pressure: 130/82, heart rate 62 BPM, respiratory rate: 20 breaths/minute

Physical Examination:

Bilateral wheezing, use of accessory muscles on inhalation, remainder of examination is within normal limits

Assessment:

MD is experiencing shortness of breath that is caused by bronchoconstriction induced by ophthalmic and systemic beta blockade.

Plan:

1. Recommend the discontinuation of the timolol ophthalmic solution and substitution of latano-prost eye drops.

2. Recommend the discontinuation of metoprolol and substitution of amlodipine 5mg daily.

3. Re-enforce proper inhaler technique with the patient and nursing staff.

Rationale:

1. The use of ophthalmic beta blockers has been shown to exacerbate reactive airway disease due to systemic absorption. Patients already taking systemic beta blockers are at an increased risk for bronchoconstriction and addition of the topical agent is likely tipping the patient into bronchoconstriction. The use of ophthalmic beta blockers should be avoided in patients with a history of asthma. If they must be used, nasolacrimal pressure should be applied for 1 minute after the instillation of the drops to minimize systemic absorption.

2. This patient has no compelling indications for the use of a beta blocker (e.g., post myocardial infarction) and has a relative contraindication (i.e., asthma). Amlodipine will not cause broncho-constriction. The dose should be titrated to achieve blood pressure goal.

3. Proper inhaler technique is difficult to achieve for many elderly patients, and periodic assessment of a patient's technique is useful to assure optimal medication management. Because nursing staff are involved in drug administration in long-term care facilities, they are helpful in evaluating and re-enforcing proper technique on a day-to-day basis.

Case Summary:

Older adults are at increased risk for adverse drug reactions and drug-induced disease. A careful assessment should be conducted before prescribing any new medications to ensure that the proposed therapy will not exacerbate other chronic conditions. It is imperative that clinicians consider any symptom in an elderly patient a medication adverse event until proven otherwise. Using this mindset the clinician will not overlook the possibility that the patient maybe suffering from a medication adverse event as oppose to worsening of the underlying asthma. Patient education is critical for effective management of asthma and other respiratory disorders. Experts have stated that management of respiratory disorders is 10% medication and 90% education. Patients need to be assessed for their abilities to comprehended self management plans and the complexities of using inhaler devices.

CASE 2: PNEUMONIA

Setting:
Emergency room

Subjective:
SM is a 65-year-old male with generalized weakness, fatigue and confusion for 7 days. He also has a productive cough and wheezing. Upon presentation to the clinic, he is afebrile and appears short of breath.

Past Medical History:
Diabetes × 5 years; HTN × 10 years

Medications:
Metformin 1000 mg BID; lisinopril/HCTZ 20/25 mg daily; ASA 81 mg daily
Allergies: NKDA

Social History:
Denies use of tobacco or illicit drug use; drinks alcohol on special occasions

Family History:
Lives at home alone, no children, and is retired.

Vitals:
BP 128/78, P 127, RR 31, T 37.7 °C, ht 70 in, wt 93 kg

Physical Exam:
Well-nourished male in moderate respiratory distress. Patient is tachypneic with labored breathing and has decreased breath sounds with rhonchi in right lung field.

Laboratory:
Chest x-ray is indicative of right middle and lower lobe disease, possible pneumonia. CBC shows WBC 14,000; Hgb 11.4 mg%; and platelets 160,000. Serum creatinine is 1.1 mg/dL.

Assessment:
SM is experiencing multilobar community-acquired pneumonia. The emergency room physician determines disease severity and admits the patient to the general ward of the hospital and initiates the community-acquired antibiotic protocol according to pharmacist recommendations.

Plan:
1. Initiation of levofloxacin 500 mg intravenously daily for 7 days. First dose to be given as quickly as possible.
2. Provide oxygen and albuterol nebulizer as needed for supportive therapy.
3. Monitor physical examination including cough, sputum production, vital signs, and mental status. Monitor white blood count and pulse oximetry. Convert to oral levofloxacin after 48 hours if patient is stable.
4. Administration of pneumococcal and influenza vaccines.

Rationale:
1. Based on SM's disease severity and clinical judgment he should be admitted to the general ward of the hospital. A respiratory fluoroquinolone is appropriate empiric therapy for elderly

patients being treated outpatient or admitted to a general ward. If renal function is diminished, appropriate dose adjustment is required. It is critical to have antibiotics administered within 4–8 hours of presentation to the hospital, especially in this patient who has likely been infected for a week. Intravenous administration is appropriate for patients who present in a confused state, but once a patient has responded to treatment with stabilization of monitoring parameters, switching to oral treatment is more cost-effective.

2. The influenza vaccine should be given yearly to all patients ≥ 50 years of age. Also, the pneumococcal vaccine should be given at least once to all patients ≥ 65 years of age.

Case Summary:

Elderly individuals with comorbid conditions have a high incidence of pneumonia. Atypical symptoms or nonspecific manifestations can mask the presence of an infection. A chest x-ray is a defined way to detect the presence and severity of pneumonia. Severity assessment (PSI or CURB-65) along with clinical judgment should be used to stratify site-of-care and determine empiric therapy. Rapid administration of appropriate empiric antibiotic therapy is an important quality indicator. The influenza and pneumococcal vaccine should be administered to appropriate individuals.

Clinical Pearls

- *Chest radiographs are recommended to confirm a diagnosis of pneumonia if at all possible, however, the patient's venue of care or advanced directives may preclude transfer to a hospital or access to this test. Due to the necessity of initiating antibiotics as quickly as possible, diagnosis may have to be based on clinical presentation, simple laboratory tests, and pulse oximetry. Scoring tools that evaluate factors such as presence of fever, elevated white cell count, respiratory rate, or cognitive status can increase the likelihood of accurately identifying pneumonia.*

- *Atypical disease presentation can make it difficult for the clinician to differentiate signs of respiratory conditions such as COPD from other conditions, such as heart failure. Older patients may be vulnerable to receiving medications directed at symptoms without a clear diagnosis of the underlying cause. When a drug regimen review reveals the use of breathing treatments such as albuterol or ipratropium nebulizers for shortness of breath in combination with medications such as furosemide for edema, a diagnostic evaluation to confirm the root cause and initiate the appropriate evidence-based therapy is necessary.*

Chapter Summary

Respiratory disorders have a significant impact on the quality of life of older adults. Whether it is a chronic condition such as asthma or COPD or an episode of pneumonia, influenza, or tuberculosis, the central issues remain common: accurate diagnosis, appropriate therapy, and adequate monitoring. The diagnosis of respiratory disorders in older adults is sometimes challenging due to differences in disease presentation such as the presentation of pneumonia and tuberculosis. Under diagnosis is also common in asthma. Regardless of the condition there is a paucity of data evaluating the treatment options for respiratory disorders in older adults particularly the frail elderly. In a majority of the cases the application and adaptation of standard adult treatment will be appropriate. However, the clinician needs to anticipate the various problems that may occur in older adults including the potential for medication adverse effects especially in those patients with multiple medical comorbidities; drug interactions in patients receiving polypharmacy, and issues of effective medication delivery, especially with reference to inhaled medications. With appropriate assessment, monitoring, and follow-up respiratory disorders can be effectively managed in older adults.

Self-Assessment Questions

1. How well are older adults with asthma and COPD represented in the medical literature? What age groups are represented? What medical comorbidities do they have?

2. How can mental status influence the use of inhaled medications?

3. What are the common risk factors that contribute to a higher incidence of pneumonia in the elderly population?

4. What are the benefits of vaccinating against pneumonia and influenza in the elderly population?

5. What is the role of antiviral therapy in the prevention and treatment of influenza in elderly patients?

6. What is the two step tuberculin skin test and why is it useful in older adults?

7. What are potential medication-related problems anticipated with the use of antituberculous drugs?

References

1. Mannino DM, Homa DM, Akinbami LJ, et al. Chronic obstructive pulmonary disease surveillance-United States, 1971–2000. *MMWR Surveill Summ.* 2002;51:1–16.

2. Global Initiative for Chronic Obstructive Lung Disease. Global Strategy for the Diagnosis, Management and Prevention of Chronic Obstructive Pulmonary Disease. NHLBI/WHO workshop report. Bethesda, MD: National Heart Lung and Blood Institute, April 2001; Updated 2008. Available at: http://www.gold-copd.com/.

3. Zeleznik J. Normative aging and the respiratory system. *Clin Geriatr Med.* 2003;19:1–18.

4. Gupta P, O'Mahony MS. Potential adverse effects of bronchodilators in the treatment of airways obstruction in older people recommendations for prescribing. *Drugs Aging.* 2008;25:415–433.

5. Diette G, Krishnan J, Dominici F, et al. Asthma in older patients; factors associated with hospitalization. *Arch Intern Med.* 2002;162:1123–1132.

6. Salpeter SR, Ormiston TM, Salpeter EE. Cardiovascular effects of beta-agonist in patients with asthma and COPD: a meta-analysis. *Chest.* 2004;125:2309–2321.

7. Ebell M. Beta agonists may slightly increase risk of adverse cardiac events. Available at http://www.aafp.org/afp/20041015/tips/1.html. Accessed September 3, 2008.

8. Calverley PMA, Anderson JA, Celli B, et al. The TORCH investigators: salmeterol and fluticasone propionate and survival in chronic obstructive pulmonary disease. *N Eng J Med.* 2007;356:775–789.

9. Salpeter SR, Aaron SD. Should we avoid beta-agonists for moderate and sever chronic obstructive pulmonary disease? *Canadian Family Physician.* 2007;53:1290–1293.

10. Gartlehner G, Hansen RA, Carson SS et al. Efficacy and safety of inhaled corticosteroids in patients with COPD; a systematic review and meta-analysis of health outcomes. *Ann Fam Med.* 2006;4:253–262.

11. Jones A, Fay JK, Burr M, et al. Inhaled corticosteroid effects on bone metabolism in asthma and mild chronic obstructive pulmonary disease. Cochrane Database of Systematic Reviews 2002.

12. Suissa S, McGhan R, Niewoehner D, et al. Inhaled corticosteroids in chronic obstructive pulmonary disease. *Proc Am Thorac Sco.* 2007;4:535–542.

13. Leone FT, Fish JE, Szefer SJ, et al. Systematic review of the evidence regarding the potential complications of inhaled corticosteroid use in asthma. *Chest.* 2003;124:2329–2340.

14. National Institute for Clinical Excellence (NICE). National Clinical Guidelines for management of Chronic Obstructive Airway Disease in primary and secondary care. Managing stable COPD. *Thorax.* 2004;59(S1):39–130.

15. Allen SC. Competence thresholds for use of inhalers in people with dementia. *Age Aging.* 1997;26:83–86.

16. Connolly M. Inhaler technique of elderly patients: Comparison of metered dose inhalers and large volume spacers. *Age Aging.* 1995;24(3);190–192.

17. Jarvis S, Ind PW, Shiner RJ. Inhaled therapy in elderly COPD patients; time for re-evaluation? *Age Aging.* 2007;36:213–218.

18. Pederson S, Steffense G. Fenoterol powder inhalation technique in children; influence of inspiratory flow rate and breath holding. *Eur Respir J.* 1986;68:207–211.

19. Allen SC, Ragab S. Ability to learn inhaler technique in relation to cognitive scores and tests of praxis in old age. *Postgrad Med J.* 2002;78:37–29.

20. Allen SC, Jain M , Regab S, et al. Acquisition and short-term retention of inhaler techniques require intact executive function in elderly subjects. *Age Aging.* 2003;32:299–302.

21. Jones V, Fernandez C, Diggory P. A comparison of large volume spacers, breath-activated and dry powder inhalers in older people. *Age Aging.* 1999;28:418–484.

22. Dolovich M, Aherns RC, Hess DR, et al . Device selection and outcomes with aerosol therapy: evidence-based guidelines. *Chest.* 2005;127:335–371.

23. Fink JB, Rubin BK. Problems with inhaler use; a call for improved clinician and patient education. *Resp Care.* 2005;50:1360–1374.

24. Corden ZM , Bosley CM, Ress PJ, et al. Home nebulized therapy for patients with COPD: patient compliance with treatment and its relation to quality of life. *Chest.* 1997;112:1278–1282.

25. Braman, SS. Drug treatment of asthma in the elderly. *Drugs.* 1996;51:415–423.

26. Braman SS. Asthma in the elderly. *Clin Geriatr Med.* 2003;19:57–75.

27. Barua P, O'Mahony MS. Overcoming gaps in the management of asthma on older patients-new insights. *Drugs Aging.* 2005;22:1029–1059.

28. Restrepo RD. Use of inhaled anticholinergic agents in obstructive airway disease. *Respir Care.* 2007;52:833–851.

29. Ruffin RE, Wolff RK, Dolovich MB, et al. Aerosol therapy with Sch 1000: short-term mucociliary clearance in normal subjects. *Chest.* 1988;93:739–41. 30. Singh S , Loke YK, Furberg CD. Inhaled anticholinergic and risk of major cardiovascular events in patients with chronic obstructive pulmonary disease. *JAMA.* 2008;300:1439–1450.

31. NAEPP Working Group Report. Considerations for diagnosing and managing asthma in the elderly. National Heart, Lung, and Blood Institute, NIH publication No. 96-3662,1996.

32. Health trends 2007: National Center for Health Statistics. Health, United States, 2007, with chartbook on trends in the health of Americans. Available at: http://www.cdc.gov/nchs/data/hus/hus07.pdf. Accessed 20 August 2008.

33. Niederman MS, Qanta AA, Ahmed MD. Community-acquired pneumonia in elderly patients. *Clin Geriatr Med.* 2003;19:101–120.

34. Niederman MS, Brito V. Pneumonia in the older patient. *Clin Chest Med.* 2007;28:751–771.

35. Mandell LA, Wunderink RG, Anzueto A, et al. Infectious disease society of America/American thoracic society consensus guidelines on the management of community-acquired pneumonia in adults. *Clin Infect Dis.* 2007;44:S27–72.

36. Ruiz M, Ewig S, Marcos MA, et al. Etiology of community-acquired pneumonia: impact of age, comorbidity, and severity. *Am J Resp Crit Care Med.* 1999;160:397–405.

37. Arancibia F, Bauer TT, Ewig S, et al. Community-acquired pneumonia due to gram-negative bacteria and *Pseudomonas aeruginosa:* incidence, risk, and prognosis. *Arch Intern Med.* 2002;162:1849–1858.

38. Ruhe JJ, Hasbun R. *Streptococcus pneumoniae* bacteremia: duration of previous antibiotic use and association with penicillin resistance. *Clin Infect Dis.* 2001;32:701–707.

39. Troy CJ, Peeling AG, Ellis JC, et al. Chlamydia pneumoniae as a new source of infectious outbreaks in nursing homes. *JAMA.* 1997;277:1214–1218.

40. Waterer GW, Kessler LA, Wunderink RG. Delayed administration of antibiotics and atypical presentations in community-acquired pneumonia. *Chest.* 2006;130(1):11–15.

41. American Thoracic Society and Infectious Disease Society of America. Guidelines for the management of adults with hospital-acquired, ventilator-associated, and healthcare-associated pneumonia. *Am J Respir Crit Care Med.* 2005;171:388–416.

42. Gutierrez F, Masia M. Improving outcomes of elderly patients with community acquired pneumonia. *Drugs Aging.* 2008;25(7):585–610.

43. Meehan TP, Fine MJ, Krumholz HM, et al. Quality of care, process, and outcomes in elderly patients with pneumonia. *JAMA.* 1997;278:2080–2084.

44. Houck PM, Bratzler DW, Nsa W, et al. Timing of antibiotic administration and outcomes for Medicare patients hospitalized with community-acquired pneumonia. *Arch Intern Med.* 2004;164:637–644.

45. Dean NC, Bateman KA, Donnelly SA, et al. Improved clinical outcomes with utilization of a

community-acquired pneumonia guideline. *Chest.* 2006;130(3):794–799.

46. Jackson LA, Neuzil KM, Yu O, et al. Effectiveness of pneumococcal polysaccharide vaccine in older adults. *N Engl J Med.* 2003;1;348(18):1747–1755.

47. Ortqvist A, Hedlund J, Burman LA, et al. Randomized trial of 23-valent pneumococcal capsular polysaccharide vaccine in prevention of pneumonia in middle-aged and elderly people. Swedish pneumococcal vaccination study group. *Lancet.* 1998;351(9100):399–403.

48. Vila-Corcoles A, Ochoa-Gondar O, Hospital I, et al. Protective effects of the 23-valent pneumococcal polysaccharide vaccine in the elderly population: the EVAN-65 study. *Clin Infect Dis.* 2006;43(7):860–868.

49. Christenson B, Hedlund J, Lundbergh P, et al. Additive preventive effect of influenza and pneumococcal vaccines in elderly persons. *Eur Respir J.* 2004;23(3):363–368.

50. Fiore AE, Shay DK, Broder K, et al; Advisory Committee on Immunization Practices. Prevention and Control of Influenza; Recommendations of the Advisory Committee on Immunization Practices (ACIP), 2008. *MMWR Recomm Rep.* 2008;57:1–60.

51. Thompson WW, Shay DK, Weintraub E, et al. Influenza-associated hospitalizations in the United States. *JAMA.* 2004;292:1333–1340.

52. Thompson WW, Shay DK, Weintraub E, et al. Mortality associated with influenza and respiratory syncytial virus. *JAMA.* 2003;289:179–186.

53. Sethi S. Bacterial pneumonia: managing a deadly complication of influenza in older adults with comorbid disease. *Geriatrics.* 2002;57:56–61.

54. Govaert TM, Thijs CT, Masurel N, et al. The efficacy of influenza vaccination in elderly individuals. A randomized double-blind placebo-controlled trial. *JAMA.* 1994;272:1661–5.

55. Ohmit SE, Arden NH, Monto AS. Effectiveness of inactivated influenza vaccine among nursing home residents during an influenza A (H3N2) epidemic. *J Am Geriatr Soc.* 1999;47:165–71.

56. Jefferson T, Rivetti D, Rudin M, et al. Efficacy and effectiveness of influenza vaccines in elderly people: a systematic review. *Lancet.* 2005;366:1165–1174.

57. Cooper NJ, Sutton AJ, Abrams KR, et al. Effectiveness of neuraminidase inhibitors in treatment and prevention of influenza A and B: systemic review and meta-analyses of randomized controlled trials. *BMJ.* 2003;326;1–6.

58. U.S. Department of Health and Human Services. Healthy people 2010 2nd ed. With understanding and improving health and objectives for improving health (2 vols.). Washington, DC: U.S. Department of Health and Human Services; 2000.

59. Zevallos M, Justman JE. Tuberculosis in the elderly. *Clin Geriatr Med.* 2003;121–138.

60. Rajagopalan S, Yoshikawa TT. Tuberculosis in long-term-care facilities. *Infect Control Hosp Epidemiol.* 2000;21:611–615.

61. Thrupp L, Bradley S, Smith P, et al. Tuberculosis prevention and control in long-term-care facilities for older adults. *Infect Control Hosp Epidemiol.* 2004;25(12):1097–1108.

62. American Thoracic Society. American Thoracic Society/ Centers for Disease Control and Prevention/Infectious Diseases Society of America: treatment of tuberculosis. *Am J Resp Crit Care Med.* 2003;167:603–662.

63. Van den Brande P. Revised guidelines for the diagnosis and control of tuberculosis impact on management in the elderly. *Drugs Aging.* 2005;22(8):663–689.

64. Gomez-Reino JJ, Carmona L, Rodriquez V, et al. Treatment fo rheumatoid arthritis with tumor necrosis factors inhibitors may predispose to significant increase in tuberculosis risk. *Arthritis Rheum.* 2003;48(8):2122–2127.

65. Keane J, Gershon S, Wise RP, et al. Tuberculosis associated with infliximab, a tumor necrosis factor α-neutralizing agent. *N Engl J Med.* 2001;345:1098–104.

66. Gardam MA, Keystone EC, Menzies R, et al. Anti-tumour necrosis factor agents and tuberculosis risk: mechanisms of action and clinical management. *Lancet Infect Dis.* 2003;3:148–155.

67. Keane J, Gershon SK, Braun MM. Tuberculosis and treatment with infliximab. *N Engl J Med.* 2002;346:625–626.

68. Ormerod LP, Milburn HJ, Gillespie S, et al. BTS recommendations for assessing risk and for managing *Mycobacterium tuberculosis* infection and disease in patients due to start anti-TNF-α treatment. *Thorax.* 2005;60:800–805.

69. Kopanoff DE, Snider DE, Caras GJ. Isoniazid-related hepatitis: a US Public Health Service cooperative surveillance study. *Am Rev Respir Dis.* 1978;117:991–1001.

70. Rello J, Rodriguez R, Juber P, et al. Severe community-acquired pneumonia in the elderly: epidemiology and prognosis. *Clin Infec Dis.* 1996;23:734–738.

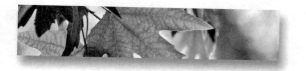

9

Renal and Urologic Disorders

NORMA J. OWENS AND ERICA L. ESTUS

Learning Objectives

1. Evaluate the changes in renal function that occur with age and determine how these changes result in an increased risk for older patients with chronic illnesses.

2. In a patient with chronic kidney disease and diabetes, develop a treatment plan to help preserve renal function.

3. Assess a pharmacotherapy regimen for drug induced causes of incontinence for an older person with a recent onset of incontinence.

4. Distinguish between older men with benign prostatic hyperplasia who would benefit from single agent versus combined therapy with alpha reductase inhibition and alpha blockade.

5. Evaluate patient signs, symptoms, and laboratory data that should be present to diagnose a urinary tract infection. Develop a treatment plan for a urinary tract infection in an older person.

Key Terms

BACTERIURIA: The presence of bacteria in the urine.

CYSTOCELE: Protrusion of the bladder into the vagina due to pelvic support defects.

DETRUSOR MUSCLE: The muscular coat of the urinary bladder that contracts to empty urine.

KEGEL EXERCISES: Pelvic muscle exercises intended to strengthen the muscles of the pelvic floor to improve urethral and rectal sphincter function.

MICTURITION: Urination or voiding.

NEUROGENIC BLADDER: Dysfunction of the bladder caused by neurologic damage. Potential causes include brain or spinal cord injuries, diabetes, acute infection, or genetic nerve complications.

PYURIA: Increased numbers of polymorphonuclear leukocytes in the urine and represents an inflammatory response in the urinary tract.

Renal Disorders

Changes in the Kidney with Age

The aging kidney gradually develops anatomic and physiologic changes that are usually not perceptible until an illness alters the body's compensatory balance. The vascular system changes in the aging kidney leading to hypertrophy of arteries with the most significant impact occurring in the cortex of the kidney.[1] Most of the size changes in the aging kidney occur in the cortex with a loss of about 35% of the number of glomeruli as well as a decrease in the surface area and a thickening of the basement membrane of the glomeruli. Glomerular atrophy in the aging kidney results in a decrease of the glomerular filtration rate (GFR) of about 0.75–1.0 mL/min/1.73 m^2 each year beginning by about 40 years of age.[2] These changes in the structure and function of the kidney in an older person also affects their ability to maintain a normal fluid and electrolyte balance, especially when challenged with drugs and illness. Older people experience a delay in compensation to a very low sodium diet as well as an exaggerated increase in blood pressure in response to an increase in sodium intake. Older people also have a decreased response to the diuretic and natriuretic effects of loop diuretics. The regulation of water balance changes with age due to the decreased ability of the aging kidney to concentrate as well as a decreased ability to excrete a water load. These changes in kidney size and physiology result in significant alterations to kidney function with age resulting in a decrease in GFR and a decreased ability to respond to changes in fluid and electrolyte balance.[1-2]

Epidemiology and Risk Factors of Chronic Kidney Disease

Chronic kidney disease is a common and important disorder in older persons and is associated with serious adverse outcomes such as kidney failure, cardiovascular disease, anemia, functional decline, and death. In 2002, The National Kidney Foundation defined chronic kidney disease as the presence of protein (albumin) in the urine for at least 3 months, or an estimated glomerular filtration rate (GFR) of less than 60 mL/min/1.73 m^2. This group also created a five-stage system to categorize the severity of renal dysfunction.[3] A national data system collects and analyses information about chronic and end-stage kidney disease and this information shows that the prevalence of chronic kidney disease is estimated to be between 14–18% of the general population and to be more than 38% in people who are over the age of 60 years.[4] Additionally, of those individuals who have progressed to end-stage renal disease, 20% are between the ages of 65 to 74 and 16% are 75 years of age or older.[4]

The National Kidney Foundation recommends evaluation of patients on the basis of their risk factors, initiation factors, and progression factors.[3] One of the most important risk factors that contributes to the development of chronic kidney disease is advanced age. Initiation factors are diseases that cause renal damage and include diabetes and hypertension, two diseases that are strongly associated with age. Progression factors accelerate the damage to the kidney and include hyperglycemia, hypertension, and proteinuria. Other progression factors that can be modified include smoking, hyperlipidemia, and obesity. Progression factors occur commonly in older individuals and are potentially modifiable by medication therapy management.[3]

Disease Progression in the Elderly

The natural course or progression of chronic kidney disease to end-stage renal disease is different between younger and older people. Chronic kidney disease progresses in association with factors such as proteinuria, hypertension, diabetes, smoking cigarettes, hyperlipidemia, and obesity. The effect of age on the progression of chronic kidney disease was evaluated in a large cohort of elderly veterans with kidney disease showing an expected inverse relationship between estimated GFR and rates of end-stage renal disease and death.[5] In the older men with initial moderate kidney disease, the percentage who experienced a further decrease in GFR each year, increased with age. For men with moderately severe disease, the percentage of men who further decreased their GFR was less with age. The older men with more severe kidney disease, were more likely to die than progress to end-stage renal disease.[5] This research suggests that older age is a strong modifier of disease course with more rapid progression from moderate to moderately severe disease and less progression of moderately severe disease to end-stage disease. This difference in progression may be due to greater disease co-morbidity in older men that leads to death; to a stabilization of moderate kidney disease in older persons; or perhaps to a difference in the underlying cause of kidney dysfunction in the elderly.

Diagnosis of Chronic Kidney Disease in the Elderly

Renal function, as defined by GFR, declines with age by approximately 0.75–1.0 mL/min/1.73 m² each year beginning by about 40 years of age.[2] Identification of chronic kidney disease in older persons is important for several reasons. Individuals with an estimated glomerular filtration rate of ≤ 60 mL/min need to have moderate adjustments of the doses of renally eliminated medications. Prevention of end-stage renal disease can become a focus of medication therapy management if chronic kidney disease is documented. Frequently, chronic kidney disease occurs in older patients with diabetes and or hypertension which highlights the importance of achievement of goal treatment values in the management of these two chronic diseases. Pharmacists who participate in medication therapy management are uniquely situated to help older people achieve goal treatment values for chronic diseases which can slow progression of chronic kidney disease.

Estimation of Renal Function

There is some controversy about the preferred method for estimation of glomerular filtration rate in older people. To estimate GFR, the serum concentration of an endogenous filtration marker, like creatinine, is measured and the clearance of creatinine is computed with a mathematical formula. The mathematical equations have been developed from patient studies that use regression formulas to correlate the serum level of creatinine

to the measured GFR. Often, patient factors are included in the formula such as age, body weight, and sex to improve the correlation between measured and estimated GFR.[6-7] Chapter three discusses the specific formulae employed for estimating GFR and discussed pros and cons of each, but in general, it is the Cockcroft-Gault equation that is used to estimate GFR for the purposes of determining the renal dose adjustment of medications. [8] The four variable Modification of Diet in Renal Disease (MDRD) equation, which adjusts for age, sex, creatinine, and race, is used to stage patients with chronic kidney disease.[7]

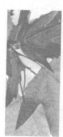

KEY POINT: Estimation of GFR through the use of the Cockcroft-Gault formulae should be performed for older patients as a part of a comprehensive medical and pharmacy assessment.

Treatment of Chronic Kidney Disease

The goals of treatment for all ages of people with chronic kidney disease are to delay or prevent the progression to more severe stages of disease including end-stage renal disease, and to prevent the occurrence of complications related to chronic kidney disease. However, because older patients generally have multiple chronic diseases and are more likely to die *with* kidney disease rather than *from* kidney disease than younger individuals, interventions should be tailored to meet the patient's lifestyle preferences, to maintain optimal physical and mental functioning, and to maintain quality of life. Interventions include non pharmacologic (dietary protein restriction) and pharmacologic. Drug therapy recommendations may be different for those with diabetic chronic kidney disease than for those with chronic kidney disease due to other causes.

Dietary restriction of protein in amounts up to 0.6 g/kg per day is recommended by the National Kidney Foundation for individuals with a GFR <

$25/mL/min/1.73 m^2$. The literature that supports this recommendation is inconsistent and suggests that a reduction in rate of decline of the GFR is small at 0.5 mL/min per year. Dietary protein restriction has not been specifically evaluated for efficacy or safety in older people. Given that the benefits are small and the risks for malnutrition and changes in quality of life with protein restriction are significant, intake levels of up to 0.75 g/kg/day are reasonable for older people.[9]

Pharmacologic Therapy

To prevent progression of chronic kidney disease, drug therapy is specifically targeted toward control of the underlying disease that initiated the kidney disease, generally either diabetes and or hypertension. Diabetes and hypertension both initiate CKD as well as contribute to disease progression A comprehensive approach to the medical management of older patients with diabetes, hypertension, and renal diseases is vital.

Glycemic Control to Prevent Chronic Kidney Disease in an Older Patient with Diabetes

In older patients with type 2 diabetes, intensive therapy that achieves goal HbA_{1c} values of ≤ 7.0% substantially reduces albuminuria[10-12] but with the risk of more frequent hypoglycemic reactions.[13-14] Clinical practice guidelines have summarized the strong evidence that exists between HbA_{1c} and the emergence of albuminuria, although the evidence that links glycemic improvement to a prevention of decline of the GFR is weaker.[15] Two important publications highlight both the risks and efficacy of intensive therapy in older patients. More than 11,000 patients with type 2 diabetes, who were 66 ± 6 years of age (mean ± standard deviation), were randomized to receive intensive therapy to achieve HbA_{1c} values ≤ 6.5% or to standard therapy where the HbA_{1c} values were generally between 7–8%.[13] This cohort represents the younger end of the age range referred to as elderly. Frail individuals of very advanced age or with multiple co-morbidities, disability or dementia were not well represented. All patients were treated with multiple oral agents that most often included a sulfonylurea with metformin. Patients in the intensive arm of the study received a modified for-

mulation of gliclazide and were more likely to be treated with insulin than the standard treatment group (40% vs. 24% respectively). After five years of treatment, patients in the intensive arm of this study had a reduction by one fifth of new or worsening nephropathy. Rates of hypoglycemia were higher in the intensive versus standard treated patients (2.7 vs. 1.5% respectively).[13] For older patients with type 2 diabetes, the risk of hypoglycemia was even higher with an even more aggressive glycemic goal regimen (HbA_{1c} < 6%) versus standard management (HbA_{1c} between 7–7.9%) resulting in significantly more deaths in the aggressive treatment arm.[14]

Older patients are more likely to experience hypoglycemia which may be due to their underlying renal disease with a decreased ability to eliminate both insulin and oral anti-diabetic drugs. Furthermore, patients with kidney disease have decreased renal gluconeogensis which reduces an important compensatory response to counter hypoglycemia.[15,16] Due to these limitations, glipizide is the preferred sulfonylurea for use in older patients with kidney disease because the drug is metabolized to inactive compounds.[17] Metformin is recommended as an effective and preferred beginning therapy for patients with type 2 diabetes due to its broad range of benefits and lack of hypoglycemia.[18] Use of metformin may be limited in older people due to prescribing guidelines that recommend individuals need adequate renal function to clear this drug and prevent lactic acidosis. In addition to recommendations to avoid metformin with serum creatinine greater than 1.4 mg/dL in women and 1.5 mg/dL in men, creatinine clearance should also be considered. Official product information recommends a minimum creatinine clearance of more than 60 mL/min, although there is some data that suggest metformin can be used in individuals with creatinine clearance as low as 30 mL/min.[18,19] Although age greater than 80 years is not an absolute contraindication for use, caution is required due to the increasing likelihood of insufficient renal function with advancing age. Other oral agents that may be preferable for use in patients with impaired renal function include repaglinide, a nonsulfonylurea secretogue. This class of oral agents is shorter acting and lowers postprandial glucose more than fasting glucose concentrations which results in less hypoglycemia. Pioglitazone may also be the preferred thiazolidinedione for use in the elderly with renal insufficiency, although concerns about weight gain and fluid retention with this class of medications warrants careful monitoring.[15-17] To avoid chronic kidney disease related to diabetes, older patients should strive to achieve HbA_{1c} concentrations that are close to 7%, while avoiding hypoglycemic reactions.

Control of Cardiovascular Risk Factors in Older Patients with Chronic Kidney Disease

Strictly focusing on chronic kidney disease, consensus guidelines suggest the appropriate blood pressure goal for people with CKD is less than 130/80 mm Hg,[15] and recommend that antihypertensive treatment that targets proteinuria is also important for patients with chronic kidney disease independent of the patient's blood pressure. Thus, present guidelines strongly recommend the use of either an angiotensin converting enzyme (ACE) inhibitor or angiotensin receptor blocker (ARB) as first-line therapy to treat hypertension or proteinuria in patients with chronic kidney disease. Although the long term outcomes of this type of drug therapy intervention is less clear in very frail individuals, the prevention of further renal compromise is important to preventing future morbidity among younger groups of the geriatric population. There are generally no significant age-related pharmacokinetic or pharmacodynamic differences between older and younger patients in the use of ACE inhibitors or ARBs.[20] To avoid renal toxicity in patients who may be volume depleted from diuretics or for those also receiving non-steroidal anti-inflammatory drugs, ACE inhibitors and ARBs should be started at low dosages and slowly titrated to effect. For those at high risk of renal toxicity, the diuretic or non-steroidal anti-inflammatory agent can be held for 2-3 days to prevent an acute decline in renal function related to any underlying dehydration.[20] Angiotensin receptor blockers may cause fewer side effects, such as cough and angioedema, and can be used as alternatives to ACE inhibitors. The combined use of ACE inhibitors with ARBs is sometimes recommended to prevent renal angiotensin escape, thus providing for a greater effect on blood pressure control and albuminuria.[20] However, elderly individuals with impaired renal function are at increased risk for hyperkalemia with this therapy, and for this reason ACE inhibitors are often cited among the classes of medications with a high prevalence of adverse effects in the long term care setting. Increased monitoring of serum potassium may be required for individuals receiving medications that alter serum potassium such as potassium supplements, potassium sparing diuretics, ACE inhibitors, and ARBs.

Hyperlipidemia increases albuminuria which accelerates the progression of chronic kidney disease. Therefore, treatment of hyperlipidemia in patients with chronic kidney disease is an important way to modify the disease course and current guidelines recommend the use of a HMG-CoA reductase inhibitor (statin) to achieve a low density lipoprotein concentration of < 100 mg/dL.[21] There is very little information available about age-related changes in either the pharmacokinetics or pharmacodynamics with the use of statins.[20] Almost all clinical trials with statins for the prevention of adverse health consequences from hyperlipidemia have included at least some older individuals with results supporting treatment.[17] This research includes individuals who are in their 60s and 70s but generally does not evaluate individuals in their 80s and 90s. And finally, the management of other complications related to chronic kidney disease, such as anemia and bone disease, is especially important in older people. As the GFR decreases, erythropoietin secretion diminishes causing anemia of chronic kidney disease. This complication and its treatment are covered in Chapter 15. Phosphate excretion decreases with worsening renal disease leading to an increase in serum phosphorus, a decrease in serum calcium, a decrease in vitamin D activation, hyperparathyroidism, and an increase in calcium resorption from bone.[22] These adverse effects on bone add further risks of bone disease and fracture to the older person who may already have coexisting osteoporosis. In this setting, serum phosphorus, calcium, and vitamin D_2 concentrations should be measured so that appropriate supplementation can occur. Phosphate binders are needed as the first step in controlling this problem although an ideal formulation or regimen does not exist.[22] Calcium containing products are often used to bind phosphate and can be taken with meals in doses that are often associated with side effects such as nausea, vomiting, and constipation. These regimens may also add to the pill burden in an older patient's medication regimen. Sevelamer is a newer non-calcium based agent that binds to phosphorus in exchange for chloride and can be used as sole therapy or in combination with other phosphate binders. Because sevelamer is a polymer that is not absorbed, older patients should be carefully monitored for constipation to prevent bowel obstruction.[22]

Fluid and Electrolyte Disorders

The renal system has a remarkable capacity to adjust to changes in our body from the environment and disease processes. However, the kidney's ability to adapt and change decreases with age, making older people more susceptible to fluid and electrolyte imbalance. In addition, older people are much more likely to have underlying diseases and drug treatments that place them at further risk for fluid and electrolyte disorders. Due to the changes in the kidney mentioned at the beginning of this chapter, older people have a reduced ability to concentrate their urine as well as a lessened ability to excrete an increased water load. Also, older people have a decreased thirst sensation and are more likely to have cognitive impairments which, when coupled with the decreased function of the kidney, place them at great risk for dehydration.[23]

Dehydration is a common problem in nursing home residents and is a frequent cause for admission to the hospital. In the community, the elderly are at great risk for dehydration and death particularly during heat waves in the summer. Even though dehydration is a common disorder, the recognition of this condition is more problematic in the elderly. For instance, older people often have diminished skin turgor due to ageing effects on the skin and dry mucus membranes can be present in those who breathe through their mouth. Autonomic reflexes decline with age diminishing the vasomotor response to heat.[23] Measurement of serum sodium is an important part of an assessment of hydration status because changes in serum sodium concentration usually reflect either an excess or deficit of water.

Sodium and Water Imbalance in the Elderly

Hypernatremia (serum sodium >145 mEq/L) is a hypertonic condition that is usually due to a deficit of water and is most common in the elderly with an impaired thirst sensation and or a lack of access to water. Older patients with dehydration usually present with a change in mental status such as lethargy, increasing confusion, and postural hypotension.[23] Treatment should focus on the repletion of water and sodium at a rate that is slow enough to allow for equilibration of water into the brain. Fluid replacement that is too rapid may cause cerebral edema and brain toxicity leading to seizures and death.[24] Fluid replacement with intravenous normal saline (or less concentrated solutions) should not exceed approximately 150–200 mL/hr to restore the intravascular volume and then at slower rates, with half-normal saline solutions, to correct the water deficit.[23-24] In older persons, hypernatremia and dehydration have often developed gradually and so the correction of this condition should, likewise, be in a slow and cautious manner.

Hyponatremia (serum sodium < 135 mEq/L) is a common disorder and can lead to impairments in brain function from cerebral edema. Chronic mild hyponatremia in the elderly is associated with an increase in falls.[25] In the older person, fluid excess, often due to an over correction of dehydration with isotonic fluids is another frequent cause of hyponatremia.[23-24] Evaluation of the serum osmolality will help determine whether or not the patient has an isotonic, hypertonic, or hypotonic variety of hyponatremia. Hypotonic hyponatremia is more common and further evaluation of the urine sodium concentration will help determine whether the patient is hypovolemic (generally due to thiazide diuretics), hypervolemic (generally due to congestive heart failure, cirrhosis, or overcorrection with isotonic fluids) or, euvolemic (generally due to low sodium intake, polydipsia, or the syndrome of inappropriate anti-diuretic hormone secretion).[24] In a patient with hyponatremia, knowledge of the volume status guides therapy.

Thiazide diuretics are a frequent cause of hypotonic hyponatremia because they block sodium reabsorption in the distal tubules of the renal cortex which increases sodium and water excretion by the kidney. Arginine vasopressin or antidiuretic hormone is released to counter the decrease in plasma volume, which increases the reabsorption of free water, resulting in a hyponatremia that is due to a net loss of more sodium than water.[24]

Treatment of hypovolemic hyponatremia should begin by addressing the cause (such as discontinuation of the thiazide diuretic) and replacement of the sodium and fluid deficit in a manner consistent with the severity of symptoms in the patient. In patients with severe central nervous system symptoms such as coma or seizures, normal saline in small amounts to slowly raise the serum sodium by 5% is a treatment goal.[24] Ringer's lactate may be a preferable replacement solution because normal saline solutions have relatively more chloride, in comparison to the plasma, and may lead to a hyperchloremic acidosis.[23]

For patients with hypervolemic hyponatremia, treatment is focused on achieving a negative water balance by increasing water excretion and limiting oral fluid intake to less than about 1,000 mL/day. If congestive heart failure is the cause for this condition, optimal treatment for the heart failure should be instituted.

Drugs can be a cause of euvolemic hyponatremia. Although the overall incidence of drug-induced syndrome of inappropriate anti-diuretic hormone is relatively low, there are many classes of drug therapy that can cause this, and drug regimen review is recommended for older individuals with signs of hyponatremia. Commonly reported drug-induced causes include antidepressants (many agents but older women are especially at risk with SSRIs), antipsychotics, anticonvulsants, and antineoplastic agents. Drug induced SIADH has also been reported with analgesics such as fentanyl and ibuprofen, antiparkinson medica-

tions, clonidine, ACE inhibitors, amiodarone, and theophylline. Discontinuation of the offending agent is recommended.[26]

Urologic Disorders
Urinary Incontinence

Urinary incontinence (UI) affects approximately 38% of women and 17% of men over age 60 and more than 50% of residents residing within long term care facilities.[27-28] Although the prevalence of urinary incontinence increases with age, it is not considered to be a normal part of aging.[29] The incidence in men is about one third that of women, but at the age of 80, men and women have similar rates of UI.[30] This disorder is expensive with an estimate of $5.5 billion being spent annually to manage urinary incontinence in long term care facilities.[28]

Before classifying the various types of urinary incontinence, review of the anatomy and physiology of the aging bladder is needed. The lower urinary tract is composed of the bladder (including the **detrusor muscle**), urethra, urinary sphincter and nearby musculofascial components including nerves, connective tissue, and blood vessels.[31] Urination is controlled by the central nervous system (CNS), the spinal cord, and the peripheral nerves. The parasympathetic nervous system (PNS), the sympathetic nervous system (SNS) and the somatic nervous system all work together to execute proper bladder control.[32]

Overall, bladder physiology and **micturition** are regulated by the action of various neurotransmitters and nervous systems (Figure 9-1).[32] Acetylcholine is the major neurotransmitter responsible for bladder contraction and it interacts with muscarinic receptors on the detrusor muscle.[33] Of the five known muscarinic subtypes M_1-M_5, M_2 subtypes predominate on the bladder smooth-muscle cholinergic receptors. The M_3 receptors are responsible for both the emptying contraction associated with urination as well as involuntary bladder contractions that can lead to UI. M_3 receptors appear to be the most clinically relevant within the human bladder and many antimuscarinic drug therapies are targeted at blocking this receptor subtype.[30,33] Disturbances in the neural regulation of micturition at any point (pelvic nerves, spinal cord or brain) may result in UI due to changes in lower tract function.[31]

Sensory receptors in the bladder are stimulated as it fills with urine, and signals are sent to the brain indicating bladder fullness. Variability exists within older adults, but approximately 100 to 200 mL of urine is required before the brain will "sense" bladder fullness. Stimulation of the SNS and inhibition of the PNS occurs during low bladder volume, and this leads to bladder filling by contraction of the internal sphincter and relaxation of the detrusor muscle. Inhibitory signals by the brain are replaced by impulses that stimulate the PNS when the bladder is full and micturition is necessary. Detrusor contraction results as well as relaxation of the internal sphincter and inhibition of the SNS. Urinary flow will occur when intravesical pressure is greater than the resistance within the urethra. Once the bladder has emptied and it is ready to be filled again, the brain signals parasympathetic inhibition and sympathetic stimulation resulting in detrusor relaxation and contraction of the internal sphincter.[34]

There are specific age-related physiological changes that occur within the urinary tract that include decreases in bladder elasticity, reduction in bladder capacity, and more frequent voiding. The detrusor muscle may contract spontaneously; in addition, reduced muscle strength can lead to incomplete bladder emptying. There is also a decrease in the urethral closing pressure and difficulty in postponing urination.[35] Sex specific changes also occur. Women experience a decline in bladder outlet and urethral resistance due to the decreased circulating estrogen levels in the genitourinary tract and the effect on the pelvic

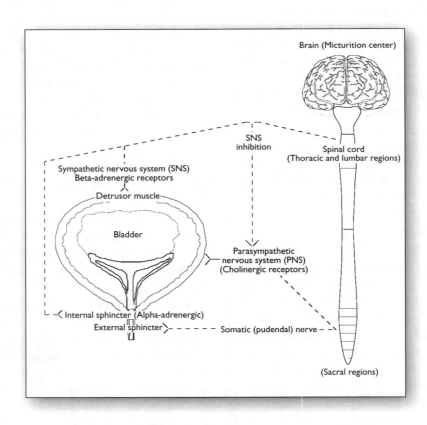

Figure 9-1. Basic bladder anatomy and physiology. *Source:* Reprinted with permission from *P&T: A Peer-Reviewed Journal for Formulary Management.*[32]

musculature. Diminished estrogen levels can lead to atrophic vaginitis and urologic complications including dysuria, urgency, and the development of urinary tract infections. Age related loss of tone in the muscles of the pelvic floor due to childbirth and/or obesity, can also contribute to incontinence. In men, prostate enlargement can lead to decreased urinary flow rates, instability of the detrusor muscle, and overflow incontinence.[36]

Urinary incontinence can be categorized by the duration of symptoms, clinical presentation, or physiologic abnormalities. In addition, transient causes of UI are a special consideration in older adults and should be differentiated from established incontinence secondary to urinary tract dysfunction. The following mnemonic (spells diapers) is used to identify some of these reversible causes: delirium, infection, atrophic vaginitis and urethritis, pharmacological agents, psychiatric disorders, excessive urine output, restricted mobility, and stool impaction.[29] Table 9-1[(29,31,33-35)] highlights some of the medication classes often implicated in causing or worsening incontinence.

Types of Urinary Incontinence

Stress incontinence typically occurs when the urinary sphincter is compromised and no longer able to resist the urine flow from the bladder, especially during physical activity. Transient increases in intra-abdominal pressure can lead to losses of small volumes of urine when laughing, sneezing, coughing, bending or lifting. This is the most common type of incontinence in women and risk factors include pregnancy, childbirth, menopause, cognitive impairment, age and obesity. Hormonal factors play a role since the prevalence increases after menopause with estrogen deficiency. Men also can experience stress incontinence, but usually only as a result of internal sphincter damage from urological procedures, including prostate surgery.[31-33]

Urge urinary incontinence (UUI) and overactive bladder (OAB) are associated with detrusor muscle over activity. The terms *overactive bladder, urge urinary incontinence,* and *detrusor over-activity* are used synonymously at times, but need to be differentiated. Overactive bladder (OAB) is a symptom complex that involves urinary urgency with or without urge incontinence, urinary frequency (> eight voiding episodes in a 24-hour period), and nocturia (≥ two nighttime awakenings to void).[34] It is important to recognize that OAB can result with or without the features of urge incontinence.[32] Individuals with UUI experience detrusor over activity that leads to forceful, early detrusor contractions before the bladder is full and results in urinary urgency and frequency.[33]

Table 9-1. **Medication Classes that Can Affect Urinary Tract Function or Urinary Incontinence**[29,31,33-35]

Drug Class	Result
Angiotensin converting enzyme inhibitor	Occurrence of cough can increase intra-abdominal pressure, aggravate stress incontinence
Acetylcholinesterase inhibitor	Polyuria, frequency
Alpha-adrenergic agonist	Increases internal sphincter tone
Alpha-adrenergic blocker	Decreases internal sphincter tone
Anticholinergic	Decreases detrusor muscle contraction, urinary retention
Calcium channel blocker	Decreases detrusor muscle contraction, urinary retention
Diuretic	Increases bladder filling
Opioid	Decreases detrusor muscle contraction, urinary retention
Sedative/hypnotic	Confusion, functional incontinence

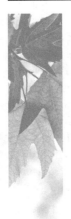

KEY POINT: Detrusor over-activity is a specific diagnosis obtained by urodynamic testing identifying involuntary detrusor contractions during the filling phase. Overactive bladder, in contrast, does not require invasive urodynamic testing and is diagnosed primarily by report of patient symptoms. These terms should not be interchanged, since the definitions are distinct.

The cause of UUI and OAB is most commonly idiopathic. Risk factors include normal aging, neurological disease, or bladder outlet obstruction. The underlying pathology for UUI and OAB may either be neurogenic or myogenic, and differing theories exist. The mechanism for the neurogenic hypothesis implies that disease related changes within the peripheral or central nervous systems lead to UUI and OAB. The myogenic hypothesis states that these conditions occur as a result of smooth muscle changes within the bladder wall. In practice, these etiologies are often related so it is difficult to differentiate.[31,34]

Overflow incontinence occurs as a result of urethral over activity and/or bladder under activity. The bladder is at maximum capacity and distended, but is unable to empty, and this leads to the leakage of urine.[31,33] Individuals usually present with symptoms of dribbling, weak urinary stream, hesitancy, or incomplete voiding. Causes can be neurogenic, such as diabetes mellitus, spinal cord injuries, or multiple sclerosis. Anticholinergic medications, conditions causing detrusor muscle under activity, or denervation of the bladder wall musculature are examples of other potential causes. In men, obstructed urinary outflow due to benign prostatic hyperplasia or prostate cancer is another common cause of overflow incontinence and an important consideration.[28,33]

Individuals with functional incontinence are unable to reach the toilet facilities in time, either due to physical (e.g., impaired mobility, poor vision) or cognitive issues (i.e., dementia, confusion, medication side effects). There are no defects within the urinary tract with the cause related to a primary disease (e.g., dementia, post operative orthopedic surgery).[28,31]

Mixed types of incontinence exist and diagnosis can be confusing due to the overlap of symptoms. The combination of bladder over activity and urethral sphincter under activity is one common form of mixed incontinence. Another mixed form characterized by bladder over activity (instability) and impaired bladder contractility may also occur in elderly men, leading to a mixed condition known as detrusor hyperactivity with impaired contractility.[28,31,36] Signs and symptoms of the mixed conditions are typical of the forms of incontinence that make up the individual diagnoses.

Neurogenic bladder, a type of overflow incontinence, involves the loss of voluntary control of bladder function due to spinal cord injury or neurological conditions. This type of incontinence is managed by intermittent catheterization or placement of a supra-pubic tube. Elderly patients may be vulnerable to inappropriate use of catheters for other types of incontinence which can lead to complications from chronic catheter use.[31]

Treatment

When treatment options are considered for UI, goals must be identified along with a plan that will be suitable for the individual, whether at home, residing in a long term care facility, or any other living situation. These goals should target a reduction in the frequency and severity of incontinence episodes and should minimize related complications. Frequently, these complications are overlooked and clinicians cannot underestimate the importance of weighing the risks and benefits of treatment options. Potential complications of not treating UI include skin breakdown, urinary tract infections, increased risk of falls, sleep disturbances, psychological effects including depression, isolation from activities, and changes in dignity relating to embarrassment.[28-30] Treating the underlying cause(s) is desirable but not always an option due to the individual's overall condition, treatment preferences, and functional ability.[28] In some cases, behavioral therapy is appropriate, and non-drug therapies may be the only choice for individuals if drugs or surgery are not desirable options. However, multiple pharmacological agents are now available with a variety of mechanisms and profiles that may suit specific needs.

Regardless of the type of urinary incontinence an individual experiences, it may be necessary to use incontinence undergarments as a means to avoid the soiling of clothing from a wetting episode. For some individuals with occasional or minor symptoms, incontinence shields or adult briefs may be the sole intervention chosen. These products may also be used in combination with drug therapy, because wetting episodes may still occur. In very frail or functionally dependent patients, adult briefs with regular changing and personal cleansing are a mainstay of incontinence care. For those individuals who are dependent on a caregiver for all toileting and personal hygiene activities, especially those with significant cognitive impairment, the decision is often made to discontinue pharmacological intervention for incontinence. If drug therapy does not result in a reduction of wetting episodes, urge discomfort, or the need for adult briefs, the side effect profile may outweigh the benefit in these individuals.

Non-drug Therapy and Behavioral/Muscle Rehabilitation

Individuals with overactive bladder or detrusor over activity often respond to behavioral therapy, and this should be implemented before any pharmacological treatment. Bladder training is a term that refers to a combination of patient education, voiding schedules, urge suppression techniques, and pelvic muscle exercises. Toileting assistance protocols are helpful in patients with cognitive or mobility impairment.[34] Using routine toileting, prompted voiding, and habit training schedules, will empty the bladder regularly to minimize leaking.[37] In addition to overactive bladder and UUI, behavioral techniques are often used for stress and mixed incontinence.[31]

Bladder training involving urge control strategies works well in individuals with higher cognition, ability to toilet, and motivation to cooperate with a training program. To retrain bladder hab-

its, scheduled toiletings are adjusted for longer or shorter times, depending on the individual voiding pattern. This may be an option for individuals who are cognitively or physically impaired and need reminders or assistance with the process. Overflow incontinence can also be managed by instructing individuals to void on a regular schedule (i.e., every 2 hours) to avoid increased volume and bladder distention.[28,31,37]

Pelvic muscle rehabilitation and exercises can be effective in stress, urge, and mixed incontinence. Examples include biofeedback, vaginal weight training, and **Kegel exercises**. Most effective in motivated individuals with adequate cognition, proper technique is required to contract the pelvic floor muscles during Kegel exercises without the use of accessory muscles.[31] The exercises strengthen the periurethral and pelvic floor muscles and must be performed regularly to be effective.[31,33] Kegel exercises or other forms of pelvic floor muscle rehabilitation may be used in combination with bladder training. Several studies in women show the combination to be more effective than either alone.[38] Older adults with cognitive impairment face additional challenges with these techniques. They may require regular reminders to urinate and dryness checks to enhance bladder training. Keeping a bed pan or commode near the bed may also prevent potential falls and subsequent injuries.

Drug Therapy

Drug therapy for urinary incontinence becomes necessary when the symptoms are not sufficiently managed with nonpharmacological therapies. Many times, the combination of drug therapy with behavioral or muscle rehabilitation is utilized for optimal results.[31] Pharmacological interventions have the potential to reduce the number of incontinence episodes experienced per day while increasing the volume of urine that the bladder can hold. Medications target specific underlying abnormalities, and it is imperative to identify the type of incontinence before beginning pharmacological treatment.[28] Table 9-2[28,31-32] summarizes possible pharmacologic options for treating various forms of urinary incontinence.

Table 9-2. **Drug Treatment of Urinary Incontinence**[28, 31-32]

Type of Incontinence	Drug Treatment Class	Specific Agent(s)	Comments
Urge or overactive bladder	Antimuscarinic/anticholinergic agents	Darifenacin, oxybutynin, solifenacin, tolterodine, trospium	Anticholinergic agents are generally first-line therapy. Various forms exist: short acting, long acting, oxybutynin patch. Differences in muscarinic receptor blocking exist.
	Tricyclic antidepressants	Imipramine, doxepin, nortriptyline, desipramine	Not preferred in elderly due to anticholinergic profile. May worsen cardiac conduction disturbances. Possibly consider if other underlying diagnoses are present (i.e., neuropathic pain)
Stress incontinence	Alpha adrenergic agonists	Pseudoephedrine phenylephrine	Avoid use with hypertension, cardiac arrhythmia. Other side effects include tremor, anxiety, or agitation.
	Topical estrogens	Conjugated estrogen vaginal cream or estradiol vaginal insert/ring	Evidence is poor, may consider in women if urethritis or vaginitis are also present
	Serotonin/norepinephrine reuptake inhibitor	Duloxetine	Not FDA approved for SUI; side effects (including nausea, dry mouth, fatigue) may limit its usefulness
Overflow incontinence	Alpha adrenergic antagonists	Alfuzosin, tamsulosin, doxazosin, terazosin	Side effects vary depending on selectivity to receptors in the bladder and/or prostate (alfuzosin and tamsulosin are more specific)
	Add-on therapy 5HT reductase inhibitors or bladder antispasmodics	Finasteride, dutasteride Tolterodine, oxybutynin	For advanced BPH or refractory symptoms. Must weigh risk of urinary retention with improvement in lower urinary tract symptoms
	Cholinomimetics	Bethanechol	May consider short term, avoid in asthma or heart disease.
Functional incontinence	Remove barriers and obstacles, provide schedules or prompted toileting, assistance may be required to transfer on/off commode		Consider therapy to remove any potential cause
Mixed incontinence	Focus on symptoms that dominate		Consider treatments for individual components (i.e., stress and urge)

Drug Therapy for Stress Incontinence

There are currently no Food and Drug Administration (FDA) approved agents to treat SUI. Alpha adrenergic agonists such as pseudoephedrine lack selectivity for the urethral alpha adrenoreceptors and cardiovascular safety concerns exist. Imipramine and estrogen are options with limited efficacy.[39] In addition, data from the Heart and Estrogen/Progestin Replacement Study demonstrated an increased risk of stress and urge incontinence in women who were randomly assigned to receive estrogen alone or the combination of estrogen and progesterone compared with placebo.[40] Using hormone therapy for the treatment of stress incontinence is generally not recommended.[41]

Duloxetine hydrochloride is a selective reuptake inhibitor of serotonin and norepinephrine. It is not currently approved for stress urinary incontinence in the United States, but it is approved by the regulatory agency in the European Union. In women it may result in stronger urethral contractions, with an improvement in sphincter tone during urine storage and physical stress.[39] Randomized, placebo controlled trials of duloxetine have been published demonstrating significant benefits in SUI, however, the emergence of adverse events such as nausea, dry mouth, and fatigue within the trials can be problematic for many healthy, non-depressed individuals. Initial manufacturer recommended doses were poorly tolerated and left clinicians with a negative perception.[31,39,42] Another weakness with the available evidence is the general under-representation of older adults within the study populations. Although a varied age range has been evaluated across many studies, the findings cannot clearly be applied to older adults.[43-44] The overall safety and efficacy, and place in treatment algorithms remains undetermined. Individuals may experience symptom relief as long as they are willing and able to tolerate the side effects, but more research is needed for an established role in therapy for older adults.[31,39,42]

Drug Therapy for Overactive Bladder

There are several muscarinic antagonists available for the treatment of urge urinary incontinence.

The anticholinergic agents used to treat overactive bladder vary in their pharmacokinetic properties, dosing and tolerability profiles. There are differences in muscarinic receptor affinities, but efficacy as reported in clinical trials appears to be similar. Oxybutynin is a lipophilic, non-specific muscarinic antagonist which is available as an immediate release, extended release or transdermal formulation. It is effective in reducing UUI symptoms, however it is associated with high incidence of anticholinergic side effects. Dry mouth, blurred vision, constipation, sedation and cognitive impairment are all concerns in the older patient. Despite similar efficacy among these formulations, it has been theorized that extended release or transdermal formulations are preferable based on tolerability considerations. For extended release oral formulations, this is based upon the idea that slow release of drug into the bloodstream avoids spikes in serum concentration associated with intermittent doses. For the transdermal formulation, this is based upon lower concentrations of the active metabolite N-desethyloxybutynin by avoidance of first pass metabolism in the liver. Data from clinical trials does suggest a reduction in adverse events, however this was primarily for dry mouth.[45]

Tolterodine is also available in both immediate release and long acting formulations and has comparable efficacy to oxybutynin for improvement of overactive bladder symptoms. It is also a non-selective muscarinic antagonist but is less lipophilic than oxybutinin, and therefore theorized to result in poor distribution into the CNS, resulting in fewer side effects. Comparisons of extended release tolterodine to either immediate release or extended release oxybutynin did show a lower incidence of adverse effects however, again, this was primarily limited to reduced incidence of dry mouth.[45]

There are two agents which are more selective for the M_3 receptor. They are solifenacin and darifenacin which are both available in formulations for once daily dosing. In one study comparing solifenacin to tolterodine, solifenacin significantly improved symptoms of urgency and urinary incontinence vs tolterodine, however, this study has been criticized because dose escalation was allowed in the solifenacin group, but not in the tolterodine group.[45] Agents with high M_3 selectivity are thought to be associated with relatively higher rates of constipation, but discontinuation rates due to adverse events were not different between the two groups. The potential sparing of M_1 receptor mediated cognitive impairment has only been minimally investigated. Darifenacin's effect on cognitive function was compared to oxybutynin ER in healthy subjects over the age of 60 years. Darifenacin-treated subjects scored similar to placebo subjects on delayed recall tests, while subjects receiving oxybutynin ER experienced memory deterioration estimated to be comparable to brain aging of 10 years. This study requires confirmation however, due to limitations such as short study duration, dropouts, differences in baseline characteristics between the groups, and questions about dose equivalence.[45-46]

Trospium is different from other muscarinic antagonists as it is a quaternary ammonium compound and is therefore thought to penetrate poorly into the central nervous system. Trospium is similar in efficacy to oxybutynin IR; dry mouth is reported to occur less often.[45]

In general, no single agent has emerged as the product of choice for treating urge urinary incontinence or overactive bladder.[45-46] Drug selection is based on the perceived side effect profile and all patients should be carefully monitored for symptom response and emergence of adverse effects. At this time, there is not a clear clinical advantage of the newer versus older agents. Tolerability, individual preference, and formulary considerations may be the deciding factor in determining the appropriate agent.[32]

Drug Therapy for Overflow Incontinence

The drug therapy for this type of incontinence will be discussed in the benign prostatic hyperplasia (BPH) section. Although women can experience this type of incontinence and there is limited data describing the use of alpha antagonists such as terazosin and doxazosin in these circumstances, the majority of the clinical data in this area has been evaluated in men with urinary symptoms associated with BPH.

Special Considerations for the Use of Drug Therapy

There are many factors to consider prior to initiating drug therapy for urinary incontinence. Comorbid conditions such as dementia, constipation, orthostatic hypotension, history of falling, or other conditions may influence choice of drug therapy. Other medications that the patient is taking may interact with an agent intended to treat incontinence. For example, adding anticholinergic medications for incontinence to a regimen that includes other anticholinergic medications can result in added side effects. Conversely, the concurrent use of acetylcholinesterase inhibitors with some of the anticholinergic drugs to treat UI may alter the efficacy of each drug and cause undesirable side effects due to a potential state of pharmacological opposition. Acetylcholinesterase inhibitors increase acetylcholine levels in the neural cleft in patients with dementia and incontinence agents target the muscarinic receptors to decrease acetylcholine. Previous studies demonstrate that bladder anticholinergic agents are associated with cognitive impairment in individuals with dementia, but literature describing concurrent use of acetylcholinesterase inhibitors and anticholinergics is limited to case reports and small observational studies.[47] In a prospective cohort of nursing home residents, the addition of either tolterodine or oxybutinin, to patients already receiving an acetylcholinesterase inhibitor, was evaluated. In individuals with higher levels of baseline functioning, the rate of decline in function (activities of daily living and cognition) was 50% faster when bladder anticholinergics were combined with acetylcholinesterase inhibitors than when acetylcholinesterase inhibitors were used alone.[47] Caution should be exercised when anticholinergics are added to a pharmacotherapy regimen in a patient with dementia as the risk for cognitive and functional decline may not outweigh any improvement in continence. It is important to evaluate the safety and efficacy of newer agents in the older adult and elderly population to determine the best choice. Although some of the newer agents may offer better side effect profiles, no clear improvement in efficacy has been demonstrated. Cost is another issue for some older adults as many of the older agents are available generically and there may be formulary and insurance restrictions. A sufficient trial should be given, at least one to two months, to determine how well any agent is working. Monitor carefully for side effects, objective evidence of incontinence frequency, and patient satisfaction with therapy. If an agent has not produced an adequate response in 2 months, consider discontinuing the drug or switching to another agent in the appropriate category.[28]

Surgery

Utilizing surgery as an option for the treatment of urinary incontinence is a consideration when behavioral modifications, pelvic muscle rehabilitation and/or drug therapy have not been successful. Surgical procedures to treat stress incontinence are intended to correct urethral closure deficiencies and to improve urethrovesical junction support. Examples in women include bladder neck needle suspension, anterior vaginal repair, or suburethral sling procedures. There are potential adverse outcomes and risks with surgery including urge incontinence, voiding difficulties, or pelvic organ prolapse.[38] In men, surgical options for SUI include collagen or an artificial urinary sphincter.[31]

For patients with overflow incontinence, there are not any effective surgical options for bladder under activity. After reversible causes are excluded, self catheterization by the patient or a caregiver several times a day is one effective management strategy to empty the bladder. Urethral over activity is typically caused by some type of anatomic obstruction. In men, this is often explained by benign prostatic enlargement.[31]

Benign Prostatic Hyperplasia

Benign prostatic hyperplasia (BPH) is a common condition affecting older men and is a cause for significant urinary symptoms that alter a man's quality of life. Age is the predominant factor in establishing the prevalence and histopathologic significance of BPH. Prostatic hypertrophy develops typically after age 40 with a 50% prevalence by age 60, and a prevalence approaching 90% by age 85. Autopsy studies show that an estimated 80% of elderly men have microscopic changes consistent with BPH. Approximately half of the individuals with these changes experience moderate to severe lower urinary tract symptoms.[48-50]

The prostate gland is surrounded by a dense fibrous capsule composed of smooth muscle cells, glandular cells, and supportive stromal cells.[51] Alpha reductase is also found within the prostate and facilitates the conversion of testosterone to dihydrotestosterone (DHT). At birth, prostate size resembles that of a pea, growing during puberty to reach an adult size by ages 25–30. A second growth spurt occurs around age 40 and growth continues through the seventh or eighth decades. The exact etiology of BPH is unknown, however, age-related hormonal changes, Type II 5-alpha reductase, and circulating androgens such as DHT are involved. The pathogenesis of BPH is due to static factors including glandular enlargement of the prostate, but also to dynamic factors such as excessive alpha adrenergic tone of the stromal component of the prostate gland, bladder neck, and posterior urethra. This leads to the narrowing of the urethral lumen by contraction of the prostate gland surrounding the urethra. Ultimately, anatomic enlargement of the prostate gland and narrowing of the urethral lumen results in obstructed urinary outflow.[48,51]

Individuals with BPH often experience a wide range of signs and symptoms of disease that are classified as obstructive or irritative. Obstructive symptoms, known as bladder outlet obstruction or prostatism, result from decreased bladder emptying and include hesitancy, urinary stream weakness, intermittency, and the sensation of incomplete bladder emptying. Irritative symptoms may occur later in the disease process, and can be attributed to long standing bladder neck obstruction. These symptoms often result in frequency, nocturia, and urgency. Symptoms of BPH are highly variable and may improve, worsen, or remain stable; it is not necessarily a progressive condition in all men.[48,51] An individual's ability to tolerate symptoms is often the motivation to seek treatment.

Men with troubling lower urinary tract symptoms (LUTS) should be evaluated to assess severity, and the potential for causes other than BPH, such as prostatitis and bladder or prostate cancer. It is important to establish that symptoms are truly due to BPH and not to other diagnoses of

LUTS.[50-51] The American Urological Association Symptom Index for BPH and the Disease Specific Quality of Life Question is a validated tool that can be used to objectively determine BPH severity in men seeking treatment (Figure 9-2)[50] and is superior to an unstructured interview in quantifying the severity and frequency of symptoms. It is recommended that symptomatic men have a digital rectal examination to determine the size and contour of the prostate and to exclude the presence of locally advanced prostate cancer.[49-50] The rectal exam should accompany a focused neurologic assessment as part of the physical exam.[51] Refer to Figure 9-3. for an algorithm for diagnosis and treatment from the American Urological Association.[50]

Patient Name: _____ DOB: _____ ID: _____ Date of assessment: _____

Initial Assessment ( ) Monitor during: _____ Therapy ( ) after: _____ Therapy/surgery ( ) _____

AUA BPH Symptom Score

	Not at all	Less than 1 time in 5	Less than half the time	About half the time	More than half the time	Almost always	
1. Over the past month, how often have you had a sensation of not emptying your bladder completely after you finished urinating?	0	1	2	3	4	5	
2. Over the past month, how often have you had to urinate again less than two hours after you finished urinating?	0	1	2	3	4	5	
3. Over the past month, how often have you found you stopped and started again several times when you urinated?	0	1	2	3	4	5	
4. Over the past month, how often have you found it difficult to postpone urination?	0	1	2	3	4	5	
5. Over the past month, how often have you had a weak urinary stream?	0	1	2	3	4	5	
6. Over the past month, how often have you had to push or strain to begin urination?	0	1	2	3	4	5	
	None	1 time	2 times	3 times	4 times	5 or more times	
7. Over the past month, how many times did you most typically get up to urinate from the time you went to bed at night until the time you got up in the morning?	0	1	2	3	4	5	
						Total Symptom Score	

The Disease Specific Quality of Life Question

The International Prostate Symptom Score uses the same 7 questions as the AUA Symptom Index (presented above) with the addition of the following Disease Specific Quality of Life Question (bother score) scored on a scale from 0 to 6 points (delighted to terrible):

"If you were to spend the rest of your life with your urinary condition just the way it is now, how would you feel about that?"

Figure 9-2. The American Urological Association Symptom Index for Benign Prostatic Hyperplasia (BPH) and the Disease Specific Quality of Life question. Reprinted with permission of the American Urological Association.[50]

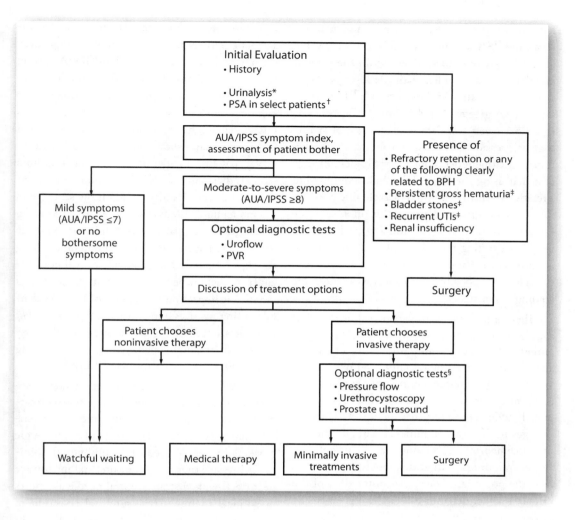

Figure 9-3. Benign prostatic hyperplasia diagnosis and treatment.

*In patients with clinically significant prostatic bleeding, a course of a 5 alpha-reductase inhibitor may be used. If bleeding persists, tissue ablative surgery is indicated.

†Patients with at least a 10-year life expectancy for whom knowledge of the presence of prostate cancer would change management or patients for whom the PSA measurement may change the management of voiding symptoms.

‡After exhausting other therapeutic options as discussed in detail in the text.

§Some diagnostic tests are used in predicting response to therapy. Pressure-flow studies are most useful in men prior to surgery.

AUA, American Urological Association; DRE, digital rectal exam; IPSS, International Prostate Symptom Score; PE, physical exam; PSA, prostate-specific antigen; PVR, postvoid residual urine; UTI, urinary tract infection.

Urinalysis is recommended for all men presenting with LUTS. Normal findings assist in ruling out bladder cancer, stones, UTI, urethral strictures or other non-BPH causes.[50] Prostate specific antigen (PSA) measurement is not part of the diagnostic workup of BPH, but it can help exclude prostate cancer as a cause of urinary tract obstruction. PSA levels should be obtained from men with at least a ten-year life expectancy where knowledge about the presence of prostate cancer would alter management, or for whom measuring PSA would change the management of their voiding symptoms.[50] This test is controversial since PSA levels are only one predictor of the natural history of BPH and the recommendations regarding PSA screening do not address the value of testing asymptomatic men within the general population. Concern lies with the test specificity since approximately 25% of men with BPH have a serum PSA greater than 4 ng/mL.[50] It is believed that PSA levels correlate with the risk of symptom progression and prostate volume which may impact treatment decisions.[49,52-53] Guidelines suggest that using the PSA and rectal exam provide a relatively sensitive method of excluding prostate cancer as a diagnosis. Perhaps this offers a better explanation of the role of utilizing both screenings. PSA testing must be explained to patients; in most cases a normal rectal exam is sufficient to exclude locally advanced cancer as a reason for voiding abnormality.[50]

There are many pharmacological agents that should be avoided in men with BPH due to the potential to worsen symptoms. Alpha adrenergic agonists used as decongestants (oral or intranasal) can lead to muscle contraction secondary to alpha adrenergic receptor stimulation in the prostate. Bladder emptying may be affected due to changes to the urethral lumen. Examples include pseudoephedrine, ephedrine, or phenylephrine. In general, drugs with anticholinergic properties have the potential to decrease contractility of the urinary bladder detrusor muscle. This is especially problematic in patients with BPH with a narrowed urethral lumen and an enlarged prostate gland. This loss of effective detrusor contraction can result in urinary retention. Example agents include antihistamines, tricyclic antidepressants, antipsychotics, or muscle relaxants. Despite this, anticholinergic drugs must be used carefully when LUTS persist despite traditional interventions. In addition, opiates may impair autonomic function and diuretics may lead to polyuria. Theoretically, testosterone replacement regimens used in primary or secondary hypogonadism should be used cautiously as these agents can be metabolized by the prostate to DHT.[48-49]

Treatment of BPH

Since BPH is a disease characterized by symptoms, treatment is focused on determining the severity of the symptoms and the individual's desire to relieve those symptoms. Treatment and management options include watchful waiting, drug therapy, and surgical interventions. The American Urology Association Guidelines on the Management of BPH is a primary tool governing treatment decisions within the United States. Within this guideline, the symptom index and quality of life questionnaire shown in Figure 9-2 is used to survey patients to identify their total symptom score. Individuals are classified as mild, moderate, or severe disease severity based on the score (mild ≤7, moderate 8-19, and severe ≥ 20). According to the guidelines, patients with mild or moderate scores should be managed using a watchful waiting strategy. Generally, these individuals will not benefit from therapy because symptoms do not have a significant impact on the quality of life.[50] Watchful waiting involves annual visits for reassessment and education about behavioral strategies that may assist with symptom management (i.e., avoiding medications that can exacerbate BPH).[48-50]

Individuals with bothersome moderate to severe symptoms and a score ≥ 8 have several treatment options available including medical watchful waiting, medical therapies (alpha adrenergic blockers or 5-alpha reductase inhibitors), minimally invasive therapies (transurethral microwave heat treatments or transurethral needle ablation), or surgical therapies (transurethral resection of the prostate or open prostatectomy). The risks and benefits of each option should be discussed with the patient to allow the most individualized therapy to be selected.[50]

Current drug treatment options for BPH generally include alpha adrenergic blockers, 5-alpha reductase inhibitors, or a combination of the two classes. Short term improvements including the relief of BPH symptoms and an increased urinary flow have been demonstrated with both alpha adrenergic blockers and 5-alpha reductase inhibitor therapy. Clear evidence is not available to prove that alpha adrenergic blockers alone can reduce the need for future prostate surgical procedures, but 5-alpha reductase inhibitors have shown reductions in the need for surgical interventions.[54] Overall, drug therapy is not as efficacious as surgical interventions, however, this option may offer symptom relief with fewer and less severe associated adverse events.[50]

Alpha adrenergic antagonists relieve symptoms in men suffering from moderate to severe BPH. Smooth muscles in the prostate gland contract in response to stimulation by alpha receptors leading to constriction of the prostatic urethra. Alpha blockers improve LUTS by encouraging smooth muscle relaxation. In addition to prostate effects, doxazosin and terazosin, considered to be non-selective alpha$_1$ adrenergic antagonists, also decrease blood pressure by their effect on vascular smooth muscle and carry an FDA labeling for hypertension. Tamsulosin and alfuzosin are newer agents that treat constriction of prostate smooth muscle.[49-50] Tamsulosin is a selective antagonist of alpha$_{1a}$ adrenoreceptors of the prostate and alfuzosin is a selective antagonist of post synaptic alpha$_1$ adrenoreceptors located in the prostate, bladder base, bladder neck, prostatic capsule, and prostatic urethra.[55-56] Alpha blockers may cause orthostatic hypotension and non-selective agents must be started at a low dose and titrated to efficacy; dose titration is not required for alfuzosin.[56] By targeting the lower urinary tract and prostatic smooth muscles, tamsulosin and alfuzosin appear to have favorable safety profiles, however, warnings for syncope and orthostatic hypotension remain in the product labeling.[54-55] The incidence of orthostatic hypotension is increased when alpha blockers are combined with drugs that can exacerbate hypotension and caution must be exercised in these situations.[49]

Alfuzosin, doxazosin, tamsulosin, and terazosin are recommended as appropriate treatment options for LUTS secondary to BPH. There are differences among these drugs regarding adverse event profiles, but in terms of clinical effectiveness, the drugs are similar. Treated patients can expect a 4–6 point improvement in the symptom index.[50] Time to peak effect on BPH symptoms differs among the agents: tamsulosin and alfuzosin generally will peak within several days, while doxazosin and terazosin may take several weeks.[48] Methodically sound trials that compare these agents against each other are needed to show superiority for any particular agent.[50] Numerous trials document that doxazosin, terazosin, alfusozin, and tamsulosin are effective as single agents in both symptom relief and increased urine flow when compared to placebo. Doxazosin monotherapy has also demonstrated decreased long-term complications of BPH including urinary incontinence, urinary retention and renal insufficiency.[57] There is insufficient data to recommend the use of the alpha$_1$ adrenergic antagonists prazosin or phenoxybenzamine as treatment options for LUTS secondary to BPH.[50]

Dihydrotestosterone is an androgenic hormone that stimulates growth of the prostate. Alpha reductase inhibitors, finasteride and dutasteride, inhibit the conversion of testosterone to dihydrotesterone.[49] These medications offer more benefit when the prostate volume is greater than 40 mL.[52] One meta analysis suggested that finasteride is more effective in men with large versus small prostate size.[58]

Alpha reductase inhibitors are appropriate and effective options for individuals with prostate enlargement and LUTS and have been shown to modify the clinical disease course and potentially reduce the risk of urinary retention and surgical interventions.[50,59] PSA levels are decreased with 5-alpha reductase inhibitor therapy so it is recommended to obtain baseline PSA levels prior to beginning treatment. Although the guidelines suggest that cancer detection is not masked, it is recommended to perform PSA and rectal exams annually and any increases in PSA should be evaluated for medication noncompliance and/or prostate cancer.[48,50]

Differences exist between finasteride and dutasteride. Finasteride competitively inhibits type II 5-alpha reductase and lowers intraprostatic DHT by 80–90% and serum DHT by 70%. On the other hand, dutasteride is a dual nonselective inhibitor of type I and II 5 alpha reductase. Intraprostatic DHT production is quickly and completely suppressed and serum DHT is decreased by about 90% with dutasteride. Despite these pharmacodynamic differences, direct comparison trials have not shown any advantage of these actions in favor of dutasteride and both agents have demonstrated comparable efficacy in reducing prostate size.[48]

One important consideration is that 5-alpha reductase inhibitors are not as effective as an alpha blocker in improving LUTS. These agents are not an appropriate treatment recommendation for men without prostate enlargement.[50] Alpha reductase inhibitors do not provide immediate symptom relief; six months of therapy is generally required to achieve clinical benefit.[60] Overall, an evidence-based review determined that 5-alpha reductase inhibitor therapy partially relieves symptoms but is less effective for symptom control than alpha blocker therapy. However, due to the more progressive disease in men with larger prostate glands or for those with higher PSA values, 5-alpha reductase inhibitors have a role in modifying BPH and its clinical course that is not found with alpha blockers.[50,61]

There are instances when combination therapy with alpha blockers and 5-alpha reductase inhibitors may be beneficial, especially in men with larger prostate size and elevated PSA.[50,57,62] These patients appear to be at an increased risk for disease progression highlighted by worsening symptoms and complications of disease.[48] Combination therapy makes sense theoretically in that the alpha blocker will begin to work for symptomatic relief until the finasteride can begin to reduce prostate size. Combination therapy with finasteride and doxazosin has been most investigated.[50] Recent studies have been conducted involving dutasteride and tamsulosin and this prompted an FDA approval for dutasteride and tamsulosin in combination for the treatment of symptomatic BPH in men with an enlarged prostate.[62-63] Two large studies, the MTOPS and the ComBAT, evaluated combination drug therapy vs. monotherapy using either doxazosin and finasteride or dutasteride and tamsulosin. Although there were baseline differences between the MTOPS and ComBAT study groups, the results of the two studies support the use of combination therapy in men with prostate enlargement and moderate to severe LUTS in achieving further symptomatic benefit.[64-66]

Alpha blockers, alpha reductase inhibitors, or even surgery (discussed below) may all improve bladder emptying or urinary flow. However, there is a potential role for the addition of an anticholinergic agent such as oxybutynin or tolterodine to improve irritative voiding symptoms such as frequency and urgency associated with BPH.[48] LUTS, BPH, and OAB are related but the mechanisms linking them are not well understood. One theory is that bladder outlet obstruction (BOO) may lead to OAB.[67] Anticholinergic agents can reduce detrusor contractions by blocking muscarinic receptors in the detrusor muscle. Since older adults are especially sensitive to the CNS adverse effects and dry mouth of anticholinergic drugs, they must be chosen carefully and used with extreme caution as discussed within the urinary incontinence portion of this chapter. In addition, the use of anticholinergic agents in individuals with BPH may also lead to acute urinary retention or increased post void residual urine volume.[48,67] The current AAU Clinical Practice Guideline does not support the use of anticholinergic agents in men with LUTS suggestive of BPH, however, these drugs have been utilized by clinicians and several recent studies have demonstrated benefits.[50,67] One recent meta analysis concluded that the addition of an anticholinergic agent may be beneficial in men with symptomatic overactive bladder and BPH who are unrelieved with alpha blocker treatment. Long-term data is lacking and the risk benefit must be considered. At minimum, it is appropriate to measure post void residual volume prior to beginning therapy to rule out baseline urinary retention.[68]

Dietary Supplements

In addition to pharmacological agents, alternative therapies may be considered by some patients. Saw palmetto plant extract (Serenoa repens) has been used to manage the lower urinary tract symptoms of BPH. The mechanism of action of saw palmetto is unknown in the management of BPH. Possible proposed mechanisms include preventing the conversion of testosterone to dihydrotestosterone, potential anti-inflammatory activity, or prostate epithelial involution similar to effects noted with other 5-alpha reductase inhibitors.[69] This proposed mechanism of saw palmetto suggests a possible drug interaction between this product and standard drug therapy for BPH. Individuals should be counseled and warned about this combination. There have been mixed opinions regarding the value of saw palmetto. A Cochrane review concluded that saw palmetto offered mild to moderate benefits in urinary flow measures and symptoms.[70] However, a recent randomized trial measuring changes in the symptom index and maximal urinary flow rates did not validate those results and found that saw palmetto did not improve symptoms or objective measures of BPH after 1 year of therapy.[71] Current practice guidelines do not recommend saw palmetto or other forms of phytotherapy for BPH.[50]

Surgery

Surgery is another intervention utilized in the management of BPH. In situations where medical treatment is ineffective, in patients with moderate to severe symptoms, or for individuals who prefer surgical intervention, surgery is an option.[48] Men experiencing complications from BPH such as acute urinary retention also may opt for surgical intervention as an initial therapy depending on individual risks versus benefits.[50] Surgical removal of the prostate, or prostatectomy, provides the highest rate of symptom improvement, but it also carries the greatest complication risk.[48] Transurethral resection of the prostate (TURP) is considered the standard surgical therapy for BPH because of the extensive success and follow-up data that are published with this procedure. Some newer surgical techniques are available, but the TURP remains the preferred technique.[49-50]

Surgery is more effective for men with moderate symptoms of BPH or in men with enlarged prostates less than 50 g compared to watchful waiting in improving genitourinary symptom and reducing treatment failure.[48,50,72] Complications reported with this procedure include sexual dysfunction, irritation with voiding, bladder neck contracture, need for blood transfusions, infection, and hematuria.[50] Newer surgical procedures include transurethral needle ablation, transurethral incision of the prostate, and transurethral microwave therapy. These procedures are minimally invasive, short, and an option for men who are poor surgical candidates for TURP.[48-49,73]

Urinary Tract Infections

Overview of Urinary Tract Infections in the Elderly

Urinary tract infection (UTI) is a frequent problem in the elderly population and represents the most common type of nosocomial infection found in long term care facilities.[74] Risk factors include benign prostatic hyperplasia, catheter use, and atrophic vaginitis. The clinical presentation is often atypical. The body's host defenses decline with age and this impacts the diagnosis, prevention, and treatment of UTI. Most UTIs in the elderly are complicated infections due to anatomical, structural or functional abnormalities of the urinary tract. In addition, older people with UTIs often have impaired renal function, concurrent disease states, and compromised immune status that adds to the complex nature of the infection.[75-76]

UTIs can be classified based on location as cystitis (bladder), urethritis (urethra), or pyelonephritis (kidney). In men, prostatitis can mimic or complicate UTIs and this is an important consideration. The prevalence of UTI increases with age in both males and females, but the female:male ratio is 2:1 in the elderly. Symptomatic UTIs are estimated to occur in as many as 10% of older adults each year, although the percentages of new infections may be lower because many of the infections are recurrent. General symptoms include dysuria, recent onset incontinence, urinary frequency, flank pain, confusion, or fever. In many instances, UTI symptoms present differently in the elderly and they may often be difficult to recognize.[75-77]

Asymptomatic **bacteriuria** (ASB) is common in the elderly; the estimated prevalence for those older than 70 years of age living in the community approaches 20%, and can reach 40–50% in long term care facilities for males and females respectively.[77] Asymptomatic bacteriuria is a term that dates back to the 1950s and was described as the presence of two consecutive clean-voided specimens yielding positive cultures ($\geq 10^5$ cfu/mL) of the same uropathogen in an individual without any urinary symptoms.[74] Newer guidelines from the Infectious Disease Society of America add further criteria to include diagnosing men with a single, clean catch urinary specimen, lowering the threshold in a catheterized sample, and describing that **pyuria** does not differentiate symptomatic from asymptomatic bacteriuria.[77]

The genitourinary tract is usually sterile, except for the distal urethra. ASB is a complex condition occurring when bacteria ascends up the urethra into the bladder with possible entrance into the kidneys. Bacteria usually originate as colonizing flora of the gut, vagina, or periurethral area. *Escherichia coli* is the most common organism, but *Klebsiella pneumoniae, Enterococcus* species, group B streptococci, and *Gardnerella vaginalis* may also be involved.[78] According to the Infectious Disease Society of America, routine screening for ASB is not suggested for older persons living in the community or institutional settings.[77] Additionally, without genitourinary localization of symptoms, bacteriuria should not be treated as discussed later in this section.[77] Screening and treatment for ASB is currently recommended in two situations: before transurethral resection of the prostate in men and before urologic procedures where mucosal bleeding is anticipated.[77]

The presence or absence of symptoms alone cannot diagnose UTIs. Also, since 30–50% of nursing home residents will have a positive urine culture at any time; a positive culture alone is not clinically significant. Symptoms of UTI are less specific in patients requiring higher levels of care in long-term care facilities. Close monitoring and reassessment of clinical status is a rational approach for these individuals since there are many inconsistencies between genitourinary findings and correlation to a UTI.[74]

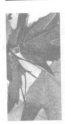 KEY POINT: Making the decision to culture a urine sample for a potential UTI is based on the presence of symptoms. Without symptoms, the recommendation is to not culture.

The diagnosis of a symptomatic UTI can be complex in older adults. Common symptoms such as dysuria, urinary frequency, recent onset incontinence, flank pain or fever may be absent or overlooked. Co-morbidities such as degenerative neurological diseases and/or neurogenic bladder are an equally important consideration in addition to the clinical presentation. Catheterization

is also a complicating factor. Although delirium or functional decline may occur with UTI, this is unlikely unless fever or sepsis is also present. This is not always the case in advanced dementia, where this type of decline may be the only obvious presenting symptom.[79] Other nonspecific symptoms including clinical deterioration are often attributed to UTI, especially in the long-term care setting, but studies have not supported this finding. The presence of foul smelling or cloudy urine may be associated with UTIs due to the polyamines produced by some urinary bacteria, and this can lead to a prescription for an antibiotic. However, not all UTIs have an unpleasant odor and not all of the cultures identified as having a foul odor are bacteriuric. Other factors such as medication use, food, continence management, and dehydration status must be considered.[80]

There is a lack of empiric data to provide criteria for surveillance, diagnosis and treatment of UTIs in long term care settings. Various infection control organizations and consensus groups provide recommendations to assist with the diagnosis of UTIs.[78] Several are based on the McGeer criteria, where three of the following conditions must be met for a suspected UTI that is not associated with an indwelling catheter.[78-79]

- Fever (>38 ºC) or chills
- New or increased burning sensation upon urination
- New flank pain or suprapubic tenderness
- Changes in urine properties
- Mental function decline
- Individuals with an indwelling catheter must have two of the following criteria for a suspected UTI. [78-79]
  - Fever (>38 ºC or chills)
  - New flank pain or suprapubic tenderness
  - Changes in urine properties
  - Mental function decline

In general, isolating significant numbers of microorganisms in an appropriate urine specimen to distinguish contamination from infection is the key to microbiological diagnosis of a

UTI.[81] In symptomatic individuals residing in long term care facilities, a quantitative count of ≥ 10^5 CFU/mL of an organism in a single specimen is diagnostic. A urine specimen may be difficult to obtain in non-cooperative individuals or in those with cognitive impairment, particularly in women. Catheterized urine specimens with a count of ≥ 10^3 CFU/mL from a single predominant pathogen is sufficient for the microbiological diagnosis of UTI.[80] Most UTIs associated with bacteremia in community dwelling older adults are due to gram negative organisms such as *E coli* and 20% are due to gram positive organisms (i.e., *enterococcus* or methicillin-resistant *Staphylococcus aureus [MRSA]*). *E coli* is still the primary pathogen cultured from institutionalized older adults, but *P aeroginosa*, vancomycin-resistant enterocci, *Candida* spp, and non-*E coli* Enterobacteriaceae are nosocomial pathogens often identified.[78] Once the organism is quantified and identified, the organism susceptibility must be determined. Knowledge of the achievable urine concentration of the antibiotic, as well as the bacterial susceptibility of the pathogen, allows the optimal agent to be selected for treatment.[81]

An additional diagnostic consideration is pyuria. Pyuria is almost always present in combination with symptomatic UTI, however, in elderly long-term care residents, 90% of asymptomatic individuals and 30% of individuals without bacteriuria have pyuria. This is presumed to be due to other causes of bladder, genital, prostate or renal inflammation. It is often possible to rule out a UTI diagnosis in the absence of pyuria, but the presence of pyuria is not sufficient for a diagnosis. If bacteriuria is present, pyuria does not allow differentiation between asymptomatic and symptomatic infection. In addition, long-term outcomes are not predictable based on the level of pyuria.[80]

Treatment of Urinary Tract Infection

The goals of treating urinary tract infections are to prevent or treat systemic consequences of infection, eliminate the invading organism, and prevent recurrence of infection. Initial antimicrobial selection is based on the site (upper or lower urinary tract) and signs and symptoms of the infection, and whether the infection is considered complicated or uncomplicated.[81] Most symptomatic urinary tract infections are considered complicated in the elderly.[74] When selecting an agent for an older adult, there are many pharmaceutical considerations including efficacy, susceptibility, adverse effects, tolerability, potential overuse leading to resistance (especially in the long term care population), as well as cost.[80,82]

Age and disease related physiological changes must also be addressed when choosing an appropriate antibiotic to treat a urinary tract infection.[83] An increased potential for adverse effects may be expected when renal dose adjustments do not occur. Elderly patients are also more vulnerable to experiencing drug side effects and drug related problems may still result, even in the absence of documented renal dysfunction.[84] Specific agents commonly used for UTI that need to be renally dosed include nitrofurantoin (avoid use in GFR < 50 mL/min), and fluoroquinolones.[85] Fluoroquinolones have been cited in a recent FDA advisory warning about the increase of tendonitis and tendon rupture in adults over age 60.[86]

As previously discussed, according to the infectious disease guidelines for asymptomatic bacteriuria, routine screening and treatment is not recommended for older adults residing within the community or long term care facilities.[77] Treatment of symptomatic UTI should not be postponed while awaiting culture and sensitivity results.[79] If empiric antibiotic therapy is initiated, previous urine cultures in the patient and, if applicable, endemic institutional pathogens should be considered when choosing an agent.[80] Limited comparative data exists and interpretation is challenging due to the heterogeneity of the study population, enrollment of both genders, asymptomatic vs. symptomatic subjects, sample size, and limited follow-up. Based on the available studies, superiority has not been demonstrated with one particular antimicrobial agent regarding efficacy or adverse effects (Table 9-3).[85,87]

In addition to selecting the appropriate agent, the proper duration of therapy must be considered. It is necessary to determine if an infection is uncomplicated or complicated prior to establish-

Table 9-3. Common Antimicrobial Agents Used in the Treatment of Urinary Tract Infections Within the Older Adult Population and Their Renal Dose Adjustment Requirements[85, 87]

Class/Agent	Dose Adjust in Mild to Moderate* Renal Impairment?	Dose Adjust in Moderate to Severe** Renal Impairment?
B-Lactam/lactamase inhibitor		
Amoxicillin/clavulanic acid	No	Yes
Cephalosporins		
cefuroxime axetil	No	Yes
cephalexin	Yes	Yes
Fluoroquinolones		
ciprofloxacin	No	Yes
levofloxacin	No	Yes
norfloxacin	No	Yes
Penicillin		
amoxicillin	No	Yes
Sulfonamide		
trimethoprim/sulfamethoxazole	No	Yes (not recommended in CrCl < 15 mL/min)
Tetracycline		
doxycycline	No	No
Miscellaneous		
nitrofurantoin	Avoid in CrCl < 50 mL/min	Avoid in CrCl < 50 mL/min

*Estimated CrCl > 40 mL/min.
**Estimated CrCl <10–40 mL/min.
Please refer to manufacturer labeling for specific dosing information.

ing the appropriate course, however, many UTIs in older adults are considered to be complicated. Especially in older adult male patients, all infections should be treated as complicated.[84,87] Additionally, patients with an atypical symptom presentation do not clearly allow for the differentiation between uncomplicated and complicated infection. Because elderly individuals are not well represented in clinical trials of short term courses of antibiotic drug regimens (such as 3-day therapy), these protocols are not generally utilized. Overall, recommendations suggest durations of at least 7–10 days, especially in the long-term care setting. Longer therapies may be advocated if known complications exist such as structural bladder abnormality (10–14 days) or pyelonephritis (14–21 days).[84] Male patients should be evaluated for prostatitis because this condition requires the selection of an agent that

will penetrate the prostate tissue effectively and the duration of therapy will be longer (30 days to 6 weeks).[87] Currently, there is no evidence to recommend post treatment urine cultures to document cure in the absence of symptoms.[80]

One study evaluated a female population of nursing home and community dwelling elderly and demonstrated that 98% of the individuals residing in a nursing home received antibiotic therapy for over seven days, compared to 77% of the community subjects. Nursing home patients in the study were five times more likely to have at least 10 days of therapy. In addition, the frequency of infection relapses and drug side effects were higher in the nursing home group.[88] Overall, although recommendations exist, data is inconclusive regarding an established duration of therapy that is appropriate for older adults, both in the nursing home and community.

Special Consideration: Catheters and Recurrent Infections

A special situation to consider involves UTIs in individuals with catheters. Within long term care facilities, up to 10% of residents have chronic indwelling catheters. Despite the use of a closed catheter system, there is an 80–95% chance of bacteriuria occurring after 30 days of catheterization, often with two to five organisms present. Criteria has been previously described for diagnosing catheter associated UTIs within this chapter. Systemic antibiotics will sterilize the urine, however, re-infection can occur and resistant organisms may become problematic.[77,80-81] Antibiotic therapy considerations are similar to individuals without catheters and similarly, the optimal duration of therapy is not known.[80]

In catheterized individuals, bacteriuria may be prevented by minimizing chronic indwelling catheter use and discontinuing the catheter if possible. Individuals with chronic indwelling catheters with symptomatic infection may benefit by limiting catheter obstruction or trauma. Closed drainage systems appear to decrease infection in the short term, however, in longer use, bacteriuria becomes inevitable. Routine irrigation of catheters has not been proven to lower rates of symptomatic UTI or catheter obstruction.[80]

Recurrent episodes of UTIs frequently occur. Most recurrent infections are considered re-infections, described as the recurrence of infection with an organism other than the organism identified from the previous infection.[81] In institutionalized older adults, catheterization, incontinence, antimicrobial exposure, and functional status are the predisposing factors most frequently related to recurrent UTI.[78] In postmenopausal women, history of UTI during premenopause, incontinence, presence of a **cystocele**, and post void residual urine increase the likelihood of UTI. Specific risk factors for older men include dementia, bladder and bowel incontinence, benign prostatic hyperplasia, and catheter use.[78] Preventing urinary tract infections is an area of concern in all older adults. Management strategies depend on predisposing factors, the number of annual episodes, and patient preferences.

The remaining recurrent infections are classified as relapses. These are persistent infections with the same organism after completion of therapy for a UTI. This usually indicates that the patient has renal involvement, a structural abnormality of the urinary tract, or chronic bacterial prostatitis. Continued therapy and/or urological evaluation may be necessary to rule out obstruction. In males, bacterial prostatitis must be considered.[81]

When considering antimicrobial prophylaxis for recurrent infection, an important indicator is the degree of discomfort that is experienced as a result of infection. The optimal method of prophylaxis is based on the frequency and pattern of recurrence.[89] In patients with infrequent episodes of UTIs (less than three infections yearly), each individual episode should be treated.[81] Continuous prophylaxis has been demonstrated in multiple studies in various population groups to decrease recurrences from two to three episodes per patient year to 0.1 to 0.2 per patient year.[89] However, this evidence is not applicable specifically to older adults because the trials focused on younger, healthy women in outpatient settings. It is not appropriate to recommend the same prophylactic regimens for older patients that have not been proven in this population. Individuals in the community and long term care facilities may be prescribed antimicrobial agents for prophylaxis, including trimethoprim-sulfamethoxazole, nitrofurantoin, and cephalexin.[89-90] There are safety concerns when introducing medications without sound justification, and a very real concern about the development of resistant pathogens that must not be overlooked when considering antimicrobial preventative therapy. This is especially problematic in the long term-care setting with infection control issues. Until definitive studies are conducted to better identify the appropriateness of antimicrobial prophylaxis in UTIs, this practice should be discouraged in older adults.[89-90] If antimicrobial prophylaxis is prescribed, monitoring is required to identify recurrent infection despite the presence of the medication. In such instances, the chronic suppressive regimen should be discontinued due to lack of efficacy.

Methenamine, a urinary antiseptic, carries a labeling from the Food and Drug Administration for UTI prophylaxis, usually when given with vitamin C to achieve an acid environment. However, achieving an acidic urinary pH is often unattainable due to the presence of *proteus, Enterobacter sp*, or *P aeruginosa*; common pathogens in long-term care facilities. Further, methenamine salts may lead to gastrointestinal side effects and should not be used in the presence of compromised renal function. Overall, preventive therapy with methenamine is not a useful approach.[90]

In postmenopausal women, there is evidence that intravaginal administration of estrogen cream prevents recurrent urinary tract infections based on a randomized, double blind, placebo controlled study performed in 93 postmenopausal women.[91] Estrogen deficiency in post menopausal women experiencing recurrent UTIs causes vaginal bacterial flora alterations that can lead to increased colonization of *E. coli*. The presumed mechanism of effect of topical estrogen is based on reversal of the microbiological changes in the vaginal flora.[90-91] Due to the risks associated with estrogen use, even in low dose topical forms, the optimal place in therapy or duration of treatment for this type of UTI intervention is not clear.

Cranberries or cranberry juice possess antibacterial activity by preventing bacterial adherence to the lining of the urinary tract, an initial step in UTI pathogenesis. Proanthocyanidin found in cranberries plays a role in compromising the function of common UTI organisms such as *E coli*, which prevents the initial attachment step from occurring. Literature evaluating the effectiveness of cranberry in the older adult population has offered mixed results. Various designs have been utilized, and the studies all have limitations. There is a low risk of harm in initiating cranberry juice as a potential method of preventing infection recurrence, and with some suggested benefits, it may be a viable option for some individuals who enjoy this beverage.[90]

Ascorbic acid, or vitamin C, has been used as a urinary acidifier in chronic and recurrent UTIs in older adults. At usual doses, the urinary acidification properties of ascorbic acid are minimal and there are insufficient well-designed studies to provide support for its place in therapy. Another consideration for older adults is that ascorbic acid is metabolized to oxalic acid, and high doses of vitamin C can lead to the development of calcium oxalate stones. If these stones are deposited in the renal tissues, bacterial overgrowth and subsequent UTIs may result leading to additional negative consequences.[90]

Non-pharmacologic Interventions for UTIs

Non pharmacological prevention of UTIs in older adults should always be employed. Observance and implementation of infection control practices are paramount, beginning with appropriate hand washing. Within long term care facilities, staff education and implementation of these practices are imperative. Elderly women who perform their own personal hygiene should be reminded to wipe from front to back after a bowel movement or urinating. Caregivers at home and long-term care facility must assist with this if necessary. If an individual is incapable of implementing appropriate infection control practices to prevent the recurrence of UTIs, then it becomes a larger burden on the part of the caregivers.[90]

Screening for medications that may worsen urinary retention is one final way to minimize the risk of UTIs, and can be considered a prevention strategy. Examples include narcotic analgesics, sedatives, and anticholinergic medications that compromise normal voiding procedures. Elderly patients, especially males with benign prostatic hyperplasia, are especially sensitive to the effects of anticholinergics.[90] While these agents may not be the cause for a UTI, it is one more reason to be selective with choosing appropriate drug therapy in older adults.

CASE 1: INCONTINENCE IN A NURSING HOME RESIDENT WITH DEMENTIA

Setting:

Quarterly care conference

Subjective:

JD is an 85 year-old Caucasian male resident of a long term care facility. He has no complaints, but the nursing staff is concerned about an increased frequency of urinary incontinence episodes.

Past Medical History:

JD was admitted to the long term care facility for care on the Alzheimer's disease and related dementia unit with a mini-mental exam score of 15/30, a decline of 2 points from the exam administered 1 year ago. His past medical history is significant for hypertension, and benign prostatic hyperplasia.

Medications:

Donepezil 10 mg once daily, hydrochlorothiazide 25 mg once daily, lisinopril 20 mg daily, a multivitamin daily, docusate 100 mg two times/day, bisacodyl 10 mg once daily as needed for constipation, and Tylenol PM one tablet at bedtime.

Allergies:

NKDA

Social History:

Unknown

Family History:

Non-contributory

Objective:

Height 5'10", weight 72 kg, blood pressure 90/65 mmHg, pulse 75 beats/minute, respiration 18 breaths/min, and temperature 37 °C.

Physical Exam:

Unremarkable and assessment of his functional abilities shows limitations in his activities of daily living requiring assistance with bathing and dressing.

Laboratory:

Normal CBC, sodium 129 mEq/L, potassium 3.4 mEq/L, chloride 100 mEq/L, and carbon dioxide 29 mEq/L, fasting glucose 85 mg/dL, creatinine 1.2 mg/dL, and blood urea nitrogen 28 mg/dL. (Calculated CrCl = 46 mL/min)

Assessment:

1. Urinary symptoms due to untreated benign prostatic hyperplasia, exacerbated by unnecessary anticholinergic medication, diuretic, and cholinesterase inhibitor.

2. Blood pressure and electrolytes such as sodium and potassium are either low or approaching the low end of the desired range, possibly associated with the thiazide diuretic.

3. Alzheimer's disease: Cognitive symptoms show a slight decline over the previous year and may be exacerbated by the anticholinergic medication. A drug interaction between donepezil and the anticholinergic is a concern. Complaints of insomnia are presumably a reason the Tylenol PM was started, however this is not formally documented and is not presenting as a current complaint.

Plan:

1. Discontinue the Tylenol PM related to urinary retention symptoms. If urinary symptoms persist, recommend initiation of tamsulosin 0.4 mg daily. Obtain urine sample to rule out possible UTI as a cause of symptoms. Monitor blood pressure with addition of alpha blocker, monitor cognition with removal of anticholinergic medication.

2. Continue lisinopril and decrease the dose of hydrochlorothiazide to 12.5 mg daily. Monitor blood pressure and serum electrolytes.

3. Discontinue Tylenol PM (above) and continue donepezil therapy at this time while observing changes in urinary symptoms and cognition. Monitor sleep patterns and level of alertness.

Rationale:

1. It is possible that urinary symptoms may resolve simply with elimination of the anticholinergic medication. If not, alpha blockers are considered first-line treatment for BPH symptoms, but nonselective agents such as doxazosin or terazosin may exacerbate his low blood pressure. This is less of a concern with tamsulosin, but can still be problematic so careful monitoring of blood pressure is required during drug initiation. Reduction in the thiazide diuretic dose may offset some of the hypotensive effect of tamsulosin.

2. JD is receiving appropriate medications for an individual with hypertension and chronic kidney disease, however his blood pressure is low and he is experiencing a mild amount of hyponatremia and hypokalemia. It is not clear the extent to which the diuretic may be exacerbating incontinence symptoms, but this can be reevaluated as therapy for BPH is initiated.

3. It is difficult to evaluate JD's true magnitude or quality of response to a cholinesterase inhibitor while there is an antagonizing medication taken concomitantly. Therefore no changes to the donepezil should be made until this complicating factor is removed. It is also unclear if the cholinesterase inhibitor is worsening urinary symptoms, but due to JD's stable cognitive status, changes to donepezil should be avoided. After the effects of the tamsulosin and diuretic reduction have been observed, possible interactions between the cholinesterase inhibitor and urinary symptoms can be evaluated. It is difficult to discern whether the lack of a documented indication for the Tylenol PM is simply oversight, or if the drug can be accurately assessed as "unnecessary". In light of his urinary symptoms and dementia with cholinesterase inhibitor use, it is more prudent to discontinue Tylenol PM at this time, while monitoring for any possible reemergence of insomnia symptoms.

Case Summary:

This patient is typical of an older man with multiple coexisting medical conditions and pharmacotherapeutic treatments. The chief complaint involves urinary symptoms; however, it is evident that the current medication regimen and any changes made to it carries implications for his other co-morbid conditions. Drug therapy interventions must be made in a careful stepwise approach considering the potential impact on the target disease state and co-morbid disease states. In this case, discontinuation of Tylenol PM and reduction of hydrochlorothiazide are the only two interventions taken initially, followed by possible initiation of tamsulosin if urinary symptoms persist. At the same time, the hope is to maximize the effectiveness of donepezil and defer making any changes to donepezil unless absolutely necessary. The two initial changes may not only impact the chief complaint but also the blood pressure, electrolytes, and cognition.

CASE 2: A COMMUNITY DWELLING WOMAN WITH NEW ONSET URINARY INCONTINENCE

Setting:
Outpatient/assisted living setting

Subjective:
MM is a 92-year-old Caucasian woman who resides in an assisted living facility. At the request of the staff, she is being evaluated today in the office of her primary care physician. Although there are no known baseline deficits in cognition and she is usually continent, she has developed new onset of confusion and urinary incontinence. The facility staff report that "she just got over this."

Past Medical History:
MM has a history of glaucoma, osteoarthritis, and osteopenia. She had an appendectomy in 1976 and was treated for a UTI 3 weeks ago.

Medications:
Timolol 0.25% solution, instill 1 drop in both eyes twice daily, acetaminophen 500 mg four times daily, calcium carbonate 500 mg three times daily, vitamin D 800 IU daily. She recently completed a course of ciprofloxacin 500 mg twice daily. She receives medication reminders from facility staff who confirm that she took all of her antibiotic and regularly prescribed medications.

Allergies:
Penicillin

Social History:
Retired music teacher, widowed 9 years ago

Family History:
Two adult children in good health
Objective: Height 5'5", weight 53 kg, blood pressure 124/75 mmHg, pulse 80 beats/min, respiration 18 breaths/min, and temperature 38 °C.

Physical Exam:
Thin confused elderly female in mild distress, otherwise physical findings unremarkable

Laboratory:
UA reveals dark cloudy urine, positive for nitrite and leukocyte esterase, with many bacteria and WBC. Culture and sensitivity data is pending. CBC reveals WBC 14.2, hemoglobin 12.1, hematocrit 36%, platelets 202.

Chemistry Panel:
Sodium 137 mEq/L, potassium 4.0 mEq/L, chloride 100 mEq/L, and carbon dioxide 28 mEq/L, glucose 92mg/dL, creatinine 1.1 mg/dL, and blood urea nitrogen 28 mg/dL. (Calculated CrCl = 27 mL/min)

MM is diagnosed with a urinary tract infection and has been prescribed nitrofurantoin 50 mg four times daily for 7 days, to be followed by nitrofurantoin 50 mg at bedtime for suppressive therapy.

Assessment:
1. Urinary tract infection that is possibly either recurrent or relapsing.

2. Sub-optimal selection of antibiotic for UTI treatment and unnecessary suppressive therapy.

3. Medication counseling and administration assistance required.

Plan:

1. Replace nitrofurantoin with trimethoprim/sulfamethoxazole 80 mg/400 mg (single strength), one tablet twice daily for 7 days. Monitor for resolution of infection, including urinary symptoms and cognition

2. Complete the acute treatment regimen but discontinue the order for suppressive therapy, monitor for future relapse or recurrence.

3. Provide careful instructions to both MM and her caregivers about medication administration instructions, self monitoring for efficacy and side effects, and precautions such as ensuring good hydration and sunscreen use while on antibiotic therapy.

Rationale:

1. MM's slightly elevated temperature, new onset confusion, and urinary symptoms (sudden incontinence) satisfy the criteria for probable UTI. Although a culture and sensitivity are pending, these presenting signs are confirmed by the UA and the elevated WBC count. The recent history of UTI treated with ciprofloxacin that was administered concomitantly with a calcium supplement might suggest a relapsing infection due to inadequate absorption of the ciprofloxacin/calcium combination. MM could also have a new urinary tract infection.

2. MM's calculated CrCl is 27 mL/min, which is below the threshold needed for optimal nitrofurantoin use. The reoccurrence of MM's infection does not warrant chronic suppressive therapy.

3. MM requires medication assistance for several reasons, including possible poor vision associated with glaucoma, current confusion associated with her infection, and the recent history of a poor drug therapy outcome for the UTI.

Case Summary:

The patient in this case presents with some of the classic features of UTI in the older woman. MM represents an individual who is vulnerable to adverse medication outcomes due to many factors. Her reduced creatinine clearance does not present a problem for her chronic medication regimen, but she must be monitored for dose adjustments when new medications are initiated. Antibiotics commonly require dosage adjustment based on renal function. As an outpatient who must self-administer medications, even with reminders from the staff of the assisted living facility, she is vulnerable to medication related problems.

Co-administration of a fluoroquinolone with calcium is perhaps an example of this. While it is difficult to confirm that a therapeutic failure associated with this interaction is the true cause of the new UTI presentation, this situation could have led to exposure to unnecessary chronic antibiotic use, as her provider has interpreted her to have recurrent UTI.

Clinical Pearls

- *Over-use of loop diuretics is an important contribution to dehydration in the elderly. Often, the dose of diuretic needed to manage acute heart failure is greater than the dose required to maintain a patient with chronic heart failure. Where possible, patients and care-givers should be taught to gauge their fluid response to a loop diuretic by using daily weights. The negative or positive change in weight, in comparison to a person's dry weight, is helpful in managing the appropriate dose of the diuretic.*

- *The two 5-alpha reductase inhibitors finasteride and dutasteride are both Pregnancy Category X and require labeling regarding risk of birth defects. While these medications are prescribed for male patients, the potential for medication handling by female caregivers should not be overlooked. In any circumstance where a caregiver is concerned about the safety of handling drug products, recommendations should be made to wash hands before and after medication administration or to wear gloves.*

Chapter Summary

Renal function declines with age and older patients will frequently develop chronic kidney disease as they enter their 80s and 90s. Older patients also often have other co-morbid diseases such as diabetes and hypertension, which may lead to further deterioration in their renal function. This decline in renal function, in addition to diuretic use, and changes in cognition and environment, increase the risk of dehydration and imbalances in serum sodium. To estimate renal function, pharmacists must calculate the patient's creatinine clearance and assess the older patient's medication regimen to be sure that appropriate renal protection therapies are being utilized and that drugs are screened for their potential to accumulate.

The prevalence of urinary incontinence increases with age although it is not considered an expected part of aging. Age related physiologic changes must be taken into consideration when diagnosing and classifying the various forms of urinary incontinence. Behavioral rehabilitation techniques, medications, and surgery are all possible treatments but must be chosen only after reviewing the goals of therapy with the individual patient. Benign prostatic hyperplasia is the most common urologic condition of aging men. A wide range of signs and symptoms occur in BPH and it is the individual's ability to tolerate the symptoms that is usually the motivating factor to seek treatment. Alpha blockers and or 5-alpha reductase inhibitors are the drugs utilized most, as well as surgical interventions. Information from future long-term studies will help define the role of medication therapy, for both symptom improvement and to delay disease progression of BPH.

Urinary tract infections are a common health concern in older adults and are associated with incontinence, BPH, and other diseases. Patients with suspected UTIs should meet accepted diagnostic criteria before treatment is initiated. Antibiotics prescribed to treat these infections should target specific organisms and be dosed based on the individuals pharmacokinetic elimination parameters.

Self-Assessment Questions

1. What are the common changes in physiology of the kidney that occur with age and how do these changes impact the development of chronic kidney disease?

2. What are the advantages and disadvantages, in an older person, of the commonly used equations to calculate creatinine clearance?

3. Explain what common electrolyte disorder might occur in an older person on a thiazide diuretic. What is the mechanism for this effect?

4. What are the major differences between the signs and symptoms of the types of urinary incontinence? Explain how these symptom differences can help to differentiate between the types of urinary incontinence in a patient.

5. Under what circumstances would an alpha-blocker cause urinary incontinence? Under what circumstances would an alpha-blocker be helpful in treating urinary incontinence?

6. In a patient with overactive bladder, how do you choose between the different anticholinergic medications approved to treat this disorder?

7. In an older man with benign prostatic hyperplasia with severe lower urinary tract symptoms, what is a recommended treatment?

8. In a man with benign prostatic hyperplasia, under what circumstances is it most justified to use the combination of an alpha-blocker and an alpha-reductase inhibitor?

9. In an 85 year old female resident of a nursing home, what signs, symptoms, and laboratory tests are needed to confirm a diagnosis of urinary tract infection?

10. In an 85-year-old female resident of a nursing home, what patient parameters should be considered prior to prescribing an antibiotic for a confirmed urinary tract infection?

References

1. Merck Manual of Geriatrics. Renal and urologic disorders. Available at: http://www.merck.com/mkgr/mmg/sec12/ch98/ch98a.jsp Accessed May 2, 2009.

2. Lindeman RD, Tobin J, Shrock NW. Longitudinal studies on the rate of decline in renal function with age. *J Am Geriatr Soc.* 1985;33:278–281.

3. Levey AS, Coresh J, Balk E, et al. National Kidney Foundation practice guidelines for chronic kidney disease: evaluation, classification, and stratification. *Ann Intern Med.* 2003;139:137–147.

4. U.S. Renal Data System, USRDS 2007 Annual Data Report: Atlas of Chronic Kidney Disease and End-Stage Renal Disease in the United States, National Institutes of Health, National Institute of Diabetes, Digestion, and Kidney Diseases, Bethesda, MD, 2007.

5. O'Hare AM, Choi AI, Bertenthal D, et al. Age affects outcomes in chronic kidney disease. *J Am Soc Nephrol.* 2007;18:2758–2765.

6. Dowling TC. Controversies in assessing kidney function. In: Dunsworth T, Richardson M, Cheng J, et al., eds. *Pharmacotherapy Self-Assessment Program.* 6th ed. Nephrology I. Lenexa, KS: American College of Clinical Pharmacy; 2007:1–10.

7. Stevens LA, Coresh J, Greene T, Levey AS. Assessing kidney function—measured and estimated glomerular filtration rate. *N Engl J Med.* 2006;354:2473–2483.

8. Lamb EJ, Webb MC, Simpson DE, Coakley AJ, Newman DJ, O'Riordan SE. Estimation of glomerular filtration rate in older patients with chronic renal insufficiency: is the modification of diet in renal disease formula an improvement? *J Am Geriatr Soc.* 2003;51:1012–1017.

9. Joy MS, Ksirsagar A, Franceshini N. Chronic kidney disease: progression-modifying therapies. In: DiPiro JT, Talbert RL, Yee GC, et al., eds. *Pharmacotherapy: A Pathophysiologic Approach.* 7th ed. New York: MCGraw-Hill; 2008:745–764.

10. Ohkubo Y, Kishikawa H, Araki E, et al. Intensive insulin therapy prevents the progression of diabetic microvascular complications in Japanese patients with non-insulin-dependent diabetes mellitus: A randomized prospective 6-year study. *Diabetes Res Clin Pract.* 1995;28:103–117.

11. Shichiri M, Ohkubo Y, Kishikawa H, Wake N. Long-term results of the Kumamoto Study on optimal diabetes control in type 2 diabetic patients. *Diabetes Care.* 2000;23(Suppl 2):B21–B29.

12. UK Prospective Diabetes Study (UKPDS) Group: Intensive blood-glucose control with sulphonylureas or insulin compared with conventional treatment and risk of complications in patients with type 2 diabetes (UKPDS 33). *Lancet.* 1998;352:837–853.

13. The ADVANCE Collaborative Group. Intensive blood glucose control and vascular outcomes in patients with Type 2 Diabetes. *N Engl J Med.* 2008;358:2560–2572.

14. The Action to Control Cardiovascular Risk in Diabetes Study Group. Effects of intensive glucose lowering in Type 2 diabetes. *N Engl J Med.* 2008; 358:2545–2559.

15. National Kidney Foundation. KDOQI Clinical Practice Guidelines on diabetes and chronic kidney disease. *Am J Kidney Dis.* 2007;49(S2):S12–154.

16. Gerich JE, Meyer C, Woerle HJ, Stumvoll M. Renal gluconeogenesis: its importance in human glucose homeostasis. *Diabetes Care.* 2001;24:382–391.

17. Chelliah A, Burge MR. Hypoglycemia in elderly patients with diabetes mellitus. *Drugs Aging.* 2004;21(8):511–530.

18. American Diabetes Association. Standards of medical care in diabetics–2009. Available at: www.diabetes.org.

19. Shaw JS, Wilmot RL, Kilpatric ES. Establishing pragmatic estimated GFR thresholds to guide metformin prescribing. *Diabet Med.* 2007;24:1160–1163.

20. Mangoni AA. Cardiovascular drug therapy in elderly patients. Specific age-related pharmacokinetic, pharmacodynamic and therapeutic considerations. *Drugs Aging.* 2005;22:913–941.

21. National Kidney Foundation. KDOQI Clinical Practice Guidelines for managing dyslipidemias in chronic kidney disease. *Am J Kidney Dis.* 2003;41(Suppl 3):S1–S92.

22. Tomasello SR. Bone metabolism and disease in chronic kidney disease. In: Dunsworth T, Richardson M, Cheng J, et al., eds. *Pharmacotherapy Self-Assessment Program.* 6th ed. Nephrology. Lenexa, KS: American College of Clinical Pharmacy; 2008:55–67.

23. Allison SP, Lobo DN. Fluid and electrolytes in the elderly. *Curr Opin Clin Nutr Metab Care.* 2004;7:27–33.

24. Coyle JD, Joy MS. Disorders of sodium and water homeostasis. In: Dipiro JT, Talbert RL, Yee GC, eds. *Pharmacotherapy: A Pathophysiologic Approach.* New York: McGraw Hill Medical; 2008:845–860.

25. Renneboog B, Musch W, Vandemergel X, Manto MU, Decaux G. Mild chronic hyponatremia is associated with falls, unsteadiness, and attention deficits. *Am J Med.* 2006;119:71.e1–8.

26. Jones E. Drug-induced syndrome of inappropriate antidiuretic syndrome. *CPJ/RPC.* 2007;140(6):397–399.

27. National Kidney and Urologic Diseases Information Clearinghouse. Kidney and urologic diseases statistics for the United States. Available at: http://kidney.niddk.nih.gov/kudiseases/pubs/kustats/ Accessed September 5, 2008.

28. American Medical Directors Association. Urinary Incontinence: Clinical Practice Guideline. 2005.

29. Merck Manual of Geriatrics. Urinary incontinence. Available at: http://www.merck.com/mkgr/mmg/sec12/ch99/ch99a.jsp Accessed July 7, 2008.

30. Marshall LL, Bailey W. Urinary incontinence management in geriatric patients. *Consult Pharm.* 2008;23:681–684.

31. Rovner ES, Wman J, Lackner T, et al. Urinary incontinence. In: Dipiro JT, Talbert RL, Yee GC, eds. *Pharmacotherapy: A Pathophysiologic Approach.* New York: McGraw Hill Medical; 2008:1399–1415.

32. DeMaagd G, Geibig JD. An overview of overactive bladder and its pharmacological management with a focus on anticholinergic drugs. *PT.* 2006;31:462–471.

33. Chutka DS, Takahashi PY. Urinary incontinence in the elderly: Drug treatment options. *Drugs.* 1998;56:587–595.

34. Ouslander JG. Management of overactive bladder. *N Engl J Med.* 2004;350:786–799.

35. Martin CM. Urinary incontinence in the elderly. Available at: http://www.ascp.com/publications/tcp/1997/aug/elderly.html. Accessed July 17, 2008.

36. Rosenthal AJ, McMurray CT. Urinary incontinence in the elderly. *Post Grad Med.* 1995;97:109–116.

37. Agency for Healthcare Research and Quality. Overview: Urinary Incontinence in Adults: Clinical Practice Guideline Update. Available at: http://www.ahrq.gov/clinic/uiovervw.htm Accessed July 17, 2008.

38. Holroyd-Ledue JM, Straus SE. Management of urinary incontinence in women: Scientific review. *JAMA.* 2004;291:986–995.

39. Sweeney D, Chancellor MB. Treatment of stress urinary incontinence with duloxetine hydrochloride. *Rev Urol.* 2005;7:81–86.

40. Grady D, Brown JS, Vittinghoff E. Postmenopausal hormones and incontinence: the Heart and Estrogen/Replacement Study. *Obstet Gynecol.* 2001;97:116–120.

41. Rogers, R. Urinary stress incontinence in women. *N Engl J Med.* 2008;358:1029–1036.

42. Duckett, J. Duloxetine as a treatment for stress incontinence: where are we now? *Int Urogynecol J.* 2008;9:1–3.

43. Schagen van Leeuwen JH, Lange RR Fianu Jonasson A, et al. Efficacy and safety of duloxetine in elderly women with stress urinary incontinence or stress-predominant mixed urinary incontinence. *Maturitas.* 2008;60:138–147.

44. Mariappan P, Alhasso A, Ballantyne Z, et al. Duloxetine, a serotonin and noradrenaline reuptake inhibitor (SNRI) for the treatment of stress urinary incontinence: A systematic review. *Eur Urol.* 2007;51:67–74.

45. Yamaguchi O, Nishizawa O, Takeda M, Yokoyama O, Homma Y, Kakizaki H, et al. Clinical guidelines for overactive bladder. *Int J Urol.* 2009;16:126–142.

46. Chughtai B, Levin R, De E. Choice of antimuscarinic agents for overactive bladder in the older patient: focus on darifenacin. *Clin Interv Aging.* 2008;3(3):503–509.

47. Sink KM, Thomas J, Xu H, et al. Dual use of bladder anticholinergics and cholinesterase inhibitors: Long-term functional and cognitive outcomes. *J Am Geriatr Soc.* 2008;56:847–853.

48. Lee, M. Management of benign prostatic hyperplasia. In: Dipiro JT, Talbert RL, Yee GC, eds. *Pharmacotherapy: A Pathophysiologic Approach.* New York: McGraw Hill Medical; 2008:1387–1397.

49. Edwards JL. Diagnosis and management of benign prostatic hyperplasia. *Am Fam Phys.* 2008;77:1403–1410.

50. American Urological Association. Guideline on the management of benign prostatic hyperplasia (2006 update). Available at: http://www.auanet.org/content/guidelines-and-quality-care/clinical-guidelines.cfm?sub=bph Accessed: August 5, 2008.

51. Zagaria M. Benign prostatic hyperplasia: Symptoms and treatment options. *US Pharm.* 2003;28(8).

52. Roehrbron CG, Boyle P, Gould AL, et al. Serum prostate-specific antigen as a predictor of prostate volume in men with benign prostatic hyperplasia. *Urology.* 1999;53:581–589.

53. Roehrborn CG, Boyle P, Bergner D, et al. Serum prostate-specific antigen and prostate volume predict long-term changes in symptoms and flow-rate: Results of a four-year, randomized trial comparing finasteride versus placebo. *Urology.* 1999;54;662–669.

54. Tangalos EG, Zarowitz BJ. Benign prostatic hyperplasia. In: *Geriatric Pharmaceutical Care Guidelines.* Covington, KY: Omnicare, Inc.; 2008:163–168.

55. Flomax (tamsulosin)[package insert]. Ridgefield, CT: Boehringer Ingelheim Pharmaceuticals, Inc; March 2008.

56. Uroxatral (alfusozin) [package insert]. Bridgewater, NJ: Sanofi Aventis U.S. LLC; April 2008.

57. McConnell JD, Roehrborn CG, Bautista OM, et al. The long-term effect of doxazosin, finasteride, and combination therapy on the clinical progression of benign prostatic hyperplasia. *N Engl J Med.* 2003;349:2387–98.

58. Boyle P, Gould AL, Roehrborn CG. Prostate volume predicts outcome of treatment of benign prostatic hyperplasia with finasteride: Meta analysis of randomized clinical trials. *Urology.* 1996;48:398–405.

59. McConnell D, Bruskewitz R, Walsh P, et al. The effect of finasteride on the risk of acute urinary retention and the need for surgical treatment among men with benign prostatic hyperplasia. *N Eng J Med.* 1998;338:557–563.

60. Logan YT, Belgeri MT. Monotherapy versus combination therapy for the treatment of benign prostatic hyperplasia. *Am J Geriatr Pharmcother.* 2005;3:103–114.

61. Trachtenberg J. Treatment of lower urinary tract symptoms suggestive of benign prostatic hyperplasia in relation to the patient's risk profile for progression. *BJU Int.* 2005;95(suppl 4):6–11.

62. Avodart (dutasteride) [package insert]. Research Triangle Park, NC: GlaxoSmithKline; June 2008.

63. Roehrborn CG, Siami P, Barkin J et al. The effects of dutasteride, tamsulosin and combination therapy on lower urinary tract symptoms in men with benign prostatic hyperplasia and prostatic enlargement: 2-year results from the CombAT study. *J Urol.* 2008;179:616–621.

64. Sherman JJ. Health issues in older men. In: Dunsworth T, Richardson M, Chant C, et al., eds. *Pharmacotherapy Self-Assessment Program.* 6th ed. Women's and Men's Health. Lenexa, KS: American College of Clinical Pharmacy; 2008:163–180.

65. Kaplan SA, McConnell JD, Roehrborn CG, et al. Combination therapy with doxazosin and finasteride for benign prostatic hyperplasia in patients with lower urinary tract symptoms and a baseline total prostate volume of 25 ml or greater. *J Urol.* 2006;175:217–221.

66. Kaplan SA, Roehrborn CG, McConnell JD, et al. Long-term treatment with finasteride results in a clinically significant reduction in total prostate volume compared to placebo over the full range of baseline prostate sizes in men enrolled in the MTOPS trial. *J Urol.* 2008;180:1030–1033.

67. Blake JB, Rashidian A, Ikeda Y, et al. Lower urinary tract: The role of anticholinergics in men with lower urinary tract symptoms suggestive of benign prostatic hyperplasia: a systematic review and meta-analysis. *Br J Urol.* 2006;99:85–96.

68. Gallegos PJ, Frazee LA. Anticholinergic therapy for lower urinary tract symptoms associated with benign prostatic hyperplasia. *Pharmacotherapy.* 2008;28:356–65.

69. Gordon AE, Shaughnessy AF. Saw palmetto for prostate disorders. *Am Fam Phys.* 2003;67:1281–83.

70. Wilt T, Ishani A, MacDonald R. Serenoa repens for benign prostatic hyperplasia. Cochrane Database of Systematic Reviews 2002, Issue 3. Art. No.: CD0014323. DOI:10.1002/14651858.CD001423

71. Bent S, Kane C, Shinohara K, et al. Saw palmetto for benign prostatic hyperplasia. *N Engl J Med.* 2006;354:557–566.

72. Wasson JH, Reda DJ, Bruskewitz RC, et al. A Comparison of transurethral surgery with watchful waiting for moderate symptoms of benign prostatic hyperplasia. *N Engl J Med.* 1995;332:75–79.

73. Keister D, Neal R. Managing BPH: When to consider surgery. *Am Fam Phys.* 2008; 77:1375–1377.

74. Wagenlehner F, Naber KG, Weidner W. Asymptomatic bacteriuria in elderly patients: Significance and implications for treatment. *Drugs Aging.* 2005;22:801–807.

75. Merck Manual of Geriatrics. Urinary Tract Infections. Available at: http://www.merck.com/mkgr/mmg/sec12/ch100/ch100a.jsp Accessed June 24, 2008.

76. Midthun SJ. Criteria for urinary tract infection in the elderly: Variables that challenge nursing assessment. *Urol Nurs.* 2004;24:157–170.

77. Nicolle LE, Bradley S, Colgan R, et al. Infectious Diseases Society of America (IDSA) guidelines for the diagnosis and treatment of asymptomatic bacteriuria in adults. *Clin Infect Dis.* 2005;40:643–654.

78. Juthani-Mehta M. Asymptomatic bacteriuria and urinary tract infection in older adults. *Clin Geriatr Med.* 2007;23:585–594.

79. Kamel HK. Managing urinary tract infections: Guide for nursing home practitioners. *Ann Long-Term Care.* 2005;13:25–30.

80. Nicolle LE. SHEA Position Paper: Urinary tract infections in long-term care facilities. *Infect Control Hosp Epidemiol.* 2001;22:167–175.

81. Coyle EA, Prince RA. Urinary infections and prostatitis. In: Dipiro JT, Talbert RL, Yee GC, eds. *Pharmacotherapy: A Pathophysiologic Approach.* New York: McGraw Hill Medical; 2008:1899–1913.

82. Loeb M, Bentley DW, Bradley S, et al. Development of minimum criteria for the initiation of antibiotics

in residents of long-term care facilities: Results of a consensus conference. *Infect Control Hosp Epidemiol.* 2001;22:120–124.

83. Elliott DP. Pharmacokinetics and pharmacodynamics in the elderly. In: Dunsworth TS, Schumock GT, Brundage DM, Chessman KH, Fagan SC, Kelly HW, et al., eds. *Pharmacotherapy Self-Assessment Program.* 5th edition. Geriatrics/Special Populations. Kansas City, MO: American College of Clinical Pharmacy; 2004:115–126.

84. Sleeper, R. Infections in the long-term care setting. In: Dunsworth T, Richardson M, Chant, C, Cheng JWM, Chessman KH, Hume AL, et al., eds. *Pharmacotherapy Self-Assessment Program.* 6th ed. Infectious Diseases. Lenexa, KS: American College of Clinical Pharmacy; 2008:115–126.

85. Micromedex® Healthcare Series (Internet Database). Greenwood Village, CO: Thomson Healthcare. Updated periodically.

86. Food and Drug Administration. Information for healthcare professionals: Fluoroquinolone antimicrobial drugs. Available at: http://www.fda.gov/cder/drug/InfoSheets/HCP/fluoroquinolonesHCP.htm Accessed July 28, 2008.

87. Tangalos EG, Zarowitz BJ. Urinary tract infection. In: *Geriatric Pharmaceutical Care Guidelines.* Covington, KY: Omnicare, Inc.; 2008: 799–806.

88. Takahashi P, Trang N, Evans J. Antibiotic prescribing and outcomes following treatment of symptomatic urinary tract infections in older women. *J Am Med Dir Assoc.* 2002;3:352–355.

89. Hooton TM. Recurrent urinary tract infection in women. *Int J Antimicrobial Agents.* 2001;17:259–268.

90. Regal RE, Pham CQ, Bostwick TR. Urinary tract infections in extended care facilities: Preventative management strategies. *Consult Pharm.* 2006;21:400–409.

91. Raz R, Stamm WE. A controlled trial of intravaginal estriol in postmenopausal women with recurrent urinary tract infections. *N Engl J Med.* 1993;329:753–756.

10

Endocrine Disorders

ANNE L. HUME AND LISA B. COHEN

Learning Objectives

1. Identify the prevalence and clinical presentation of endocrine disorders including diabetes mellitus, thyroid disorders, and sexual dysfunction among older adults;

2. Evaluate the management of older adults with endocrine disorders compared with younger patients;

3. Assess the potential effects of major endocrine disorders on common comorbid diseases in older adults and on quality of life issues;

4. Critique major studies of diabetes mellitus that enrolled older adults with respect to their application to clinical practice; and

5. Develop a treatment plan appropriate for older adults with selected endocrine disorders.

Key Terms

GRAVES' DISEASE OPHTHALMOPATHY: The characteristic finding is the presence of painful, red eyes due to inflammation. Eyelids and tissues around the eyes are swollen with the eyeballs bulging out of their sockets.

HEMOGLOBIN A$_{1c}$ CONCENTRATION: Hemoglobin A$_{1c}$ (A1C) is a minor component of hemoglobin to which glucose is bound. A1C also is referred to as glycosylated hemoglobin and provides a measure of glucose control over the past 3 months.

MACROVASCULAR COMPLICATIONS: Diseases of the larger blood vessels resulting in atherosclerotic vascular disease.

MICROALBUMINURIA: Microalbuminuria is defined as urinary albumin excretion between 30 and 300 mg in a 24-hour period.

MICROVASCULAR COMPLICATIONS: Diseases of the small blood vessels may lead to loss of sensation and to foot ulcers.

SECRETAGOGUES: A substance or hormone that causes or stimulates secretion.

T3: Triiodothyronine is an iodine-rich thyroid hormone formed from one molecule of monoiodotyrosine and one of diiodotyrosine. Most of the circulating T3 is the result of the enzymatic degradation of T4 in extrathyroidal peripheral tissues. T3 is extensively bound to albumin, thyroxine-binding globulin, and transthyretin.

T4: Thyroxine is an iodine-rich thyroid hormone formed from two molecules of diiodotyrosine in the thyroid gland. **T3** is extensively bound to albumin, thyroxine-binding globulin, and transthyretin.

THYROIDITIS: An inflammation of the thyroid gland in which there is a release of thyroid hormone resulting in a temporary hyperthyroid state.

TSH: Thyroid stimulating hormone is secreted by the pituitary gland and stimulates thyrotropin receptors to regulate the activity of the thyroid gland.

Introduction

The endocrine system has physiologic effects that affect almost every organ in the body. These effects range from regulation of glucose and thyroid metabolism to the maintenance of muscle and skeletal mass to normal gonadal functioning in men and women, as well as many other physiologic roles. Similar to other systems, the endocrine system may undergo diverse changes due to aging. The best recognized age-related endocrine change occurs within the hypothalamic-pituitary-adrenal axis with the onset of menopause in middle-aged women. The secretion of growth hormone and the serum concentration of insulin-like growth factor may decrease with age.[1] The secretion of dehydroepiandrosterone from the adrenal cortex may also decline with advancing age[2] and older adults may have greater variability in serum cortisol concentrations throughout a 24-hour period.[3] Although the secretion of other hormones may differ in older versus younger adults, it is frequently difficult to establish if the differences are truly age-related or are due instead to disease-related processes that may be present. In addition, endocrine diseases such as diabetes mellitus and thyroid disorders together affect approximately 12% of the American population. This chapter will focus on diabetes mellitus, thyroid disorders, sexual dysfunction, and other endocrine diseases in older adults.

Diabetes Mellitus

Etiology, Epidemiology, and Clinical Presentation in Older Adults

According to the Centers for Disease Control and Prevention, the prevalence of diabetes has risen to almost 25% of people 60 years of age and older.[4] Because the prevalence of the disease increases with advancing age, diabetes will become even more common with the aging of the American population. Interestingly, nondiabetic patients have been noted to have higher **hemoglobin A$_{1C}$ (A1C)** levels as they age. The A1C levels have been reported to increase approximately 0.012% per year.[5] Also, the prevalence of diabetes continues to rise among minority groups.[6] Among older adults with diabetes, about 40% were diagnosed at 65 years of age or older.[7] Patients with type 1 diabetes have increased their life expectancy and, as a result, more older adults will likely have type 1 diabetes in the near future. Case reports of older adults diagnosed with type 1 diabetes have been published,[8] although the true prevalence of type 1 diabetes in the older adults is uncertain.

An estimated 26% of adults have impaired glucose tolerance and this estimate increases to more than 35% in individuals over 60 years of age.[4] Diabetes, both diagnosed and undiagnosed, is present in approximately 7.8% of Americans. This figure increases to 23.8% among people over the age of 60.[9,10] (See Figure 10-1.) The American Diabetes Association (ADA) recommends screening all adults over the age of 45 years for diabetes every 3 years. About 20–25% of patients in this age group have impaired glucose tolerance and a twofold increase in the risk of **macrovascular complications.**[11] Older adults with diabetes, compared with individuals of the same age who do not have the disease, are two to three times more likely to report an inability to walk ¼ of a mile or to perform activities such as climbing stairs, using a cane or walker, or doing housework.[9]

The etiology of type 2 diabetes includes both genetic and environmental factors with obesity and physical inactivity comprising the latter group. Several genes have been identified as increasing the risk of developing type 2 diabetes independent of the environmental factors.[12] Predictors for the development of type 2 diabetes include a reduction in insulin secretion, insulin resistance, elevated body mass index (BMI), being a current smoker, and elevated liver enzymes.[13] Insulin resistance is the result of increased inflammation secondary to high concentrations of free fatty acids and tumor necrosis factor-α, an increase in obesity, increasing age, and decreased physical activity.[13] Several factors increase the likelihood of older adults developing type 2 diabetes. One of the age-related factors in diabetes is the altera-

tion of insulin secretion in response to an oral glucose load.[14] Older adults may also have an increase in insulin resistance due to central obesity, high saturated fat intake, and inactivity. The poor food choices in some older individuals may be due to financial stressors and an inability to chew certain foods. Research has identified differences between older obese and lean individuals. While older adults with diabetes often have normal hepatic glucose production, lean older adults may have decreased insulin secretion, but normal insulin-mediated glucose disposal.[14] These patients have recently been referred to as having "diabetes type 1 ½".[14,15] Conversely, obese older adults with diabetes often have normal insulin secretion, but increased insulin resistance.[14]

Older adults with diabetes may not have the typical symptoms of hyperglycemia. As people age, the renal threshold for glucose increases and, as a result, older persons may not have the polyuria and nocturia that younger patients may experience.[11] In addition, the normal thirst mechanism declines with advancing age. Older persons may have only vague symptoms of fatigue, weight loss, vision disturbances, urinary incontinence, or other symptoms that are easily mistaken for common co-morbid conditions.[11] Older adults with

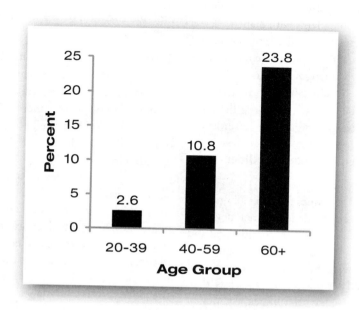

Figure 10-1. Estimated prevalence of diagnosed and undiagnosed diabetes in people aged 20 years or older, by age group, United States, 2007.

diabetes may have an abnormal random glucose, such as 207 mg/dL, as their only presenting sign of diabetes.

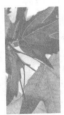

KEY POINT: Older patients often lack the classic symptoms of diabetes and instead present with urinary incontinence, confusion, and fatigue which may be confused with other diseases.

Summary of Standard Treatment

Based on the American Diabetes Association clinical practice guidelines, the recommended optimal glycemic control for an adult with diabetes is to achieve an A1C less than 7%.[16] This would include preprandial glucose concentrations between 70–130 mg/dL and postprandial concentrations less than 180 mg/dL.[16] Although a target A1C of less than 6% may reduce some diabetes-related complications, the risk of hypoglycemia increases. In addition, recent trials have shown that decreasing A1C levels below 7% may increase the risk of cardiovascular complications as well as increased hypoglycemic episodes.[17,18] The recommendation for goal blood pressure in patients with diabetes is less than 130/80 mmHg.[16] Overall treatment should include medical nutrition therapy (MNT), metformin with lifestyle changes such as MNT and exercise, and early insulin initiation, if necessary (Table 10-1 describes the standard drug therapies for diabetes as well as other endocrine disorders).

Treatment Recommendations for Older Adults

Potential quality of life issues for older adults with diabetes should be acknowledged, when developing a treatment plan that may be complicated and expensive. An older person who is cognitively intact and is otherwise functional in activities of daily living should have a target A1C less than 7%. Frail older persons with a life expectancy of less than 5 years or individuals at otherwise high risk of adverse outcomes from hypoglycemia may

have a higher goal such as an A1C less than 8%, as long as the risk of acute hyperglycemia is reduced.[6,16] The complication from diabetes mellitus with the highest morbidity and mortality is cardiovascular disease. It is the consensus of the American Geriatric Society Panel on Improving Care for Elders with Diabetes that, similar to younger individuals, most older persons who have diabetes also benefit from treatment of their hypertension and dyslipidemia if present, although clinical trials evaluating treatment outcomes in specific subgroups of frail individuals with these combinations of comorbidities are lacking.[6] The use of low-dose aspirin for primary prevention should also be considered on an individual basis.

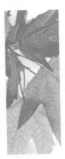

KEY POINT: Older patients must have individualized treatment goals taking into consideration their life expectancy, comorbid conditions, level of frailty, acute risk of hypoglycemia, care setting, and quality of life issues.

Individualization of Treatment in Type 2 Diabetes

Treatment of older adults with diabetes is similar to that of younger patients and involve the same stepwise approach to medication management.[19,20] Nonpharmacologic treatments involving diet and exercise should be carefully tailored to the needs of the individual older adult. An older adult who is malnourished will need adequate calories and protein. The presence of comorbid conditions such as severe cardiovascular disease and mobility problems will require careful consideration in the development of an exercise plan. An interdisciplinary team that includes a dietician or nutritionist, as well as a physical therapist, may be important in developing an optimal care plan for the older person with diabetes.

The selection of drug therapy for diabetes in older adults also requires consideration of goals

Table 10-1. Endocrine Treatments and Geriatric Considerations

Class	Medication Examples	General Adult Treatment Principles	Geriatric Considerations
Antidiabetic agents			
Alpha-glucosidase inhibitors	Miglitol (Glyset) Acarbose (Precose)	Monotherapy adjunct to diet to improve glycemic control in type 2 diabetes; combination therapy with a sulfonylurea	No specific trials in older adults have been conducted in patients on acarbose; dosage adjustments not necessary; elderly patients had 1.5 times serum concentrations as compared with younger adults
Biguanides	Metformin (Glucophage)	Monotherapy for type 2 diabetes or used concomitantly with a sulfonylurea or insulin to improve glycemic control	AUC and half-life increased in elderly; Initial dose and maintenance dosing should be conservative; should not titrate to maximum dosage; not recommended to use in elderly patients ≥ 80 years
Dipeptidyl peptidase IV inhibitors	Sitagliptin (Januvia) Saxagliptin (Onglyza)	Monotherapy for type 2 diabetes or in combination with other antidiabetic agents	One clinical trial showed no difference in safety or efficacy as compared to younger adults; less risk of hypoglycemia than other medications
Incretin mimetics	Exenatide (Byetta)	Adjunctive treatment of type 2 diabetes in patients receiving sulfonylurea, metformin, or TZD or a combination of these medications	Not recommended to use in patients with creatinine clearance < 30 mL/min; less risk of hypoglycemia than other medications
Meglitinides	Repaglinide (Prandin) Nateglinide (Prandin Starlix)	Monotherapy for type 2 diabetes or adjunctive therapy in patients on metformin or TZD	No changes in safety and efficacy were seen in patients ≥ 65 years on nateglinide; one trial showed that patients ≥ 65 years taking repaglinide had less hypoglycemia as compared with a sulfonylurea
Sulfonylureas	Glyburide (Micronase, Diabeta) Glipizide (Glucotrol) Glimepiride (Amaryl) Chlorpropamide (Diabinese) Tolbutamide (Orinase) Tolazamide (Tolinase)	Management of type 2 diabetes; may be used as monotherapy or in combination with metformin or insulin	Differences between each sulfonylurea; may cause rapid and prolonged hypoglycemia despite glucose administration; use with caution in patients with renal insufficiency; glipizide preferred due to less drug interactions and drug elimination is not dependent on renal function; chlorpropamide not recommended for use in the elderly.

(continued)

Table 10-1. Endocrine Treatments and Geriatric Considerations (cont'd)

Class	Medication Examples	General Adult Treatment Principles	Geriatric Considerations
Thiazolidinediones (TZDs)	Pioglitazone (Actos) Rosiglitazone (Avandia)	Monotherapy for type 2 diabetes or in combination therapy with sulfonylureas, metformin, or insulin; rosiglitazone is not recommended in combination with insulin.	No dosage adjustments recommended with either rosiglitazone or pioglitazone; with rosiglitazone there may be an increased risk of fractures in hand, upper arm, and foot; rosiglitazone should be used cautiously in patients with low bone density, history of fractures or history of falls.
Insulin	Various	Treatment of type 1 or type 2 diabetes.	Initial doses may require consideration for renal function; elderly may need assistance to draw up insulin in a syringe due to dexterity and vision issues; may need to use prefilled syringes or pen devices; patient needs to be able to recognize hypoglycemic and hyperglycemic symptoms.
Drugs for Thyroid Disorders			
Thioureas	Methimazole (Tapazole) Propylthiouracil	Adverse effects include rash, urticaria, arthralgias, hepatotoxicity, and agranulocytosis.	Older adults may be at increased risk of agranulocytosis.
Thyroid replacement drugs	Levothyroxine (Synthroid) Triiodothyronine (Cytomel) T3+T4 (Liotrix) Dessicated thyroid (Armour thyroid)	Levothyroxine preferred due to its stable conversion to T3 and a half life of approximately 4 to 7 days. T3 has a shorter half-life and requires multiple daily dosages. Combination T3+T4 products are more expensive and require monitoring of both T3 and T4 concentrations unlike levothyroxine preparations. Dessicated thyroid has had standardization problems, as well as with adverse cardiac effects.[3]	A primary concern is the precipitation of cardiac events when beginning replacement therapy. Dosages should be started low and gradually titrated upwards especially in the presence of known cardiovascular disease.
Sexual Dysfunction			
Oral phosphodiesterase type 5 (PDE-5) inhibitors	Sildenafil (Viagra) Tadalafil (Cialis) Vardenail (Levitra)	PDE-5 inhibitors are considered the first-line treatment for erectile dysfunction when contributing factors for ED have been evaluated. The drugs are generally safe.	Older men should be evaluated for use of nitrates (and other potentially interacting drugs) as well as for overall cardiovascular disease before using PDE-5 inhibitors. Older men may be at increased risk of nonarteritic anterior ischemic optic neuropathy (NAION).

and the presence of comorbid conditions especially in the frail older adult. (See Table 10-2.) A primary consideration in selecting drug therapy for the older person with diabetes is the risk of hypoglycemia, such as a patient with renal insufficiency or inconsistent oral calorie intake. A patient with cognitive impairment may not be able to communicate symptoms of hypoglycemia. Other considerations include life expectancy, baseline glycemic control, adverse effects, tolerability, and previous diabetes medication use.[19] For example, an older adult with previous falls and hospital admissions secondary to sulfonylurea therapy should be switched to alternative agents with a lower potential for hypoglycemia. Biguanides, thiazolidinediones, alpha-glucosidase inhibitors, exenatide, and dipeptidyl peptidase IV inhibitors generally do not cause hypoglycemia unless they are used in combination with medications that stimulate insulin release.[19,21]

Diabetes mellitus generally requires the addition of more medications over time in order to maintain glycemic control. Additional medications should be considered within 2 to 3 months after initiation of a therapy or any time that the A1C is not at goal. Of course, individualization of treatment is always recommended. Lifestyle interventions remain essential and may significantly decrease hyperglycemia if implemented into the treatment regimen.[22] Implementing lifestyle changes such as weight loss and exercise programs may improve blood glucose concentrations and may also improve cardiovascular risk factors such as hypertension and dyslipidemias. However, development of lifestyle recommendations must consider the individual's functional status, level of frailty, and comorbid conditions. Maintenance of lifestyle modifications is difficult in all patient groups, and risks with exercise in older patients with diabetes may include musculoskeletal injuries or worsening foot ulcers or wounds, so the exercise plan should be carefully tailored to the individual.

Common Oral Medications

Along with lifestyle interventions, initial treatment with metformin is the preferred drug therapy for type 2 diabetes. Metformin is generally well tolerated if slowly titrated upwards.

Metformin also has the advantage of potentially causing weight loss which may benefit the lipid profile. Data from a recent systematic review indicates that the use of metformin may decrease the risk of cardiovascular mortality in older adults.[7] Several cautions exist when using metformin in older adults (Table 10-2). Metformin may have a reduced total body clearance and has a prolonged half-life in older patients. Clinical trials of metformin did not include enough older patients to specifically evaluate its use in this age group. Recent data obtained from relatively younger study subjects has shown that metformin may be used in patients until the glomerular filtration rate falls below 30 mL/min.[23]

Clinically significant responses to metformin usually occur at dosages over 1500 mg daily. The dosage of metformin should not be increased to the maximum due to the potential risk for lactic acidosis in older adults with impaired kidney function. Metformin decreases hepatic glucose production and increases insulin sensitivity and should be used only after careful calculation of the creatinine clearance in older adults and after ensuring the creatinine clearance is greater than 30 mL/min.[19] Dosages may need to be titrated more slowly than in younger adults. Metformin may cause loss of appetite, stomach upset, and diarrhea to which older adults may be more sensitive. In addition, a study of older adults comparing tolbutamide and metformin showed that, while each drug was equally effective, metformin caused weight loss whereas tolbutamide caused weight gain.[23] Lastly, vitamin B12 deficiency is associated with the use of metformin especially in older adults due to its effect on the ileal absorption of the vitamin; the use of metformin may be overlooked as a potential contributing factor for vitamin B12 deficiency.[24]

KEY POINT: Patients should start with lifestyle changes, individualized to their own needs, and metformin if their renal function is adequate.

Table 10-2. Comparison of Pharmacotherapy Options for Type 2 Diabetes in Older Adults

Medication	Advantages	Disadvantages
Metformin	Hypoglycemia adverse effect usually does not occur if monotherapy. May help with weight loss. May be beneficial to lipid profile. Available as a generic drug May improve insulin resistance.	Not recommended in patients over 80 years of age. Generally, should not be dosed to maximum dosages in older adults. Gastrointestinal side effects may be common. Rare risk of lactic acidosis. Should not use in patients with moderate-severe heart failure due to risk of lactic acidosis.
Sulfonylureas	Least expensive, available generically. Works well in lean patients.	High risk of hypoglycemia. Weight gain.
Thiazolidinediones	No hypoglycemia, if monotherapy. Improves insulin resistance.	Weight gain. Edema. Expensive. Increased risk of fractures of the hand, upper arm, and foot. Risk of cardiovascular events with rosiglitazone.
Alpha-glucosidase inhibitors	No hypoglycemia, if monotherapy. No weight gain. Lowers postprandial glucose levels.	High incidence of gastrointestinal side effects. Hypoglycemia must be treated with dextrose or lactose. Weak, lowers HbA1c 0.5%. Must be dosed prior to each meal.
Meglitinides	Slight decreased risk of hypoglycemia compared with sulfonylureas. Reduces postprandial glucose levels.	Expensive medication. Risk of hypoglycemia. Must be taken with each meal: multiple doses. Can cause weight gain.
Dipeptidyl peptidase IV inhibitors	No hypoglycemia if monotherapy. Few side effects.	Caution use in renal impairment. Weak, lowers HbA1c 0.5%. Expensive.
Incretin mimetics	No hypoglycemia, if monotherapy.	Injectable medication. Nausea, vomiting. Expensive. Should not use in patients with creatinine clearance < 30 mL/min.
Amylin analog	Effective at lowering blood glucose levels.	High risk of hypoglycemia. Must be used with insulin. Expensive medication. Injectable.
Insulin	Relatively inexpensive. Effective at lowering blood glucose levels.	High risk of hypoglycemia. Injectable.

First and second generation sulfonylureas are equally effective and are available as generic drug products. In general, the second generation sulfonylureas including glyburide, glipizide, and glimepiride are preferred, although glyburide may accumulate in renal insufficiency and a meta-analysis comparing glyburide with other secretagogues showed an increased risk of hypoglycemia with glyburide treatment.[25,26] Patients should be initiated on the lowest dosage such as glipizide 2.5 mg per day and increased by 2.5–5 mg every 1–2 weeks. Some first generation sulfonylureas require more frequent dosing and others have longer half-lives such as chlorpropamide which significantly increases the risk of hypoglycemia and are generally not considered optimal choices for older adults.

The thiazolidinediones (TZDs), pioglitazone and rosiglitazone, act by improving insulin resistance. Pioglitazone is preferred because rosiglitazone has been shown to increase the risk of myocardial infarction and death from cardiovascular disease.[27] The use of rosiglitazone should be avoided in older adults because of the higher prevalence of cardiovascular diseases such as myocardial infarction and heart failure. Pioglitazone is effective in the treatment of type 2 diabetes in older adults and may also have a beneficial effect on lipids. Pioglitazone should be started at a dosage of 15–30 mg per day and titrated to a maximum of 45 mg daily. The beneficial effects of pioglitazone on glucose concentrations may take at least several weeks. Adverse effects with TZD include weight gain, leg edema, and a twofold increase in the risk of heart failure. These drugs should generally be avoided in older adults with heart failure.[19]

Insulin

If the patient's diabetes does not respond to combinations of oral medications, insulin should be considered. In the past, the initiation of insulin was delayed for years after diagnosis or for very poor glycemic control. Often, insulin is deferred because of a perception that older adults are unable to manage insulin therapy. Insulin can be used safely in older adults by initiating the therapy slowly and titrating carefully. Treatment with insulin and additional medications is now recommended within 2–3 months of failed monotherapy.[19] Newer basal insulin products such as insulin glargine may have advantages in older adults, but they have not been studied in these patients.

Basal insulin may be added to oral combination therapy in older adults. For example, intermediate-acting insulin NPH may be initiated at 10 units daily in addition to combination treatment with metformin and glipizide. The dosage of the insulin may be slowly titrated up by 1–2 units every 3 days to avoid hypoglycemia and maintain premeal and bedtime blood glucose concentrations of 80–140 mg/dL. Titrating insulin NPH to achieve an A1C of less than 7% may take several weeks to months. Once target fasting blood glucoses are achieved, pre-lunch, pre-dinner, and pre-bedtime readings can be checked. Basal or bolus insulin can be added to the regimen with continued monitoring.[19] If basal insulin therapy becomes inefficient or the targets are not achievable, the patient may alter their insulin regimen with basal and bolus combinations in fixed regimens (i.e., insulin 70/30 twice daily therapy) or multiple daily doses of insulin (i.e., insulin glargine daily with mealtime boluses of insulin lispro). Monitoring hypoglycemia is especially important in older adults, as this may increase their risk of falling.

KEY POINT: Medications should be started with the lowest dosage and titrated slowly to minimize adverse effects.

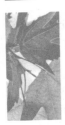

KEY POINT: Insulin treatment should be considered when the A1C remains above the desired goal, despite taking combination therapy with the recommended dosages.

Assistive devices for insulin therapy may help older patients with vision, hearing, and dexterity problems successfully manage their therapy. One product attaches to an insulin syringe to magnify the markings on the syringe for those with impaired vision. Insulin pen devices have also made insulin delivery easier for individuals who are visually impaired or who have dexterity problems. Although no insulin pen devices are specifically promoted for use by individuals who are visually impaired, patients can be trained to use these devices successfully, if they are provided with appropriate opportunities to practice their use. Another product called Count-A-Dose attaches up to two vials of insulin and uses a low-dose syringe (< 50 units). The product clicks with each unit of insulin withdrawn from the vial and also allows for mixing different types of insulin.

Adjunctive Medications

Other medications may be used as adjunctive therapies in the treatment of diabetes although they have not been well studied in older adults. The primary goal of adding these medications to existing regimens is to control blood glucose with little or no hypoglycemia or other adverse effects.[16] Clinicians should recognize that many older adults may have a limited income and that each additional medication should be evaluated for cost, ease of use, adverse effects, and actual effects on glycemic control.

Meglitinides including repaglinide and nateglinide are similar to the sulfonylureas and stimulate beta-cells to increase insulin secretion, although they bind to a different receptor. These drugs have a shorter half-life than sulfonylureas and should be dosed with meals.[20] The primary benefit of the meglitinides is that the risk of hypoglycemia is lower because the patient takes the medication only if they are eating food containing carbohydrates and they may skip doses if they are not eating.[11]

The alpha-glucosidase inhibitors include acarbose and miglitol. Their mechanism of action involves slowing the absorption of polysaccharides in the brush border of the small intestine, thereby delaying glucose absorption and lowering postprandial blood glucose concentrations. The A1C level is lowered approximately 0.5% and the medication should be used cautiously in patients with serum creatinine over 2.0 mg/dL even though less than 2% of the drug is absorbed. The initial dosage of acarbose would be 25 mg three times a day with the first bite of each meal. If the patient forgets to take acarbose with the first bite of the meal, they should skip that dose. Increased gastrointestinal gas and belching occur in about 25–45% of patients.[20] Patients who become hypoglycemic while taking a combination of antidiabetic drugs that include acarbose or miglitol should be advised to take glucose tablets or skim milk and not sucrose products such as orange juice. This can be an important counseling point in long term care environments where nursing protocols may include orange juice as among interventions for hypoglycemia.

Glucagon-like peptide-1 (GLP-1) agonists are produced by the L-cells in the small intestine and enhance glucose-stimulated insulin secretion. Exenatide is an analog of GLP-1 and has a longer half-life than the naturally occurring peptide.[19] Exenatide slows gastric motility and suppresses the secretion of glucagon. Although hypoglycemia does not occur, gastrointestinal symptoms such as nausea, vomiting, and diarrhea may develop with the use of exenatide.[19] Patients taking exenatide may be able to decrease their nausea by ingesting smaller meals. The nausea from exenatide may also be due to previously unrecognized diabetic gastroparesis. The initial dosage is 5 mcg injected subcutaneously twice daily and slowly titrated after a month to a maximum of 10 mcg twice a day prior to meals. Although exenatide trials have enrolled older adults, its use in this patient group has not been specifically evaluated.

The amylin agonist, pramlintide, is dosed three times daily before meals in patients using mealtime insulin. It works by inhibiting glucose-dependent glucagon secretion and slowing gastric emptying, ultimately lowering postprandial glucose values.[19] Adverse effects include nausea, anorexia, and weight loss. Severe hypoglycemia may occur if the insulin dosage is not halved when pramlintide is first started. Pramlintide is usually dosed 60–120 mcg subcutaneously prior to meals in patients with type 2 diabetes.

The dipeptidyl peptidase-IV (DPP-IV) enzyme rapidly breaks down GLP-1 and glucose-dependent insulinotropic peptide (GIP). Sitagliptin and saxagliptin are DPP-IV inhibitors that enhances the activity of GLP and GIP.[19,28] Although generally well tolerated and orally dosed, the A1C is only lowered by 0.6–0.9%. Sitagliptin is dosed 100 mg daily and saxagliptin is dosed 2.5 mg or 5 mg daily, but if the creatinine clearance is between 30–50 mL/min the dosage should be reduced to 50 mg or 2.5 mg daily, respectively. If the creatinine clearance is less than 30 mL/min, sitagliptin 25 mg daily should be used.[19,28]

Special Considerations in Older Adults
Team Approach

Patients with diabetes should be managed using an individualized team-based approach that includes physicians, pharmacists, nurses, and dieticians among others. All patients need education about their disease, as well as problem-solving skills to manage their diabetes on a day-to-day basis. A patient's age, activity level, eating patterns and preferences, dental issues, cultural and social factors, personality, financial situation, eyesight and other medical conditions should be considered in developing an individualized care plan. Collaboration between the patient, family or other caregivers, and health professionals is essential for optimal care.

Comprehensive Care

Older adults with diabetes are a heterogeneous group. While some may have had diabetes for several years with mild-to-severe **microvascular and macrovascular complications** already present, other individuals may have just been diagnosed with diabetes and have no complications. According to the ADA[16] and the American Ge-

riatrics Society[6] clinical practice guidelines, frail patients and patients who have complications that lead to shortened life expectancy should have a less intensive glycemic goal. Even if the therapeutic plan does not include tight control of blood glucose, other disease states should be assessed independently from this decision. For example, aggressive treatment to target LDL-cholesterol of 70 mg/dL or anticoagulation in atrial fibrillation may still be appropriate even if the A1C target for a patient is 8%. Another example is control of hypertension which has demonstrated benefit in healthy older adults with diabetes. In the Systolic Hypertension in the Elderly Program trial, older persons with diabetes and isolated systolic hypertension treated with antihypertensive therapy had a significantly decreased risk of coronary events compared with their nondiabetic counterparts.[29] In addition, older persons often have more disability due to their diabetic complications which may lead to depression in patients over 55 years old with diabetes. Their depression should be managed aggressively.[30]

In managing diabetes in older adults, the effect of concomitant diseases and drug therapy, vision and hearing problems, poor nutritional intake, financial issues related to medications and other diabetic supplies should be carefully considered, as well as cognitive problems and depression. A frail older adult with unrecognized cognitive impairment and who is living alone will have difficulty adhering to complicated lifestyle interventions and complex drug regimens. Also, adults aged 18–44 years old with diabetes have approximately a 15% prevalence of blindness, whereas about 27% of adults 75 years and older with diabetes are blind.[9] The management of diabetes requires patients to have adequate vision and dexterity to use devices such as an insulin syringe and a glucometer for self-monitoring of blood glucose concentrations. Drawing up insulin from a vial requires adequate vision to accurately read the markings on the syringe. Dexterity is also important for insulin administration and blood glucose monitoring which requires fine motor skills and dexterity to get test strips out of storage vials. Even the simple act of recording blood glucose concentrations in a logbook requires dexterity, vision, adequate cognition, and other steps in order to successfully accomplish the task.

A pharmacist can not only provide patient counseling or assessment of self-administration abilities, but can provide support to caregivers who provide insulin administration assistance. In the long term care setting, the consultant pharmacist's observance of an "insulin pass" by the nursing staff is one way of providing ongoing quality assurance regarding administration procedures.

Blood Glucose Monitoring

Self-monitoring of blood glucose is recommended for all patients who have been prescribed an intensive insulin regimen consisting of multiple injections per day.[16] In other patients, including younger adults, self-monitoring of blood glucose is considered an important tool in managing the disease. Although improving glycemic control via blood glucose monitoring has not been consistently demonstrated in studies, testing blood glucose in the older adults might help to improve long-term outcomes and prevent hypoglycemic reactions.

The preferred frequency and timing of blood glucose measurements in older adults is not known, however, individual patients may be assessed to evaluate their interest and ability to monitor blood glucose concentrations. As their diabetes therapy intensifies, blood glucose monitoring should also be increased either by the patient or a qualified caregiver. Patients who are taking medications that increase insulin secretion such as sulfonylureas and meglitinides or insulin may require more testing than patients receiving other therapies. Frail older adults are at an increased risk of severe hypoglycemia and blood glucose monitoring by caregivers may reduce this risk.[31]

Blood glucose monitors have helped to improve a patient's autonomy in the management of their diabetes. All patients should be shown how to use their glucose monitors and should have routine follow up to ensure proper technique.[16] However, the use of glucose monitors can be difficult for patients who have cognitive impairment, visual impairment, or dexterity problems. Blood glucose monitors vary in size, amount of blood needed for obtaining sample, visual acuity to perform the test, dexterity to handle test strips and supplies, and cognitive ability to accomplish a successful test. Some glucose monitors are able to "talk" to the patients to assist them in testing their blood glucose (i.e., ACCU-CHEK® Voicemate System). Other systems also help patients maintain independence in their diabetes self-care.

For older patients with good vision, but dexterity problems, several glucose meters can be used. Test strips for glucose meters are small and removing them from the vial to insert into the meter can be difficult if the patient has arthritis of the hands. Some glucose monitors have cartridge or drum systems that contain several test strips in a disk and allows for multiple tests to be done (i.e., Accu-Chek Compact®). Coding the meter, code keys, and setting meters can also be difficult. Several meters do not require changing codes or code keys which allows the patient to test their blood glucose with fewer steps.

Ongoing self-management of diabetes is a key component in the successful treatment of the disease. Many older adults with diabetes, either newly diagnosed or those with long-standing disease, will have challenges in effectively managing their diabetes. Health professionals, particularly pharmacists, must be aware of these barriers and be able to offer potential strategies for overcoming the specific challenges.

Prevention of Diabetes-Related Complications

A primary goal in treating diabetes is to prevent the long-term complications which include cardiovascular disease, nephropathy, retinopathy, neuropathy, impaired wound healing, and dental disease. As discussed previously, the long-term complications may or may not be relevant to a newly diagnosed older adult with diabetes especially considering the patient's predicted life expectancy. Few large placebo-controlled prospective studies of diabetes have enrolled older adults. The United Kingdom Prospective Diabetes Study (UKPDS) examined the effect of different treatments on the chronic complications from type 2 diabetes mellitus and only enrolled patients between 25 and 65 years old.[32] As a result, the findings from UKPDS are difficult to apply to older adults especially to frail individuals in their 80s or older.

The Action to Control Cardiovascular Risk in Diabetes (ACCORD) trial randomized patients between the ages of 40 and 79 into either intensive glucose control (targeting A1C less than 6%) or standard treatment (A1C 7% to 7.9%).[17] The mean age of participants was 62 years old. The primary and secondary outcomes of the AC-CORD trial were nonfatal myocardial infarction, nonfatal stroke, death from cardiovascular causes or death from any cause. Overall, the primary and secondary outcomes were increased in patients receiving intensive treatment compared with the group receiving standard therapy. The worse outcomes in the intensive group may have been due to the rapidity of the decrease in blood glucose concentrations early in therapy.[17] Hypoglycemia requiring medical assistance was three times higher in the group receiving intensive versus standard therapy.[17] A significant weight gain of 10 kilograms occurred twice as frequently in the group receiving intensive therapy.[17] Although older adults were enrolled in this study, few participants had common concomitant diseases such as heart failure or were otherwise frail.

Participants in the Action in Diabetes and Vascular Disease: Preterax and Diamicron in Controlled Evaluation (ADVANCE) trial had a mean age of 66 years and only included patients over 55 years of age.[18] This study evaluated if intensive management of blood glucose versus standard treatment decreased microvascular or macrovascular outcomes. Primary outcomes were composites of macrovascular and microvascular events and secondary outcomes included death from any cause, death from cardiovascular causes, and major coronary events. The outcome was not influenced by age.

Diabetic nephropathy is the leading cause of end-stage kidney disease and is increased in patients who have **microalbuminuria**. Several trials have demonstrated the benefit of reducing nephropathy in patients with type 2 diabetes.[33] The ADVANCE trial showed a 21% relative risk reduction of nephropathy in patients intensively managed using sulfonylureas and other medica-

tions and the average age of participants was 66.[18] The presence of microalbuminuria should be tested in all patients at the time of diagnosis of type 2 diabetes and annually thereafter.[6]

Approximately 60% of patients with type 2 diabetes and proteinuria will also have retinopathy. Patients with newly diagnosed type 2 diabetes should have a dilated eye exam immediately and annually thereafter.[16] Older adults with diabetes and nephropathy are also likely to have dental disease and peripheral neuropathy. Appropriate dental care for older adults with diabetes should include brushing teeth twice daily and flossing every day. Patients with diabetes should visit their dentist every 6 months for routine scaling and check-up.[16] Of note, many older adults will not have insurance for dental care and in the nursing home setting, it may be quite difficult to arrange appropriate dental monitoring.

Complications from neuropathies are common in older adults and are often undertreated.[6] Older adults should be assessed at diabetes diagnosis and periodically. They should be asked about pain as well as using other words to adequately assess the patient. Some cultures may not use words such as pain, but rather discomfort or "aching in legs." Postural hypotension from autonomic neuropathies and weakness secondary to peripheral neuropathies can lead to falls in older adults.[34] Although low-dose tricyclic antidepressants, anticonvulsants, and other medications treat peripheral neuropathies, adverse effects commonly occur in older adults. Adverse effects may include fatigue, urinary retention, dizziness, constipation, delirium, and confusion.[35] Treatment options for peripheral neuropathy are discussed more fully in Chapter 13.

Hypoglycemia

Hypoglycemia is a potentially dangerous side effect in any patient with diabetes. Although hypoglycemia is usually mild and includes symptoms of shakiness, nervousness, dizziness, sweating, weakness, and confusion, a loss of consciousness may occur. Older adults may lose the ability to feel certain symptoms of hypoglycemia; they can be educated to recognize symptoms such as sweating, weakness, and fatigue. They or their caregivers should be encouraged to test their blood glucose when feeling these symptoms. Patients should also be encouraged to wear medical identification and carry glucose tablets or other 15-gram carbohydrate sources.

Cognitive impairment often prevents an individual from being able to articulate symptoms of hypoglycemia. In 24-hour care settings such as long term care, regular blood glucose monitoring should be coupled with monitoring of dietary intake patterns. Facility protocols should include orders for hypoglycemia interventions including parameters instructing the nursing staff when to react.

Most studies of diabetes and hypoglycemia have excluded older adults. In a recent trial, severe hypoglycemia requiring hospitalization was evaluated in patients over 80 years old with type 2 diabetes. Most patients had several comorbid conditions and the A1C averaged 5.1% indicating very tight control of their diabetes. Approximately 75% of the patients had been prescribed glyburide by a primary care provider and only a few were self-monitoring blood glucose concentrations on a regular basis. This study indicated that older adults who are aggressively managed are likely to experience severe hypoglycemia requiring hospitalization. Older patients who are taking medications that can cause hypoglycemia should be closely monitored and have their medications and their dosages adjusted when the A1C is within the target range.[36] As discussed previously, insulin and sulfonylureas are common causes of hypoglycemia in frail older adults.

Another trial examined the risk of sulfonylureas and insulin in causing severe hypoglycemia in older adults. Combining both treatment groups, the incidence of severe hypoglycemia was 2 per 100 person-years which would indicate a certain safety in treating older adults with hypoglycemic agents. The patients who were at a higher risk of developing severe hypoglycemia were the very elderly, patients who were frequently admitted to the hospital, and those patients with multiple medications.[37] If a patient is likely to have hypoglycemia, they should have less stringent glycemic goals such as an A1C of less than 8% as compared with a goal of less than 7%.

Hyperosmolar Hyperglycemic Nonketotic Syndrome

In contrast to diabetic ketoacidosis which is more common in type 1 diabetes, hyperosmolar hyperglycemic nonketotic syndrome (HHNS) is more common in adults with type 2 diabetes and has a peak incidence in the seventh decade of life. Patients who develop HHNS have severe hyperglycemia and dehydration, as well as increased serum osmolality. Individuals who have dementia are at the highest risk of developing HHNS.[38] Older patients presenting with HHNS often have other acute conditions such as pneumonia, pancreatitis, and cardiovascular events. They may have had a severe osmotic diuresis and their dehydration is due to both extracellular and intracellular water loss.[38] Fluid replacement can be initiated with 0.9% NaCl until vital signs have stabilized, and then switch to 0.45% NaCl. A regular insulin bolus of 10–15 units followed by continuous infusion of 0.1 unit /kg/hour should be also initiated. Frequently patients who present with HHNS may be managed on oral agents when they are discharged from the hospital.[38]

Summary of Diabetes in Older Adults

Diabetes is an increasingly important condition affecting many older adults. Older patients with diabetes may initially present with vague symptoms that are easily overlooked. The development of an individualized treatment plan should consider their life expectancy, comorbid conditions, acute risk of hypoglycemia, and quality of life issues. Nonpharmacologic therapy should be tailored to the individual's nutritional and exercise needs. Metformin is a first line therapy if the individual's estimated kidney function is greater than 30 mL/min. Insulin treatment should be considered when the A1C remains above the desired goal, despite taking combination therapy with the recommended dosages.

Thyroid Disease

Individuals with thyroid disease comprise approximately 7.35% of the total population. This statistic includes hypothyroidism, hyperthyroidism, and **thyroiditis.**[10] Thyroid diseases are common in older adults especially among women. Despite their frequency, thyroid diseases may be a challenge because their presentation may differ from that in young or middle-aged adults. The symptoms of hyperthyroidism and hypothyroidism in older adults are easily misinterpreted as part of the aging process and usually develop slowly over time. Clinicians should routinely consider thyroid diseases as a potential diagnosis in older adults. For example, a patient with new onset atrial fibrillation due to a thyroid disorder has no symptoms from the arrhythmia nor does the patient have other signs or symptoms of thyroid disease. Thyroid function tests may also be altered by nonthyroidal diseases in older adults. Treatment of thyroid diseases such as hypothyroidism may also be a challenge due to the presence of cardiovascular diseases in older adults.

Etiology, Epidemiology, and Clinical Presentation in Older Adults

Hyperthyroidism

In the United States, the most common causes of hyperthyroidism are **Graves' disease,** uni- or multinodular goiters, and iodine-induced disease.[39-41] Between 50% to 80% of patients with hyperthyroidism have Graves' disease caused by thyroid stimulating antibodies.[39,40] The peak incidence of hyperthyroidism is in the second to fourth decade of life, although hyperthyroidism including Graves' disease occurs in older adults as well. The prevalence of multinodular goiter and toxic nodules as a cause of hyperthyroidism is increased in older adults.[41] Women are at higher risk of Graves' disease than are men, however, older men have the highest risk of severe **ophthalmopathy** from Graves' disease.[40]

Although some older adults will have the classic symptoms of hyperthyroidism such as tremor, nervousness, increased appetite, heat intolerance, and diarrhea, many will lack these presenting complaints. Palpitations, angina, and especially atrial fibrillation with a slow ventricular response may be more common presenting cardiovascular symptoms in older adults.[39,40] Muscle wasting especially of the quadriceps muscle in the thigh

may be present and increases the risk of falling in older adults.[41] One form of Graves' disease, apathetic hyperthyroidism, is more common in older adults and may actually present with symptoms of apathy, weakness, lethargy, and severe depression which can make the diagnosis of thyroid storm very difficult.[42] One report identified the presence of apathy, tachycardia, or weight loss as strong predictors of thyrotoxicosis in older adults.[42]

Hypothyroidism

The incidence of hypothyroidism increases with advancing age and the disease is also more common in women than in men. Hypothyroidism is divided into primary (in which the thyroid gland is unable to respond to stimulation by **thyroid stimulating hormone [TSH]**) or secondary (due to a pituitary or hypothalamic cause). The latter type is rare in older adults. Hypothyroidism in older adults is frequently due to autoimmune disease such as Hashimoto's thyroiditis or chronic lymphocytic thyroiditis.[39,43] Hypothyroidism may also commonly be the result of the treatment of Graves' disease especially following the use of radioactive iodine or thyroidectomy.[44] It is recommended to measure TSH every 6–12 months in individuals treated with radioactive iodine for the patient's lifetime as the risk for hypothyroidism after its use remains 2–3% per year after the first year. Drugs such as amiodarone, lithium, interferon, propylthiouracil, and methimazole may also cause hypothyroidism.

Many of the classic signs and symptoms of hypothyroidism are easily attributed to the aging process. Older adults may present less frequently with weight gain, cold intolerance, muscle cramps, and paresthesias than younger adults with hypothyroidism. Hypertension, hyperlipidemia, bradycardia, as well as both pitting and nonpitting edema may be present in older adults with hypothyroidism and may be attributed to comorbid diseases and drug therapies. Most importantly, neuropsychiatric symptoms including depression and impaired cognition may be present in older adults with hypothyroidism. A recent cohort study from the Framingham study indicated that women who had TSH concentrations less than 1.0 mIU/L (lowest tertile) and over 2.1

IU/L highest tertile) were at increased risk of incident Alzheimer's disease.[45]

KEY POINT: A TSH concentration should be obtained to rule out potentially reversible causes of dementia in older adults.

Subclinical Hypothyroidism

Subclinical hypothyroidism is one of the most common thyroid disorders in older adults with an estimated prevalence of over 15% among older women.[39,46] The serum concentration of TSH is elevated although the free **thyroxine (T4)** concentrations are within the normal range. Frequently, individuals may have antithyroid antibodies present suggesting an autoimmune basis for the condition. Patients may have a history of Graves' disease and/or the prior use of lithium or an iodine-containing medication such as amiodarone. The likelihood of developing hypothyroidism may be as high as 20% per year.[39,46] Screening for the development of clinical hypothyroidism is recommended every 5 years. In general, if the serum TSH concentration is greater than 10mU/L, replacement therapy with levothyroxine is initiated whether or not the patient is symptomatic.[46] For individuals who are asymptomatic and who have serum TSH concentrations between 4 and 10 mU/L, monitoring is generally recommended.[46]

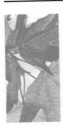

KEY POINT: Initiation and dosage adjustment of levothyroxine should be made based upon assessment of T4 and TSH, rather than TSH alone to avoid inappropriate treatment.

Euthyroid Sick Syndrome

The euthyroid sick syndrome (ESS) has been described as abnormal thyroid function tests in patients with serious nonthyroidal diseases such as gastrointestinal, pulmonary, renal, or cardiovascular illnesses.[39,47] These patients lack a prior history of hypothalamic, pituitary, or thyroid disease. In general, serum T3 concentrations are low and the reverse T3 uptake is elevated. Serum concentrations of T4 are usually in the normal range and TSH may be slightly decreased. In severe nonthyroidal illnesses associated with a high risk of death such as sepsis, concentrations of T3, T4, and TSH may be reduced with an elevated reverse T3 uptake. After recovering from the illness, thyroid function tests return to baseline values. It is unknown if the nonthyroidal disease is causing an artificial effect on the thyroid function tests or if it reflects a true change in thyroid functioning. Although advancing age is not necessarily a risk factor for ESS, older adults have an increased prevalence of ESS due to the increased risk of having multiple chronic systemic diseases. The primary treatment approach is focused on managing the underlying illness and monitoring thyroid function tests during and after recovery.

Summary of Standard Treatment

The recommended treatment for hyperthyroidism consists of the use of antithyroid drugs, radioactive iodine (I-131) or thyroidectomy.[40,48] The antithyroid drugs, propylthiouracil and methimazole, inhibit thyroid peroxidase and the resulting synthesis of thyroid hormone. Propylthiouracil (PTU) also inhibits the peripheral conversion of thyroxine (T4) to triiodothyronine (T3) so that symptoms may resolve more quickly.[48] Methimazole has a longer half-life that permits once daily dosing of the drug compared with propylthiouracil which requires multiple daily doses. In a comparative study of once daily methimazole and once daily PTU, methimazole induced euthyroidism more quickly than PTU.[44] Therapy with antithyroid drugs is continued for 6 to 18 months.[48] The use of I-131 results in radiation-induced destruction of the thyroid gland, while thyroidectomy removes all or part of the thyroid gland. Adjunctive therapy includes beta-adrenergic blockers to control the tachycardia, tremor, and other symptoms of adrenergic excess, as well supersaturated potassium iodine and glucocorticoids in preparation for thyroid surgery.[40]

The recommended first-line treatment for hypothyroidism is levothyroxine. Although other preparations such as dessicated thyroid, triiodothyronine, and combination products containing T4 and T3 are available, these formulations do not offer clinical advantages over levothyroxine for most patients. (Dessicated thyroid is a potentially inappropriate drug to use in older adults due to its potential cardiac effects. This drug is on the list of Beers criteria drugs.[49]) A meta-analysis of 11 studies consisting of 1216 patients evaluated the combination of T4+T3 versus T4 monotherapy in clinical hypothyroidism. Bodily pain, quality of life, depression, fatigue and anxiety were similar between the two treatments. In addition, cognitive functioning, lipids and lipoproteins, and adverse effects were similar. Based on this evidence, a combination product of T3 and T4 does not offer compelling advantages in clinical hypothyroidism.[50]

Treatment Recommendations for Older Adults

Hyperthyroidism

The treatment of hyperthyroidism in older adults usually involves the use of radioactive iodine and antithyroid drugs. Radioactive iodine is the preferred therapy in older adults because the treatment is effective and the long-term risks with the radiation are of less concern. In addition, if hyperthyroidism recurs such as following the use of antithyroid drugs, older adults may have an increased risk of atrial fibrillation.[40] Patients generally become euthyroid within 6 to 12 weeks after receiving radioactive iodine with many individuals eventually becoming hypothyroid.[41] The use of radioactive iodine in older adults with underlying ischemic heart disease may increase the risk of radiation-induced thyroiditis due to the release of preformed thyroid hormone from the gland. To prevent this effect of radioactive iodine, antithyroid drugs may be administered for 1 to 2 months and then discontinued for 3 to 5 days before administering the radioactive iodine.[48]

Another approach to the treatment of hyperthyroidism is to use antithyroid drugs as the first-line treatment. PTU is dosed 50 mg to 100 mg every 8 hours and methimazole 15 mg to 30 mg once daily. Antithyroid drugs are administered for 6 to 18 months with thyroid function tests being monitored every 2 months at least early in therapy. Adverse effects include skin rashes, arthralgias, and myalgias. The most important, although rare, potential adverse effect is agranulocytosis which may be more common in older adults.[40,47] Agranulocytosis has been reported early in therapy in the first 90 days, although it may occur at any time in therapy.[51,52]

Hypothyroidism

The treatment of hypothyroidism should begin with a dosage of 12.5 to 25 mcg of levothyroxine daily, especially in older adults with underlying ischemic heart disease or heart failure.[39] Serum TSH concentrations should be monitored 4 to 6 weeks after starting levothyroxine and after any subsequent dosage adjustment.[41] Dosage adjustments should be between 12.5 and 25 mcg generally and symptoms should be carefully assessed. The goal is to have the TSH within the normal reference range and to prevent overreplacement which might increase the risk of precipitating cardiac symptoms and of worsening osteopenia (or osteoporosis).

Levothyroxine should be dosed once daily on an empty stomach. In addition to foods such as fiber decreasing the absorption of levothyroxine, many drugs and minerals may also prevent its absorption. Bile acid sequestrants such as colestipol and minerals such as calcium and iron may decrease levothyroxine absorption. Other drugs such as phenobarbital, phenytoin, carbamazepine, and rifampin may increase the hepatic metabolism of levothyroxine. A thorough medication history is essential for older adults who are taking levothyroxine.

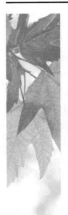

KEY POINT: As patients become euthyroid after treatment of hyperthyroidism or hypothyroidism, their entire drug regimen should be carefully reviewed. The clearance of some medications may have been increased or decreased and dosage adjustments may be indicated to maintain the safety and efficacy of the drug regimen.

Amiodarone-induced Thyroid Dysfunction

Although considered a potentially inappropriate medication in older adults (i.e., Beers drug),[49] amiodarone has been used in many older adults with tacharrhythmias.[53] A meta-analysis reported that the odds ratio of developing a thyroid disorder with amiodarone in a dosage of 152 mg to 330 mg daily was 4.2.[53] Amiodarone has multiple effects on thyroid function due its high iodine content which is about 37% by weight.

Amiodarone may decrease the peripheral conversion of T4 to T3 resulting in reduced concentrations of T3.[53,54] The drug may also decrease the entry of T4 and T3 into peripheral tissues and antagonize the effects of T3 on cardiac cells.[54] Older adults taking amiodarone should probably have thyroid function tests monitored every 6 months.

Amiodarone causes hypothyroidism more commonly in older adults and women probably due to the high prevalence of thyroid disease in these two groups. The onset of amiodarone-induced hypothyroidism is usually slow and occurs in the first 18 months of therapy.[53] In individuals with prior thyroid disease, hypothyroidism from amiodarone may resolve with the discontinuation of the drug, although this may take many months. If the antiarrhythmic is continued due to the underlying cardiac disease or the lack of alternative drugs, larger dosages of levothyroxine may be needed.

Amiodarone may also cause hyperthyroidism. Type 1 thyrotoxicosis develops in individuals with subclinical thyroid disease and low iodine intake, while type 2 occurs in people with normal thyroid glands and is caused by a thyroiditis. The onset of thyrotoxicosis is rapid and may result in new onset angina and tachyarrhythmias. Type 1 hyperthyroidism is treated with high dosages of either methimazole or PTU. In addition to discontinuation of amiodarone, glucocorticoids may have some benefit in type 2 hyperthyroidism by inhibiting the conversion of T4 to T3.

Pituitary Gland Dysfunction

The pituitary gland is responsible for the secretion of many hormones such as adrenocorticotropic hormone (ACTH) and GH. Although little data exist on the prevalence of disorders of the pituitary gland in older adults, deficiency of GH may occur in some older adults. One study demonstrated that GH replacement can increase lean muscle mass, reduce adipose tissue, and increase markers for bone metabolism in older adults with pituitary disease.[55] More importantly, GH has been promoted as an anti-aging therapy, however, evidence of its safety and efficacy in older adults remains limited.[56] A 26-week study of 131 healthy community dwelling adults between 65 and 88 years of age demonstrated increased lean body mass and decreased fat mass, however, muscle strength did not improve.[56] The long-term safety of GH remains unknown with concerns existing about the possible development of adverse effects such as diabetes and glucose intolerance,[57] peripheral edema, joint pain, carpal tunnel syndrome, gynecomastia, and potentially an increased risk of cancer in older adults.[58]

Changes in Sex Hormones in Older Adults
Menopause

Most women will experience the menopause between the ages of 45 and 55 years of age. With this "change of life," women may experience vasomotor symptoms such as hot flashes and also vaginal atrophy and dryness. Although occurring in middle age, most American women can expect to live the last third of their lives in the postmenopausal state. During this time period, the risks of developing coronary heart disease (CHD), osteoporosis, breast and colorectal cancer, and cognitive impairment increase significantly. Since the mid 1960s, the menopause has at times almost been considered an "endocrinopathy" which should be treated with estrogen either alone or in combination with a progestin, when in fact it is a normal part of aging in women.

Over the past 40 years, many observational studies and several small clinical trials suggested that hormone therapy (HT) with either estrogen alone or in combination with a progestin had many health benefits in older women. Although the findings from the observational studies were consistent, the studies were seriously flawed. Women who were using HT in cohort studies were quite different from women who chose not to use hormones in that they were generally much healthier and more adherent.[59] In addition, the women in cohort studies typically had begun using HT shortly after the menopause.[59]

The implementation and subsequent publication of the Women's Health Initiative (WHI) challenged traditional beliefs about the risks and benefits with HT. [60,61] This study enrolled over 162,000 postmenopausal women between the ages of 50 and 79 years into three clinical trials and an observational study. One clinical trial evaluated the risks and benefits of hormone therapy in 16,608 women without CHD.[60] The active treatment included conjugated equine estrogens 0.625 mg plus medroxyprogesterone 2.5 mg daily in women who had an intact uterus. A second WHI study of 10,739 women used conjugated equine estrogens 0.625 mg daily in women who had undergone a hysterectomy.[61] Nonfatal myocardial infarction and death due to CHD was the primary outcome measure and the development of invasive breast cancer was the primary adverse outcome. The study also used a global index to evaluate overall risks such as thromboembolism and benefits such as osteoporosis. Table 10-3 lists the risks and benefits with oral HT from the WHI studies.

Although many middle-aged and older women discontinued the use of HT after the publication of WHI, some elderly women have continued to take HT even after decades of use. Given the risk of breast cancer and the effect of age itself on risk for CHD and stroke, HT should be discontinued whenever possible. Evidence from clinical trials of the risks and benefits of HT after decades of use in elderly women does not exist and such a trial is unlikely to ever be done. As a result, clinicians frequently have little evidence to guide their decision-making regarding HT in women in their 80s and 90s and little informa-

Table 10-3. Selected Potential Risks and Benefits of Oral Hormone Therapy (Estrogen plus Progestin) in Older Women

Risks
- Increased risk of thromboembolic disease in the first year of HT usage.
- Increased risk of coronary heart disease and stroke within the first several years of HT usage with the risk highest among older postmenopausal women.
- Increased risk of breast cancer with longer duration of HT usage which rapidly decreases with cessation of therapy.
- Potentially increased risk of ovarian cancer with HT.
- Potentially increased risk of dementia possibly due to silent small strokes and no benefit on mild cognitive impairment.

Benefits
- Decreased risk of hip and related fractures.
- Decreased risk of invasive colorectal cancer although it is diagnosed at a more advanced stage.
- Decreased moderate-to-severe vasomotor symptoms although no overall benefit on health-related quality of life.

tion to discuss with these women (and potentially with their caregivers).

From one study of women ages 65 to 102 years, discontinuation of HT had variable effects on their health-related quality of life (HRQOL).[62] Among women 65 to 74 years of age, multiple adverse effects on HRQOL were noted including an increase in bodily pain and poorer mental health. Women 75 to 84 years of age reported an increase in the number of days when their physical health was worsened with the discontinuation of HT. In addition, when HT is discontinued, its beneficial effects on bone begin to decrease within several months. If the woman has risk factors for or documented osteoporosis, alternative therapy should be identified to prevent fractures.

Among women 85 years or older, however, an improvement in HRQOL was actually noted with the discontinuation of HT with increases in the number of healthy days among other benefits reported by these women.[62] The optimal way to discontinue HT remains unclear, although the therapy is usually tapered over at least 3 to 6 months if the clinical situation permits.[63,64] This can be accomplished by either slowly decreasing the daily dosage or extending the dosing interval. Of note, studies evaluating different regimens for discontinuing HT have not shown clear benefits of tapering versus abrupt discontinuation and few have evaluated different regimens in very elderly women who have been taking HT for decades.[65]

Andropause

While women have a clearly defined and consistent pattern of hormonal changes during the menopause, it remains controversial as to whether a similar condition occurs in men since some are able to father children even into their 90s. Despite this, the term, andropause, has been used to describe a syndrome in some older men that includes decreased energy, impaired libido and erectile dysfunction, muscle weakness, and depression. Unlike women, men have variable declines in hormone concentrations which may also be influenced by concomitant disorders and drug therapies.[66] There are many potential causes of reduced testosterone concentrations in older men including decreased

bioavailability of the hormone due to increased binding sex-hormone-binding globulin.[66]

Large scale studies evaluating the effect of supplemental testosterone on the musculoskeletal system, cognition, and cardiovascular system in older men are not available. The Endocrine Society's guideline on the use of testosterone products did not recommend a general policy of offering hormone supplementation to all older men with low testosterone concentrations (as compared to levels found in healthy young men) based largely on the lack of the safety and efficacy data.[67,68] The members of the task force for this guideline disagreed as to the specific testosterone levels in older men which would justify replacement, with some indicating concentrations below 300 ng/mL and others favoring below 200 ng/mL. The available testosterone products have the Food and Drug Administration (FDA) labeled indication for the treatment of classical hypogonadism in which testosterone concentrations are very low (discussed as a potential cause of sexual dysfunction below) and not for the management of symptoms associated with andropause.[67]

Sexual Dysfunction

Sexual intimacy and activity remains important even into late life. A recent nationally representative survey reported the prevalence of sexual activity among 3005 community-dwelling older Americans between the ages of 57 and 85 years of age. Sexual activity was defined as a mutually voluntary activity with another person that involved sexual contact regardless of whether or not intercourse or orgasm occurred. Among respondents ages 57 to 64, the prevalence of sexual activity was 73%, while among those 65 to 74 years and 76 to 85 years the prevalence was 53% and 26%, respectively.[69] Among sexually active adults between the ages of 75 and 85, 54% reported sexual activity at least two to three times per month and 23% indicated sex at least once a week. Although a lack of a partner or the presence of a partner with serious health-related issues may limit the frequency of sexual function, older adults, similar to younger individuals, value sexual activity as a part of maintaining close personal relationships.

Etiology, Epidemiology, and Clinical Presentation in Older Adults

Erectile problems are the most commonly reported form of sexual dysfunction, with an estimated prevalence of 37% of older men.[69] The annual incidence of erectile dysfunction was 12.4 per 1,000 person-years among men 40 to 49, 29.8 among men 50 to 59, and 46.4 among men 60 to 69 years old. After adjusting for age, the risk of erectile dysfunction was higher among men with hypertension, diabetes, and heart disease.[70] Normal erectile functioning is the result of a complex interplay between endocrine, vascular, neurologic, and psychosocial factors. Erectile dysfunction, defined as the inability to attain or maintain an erection sufficient for satisfactory sexual intercourse, may be due to many factors. Vascular causes such as atherosclerosis from diabetes, as well as neurological problems following a stroke may result in erectile dysfunction. Many drugs may also contribute to the development erectile dysfunction.

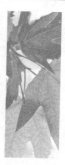

KEY POINT: Erectile dysfunction in older men is a multifactorial condition. Attention should be focused on optimal treatment of underlying diseases such as hypertension and diabetes, rather than considering it solely to be a drug side effect.

Sexual dysfunction in men may also include changes in libido, ejaculation, and orgasm and commonly occur with advancing age. Testosterone concentrations may decline by 1% to 2% per year with levels of free testosterone decreased by up to 30% in men in their seventh decade of life. Luteinizing hormone is reported to be higher than among younger men.[71]

Women have reported less sexual activity across all age groups compared with men. Among women ages 75 to 85, only 16.7% reported sex with a partner in the prior 12 months, while 38.5% of men had engaged in sexual activity.[69] In the recent survey, decreased libido, difficulty with vaginal lubrication, and the inability to climax was reported by 43%, 39%, and 34% respectively.[69] Female sexual dysfunction has been classified as disorders of desire, arousal, orgasm and sexual pain or dyspareunia. Sexual dysfunction among women may be caused by many factors including physiological and hormonal changes resulting from the menopause, as well as relationship, physical and mental health problems. In addition, older women frequently may lack a partner or have a partner with serious health-related issues which limits their sexual activity.

Summary of Standard Treatment

The first-line pharmacotherapy of erectile dysfunction in men consists of the use of oral phosphodiesterase type 5 (PDE5) inhibitors including sildenafil, tadalafil, and vardenafil. The transurethral or intracavernosal administration of alprostadil also enhances the smooth muscle relaxation needed to attain an erection. Testosterone therapy, especially as in a transdermal formulation, is reserved for in men with documented hypogonadism. Other drug therapies such as yohimbine and trazodone are not recommended.[72] Penile devices including a vacuum pump and a penile prosthetic implant that is surgically implanted have been used in men who either do not respond or who have contraindications to drug therapy. Psychotherapy may be used when the erectile dysfunction is believed to have a psychogenic etiology.[73]

The treatment of sexual dysfunction in women is dependent on the potential underlying cause and the specific sexual disorder. For example, symptoms of vaginal dryness can be treated with topical lubricants. The treatment of hypoactive sexual desire disorder has included nonpharmacologic and educational approaches, as well as drug therapy. Transdermal testosterone in a dosage of 300 mcg daily has been used although this is not commercially available for arousal disorders and is not an FDA-approved labeled indication. A recent 6-month study of 814 postmenopausal women ages 20 to 70 with hypoactive sexual desire disorder evaluated the effectiveness of 150 mcg and 300 mcg testosterone patches compared with a placebo patch. Although the higher dose patch demonstrated some benefit, the effects were modest.[74]

PDE-5 inhibitors have also been studied for disorders in desire, arousal, and orgasm, but have not demonstrated consistent benefits and are also not FDA-approved for this use. Sexual pain disorders have been treated with psychotherapy and other nonpharmacologic approaches. Dyspareunia due to vaginal atrophy has been managed with oral and topical estrogens among other therapies.

Treatment Recommendations for Older Adults

The treatment of sexual dysfunction in older men and women involves first identifying and appropriately managing the potentially contributing factors. Many diseases and drugs may adversely affect sexual functioning, however, the cause of sexual dysfunction is frequently due to multiple factors. Although different drug therapies have been used for treating sexual dysfunction in middle-aged men and women, little evidence is available to specifically guide therapy in elderly women.

Contraindications to the use of PDE-5 inhibitors may be more likely to be present in older men than in younger individuals due to the presence of underlying cardiovascular disease. Although PDE-5 inhibitors are generally safe, their use in older men raises several potential concerns. All PDE-5 inhibitors are contraindicated in individuals taking nitrates due to the risk of severe hypotension, as vasodilation from the anti-ischemic therapy may be significantly increased due inhibition of phosphodiesterase. In general, nitrates should be avoided for at least 24 and 48 hours following the use of sildenafil and tadalafil, respectively. The 2007 American Heart Association guidelines on the management of patients with unstable angina/non-ST segment myocardial infarction specifically stated that nitrate use should be avoided for 24 hours after sildenafil use and for 48 hours after tadalafil to prevent severe hypotension.[75]

Older men should also be carefully evaluated with regard to underlying coronary artery disease (CAD) due to concern that increased sexual activity theoretically might increase the risk of coronary ischemia. Patients who are considered to be at intermediate risk include those who have CAD and at least three other risk factors such as a recent myocardial infarction or a cerebrovascular accident. Individuals at high risk include those men with unstable angina and uncontrolled risk factors such as class III or IV heart failure or a myocardial infarction in the past 2 weeks.[76]

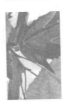

KEY POINT: Older men should be carefully evaluated for their history of CAD and concomitant drug therapy such as nitrates before using a PDE-5 inhibitor.

In 2005, the association between the use of PDE-5 inhibitors and the development of non-arteritic anterior ischemic optic neuropathy (NAION) was reported by the Food and Drug Administration. This disorder is a common cause of sudden visual loss in older adults with an estimated incidence among Caucasian older adults of approximately 5700 cases yearly.[77] Several risk factors, in addition to age, include the presence of diabetes, hypertension, hypercholesterolemia and atherosclerosis. The disorder is believed to be caused by a decreased blood flow to the optic nerves. Whether older men especially in their 70s and 80s are at increased risk of NAION from PDE-5 inhibitors is unknown. A recent review of the available data from clinical trials with PDE-5 inhibitors and postmarketing case reports of NAION did not substantiate this association.[78]

Older men with documented hypogonadism as the cause of their erectile dysfunction may be candidates for testosterone therapy, although the testosterone concentration should be below 200 to 300 ng/mL.[67] Multiple testosterone products are available including depot injectable formulations, patches, gels and buccal tablets. Testosterone enanthate or cypionate is started at a dosage of 75 to 100 mg intramuscularly weekly or 150 to 200 mg every 2 weeks. Testosterone patches may be started at one to two 5-mg patches applied to the back, neck or upper arm every night. The testosterone gel (Androgel, Testim) is applied in the morning to clean, dry nonscrotal skin in a starting dosage of 5 g of gel which delivers 5 mg of testosterone daily. A self-adherent buccal tablet of 30 mg of testosterone is also available and dosed twice daily. The tablet is placed between the inner check and the gums above the incisor tooth and held firmly in place for 30 seconds using a finger. The rounded side of the tablet should be against the gums. The tablet remains in place until the epithelial cells are shed in 12 to 15 hours. The dosage of these testosterone products is increased based on the serum testosterone concentrations obtained 2 to 3 months after starting the products. The testosterone gel package inserts recommend checking testosterone concentrations after 2 weeks of therapy.

Adverse effects from testosterone therapy include the development of polycythemia vera and therapy should be stopped if the hematocrit exceeds 55%. Sleep apnea may worsen especially if risk factors such as obesity and chronic lung disease are present and gynecomastia may also occur with testosterone therapy. Older men receiving testosterone should be carefully monitored for worsening of their benign prostatic hyperplasia if present. The prostate specific antigen concentrations should also be carefully monitored and a digital rectal exam performed at least on a yearly basis.[67]

Other monitoring of testosterone therapy is product specific.[67] In men receiving the buccal formulation, potential changes in taste and irritation of oral mucosa should be evaluated. For the injectable products, men should be asked about any fluctuations in mood and libido in the interval between injections. The development of skin irritation should be carefully monitored with the use of testosterone patches. Although testosterone gels may also cause skin irritation, the most important education issue is to assure that the skin-to-skin transmission of the testosterone to women and children is avoided to minimize potential exposure to the hormone.[79]

CASE 1: DIABETES MELLITUS

Setting:
Outpatient diabetes endocrine treatment center.

Subjective:
JP is a 76-year-old man who presents as a referral from his primary care physician (PCP) for treatment of his diabetes.

Past Medical History:
Hypertension x12 years, newly diagnosed type 2 diabetes mellitus, osteoarthritis in left knee.

Medications:
Atenolol 50 mg qd, hydrochlorothiazide 25 mg qd, acetaminophen 1000 mg qid prn, EC aspirin 81 mg qd, multivitamin qd, chamomile tea every night for sleep.

Allergies:
NKDA

Family History:
Mother died of diabetes complications at age 71, father is 96 years old and living in an assisted living; his daughter had gestational diabetes during her pregnancy.

Social History:

No tobacco, occasionally has 1 alcoholic beverage at a social event. Does not follow any particular diet and patient admits to no desire to change his current eating habits; does not exercise except that he walks his dog for about 5 minutes twice a day. Lives alone and cooks his own meals.

Objective:

Height: 5'9" weight: 247 pounds, blood pressure: 138/92 HR 72, fasting blood glucose: 157mg/dL (2 weeks ago), fasting blood glucose last week: 154 mg/dL. HBA1c today: 8.3%, serum creatinine: 1.2mg/dL

Assessment:

JP is a 76-year-old man with type 2 diabetes and has an increased risk of diabetes complications due to inadequate achievement of target goals for HBA1c and blood pressure.

Plan:

1. Encourage JP to make an individual appointment with a dietician for meal planning assessment and education. Also, offer JP diabetes self-management education referral. Encourage JP to increase exercise. JP may be willing to take longer walks with his dog, for example.

2. Start JP on an oral agent for his elevated blood glucose, consider metformin 500 mg bid for 1–2 weeks and increase by 500 mg every other week until blood glucose is reaching the target goals. The maximum dosage of metformin is 2550 mg of intermediate release, or 2000 mg of XR formulation, but dosages should not be titrated to maximum in older adults.

3. JP should check home blood sugar readings a few times per week in a pattern. Reassess home blood glucose readings in 2–4 weeks, and recheck HBA1c in 3 months.

4. Consider changing atenolol to an angiotensin-converting enzyme (ACE) inhibitor such as lisinopril 10 mg qd for renal protection.

Rationale:

Older adults are at increased risk of hypoglycemic reactions and hypoglycemic unawareness, and metformin does not generally cause hypoglycemia. The drug can be used safely in patients with normal renal function, but should be dosed cautiously in older patients. The incremental increases in dosages are slower than the approach used for a younger adult. Metformin should not be titrated to the maximum dosage in older adults. Metformin generally lowers A1C values by approximately 1.5% which would achieve a target of less than 7%. Hydrochlorothiazide may cause elevations in blood glucose, but does not cause diabetes mellitus. Therefore the hydrochlorothiazide 25mg qd can be continued for hypertension, but the patient also needs renal protection and may benefit from the addition of an ACE inhibitor.

Summary:

This case illustrates the appropriate interventions for an older patient with diabetes, with special attention to age-related considerations for agent choice and dosing. This individual lives alone and manages his own medications, but consider how the approach might differ if he were functionally dependent, cognitively impaired, or living in an institutional setting.

CASE 2: HYPOTHYROIDISM

Setting:
Ambulatory care center

Subjective:
EP is a 78-year-old woman presenting to the ambulatory care center complaining of "tiredness that makes me want to sit around all day." She describes the tiredness as worsening over the past 3 months. She is normally extremely active at her local community senior center. EP also feels that she is somewhat sad and lonely, although she normally has a very active life. She states that she has never experienced anything like this in the past. She also can't tolerate the air conditioning and she normally has her air conditioning on all day during the summer.

Past Medical History:
Hypertension x18 years, osteoporosis x10 years, hyperlipidemia x11 years.

Medications:
Hydrochlorothiazide 25 mg qd, EC aspirin 81 mg qd, lisinopril 10 mg qd, alendronate 70 mg once a week, pravastatin 20 mg q pm, calcium/vitamin D.

Allergies:
Penicillin rash

Family History:
Noncontributory

Social History:
No tobacco, occasionally has 1 alcoholic beverage at a social event
Objective: Height: 5'1" weight: 183 pounds, blood pressure: 124/86 HR 68, T4 =7.2, TSH = 12.1

Geriatric Depression Scale:
4/15, MMSE 28/30

Assessment:
EP is a 72-year-old female with primary hypothyroidism.

Plan:
1. Start EP on a medication for her low thyroid function. Recommend levothyroxine due to its once daily dosing and long half-life. The initial starting dose of levothyroxine is 25 mcg once daily or every other day. Thyroid panel should be monitored in 6–8 weeks after initiating treatment with maximum titration increments of 25 mcg if needed. Cousel EP to take her levothyroxine on an empty stomach at the same time each day, avoiding coadministration with her calcium and vitamin D. Reassess lipids once TSH and T4 are in the normal reference ranges.

Rationale:
EP's symptoms are most likely related to hypothyroidism. The levothyroxine intervention in this case employs a conservative dose and titration schedule. Older adults are at increased risk of overreplacement of thyroid replacement and this may lead to cardiovascular effects as well as worsening osteoporosis. There are several medications that can interact with thyroid replacement treatment. Recommend that any new medications or over-the-counter products first be reviewed by a pharmacist.

Summary:
This patient is presenting with some, but not all, of the classic signs of hypothyroidism. Elderly patients can be vulnerable to misinterpretation of presenting symptoms; for instance her mood symptoms could be interpreted as depression so careful assessment of all possible causes is necessary. Of note, evaluation of both TSH and T4 was used to confirm the diagnosis.

Clinical Pearls

- *Older adults taking antipsychotic medications should be closely monitored for signs and symptoms of hyperglycemia. The risk of developing new onset diabetes from antipsychotic medications appears to be inversely related to age.[80] However, glucose dysregulation may be problematic among older users of antipsychotics with pre-existing diabetes.*

- *Assessment of blood glucose can be difficult for an individual with cognitive impairment who resists fingerstick testing. If monitoring activites routinely turn into a battle resulting in acute agitation, caregivers may find themselves facing tough choices regarding whether to monitor less frequently, reduce or withdraw drug therapy, turn to psychoactive drug therapy, or employ alternate testing methods such as urine dipstick. The risk benefit and the rationale for the strategy employed should be carefully documented.*

Summary

Endocrine diseases such as diabetes mellitus and hypothyroidism are common among older adults. Although they can be safely and effectively treated with standard approaches such as drug therapy, careful attention must be focused on establishing appropriate goals for the individual patient which take into consideration factors such as life expectancy and level of frailty, comorbid conditions and concomitant drug therapy. The old aphorism of "start low and go slow" remains particularly applicable to the management of endocrine disorders in older adults.

Self-Assessment Questions

1. What are the advantages and disadvantages of the available drug therapy to manage diabetes mellitus in older adults?

2. What are common risk factors, presenting symptoms, and management approaches for hypoglycemia due to drug therapy in older adults with diabetes?

3. What are common risk factors, presenting symptoms, and management approaches for hyperosmolar hyperglycemic nonketotic syndrome?

4. Compare and contrast hypothyroidism, subclinical hypothyroidism, and euthyroid sick

syndrome in terms of underlying etiology, presentation, laboratory tests, and management?

5. What are the advantages and disadvantages of the three primary treatments of hyperthyroidism in older adults?

6. How do the available oral medications for hypothyroidism differ?

7. Describe the mechanism and management of amiodarone-induced hyperthyroidism and hypothyroidism in older adults?

8. What are the primary risks with the use of PDE-5 inhibitors and testosterone products in older men who have erectile dysfunction?

9. What are the primary types of female sexual dysfunction and the potential treatments?

References

1. Perry H. The endocrinology of aging. *Clin Chem.* 1999;45:1369–1376.

2. Davison SL, Bell R, Donath S, et al. Androgen levels in adult females: changes with age, menopause, and oophorectomy. *J Clin Endocrinol Metab.* 2005;90:3847–3853.

3. Bergendahl M, Iranmanesh A, Mulligan T, et al. Impact of age on cortisol secretory dynamics basally and as driven by nutrient-withdrawal stress. *J Clin Endocrinol Metab.* 2000;85:2203–2214.

4. Centers for Disease Control and Prevention. Number of people with diabetes increases to 24 million. June 28, 2008. Available at: http://www.cdc.gov/media/press-rel/2008/r080624.htm. Accessed September 29, 2008.

5. Pani LN, Korenda L, Meigs JB, et al. Effect of aging on A1C levels in individuals without diabetes: evidence from the Framingham Offspring Study and the National Health and Nutrition Examination Survey 2001–2004. *Diabetes Care.* 2008; 31(10):1991–1996.

6. Care California Healthcare Foundation/American Geriatrics Society Panel on Improving Care for Elders with Diabetes. Guidelines for improving the care of the older person with diabetes mellitus. *JAGS.* 2003;51:265–280.

7. Selvin E, Bolen S, Yeh H-C, et al. Cardiovascular outcomes in trials of oral diabetes medications. *Arch Intern Med.* 2008;168:2070–2080.

8. Kumar J, Laji K, Page M. Type 1 diabetes in the elderly. Presented at British Endocrine Societies Joint Meeting. *Endocrine Abstracts.* 2002;3:16.

9. Centers for Disease Control and Prevention National Diabetes Fact Sheet, 2007. Available at: http://www.cdc.gov/diabetes/pubs/pdf/ndfs_2007.pdf. Accessed September 29, 2008.

10. Department of Health and Human Services. Data and Statistics 2008. Available at: www.hhs.gov. Accessed September 29, 2008.

11. Meneilly GS. Diabetes in the elderly. *Med Clin North Am.* 2006;90:909–923.

12. Lyssenko V, Jonsson A, Almgren P, et al. Clinical risk factors, DNA variants, and the development of type 2 diabetes. *N Engl J Med.* 2008;359(21):2220–2232.

13. Mazza AD. Insulin resistance syndrome and glucose dysregulation in the elderly. *Clin Geriatr Med.* 2008;24(3):437–454.

14. Meneilly GS, Tessier D. Diabetes in elderly adults. *J Gerontol A Biol Sci Med Sci.* 2001;56(1):M5–13.

15. Morley JE. Diabetes mellitus: a major disease of older persons. *J Gerontol A Biol Sci Med Sci.* 2000;55(5):M255–256.

16. American Diabetes Association. Clinical Practice Recommendations. *Diabetes Care.* 2009;32:S1–61.

17. The Action to Control Cardiovascular Risk in Diabetes Study Group. Effects of intensive glucose lowering in type 2 diabetes. *N Engl J Med.* 2008;358:2545–2559.

18. The ADVANCE Collaborative Group. Intensive blood glucose control and vascular outcomes in patients with type 2 diabetes. *N Engl J Med.* 2008:358:2560–2572.

19. Nathan DM, Buse JB, Davidson MB, et al. Medical management of hyperglycemia in type 2 diabetes: A consensus algorithm for the initiation and adjustment of therapy: A consensus statement of the American Diabetes Association and the European Association for the Study of Diabetes. *Diabetes Care.* 2009;32:193–203.

20. Rosenstock J. Management of type 2 diabetes mellitus in the elderly: Special considerations. *Drugs Aging.* 2001;18(1):31–44.

21. DeFronzo RA, Goodman AM. Efficacy of metformin in patients with non-insulin-dependent diabetes mellitus. The Multicenter Metformin Study Group. *N Engl J Med.* 1995;333(9):541–549.

22. The Diabetes Prevention Program Research Group. Impact of intensive lifestyle and metformin therapy on cardiovascular disease risk factors in the Diabetes Prevention Program. *Diabetes Care.* 2005;28:888–894.

23. Shaw JS, Wilmot RL, Kilpatrick ES: Establishing pragmatic estimated GFR thresholds to guide metformin prescribing. *Diabet Med.* 2007; 24: 1160–1163.

24. Ting RZW, Szeto CC, Chan MHM, et al. Risk factor of vitamin B12 deficiency in patients receiving metformin. *Arch Intern Med.* 2006;166:1975–1979.

25. Rosenstock J, Corrao PJ, Goldberg RB, Kilo C. Diabetes control in the elderly: a randomized, comparative study of glyburide versus glipizide in non-insulin-dependent diabetes mellitus. *Clin Ther.* 1993;15(6):1031–1040.

26. Gangji AS, Cukierman T, Gerstein HC, Goldsmith CH, Clase CM. A systematic review and meta-analysis of hypoglycemia and cardiovascular events: A comparison of glyburide with other secretagogues and with insulin. *Diabetes Care.* 2007; 30:389–394.

27. Nissen SE, Wolski K. Effect of rosiglitazone on the risk of myocardial infarction and death from cardiovascular causes. *N Engl J Med.* 2007;356(24):2457–2471.

28. Saxagliptin. In: DRUGDEX® System [Internet database]. Greenwood Village, Colo: Thomson Reuters (Healthcare) Inc. Updated periodically. Accessed October 5, 2009).

29. Prevention of stroke by antihypertensive drug treatment in older persons with isolated systolic hypertension. Final results of the Systolic Hypertension in the Elderly Program (SHEP). SHEP Cooperative Research Group. *JAMA.* 1991; 265(24):3255–3264.

30. de Jonge P, Roy JF, Saz P, Marcos G, Lobo A. Prevalent and incident depression in community-dwelling elderly persons with diabetes mellitus: results from the ZARADEMP project. *Diabetologia.* 2006;49(11):2627–2633.

31. Ben-Ami H, Nagachandran P, Mendelson A, Edoute Y. Drug-induced hypoglycemic coma in 102 diabetic patients. *Arch Intern Med.* 1999;159(3):281–284.

32. Intensive blood-glucose control with sulphonylureas or insulin compared with conventional treatment and risk of complications in patients with type 2 diabetes (UK-PDS 33). UK Prospective Diabetes Study (UKPDS) Group. *Lancet.* 1998;352(9131):837–853.

33. Gall MA, Nielsen FS, Smidt UM, Parving HH. The course of kidney function in type 2 (non-insulin-dependent) diabetic patients with diabetic nephropathy. *Diabetologia.* 1993;36(10):1071–1078.

34. Sima AA, Greene DA. Diabetic neuropathy in the elderly. *Drugs Aging.* 1995;6(2):125–135.

35. Belmin J, Valensi P. Diabetic neuropathy in elderly patients. What can be done? *Drugs Aging.* 1996;8(6):416–429.

36. Greco D, Angileri G. Drug-induced severe hypoglycaemia in Type 2 diabetic patients aged 80 years or older. *Diabetes Nutr Metab.* 2004;17(1):23–26.

37. Shorr RI, Ray WA, Daugherty JR, Griffin MR. Incidence and risk factors for serious hypoglycemia in older persons using insulin or sulfonylureas. *Arch Intern Med.* 1997;157(15):1681–1686.

38. Levine SN, Sanson TH. Treatment of hyperglycaemic hyperosmolar non-ketotic syndrome. *Drugs.* 1989;38(3):462–472.

39. AACE Thyroid Task Force. American Association of Clinical Endocrinologists medical guidelines for clinical practice for the evaluation and treatment of hyperthyroidism and hypothyroidism. *Endocrine Practice.* 2002;8:457–469.

40. Brent GA. Graves' disease. *N Engl J Med.* 2008; 358:2594–2605.

41. Greenspan SL, Resnick NM. Geriatric endocrinology. In: Gardiner DG, Shoback D, eds. Greenspan's Basic & Clinical Endocrinology. New York: McGraw Hill Medical, 2007:844–858.

42. Trivalle C, Doucet J, Chassagne P, et al. Differences in the signs and symptoms of hyperthyroidism in older and younger patients. *JAGS.* 1996;44(1):50–53.

43. Laurberg P, Andersen S, Pedersen IB, et al. Hypothyroidism in the elderly: pathophysiology, diagnosis, and treatment. *Drugs Aging.* 2005;22:23–38.

44. Homsanit M. Efficacy of single daily dosage of methimazole vs. propylthiouracil in the induction of euthyroidism. *Clin Endocrinol (Oxf).* 2001;54(3): 385–390.

45. Tan ZS, Beiser A, Vasan RS, Au R, et al. Thyroid function and the risk of Alzheimer disease. *Arch Intern Med.* 2008;168:1514–1520.

46. Surks MI, Ortiz E, Daniels GH, et al. Subclinical thyroid disease: scientific review and guidelines for diagnosis and practice. *JAMA.* 2004;291:228–238.

47. Cooper DS. Antithyroid drugs. *N Engl J Med.* 2005; 352:905–917.

48. Abraham P, Avenell A, Watson WA. Antithyroid drug regimen for treating Graves' hyperthyroidism. *Cochrane Database Syst Rev.* 2005;2:CD003420.

49. Fick DM, Cooper JW, Wade WE, et al. Updating the Beers criteria for potentiallyinappropriate medication use in older adults. *Arch Intern Med.* 2003;163:2716–2724.

50. Grozinsky-Glasberg S, Fraser A, Nahshoni E, et al. Thyroxine-triiodothyronine combination therapy versus thyroxine monotherapy for clinical hypothyroidism: Meta-analysis of randomized controlled trials. *J Clin Endocrinol Metab.* 2006;91:2592–2599.

51. Cooper DS, Goldminz D, Levin AA, et al. Agranulocytosis associated with antithyroid drugs: effects of patient age and drug dose. *Ann Intern Med.* 1983;98:26–29.

52. Pearce SH. Spontaneous reporting of adverse reactions to carbimazole and propylthiouracil in the UK. *Clin Endocrinol.* 2004;61:589–594.

53. Vorperian VR, Havinghurst TC, Miller S et al. Adverse effects of low dose amiodarone: a meta-analysis. *J Am Coll Cardiol.* 1997;30:791–798.

54. Basaria S, Cooper DS. Amiodarone and the thyroid. *Am J Med.* 2005; 118:706–714.

55. Fernholm R, Bramnert M, Hagg E, et al. Growth hormone replacement therapy improves body composition and increases bone metabolism in elderly patients with pituitary disease. *J Clin Endocrinol Metab.* 2000;85:4104–4112.

56. Vance ML. Growth hormone for the elderly? *N Engl J Med.* 1990;323:52–54.

57. Blackman MR, Sorkin JD, Munzer T, et al. Growth hormone and sex steroid administration in healthy aged men and women: a randomized controlled trial. *JAMA.* 2002;288:2282–2292.

58. Liu H, Bravata DM, Olkin I et al. Systematic review: the safety and efficacy of growth hormone in the health elderly. *Ann Intern Med.* 2007;146:104–115.

59. Grodstein F, Clarkson TB, Manson JE. Understanding the divergent data on postmenopausal hormone therapy. *N Engl J Med*. 2003;348:645–650.

60. Writing Group for the Women's Health Initiative Investigators. Risks and benefits of estrogen plus progestin in healthy postmenopausal women. Principal results from the Women's Health Initiative randomized controlled trial. *JAMA*. 2002;288:321–333.

61. Women's Health Initiative Steering Committee. Effects of conjugated equine estrogen in postmenopausal women with hysterectomy. The Women's Health Initiative randomized controlled trial. *JAMA*. 2004;291:1701–1712.

62. Heller DA, Gold CH, Ahern FM, et al. Changes in elderly women's health-related quality of life following discontinuation of hormone replacement therapy. *BMC Women's Health*. 2005;5:1–13

63. Nelson HD. Assessing benefits and harms of hormone replacement therapy. *JAMA*. 2002;288:882–884.

64. Grady D. A 60-year-old woman trying to discontinue hormone replacement therapy. *JAMA*. 2002;287:2130–2137.

65. Haskell SG, Bean-Mayberry B, Gordon K. Discontinuing postmenopausal hormone therapy: an observational study of tapering versus quitting cold turkey: is there a difference in recurrence of menopausal symptoms? *Menopause*. 2009;16(3):494–499.

66. Travison TG, Araujo AB, Kupelian V, et al. The relative contribution of aging, health, and life style factors to serum testosterone decline in men. *J Clin Endocrinol Metab*. 2007;2:549–555.

67. Bhasin S, Cunningham GR, Hayes FJ, et al. Testosterone therapy in adult men with androgen deficiency syndromes: An Endocrine Society Clinical Practice Guideline. *J Clin Endocrinol Metab*. 2006;91(6):1995–2010.

68. Calof OM, Singh AB, Lee ML, et al. Adverse events associated with testosterone replacement in middle-aged and older men: a meta-analysis of randomized, placebo-controlled trials. *J Gerontol A Biol Sci Med Sci*. 2005;60:1451–1457.

69. Lindau ST, Schumm LP, Laumann EO, et al. A study of sexuality and health among older adults in the United States. *N Engl J Med*. 2007;357:762–774.

70. Johannes CB, Araujo AB, Feldman HA, et al. Incidence of erectile dysfunction in men 40 and 69 years old: longitudinal results from the Massachusetts Male Aging Study. *J Urol*. 2000;163:460–463.

71. Camacho ME, Reyes-Ortiz CA. Sexual dysfunction in the elderly: age or disease? *Int J Impot Res*. 2005;17:S52–56.

72. American Urologic Association Erectile dysfunction guidelines update panel. Management of erectile dysfunction. 2006 http://www.auanet.org/guidelines/main_reports/edmgmt/chapter1.pdf

73. McVary KT. Erectile dysfunction. *N Engl J Med*. 2007;357:2472–2481.

74. Davis SR, Moreau M, Kroll R, et al. Testosterone for low libido in postmenopausal women not taking estrogen. *N Engl J Med*. 2008;359:2005–2017.

75. Anderson JL, Adams CD, Antman EM, et al. ACC/AHA 2007 guidelines for the management of patients with unstable angina//non-ST-elevation myocardial infarction: a report of the American College of Cardiology/American Heart Association Task Force on Practice Guidelines. *J Am Coll Cardiol*. 2007;50:e1–157.

76. Jackson G, Rosen RC, Kloner RA, et al. The second Princeton consensus on sexual dysfunction and cardiac risk: new guidelines for sexual medicine. *J Sex Med*. 2006;3:28–36.

77. Hattenhauer MG, Leavitt JA, Hodge DO, et al. Incidence of nonarteritic anterior ischemic optic neuropathy. *Am J Ophthalmol*. 1997;123:103–107.

78. Laties AM. Vision disorders and phosphodiesterase type 5 inhibitors: A review of the evidence to date. *Drug Safety*. 2009;32(1):1–18.

79. FDA News. Testosterone gel safety concerns prompt FDA to require label changes, medication guide. http://www.fda.gov/bbs/topics/NEWS/2009/NEW02011.html Accessed 5/24/09.

80. Hammerman A, Dreiher J, Klang SH, et al. Antipsychotics and diabetes: an age-related association. *Ann Pharmacother*. 2008;42(9):1316–1322.

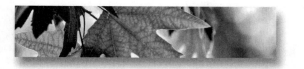

11

Gastrointestinal Disorders and Nutrition

JEANNIE KIM LEE

Learning Objectives

1. Identify the prevalence of GI disorders and nutritional problems among different subgroups of elderly patients.

2. Assess the applicability of general adult treatment guidelines and management strategies for GI disorders to different age strata of elderly patients.

3. Recommend treatment goals and appropriate drug therapy for GI disorders in elderly patients.

4. Recommend treatment goals and strategies for maintaining optimal oral health and nutrition in elderly patients.

Key Terms

ANASTOMOSIS: Surgical connection of two tubular structures (e.g., intestines).

AUERBACK'S PLEXUS: A plexus of sympathetic nerve fibers located in the muscle coat of the stomach and intestine.

BARRETT'S ESOPHAGUS: A complication of GERD in which the tissue lining the esophagus is replaced by tissue that is similar to the lining of the intestine (intestinal metaplasia); can progress to esophageal cancer.

DENTURE STOMATITIS: Inflammation of the mouth caused by painful or ill-fitting dentures.

HYPOCHLORHYDRIA: Decreased or diminished secretion of hydrochloric acid.

POLYPHARMACY: Use of multiple medications concurrently.

PYROSIS: Heartburn.

XEROSTOMIA: Dry mouth.

Introduction

Gastrointestinal (GI) disorders are prevalent in the elderly and GI complaints common. Ranging from mild reflux symptoms to major bowel ischemia, GI diseases such as diverticulitis are more common, while other conditions such as acid reflux often present and progress differently in this population. Aging imparts various physiologic changes in the oropharynx, esophagus, and stomach that lead to increased risk of esophageal and gastrointestinal disorders. Age-related changes in intestinal innervation may contribute to gastrointestinal disorders that are seen with increased incidence in the elderly such as dysphagia, gastroesophageal reflux disease (GERD) and constipation. Special nutritional needs required by age and disease processes must be met in order for patients to experience optimal quality of life and longevity. This chapter discusses etiology, epidemiology and clinical presentation of various GI disorders and nutritional conditions commonly seen in the aging patient population; summarizes standard treatment and management strategies seen in the general population; reviews evidence base for recommendations specific to the older patients; and explores special considerations affecting desired clinical outcomes.

Gastroesophageal Reflux Disease

Etiology, Epidemiology, and Clinical Presentation

Gastroesophageal Reflux Disease (GERD) symptoms are increased in the older adults partly due to physiologic changes, such as slow gastric emptying and decreased saliva production, brought on by the aging process. GERD, the most prevalent GI disorder affecting the elderly in the U.S., causes monthly symptoms in more than 40% of patients and daily symptoms in nearly 10%.[1] Persistent symptoms, often require chronic maintenance therapy and decrease quality of life. If left untreated or undertreated, GERD can lead to complications, including esophagitis, ulceration, bleeding, and Barrett's esophagus.[1] In fact, elderly patients typically have milder symptoms, yet more severe esophagitis compared to the younger patients.[2] The older adults also have reduced intra-abdominal length of the lower esophageal sphincter and increased incidence of hiatal hernia (over 60% for patients over 60 years of age) contributing to higher rates of GERD.[3] Due to decreased visceral sensation or taking medications that blunt sensation, the typical symptoms of GERD may be masked in older adults.

Medications causing GERD are associated with higher risk of GERD in the elderly[4] and include bisphosphonates (e.g., alendronate, risedronate), potassium chloride, nonsteroidal anti-inflammatory Drugs (NSAIDs), aspirin, tetracycline derivatives, clindamycin, ferrous compounds, calcium channel blockers (e.g., verapamil), narcotics (e.g., codeine, morphine), anticholinergics (e.g., diphenhydramine, amitriptyline), phosphodiesterase-5 inhibitors (e.g., sildenafil), and theophylline. Lesser known causes of these symptoms may also include acetylcholinesterase inhibitors or antipsychotic medications. In addition, foods such as tomato, dairy products, fatty meat, peppermints, fruit juices, alcohol and caffeine can exacerbate or worsen GERD symptoms. Therefore, dietary habits should be assessed for these patients. Other reasons for higher risk of GERD in the elderly include taking more medications, spending more time in a recumbent position, having reduced salivary production in association with poor oral fluid intake, predisposition to motility or anatomic disorders of the esophagus.[3]

A 2006 study found patients with mean age of 88 years experiencing highest rates of dysphagia, anorexia, anemia, weight loss and vomiting related to reflux esophagitis, followed by patients with mean age of 77 years, compared to adults younger than 60 years of age.[4] Older patients often present with atypical or alarm symptoms, including chest pain, hoarseness, cough, wheezing, dysphagia, and poor dentition. A clinician's ability to recognize these symptoms and relate them to GERD is vital, and can prevent delayed diagnosis and treatment. Esophagogastroduodenoscopy (EGD) is safely performed even in the very old, and biopsies can be obtained during the procedure. Additionally, elderly patients may not seek medical attention for bothersome GERD symptoms simply attributing them to being part of the normal aging. Thus, probing to obtain accurate symptom history may be required for proper diagnosis.

Standard Treatment and Management Strategies in General Adult Population

According to the American College of Gastroenterology, GERD can be diagnosed when patients presenting with typical symptoms of pyrosis and regurgitation improve after completion of a short course proton pump inhibitor (PPI) therapy (e.g., omeprazole 20 mg daily for 1 week).[5] Goals of therapy include alleviating symptoms, decreasing frequency of recurrent disease, promoting healing of the mucosal injury, and preventing complications. Either "step up" or "step down" therapy is chosen depending on patient's clinical presentation and associated risk factors as well as patient preference (see Table 11-1). Lifestyle modification, shown in Table 11-1, should be part of all management strategies employed for treating GERD.[5] Although over-the-counter antacids can

Table 11-1. Therapeutic Strategies in GERD

Lifestyle Modification			Therapy Strategy	
Always Done	Medication Class	Medication Regimen	Step Down	Step Up
• Elevating head of bed • Smoking cessation • Avoid recumbency for 3 hours after meals • Eat low-fat meals in small portions • No eating before sleep • Weight loss • Avoid irritating medications (NSAIDs,* etc) • Avoid irritating foods (chocolate, tomato, alcohol, coffee, etc)	PPI	**Esomeprazole** 20 mg daily **Lansoprazole** 15 mg daily **Omeprazole** 20 mg daily **Pantoprazole** 40 mg daily **Rabeprazole** 20 mg daily		
	H2RA	**Cimetidine** 400 mg twice daily **Famotidine** 20 mg twice daily **Nizatidine** 150 mg twice daily **Ranitidine** 150 mg twice daily		
	OTC PPI‡	**Omeprazole** 20 mg daily		
	OTC H2RA†	**Cimetidine** 200 mg twice daily **Famotidine** 10 mg twice daily **Nizatidine** 75 mg twice daily **Ranitidine** 75 mg twice daily		
	Antacid	**Aluminum/magnesium, Regular dose** 30 mL as needed or after meals and at bedtime **Aluminum/magnesium, High dose** 15 mL as needed or after meals and at bedtime **Antacid with alginic acid,** 2 tablets after meals and at bedtime **Calcium carbonate** 500 mg, 2–4 tablets as needed		

*Nonsteroidal anti-inflammatory drugs.
†Over-the-counter H$_2$-receptor antagonists.
‡Over-the-counter proton pump inhibitor.

be used for mild intermittent disease, acid suppression therapy is the mainline treatment for GERD, with PPIs having better efficacy rates than Histamine$_2$ Receptor Antagonists (H$_2$RAs).[5]

Evidence Base Supporting Treatment Recommendations in Elderly Patients

One of the treatment goals specific to older patients with GERD include using the most appropriate antireflux therapy administration option for patient's ability to swallow. Another goal is to provide optimal acid suppression to prevent complications. Clinicians should keep in mind that older patients are more prone to erosive esophagitis and complications of GERD, usually calling for more aggressive therapy. PPI therapy is warranted in patients older than 60 years of age due to superior efficacy evidenced and more convenient once daily dosing compared to the traditional agents for treating GERD.[3] Because GERD is a chronic, relapsing disease for the aging population, in whom symptoms and esophagitis can rapidly recur if therapy is discontinued, long-term treatment may be necessary to ensure effective management.

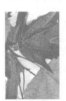

KEY POINT: Older patients require more potent and sustained acid inhibition to effectively achieve and maintain optimal clinical outcomes.

Promotility agents such as metoclopramide and bethanechol are associated with increased risk of adverse drug reactions (ADRs) in older adults. The elderly are especially sensitive to CNS effects of metoclopramide such as fatigue, lethargy, anxiety, and extrapyramidal side effects. Metoclopramide also carries several drug interaction potentials with anticholinergics, sedatives, narcotics, antipsychotics, and alcohol. Thus, use in older patients is generally discouraged.[6] Bethanechol is a cholinergic agonist that increases LES pressure and gastric contractility but decreases frequency of contractions and does not improve gastric emptying. It also has an adverse effect profile that greatly limits its usefulness, particularly in the elderly. Side effects include abdominal cramps, urinary frequency, malaise, blurred vision, diarrhea, and increased gastric acid secretion.[7] Antireflux surgery, an option for adult patients with refractory disease,[5] may not be a safe option for the elderly who are at increased risk for surgery and having multiple comorbidities.

Special Considerations Affecting Desired Clinical Outcomes

Because older adults often take multiple medications, it is important to stress the specific recommendation of antireflux therapy (e.g., take omeprazole 30 minutes before the first meal of the day). Repeated counseling on the indication for the drug can improve adherence, since many older patients stop taking their medications simply because they forget what the drugs are for.

The benefit of controlled GERD may extend to asthma control. A review of 8 studies found a correlation between patients with GERD symptoms and asthma, where improved asthma symptoms (by 69%) as well as clinical outcome (by 26%) were noted after anti-GERD therapy initiation.[8] However, despite the therapeutic effectiveness of controlling GERD, there are some findings regarding potent acid suppression therapy that may be of concern, especially for the elderly. The evidence connecting acid suppression to community-acquired pneumonia (CAP) is alarming. A cohort study of 364,683 patients taking either PPI or H$_2$RA found to have increased risk for acquiring CAP.[9] Because elderly are among the patients at risk for developing CAP, acid suppression therapy should be used at lowest possible dose only when necessary. At the same time, there is evidence showing higher incidence of hip fractures in patients receiving long-term, high-dose PPI treatment, which may result from reduced calcium absorption in the setting of potent acid suppression.[10] Since older adults are already at higher risk for falls resulting in various fractures, caution should be exercised when prescribing high-dose PPI to a frail elderly patient. In addition, gastric acid suppression using PPIs in particular have been associated with hospital-acquired and community-acquired *Clostridum difficile* infection and diarrhea.[11,12] Lastly, recent discovery of omeprazole and clopidogrel interaction has been concerning for cardiac patients undergoing stent placement when a study found significantly decreased effect of clopidogrel on platelet activation by omeprazole.[13] Currently, FDA warns against acid suppression therapy with PPI in patients taking dual aspirin and clopidogrel antiplatelet regimen after cardiac stent placement, but this is still controversial.[14]

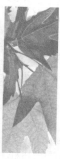

KEY POINT: Based on these findings, an accurate diagnosis and appropriate dose need to be assured, along with properly weighing the risk versus benefit when considering long-term therapy with a PPI in older patients.

Diverticular Disease

Etiology, Epidemiology, and Clinical Presentation

Diverticula are acquired sac-like mucosal projections through the muscular layer of the GI tract. They cause symptoms by trapping feces, becoming infected, bleeding, or rupturing. They develop in areas where circular smooth muscle has been weakened by the penetration of blood vessels to the submucosa. Diverticula are commonly found in the sigmoid and descending colons and rarely in the rectum.[1] Aging leads to structural weakening of colonic muscle and the development of diverticula. In Western countries, diverticular disease occurs in more than 60% of people older than 70 years and nearly 80% of those older than 80 years.[1] Higher prevalence in Western populations is most likely due to increased longevity and insufficient dietary fiber intake, since a low-fiber diet may increase colonic motor activity and intraluminal pressure.[1] More recent studies suggest, however, that with increasing globalization, factors previously uncommon in developing countries, such as the availability of highly processed food products and obesity, may be operating to cause a prevalence rate of diverticular disease in Eastern populations similar to those in Western European and American populations.[15] Of the patients with diverticula, 80–85% remain asymptomatic, however the prevalence is thought to be slightly higher in women. Asymptomatic diverticular disease can mimic a variety of other diseases, such as the following: colorectal cancer, acute appendicitis, ischemic colitis, pseudomembranous colitis, renal disease, cystitis, ovarian cyst, abscess, tumor, gallbladder disease, pancreatic disease, mucosal prolapse, small bowel obstruction, and peritonitis.[16]

Aging is accompanied by a change in bowel wall architecture that increases the wall thickness and inelasticity and tends to increase intraluminal pressure, favoring the formation of diverticula.[16] The increasing prevalence of symptomatic diverticular disease as people age may reflect an increased prevalence of constipation[16], which often is aggravated by a sedentary lifestyle and polypharmacy. An overall lack of physical activity is associated independently with an increased risk of symptomatic diverticular disease.

Clinically, patients with diverticular disease usually present with abdominal pain with or without alterations in bowel habit, but without evidence of inflammation, such as fever and leukocytosis, or peritoneal signs on physical exam.[16] The hallmark of painful diverticular disease is "attacks" of abdominal pain without any indication of an inflammatory process. The abdominal pain is most commonly described as colicky but also can be steady. It is usually exacerbated by eating and typically is relieved by a passage of flatus or a bowel movement. In two thirds of cases, there is accompanying alteration of bowel habits, more often constipation than diarrhea, and occasionally repeated bouts of constipation followed by diarrhea.[15] During these attacks of painful diverticular disease, physical exam may reveal fullness or mild tenderness in the left lower quadrant and occasionally a tender palpable loop of distended sigmoid colon.[16]

On the other hand in diverticulitis, the most common complication of diverticular disease, patients present with evidence of inflammation and clinical signs including pain, bleeding, obstruction, abscess, fistula and perforation.[1] Patients with diverticular disease have a 10–20% chance of developing diverticulitis.[16] Because the incidence of diverticulitis increases with a longer duration of diverticulosis as well as a greater number of diverticula, there is a direct correlation between diverticulitis and increasing age. Although some older patients may present with the classic symptoms, others may display only mild symptoms, no fever or elevation of the leukocyte count, and only vague abdominal signs. In an elderly or a debilitated patient, the absence of fever, leukocytosis, or rebound tenderness does not exclude diverticulitis. Consequently, diverticulitis must be approached with caution in this population, and health care professionals must be particularly careful not to underestimate the severity of disease on the basis of minimal symptoms or a normal laboratory evaluation.[15] As with many disease processes in the elderly, the pathology may be extensive and severe despite an unimpressive clinical picture. A study that assessed the effect of age and location on the severity of diverticular disease found that patients with right-sided diverticulitis, who tend to be younger, were more likely to be treated surgically and on an emergency basis out of concern for a mistaken diagnosis, since this presentation can mimic acute appendicitis.[17] Whereas, patients with left-sided diverticulitis were usually much older than those with right-sided diverticulitis, and did not attract the emergency surgeries.[17] Adopting an age cutoff of 60 years, the authors also found that older patients who were treated conservatively were more likely than younger patients to experience recurrent abdominal pain.[17]

Standard Treatment and Management Strategies in General Adult Population

The most important treatment goal is to eliminate bacterial infection. Other goals of therapy include improvement of symptoms, reduction of recurrent attacks in symptomatic uncomplicated disease, and prevention of complication of the disease such as diverticulitis.[1] Several therapies have been proposed for treatment of diverticular disease, including: high-fiber diet and/or fiber supplementation, spasmolytics, probiotics, antibiotics, and mesalamine.[15] In patients with uncomplicated diverticulitis who are clinically stable and able to tolerate fluids, outpatient treatment with broad-spectrum antibiotics covering anaerobes and gram negative rods for 7–10 days along with a clear liquid diet is adequate.[1,15] Patients should improve within 2–3 days, at which time solid foods may be introduced very cautiously. Antibiotics used in outpatient setting include, Amoxicillin-clavulanate, trimethoprim-sulfamethoxazole plus metronidazole, fluoroquinolone plus metronidazole.[15]

More acutely-ill patients are hospitalized. If a patient experiences increasing pain, fever, or inability to tolerate fluid intake, hospitalization is appropriate for his or her care. These patients need IV antibiotic therapy with either a clear liquid diet or nothing by mouth. IV fluids should be provided for hydration.[15] Improvement of symptoms should be expected within 2–4 days, at which point a solid diet can be slowly introduced. Patients can then be discharged to complete a 7–10-day course of oral antibiotics. IV Antibiotics used in inpatient setting include penicillin/beta lactase combination antibiotics, cefoxitin or cefotetan, or a combination of either third-generation cephalosporin, or aminoglycoside, or a monobactam plus metronidazole or clindamycin.[15]

Most patients admitted with acute diverticulitis respond to medical therapy, but 15–30% of them require surgery.[18] The risk of recurrent symptoms after an attack of acute diverticulitis has been reported to be between 7% and 45%. Recurrent attacks are less likely to respond to medical treatment and have a high mortality rate. Thus, most agree that elective resection is indicated after two attacks of uncomplicated diverticulitis.[18] Risk of resection is an evolving factor, with reports of increasingly favorable experiences with laparoscopic resections for diverticular disease.[19] The preferred procedure is a one-stage operation in which the diseased segment of bowel is resected and continuity restored by a primary **anastomosis**.

A significant inverse association has been reported between dietary fiber intake and risk of development of clinically evident diverticular disease in the general adult population, although studies in frail elderly are lacking. Insoluble fiber from fruits and vegetables was noted to be more protective than cereal fibers.[20]

Medications and probiotics have been tested for use in diverticular disease as well. Antispasmodics are often employed to alleviate cramping and bloating associated with symptomatic diverticular disease, however no good evidence supports the use of these anticholinergic drugs, particularly among frail elderly patients.[15] The role of probiotics in the treatment of diverticular disease remains unclear also. Rifaximin, a broad-spectrum, poorly-absorbed antibiotic, and mesalamine, appear to be of some advantage in obtaining symptom relief in uncomplicated diverticular disease, and in reducing the incidence of the primary complications.[15] However, a wide use of the above mentioned agents for diverticular disease in clinical settings has not been realized.

Evidence Base Supporting Treatment Recommendations in Elderly Patients

Given the relative safety of colonoscopy in elderly patients, as well as the exponential increase in the prevalence of colorectal cancer in patients older than age 70, performing colonoscopy in generally health ambulatory elderly patients who present for the first time with painful diverticular disease is indicated.[16] The need for hospital admission is the initial decision to be made in the treatment of uncomplicated diverticulitis. Hospitalization is recommended if patients show signs of significant inflammation, are unable to take oral fluids, are older than 75 years of age, or have significant comorbidity.[16]

KEY POINT: Based on these criteria, older patients have a high probability of needing hospital admission for adequate treatment of their diverticular disease.

Treatment strategies for diverticulitis in the elderly are similar to the standard treatment used for adult population. An older patient treated at home should have a close follow-up, and they or their caregiver should be instructed to contact the provider for increasing pain, fever, or inability to tolerate oral fluids, which may necessitate hospitalization.[16] Although it was reasonable in the past to prescribe a high-fiber diet for elderly patients for its other potential health benefits, most notably the belief that the risk of colorectal cancer may be reduced, more recent large-scale epidemiologic studies have not supported this claim.[21]

Complicated diverticulitis generally requires surgery in addition to intravenous broad-spectrum antibiotics, bowel rest, and intravenous hydration. Surgery, at times urgent, usually can be delayed pending the control of sepsis. Laparoscopic resection is preferred in older patients. Several large series of laparoscopic resections in patients with complicated diverticular disease, some of whom were very elderly, have been published, with generally favorable results.[19]

Special Considerations Affecting Desired Clinical Outcomes

Diverticular perforation with peritonitis is rare, but it carries a mortality rate as high as 35% and requires urgent surgical consultation. If generalized peritonitis develops, the mortality rate is even higher.[15] Older adults with generalized peritonitis require immediate excision of the perforation site. Giving antibiotics and waiting for resolution can result in an extremely high mortality. Glucocorticoids may increase the risk of perforation, mask symptoms, and delay appropriate therapy.[15] Thus, glucocorticoids should be used with caution in older patients for whom we know higher prevalence of diverticular disease exists. Perforation has been linked to NSAIDs use as well. Diverticular sources have been reported to be the most typically identified cause of lower GI bleeding in the elderly, accounting for over 40% of the episode.[15] In a large prospective study evaluating patients with lower GI bleeding (of whom 50% were diverticular), the bleeding risk with NSAIDs was reported to be equal to that of duodenal ulcer risk.[15] In the Health Professional Follow-Up Study, regular NSAID use was associated with an increased risk of diverticular bleeding.[22] Since many older patients take NSAIDs, prescription and over-the-counter, for arthritis and other conditions, close monitoring of above complications should be employed in managing diverticular disease in this population. More recently, a protective association has been found between calcium channel blockers and perforated colonic diverticular disease.[23] Therefore, calcium channel blockers may be considered for elderly patients with concurrent hypertension and diverticulosis.

Constipation and Fecal Incontinence
Etiology, Epidemiology, and Clinical Presentation

Chronic constipation is extremely prevalent among older adults. The meaning of the term "constipation" may vary among patients and providers. The most commonly accepted medical definition of constipation, a stool frequency of less than three times per week, may underestimate the complaints among the geriatric population.[24] Elderly patients do not always equate constipation with the frequency of the event as they may perceive straining during bowel movement as being constipated. As a result of the discrepancies in the term "constipation," two broad definitions are now utilized: (1) functional constipation and (2) outlet delay constipation. Functional constipation is defined as having any two of the following complaints[24] straining to defecate, passing hard stools, having the sensation of incomplete evacuation, defecating fewer than three times a week. In absence of above symptoms, having fewer than two bowel movements per week is also considered functional constipation. On the other hand outlet delay constipation describes patients who experience sense of anal blockage, prolonged defecation (longer than 10 minutes) or having to digitally assist bowel movement due to inappropriate contraction of the external anal sphincter on straining or anal obstruction.[24]

At the same time, there is a third group of patients, who use routine laxatives for regular bowel movement and describe themselves as being chronically constipated. Older patients are likely to self-medicate for constipation with over-the-counter medications and/or herbal products prior to discussing the options with their providers. It is estimated that 10–18% of community-dwelling elderly use laxatives routinely.[25] The prevalence of functional constipation in community-dwelling patients older than 65 years was estimated to be around 24%.[26] But, when the patients with symptoms of outlet delay constipation, self-reported constipation, and laxative use were added, the prevalence increased to approximately 40%.[26] Unfortunately, the existing prevalence estimation of constipation for this age group did not include nursing home patients; thus, the burden of this disease on the oldest old and the most frail are underestimated.[24] The estimation is still nearly twice that of the middle-aged population.

An older adult's constipation usually results from inadequate hydration, decreased activity, and using polypharmacy. For many elderly, functional decline leading to decreased mobility and poor dietary status contribute to constipation. These patients may be taking diuretics but not drinking enough fluids due to decreased sense of thirst or problems with urinary incontinence, which consequently lead to dehydration and constipation.[27] The use of polypharmacy in this population is often unavoidable given the multiple chronic conditions they treat. Constipation is a major side effect of numerous medications often prescribed in the elderly.

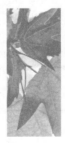

KEY POINT: Multiple medications commonly prescribed in the elderly such as narcotics, calcium channel blockers, beta blockers, diuretics, anticholinergics, hypnotics, iron, and calcium can trigger or worsen constipation.

Also, neurological conditions, commonly found in the older population, such as dementia, stroke, multiple sclerosis, spinal cord injury, diabetes, Alzheimer's disease and Parkinson's disease, can instigate neurogenic bowel (constipation and fecal incontinence).[28] In addition, common systemic diseases suffered by elderly can lead to bowel dysfunction as well[28]:

- Hypothyroidism can cause hypomotility and slow gut transit
- Heart failure can lead to bowel edema
- Autonomic or sensory neuropathies from diabetes can increase the risk of constipation
- Metabolic diseases including hyperparathyroidism and Addison's disease can affect bowel function
- Metabolic disturbances, such as hypercalcemia and hypokalemia, can affect smooth muscle function

Fecal incontinence, defined as the involuntary loss of liquid or solid stool, is understandably disabling for patients and results in anxiety, fear of public embarrassment, and having to wear a pad routinely.[24] Temporary fecal incontinence can develop in the presence of a GI infection.[24] Patients with functional incontinence possess the functional ability, but due to the decreased mobility, vision or cognitive dysfunction, are unable to use the toilet on time.[24] The most common cause of fecal incontinence in the nursing home residents and hospitalized patients is overflow incontinence secondary to constipation and stool impaction.[24] Age-related anal sphincter dysfunction contributes to the increasing prevalence of fecal incontinence in patients aged 80 years and older. According to a population-based study, the prevalence of fecal incontinence increases with age, affecting 7% of women aged 20–29 years to 21% of women aged 80 years.[29] Among most women in this study, the incontinent episodes were less than monthly regardless of age; however, 33–66% of nursing home residents had daily incontinence.[29] Another study on fecal incontinence, defined as loss of control anytime in the last year, in community-dwelling older adults reported the estimated prevalence of 12%.[30] This rate would have been much higher if the study had included older adults residing in long term care facilities.

This condition is exacerbated by chronic diarrhea, chronic constipation with overflow diarrhea, or acute infection. For example, 42% of patients having fecal incontinence reported having chronic diarrhea, and 17% chronic constipation.[24] Clinical consequences of fecal incontinence include skin breakdown, depression from social isolation, and decreased functional status, precipitating the decision to move into a long-term care environment. As with constipation, diarrhea in older adults can also be caused by medications they take. Examples include antibiotics, digoxin, metformin, colchicine, NSAIDs, cholinergic agents, cholinesterase inhibitors, magnesium-containing antacids and phosphorus. Diet high in fat as well as eating and drinking spicy foods, fruit juices, caffeine or enteral feedings can exacerbate diarrhea also.

Standard Treatment and Management Strategies in General Adult Population

Constipation

Patient assessment for constipation can been done by asking a few simple questions[24]:

- Do you often have fewer than three bowel movements a week?
- Do you often have a hard time passing stools?
- Are stools often lumpy or hard?
- Do you have a feeling of being blocked or of not having fully emptied your bowel?

After mechanical causes of constipation have been excluded, initiation of the treatment should be based on the patient's primary complaint. Patients experiencing straining and incomplete evacuation usually respond to adequate fluid intake and scheduled bathroom visits, along with taking bulk-forming agents. On the other hand, patients with infrequent bowel movements generally respond to osmotic agents such as lactulose.[1] A typical bowel regimen for a patient suffering neurogenic bowel with constipation may consist of taking stool softener at meal times (two to three times daily) plus two senna tablets at bedtime. With this regimen, the patient is expected to have a bowel movement in the morning. The patient may also require bisacodyl, use as needed daily or every other day, if above regimen does not regulate routine bowel movement. Other available agents that are generally used as needed include glycerin suppositories, phosphate enema and osmotic laxatives (e.g., lactulose and polyethylene glycol). All patients should be counseled on lifestyle modification. High-fiber diet should be initiated to help prevent constipation, whereas high-fat meats, rich and sugary deserts, processed foods should be avoided. Importance of adequate fluid intake, avoiding heavy use of laxatives or enemas, and increasing exercise should be emphasized.

The five pharmacological treatment classes for constipation are as follows[31]:

1. Bulk laxatives: psyllium, methylcellulose, polycarbophil

2. Osmotic laxatives: lactulose, sorbitol, glycerin, polyethylene glycol

3. Saline laxatives: magnesium hydroxide, magnesium citrate, sodium phosphate

4. Stimulant laxatives: bisacodyl, senna, cascara

5. Surfactant laxatives: docusate sodium, castor oil

Fecal Incontinence

Identification of the cause of fecal incontinence drives the therapy. The evaluation of incontinence for patients should start with a complete history inquiring about symptoms: (1) frequency, (2) duration, (3) severity, and (4) characteristics of incontinence (liquid vs. solid).[27] Obtaining past medical history as well as surgical history can help determine the prevalence and risk for patient's condition. Because a total of 90% of the deaths from acute diarrheal diseases, including *Clostridium difficile* infection, occur in the elderly, changes in fecal continence or diarrhea, even in neurogenic bowel, should be further explored.[28] Patients experiencing overflow incontinence resulting from constipation or fecal impaction should be managed to relieve impaction and treat constipation. Regular clearing of stool in the bowel, along with avoiding increased abdominal pressure and wearing tight undergarments, can help prevent bowel incontinence.[28] Patients should be taught to implement a routine bathroom schedule into their day, recommended to be 30 to 40 minutes after each meal to take advantage of the natural gastrocolic reflex. In order to prevent skin breakdown and infections from frequent bowel movement or leakage, gentle but thorough cleansing, pat drying, and applying a moisture barrier product, such as the Vitamin A & D Ointment, should be part of the routine care. Medication review in order to discontinue offending or aggravating agents should be performed. If idiopathic in origin, use of an antidiarrheal such as loperamide and incontinence pads can be helpful.[27]

After impaction causing overflow diarrhea is ruled out, taking fiber bulking agent, such as psyllium, in small amount of water (unlike in treatment for constipation where patients should mix the powder in 8 oz of fluid), daily can help create more firm stool and increase evacuation if patient suffers from diarrhea related to fecal incontinence. Loperamide can be used simultaneously in small doses to slow colonic transit. Patients should be directed to exercise their external anal sphincter to strengthen the muscle. In combination with the adult pad, an anal plug (an occlusive device used to block fecal leakage) can enable patients to go out in public with more confidence. Surgeries for fecal incontinence include sphincter repair, postanal repair, and newer technologies involving implantable artificial sphincters.[31] For patients with severe incontinence, refractory to medical management and corrective surgeries, a diverting colostomy or ileostomy should be considered to improve quality of life for the patient and their caregivers.[1]

Evidence Base Supporting Treatment Recommendations in Elderly Patients

Even though there is ample literature on the causes of bowel dysfunction in people with neurologic diseases, only a few studies focus on the practical management of constipation and fecal incontinence. A 2005 Cochrane review concluded the impossibility of drawing recommendation for bowel care for patients with neurologic diseases from the current studies available.[32] Empiric bowel management for such patients should remain in place until well-designed controlled trials measuring clinically relevant outcomes in adequate numbers of subjects are available for review.

Nevertheless, there are some older studies that report medication use in the elderly for constipation. Mineral oil, should not be used in elderly due to risk of aspiration that can result in lipoid pneumonia.[31] It can also decrease absorption of fat-soluble vitamins. Although safe when used for short-term, stimulant laxatives such as bisacodyl, castor oil, cascara and senna, can cause dehydration, malabsorption and increase the need for escalating doses in older patients.[31] However, for patients taking chronic narcotics, daily stimulant laxative regimen is essential in preventing opioid-induced constipation. Saline laxatives such as magnesium containing compounds have been shown to relieve constipation safely in the elderly, but caution should be exercised when using it in patients with renal dysfunction or cardiovascular disease who may not tolerate the salt content.[31]

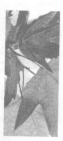

KEY POINT: Lactulose and sorbitol are osmotic agents which are most likely the safest agents for chronic use in the elderly, with sorbitol being less expensive and having less adverse reactions such as bloating.[31]

Suppositories and saline enemas have been used fairly safely long-term in treating older patients. Metoclopramide has been employed for regulating bowel but is no longer recommended for this indication among the older patients in whom the risk of adverse reactions outweigh the benefit.[31]

Two new alternatives, although expensive, offer additional alternatives. Lubiprostone is a locally-acting type-2 chloride channel activator and is indicated for chronic idiopathic constipation in adults. Two double-blind, randomized, placebo-controlled trials included 13.2%[33] and 10%[34] of patients 65 years and older. Lubiprostone promotes fluid secretion, increases the liquid content of the stool and accelerates bowel transit;

thus, improving symptoms of constipation.[33,34] It is generally well tolerated with the most common adverse reactions being headache, nausea and diarrhea.[33,34] Another new agent, methylnaltrexone, has received the approval for treating opioid-induced constipation in advanced illness. The double-blind, randomized, placebo-controlled trial was not conducted exclusively in the elderly population, but older patients, even the patients in their 90s, were included as subjects in the study.[35] Median time to laxation was 6.3 hours for patients in the methylnaltrexone group versus 48 hours for patients in the placebo group (p<0.001). Most of the patients had laxation in 30 minutes to 1 hour with the study medication, and pain scores as well as opioid withdrawal remained stable throughout the study period.[31] Methylnaltrexone may be a potentially useful medication for elderly patients suffering terminal illness and consequently constipation from opioid use. Patients should be warned about severe abdominal pain that may proceed the bowel movement. Also, providers should be warned not to use methylnaltrexone in patients suffering from complete obstruction. Dosing must be adjusted for renal impairment and body weight.

A randomized controlled trial in stroke patients, with a mean age of 72 years, showed that single clinical/educational nurse intervention improved symptoms of constipation and fecal incontinence, and changed bowel-modifying lifestyle behaviors up to 6 months and 12 months, respectively.[36] The intervention also influenced patient-provider interaction and provider's prescribing pattern. The trained nurse focused on patient and caregiver education, providing reading material, forwarding diagnostic summary and treatment recommendations to patients' general practitioners. Focus areas for obtaining history during the study were medications, bowel symptoms and access to toilets.[36] Biofeedback training to increase the strength of the sphincter muscle and the ability to hold a prolonged squeeze upon impending bowel movement can help patients suffering fecal incontinence that are not surgically correctable. A recent 10-year retrospective review found that more than 70% of patients with fecal incontinence demonstrated improvement in the short-term outcomes.[37] The treatment successes were seen more often in participants who completed six training sessions, were females, older, or had more severe incontinence.[37]

Special Considerations Affecting Desired Clinical Outcomes

With depression and social isolation, a significant concern for this population is the effect bowel dysfunction, especially fecal incontinence, has on their quality of life. In a population based-study in women, 82% of the patients with severe symptoms of fecal incontinence reported the condition having significantly negative impact on their quality of life.[29] Very low quality of life was detected by another questionnaire study[38]: 248 patients above 75 years of age who reported difficulties controlling feces also reported that 56.4% had leakage; 54.7% did not reach the toilet in time; 55.6% had incomplete emptying; 27.9% had hard stool; 36.8% were bothered from moisture from the anus; 32.2% could not withstand urgency for 5 minutes; and 17% had erythema or wounds in skin. This study also found women and patients dependent with activities of daily living being most affected by fecal incontinence.[38]

In the previously mentioned study, less than half of the patients sought help for their highly debilitating problem.[38] Therefore, healthcare providers need to become knowledgeable about the overwhelming distress bowel dysfunction has on patients, especially older adults, and initiate assessment in order to provide appropriate care.

Clostridium difficile–associated Diarrhea

Etiology, Epidemiology, and Clinical Presentation

Older adults are at risk for increased morbidity and mortality due to diarrheal diseases because of their weakened immune system, hypochlorhydria, intestinal motility disorders, poor nutritional status, and other underlying chronic medical diseases.[39] For the community-dwelling elderly, diarrhea poses a significant problem, ranging from the burden of incontinence, social embarrassment and isolation to dehydration, delirium, increased fall and fracture risk, and hospitalization. For the elderly residing in a long term care facility, diarrhea represents a more serious threat, increasing mortality in those already crippled with multiple medical comorbidities and functional loss.

Since March 2003, escalating rates of *Clostridium difficile*-associated diarrhea (CDAD) have been reported throughout the U.S. and Canada.[1] This escalation disproportionately increases in patients aged 65 years and older, with incidence estimated to be more than fivefold higher (228 cases per 100,000 population) than in other age groups.[1] In fact, the incidence of CDAD has doubled in recent years and accounts for approximately 3 million cases of diarrhea and colitis each year.[1] *Clostridium difficile (C. difficile)*–associated diarrhea and colitis are more prevalent in the elderly because of more frequent hospitalizations, increased antibiotic use, and increased numbers of patients in institutions. *C. difficile* is a large, obligate, anaerobic, spore-producing gram-positive rod. It is possible to culture *C. difficile* from various surfaces (furniture, bedpans, toilets, bathtubs, weighing scales, floors in hospitals, mops, stethoscopes, clothing, and hands) in about 50% of rooms occupied by patients who have CDAD.[39] Roommates of patients who have CDAD are more likely to acquire *C. difficile*-positive stool cultures and diarrhea. Furthermore, transmission of nosocomially acquired CDAD may be facilitated by way of health care workers. This was shown by the reduction in the spread of CDAD cases in hospitals after the institution of contact precautions, with the use of gloves and careful hand-washing techniques after examination of affected patients.[40] Additionally, *C. difficile* spores are not eradicated with alcohol-based cleaning solutions. Therefore, hospital rooms occupied by CDAD-infected patients must be cleaned thoroughly with a solution containing bleach to properly disinfect all potentially contaminated environmental surfaces.[40]

The rate of colonization with *C. difficile* in the aging population is approximately 2% of healthy older adults, 7% of healthy residents of a retirement facility, 9% of nursing home residents, and

16–56% of hospitalized older patients.[39] *C. difficile* is currently recognized as the most common cause of nosocomial infectious diarrhea in the nursing home setting.[40] Antimicrobial agents are among the most frequently prescribed medications in long-term–care facilities (LTCFs).[41] Therefore, it is not surprising that *C. difficile* colonization and CDAD occur commonly in elderly LTCF residents.[41] CDAD represents a growing concern, with epidemic outbreaks in some hospitals where very aggressive and difficult-to-treat strains have been found recently.[42] This *C. difficile* strain, North American Pulsed-field gel electrophoresis type 1 (NAP-1) prevalent in the U.S., Canada, and northern Europe, generates 16–23 times larger amounts of toxins A, B, and additional binary toxins.[43] Studies have shown high treatment failure rates to NAP-1 which is associated with poor antibiotic response and higher morbidity.[43]

KEY POINT: Outbreaks of CDAD have been reported in geriatric hospital units, rehabilitation hospitals, and freestanding skilled nursing facilities.[40]

During outbreaks, up to 30% of LTCF residents have been found to harbor *C. difficile* or its toxin.[40] Transmission of the organism in LTCFs is likely facilitated within a closed environment with a high rate of exposure to antibiotics. Control of a rapidly developing outbreak of CDAD has to be obtained with early implementation of cohorting and ward closure and reinforcement of environmental disinfection, hand hygiene, and enteric isolation precautions. Length of hospital stay of in-patients with CDAD is prolonged from 18 to 30 days.[39] Overall mortality associated with *C. difficile* infectious diarrhea is estimated to be 17% but is even higher in the older population.[39]

Risk factors for CDAD include[39] history of antibiotic-associated diarrhea, antibiotic therapy (see Table 11-2), immunosuppressive therapy (e.g., chemotherapy, long-term corticosteroid, immunosuppressant), age 65 years or older, nursing home residence, diuretic use, acid-suppressive therapy (e.g., proton pump inhibitor), ICU stay, GI surgery, nasogastric intubation, enteral tube feeding, and contact with a *C. difficile*–infected patient.

All antibiotics have the potential to cause CDAD, including macrolides and those used to treat CDAD (metronidazole and vancomycin) as shown in Table 11-2. The most likely culprits are clindamycin, broad-spectrum penicillins, fluoroquinolones and third generation cephalosporins.[39] Other penicillins and erythromycin are involved less often.[41] As mentioned in the GERD section of this chapter, it has been theorized that the use of gastric acid suppressive medications that decrease the acid concentration of the stomach, permits *C. difficile* to pass unharmed into the duodenum and

Table 11-2. Antimicrobials Predisposing to Clostridium difficile-associated Diarrhea

High Association	Common Association	Uncommon Association
Ampicillin	Cotrimoxazole	Aminoglycosides
Amoxicillin	Other penicillins	Carbapenems
Cephalosporins	Sulfamethoxazole	Chloramphenicol
Clindamycin	Trimethoprim	Daptomycin
Fluoroquinolones		Macrolides
		Metronidazole
		Rifampin
		Tetracyclines
		Tigecycline
		Vancomycin

to the colon. Also, consumption of nonsteroidal anti-inflammatory agents, but not aspirin, has been linked to an increase in CDAD rates[39] This association, however, may be linked to the patient's comorbidities, which may not have all been taken into account when the data were analyzed. Genetic factors also may play an important role in ascertaining who is predisposed to developing CDAD. One study looked at 125 hospitalized patients and discovered a possible link between genetically determined variations in the production of interleukin-8 and the predisposition to developing CDAD.[39] Alternatively, decreased serum levels of antibody to toxin A have been associated independently with an increased likelihood of acquiring moderate to severe *C. difficile*.[39]

C. difficile is responsible for a broad spectrum of enteric conditions, ranging from an asymptomatic carrier state to mild – moderate diarrheal disease to pseudomembranous colitis to fulminant colitis that can include the presence of toxic megacolon or sepsis and may progress to intestinal perforation, peritonitis, sepsis, and death.[39] The typical presentation consists of acute onset of watery diarrhea with lower abdominal cramping relieved by defecation, a low-grade febrile state, and leukocytosis. Moderate to severe CDAD may present with abdominal distention accompanied by pain and profuse watery diarrhea. Occasionally it presents with occult colonic bleeding. Systemic symptoms may include generalized malaise, fever, anorexia, and nausea. If the disease is localized to the cecum and ascending colon, the patient may have marked leukocytosis and abdominal pain with little or no diarrhea. It is also possible for patients who have CDAD to have no additional clinical symptoms other than being febrile with an increased white blood cell count.[39]

The clinical picture of an older adult, however, may be different. Elders often do not present with fevers; therefore, the presence of a fever in an elderly person is generally associated with a more severe underlying infection.[44] Instead, their first symptom may be acute confusion or altered mental status. They also may present with other nonspecific symptoms of infection, such as weakness, anorexia, weight loss, history of more frequent

falls, and overall loss of functional capacity.[44] Such atypical presentation makes the diagnosis of *C. difficile* more challenging in the older population and can delay proper diagnosis.

Standard Treatment and Management Strategies in General Adult Population

Diagnosis is typically accomplished by testing the stool for the cytotoxins produced by *C. difficile* (toxins A and B).[40] Detection of toxin B is considered the gold standard because of the assay's high specificity (99–100%). Both stool culture and cytotoxin assay may require a minimum of 48 hours for the results to become available. Other available tests include enzyme immunoassays (EIAs) that can deliver results in 2 hours. The EIA has a specificity and sensitivity most comparable to that of the cytotoxicity assay and tests for the production of toxins A and B. EIA has a reported sensitivity of 85% and a specificity of 100%.[41] The diagnosis can also be made by visualization of pseudomembranes or raised yellow plaques on sigmoidoscopy or colonoscopy for those with a clinical suspicion of CDAD but have a negative stool testing result.[39] The Infectious Diseases Society of America and the Society for Health Care and Epidemiology of America have published guidelines for the correct use of detection techniques of *C. difficile*.[42] Some key points from the guidelines are important to note. The first is there should be a high suspicion of C. diff in elderly patients with previous antibiotic exposure. The second is that microbiological tests are not needed to confirm cure once the symptoms have subsided. In addition, a *C difficle* culture may be indicated if diarrhea persists despite repeated negative toxin test.

The first line of therapy for CDAD involves cessation of the suspected offending antibiotic.[41] If symptoms persist after discontinuation of the offending antibiotic or if the disease is clinically severe, current guidelines from the American College of Gastroenterology recommend the use of either oral metronidazole (250 mg 4 times/day or 500 mg 3 times/day for 10–14 days) or oral vancomycin (125 mg 4 times/day for 10–14 days).[40] Vancomycin is not secreted into the bowel, thus IV administration is not effective. Treatment with either one of these agents leads to symptomatic improvement in 85–95% of patients within 2–4 days.[42] If oral administration is not possible, metronidazole 500 mg IV q6h should be given until oral administration can be resumed. Metronidazole and vancomycin appear to be therapeutically comparable in mild cases. In patients who are not critically ill, metronidazole is preferred to vancomycin because of metronidazole's lower cost, and because it minimizes the risk of the vancomycin-resistant enterococci. However, if the patient is seriously ill, oral vancomycin is usually recommended.[42] In a Cochrane analysis that included nine prospective and comparative studies in patients with CDAD, metronidazole, bacitracin, teicoplanin, fusidic acid, and rifaximin were each as effective as vancomycin for initial symptomatic resolution.[42] Fever usually resolves within 24hrs, and diarrhea decreases over 4 to 5 days. A worse prognosis has been reported in patients with a serum albumin <25 g/L, a fall in albumin >11g/L, and persistent toxin in the stools ≥ 7 days after therapy.[41] Supportive measures include oral and intravenous rehydration along with electrolyte replacement. Antiperistaltic agents, such as loperamide, diphenoxylate, and opiates, should not be used during the initial days of therapy.[39]

Relapse rates average around 20–50% after successful treatment with either metronidazole or vancomycin.[41] 12–24% of patients develop a second episode of CDAD within 2 months of the initial diagnosis, and if a patient has two or more episodes of CDAD, the recurrence risk increases to 50–65%.[41] The reasons for relapse include failure to eradicate the organism from the colon and reinfection from environmental sources. Independent predictors of relapsed disease identified in a study are age above 65 years and continued hospital stay longer than 16 days after the initial episode.[44] Patients with the relapsed disease are at higher risk for developing at least one CDAD-related complication. The complications include toxic megacolon, peritonitis, sepsis, septic shock, hypotension, intestinal perforation, or death

within 30 days of diagnosis.[44] Likewise, recurrent CDAD disease has been linked significantly to age, renal failure, and leukocytosis with a white blood cell count of more than 20,000 cells/μL.[44] Patients who have one relapse are more likely to have another, which cannot be explained by antibiotic resistance but may involve sporulation. Sporulation can cause a patient to relapse within 4 weeks after a successful treatment.[44] Metronidazole remains the drug of choice for treatment of an initial recurrence, even if this was the original drug used. A second course of metronidazole has cured more than 90% of patients with an initial recurrence.[42]

Severe CDAD can manifest as occurrence of paralytic ileus or toxic megacolon, which would lead to decreased or diminished diarrhea.[39] Severe CDAD, therefore, has a poor prognosis with a high mortality risk. Emergent subtotal or total colectomy may need to be performed. Less than 1% of patients with C. difficile–associated colitis require surgical intervention for the management of perforation or toxic megacolon.[39]

The theory behind the development of probiotic therapy involves the use of live microorganisms to repopulate the colon with normal colonic flora in the hopes of preventing the colonization or infection with C. difficile. Two such probiotics are Lactobacillus and Bifidobacterium. A meta-analysis from six randomized trials showed that probiotics had significant efficacy for CDAD.[42] However, prophylactic administration of Lactobacillus species does not appear to be effective in preventing the development of antibiotic-associated diarrhea.[42]

Another such organism is the nonpathogenic yeast Saccharomyces boulardii (S boulardii), which is used throughout Europe to prevent antibiotic-associated diarrhea. It is available in the United States as an over-the-counter product, Florastor (250-mg capsules). Commercial preparations of S boulardii are not regulated by the U.S. Food and Drug Administration (FDA); therefore, they are not standardized and may lack quality control testing. The efficacy of S boulardii to decrease recurrence of CDAD has been shown in several studies including two randomized trials.[42] A recently published study focused on a complication of *S boulardii*, fungemia, that may present as small epidemic outbreaks, particularly in intensive care unit patients with intravascular catheters.[45] Therefore, the administration of *S boulardii* in the elderly and the immunocompromised should commence only after careful considerations of the associated risks.

Evidence Base Supporting Treatment Recommendations in Elderly Patients

Diarrhea in the elderly population is a disease that needs special attention in treatment and management, especially in acute care patients and long-term care residents. Because of their multiple comorbidities, decreased immunity, frailty, and poor nutritional status, these patients are at higher risk for acquiring complications from prolonged diarrhea.

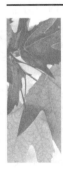

KEY POINT: Close follow-up to ensure adequate hydration and electrolyte replacement, along with infection control measures to contain outbreaks should be emphasized to caregivers and nursing staff in acute and long term care facilities.[46]

Although *C. difficile* colitis causes significant morbidity and mortality in this population, judicious use of antibiotics can decrease the incidence and recurrence of the disease.[47] As noted above, probiotic agents have been evaluated for the treatment of patients with recurrent CDAD. There have also been several studies of the prophylactic administration of probiotics to prevent the development of CDAD in patients receiving antibiotics. In one study, the prophylactic use of *S. boulardii* appeared to prevent antibiotic-associated diarrhea in hospitalized patients, but was found to be ineffective in elderly patients in another study.[44] Thus, the effectiveness of probiotics for CDAD in older adults has not been confirmed.

Special Considerations Affecting Desired Clinical Outcomes

Infections in nursing homes are expected to increase as pathogens become more resistant to antibiotic therapy, and *C. difficile* will continue to be a significant problem.[40] Diligent infection control practices, staff education, family education, and the identification of new prevention and control strategies are vital to limiting its spread. Family members and other health care consumers must understand that prevention of the spread of *C. difficile* goes hand in hand with prevention of additional weight loss, fall, and loss of function in these vulnerable elders.[46]

As mentioned above, most common causes of CDAD have been the use of clindamycin, fluoroquinolones, broad-spectrum penicillins and cephalosporins.[41] Restricting the use of clindamycin was associated with a marked decrease in the rates of nosocomial CDAD at two hospitals and restrictions on the use of broad-spectrum antibiotics were shown to reduce the frequency of CDAD in a long-term care unit.[46] Therefore, development of programs that encourage the proper use of antibiotics is essential, particularly in LTCFs.

The prevention and control guidelines should include the following[41]:

1. Implement policies in the institution for the prudent use of antimicrobial agents.

2. Surveillance of antimicrobial utilization in the facility should be conducted.

3. Healthcare providers in the facility should be educated about the clinical features, transmission, and epidemiology of CDAD.

4. Care for patients/residents with CDAD and fecal incontinence should be in a private room. If facilities are available, a private room should be considered for all residents with CDAD until the diarrhea has resolved.

5. Meticulous hand hygiene with soap or an antimicrobial agent is recommended after contact with residents, their body substances, or their potentially contaminated environment in the facility.

6. Healthcare providers should wear gloves for contact with patients/residents with CDAD, and for contact with their body substances and environment.

7. Use of disposable, single-use thermometers (rather than shared electronic thermometers) is recommended.

8. For a resident with CDAD, patient care items and equipment such as stethoscopes and blood pressure cuffs should be dedicated and not shared with other residents. If such items must be shared, they should be carefully cleaned and disinfected between residents.

9. Disinfection of the environment (e.g., room surfaces) of a patient/resident with CDAD should be done using sporicidal agents, such as a diluted hypochlorite solution.

10. Residents may be removed from isolation when their diarrhea has resolved.

Nausea and Vomiting

Etiology, Epidemiology, and Clinical Presentation

Nausea and vomiting that occur commonly near the end of life are substantial source of physical and psychological distress for patients and families involed.[48] Up to 40% of opioid-treated patients experience nausea and vomiting, triggered by constipation, chemoreceptor trigger zone (CTZ), gastroparesis, and sensitization of the labyrinth.[48] Nausea and vomiting are present in up to 62% of cancer patients.[48]

Standard Treatment and Management Strategies in General Adult Population

In most instances, acute nausea and vomiting can be readily diagnosed on clinical grounds alone; however, chronic nausea and vomiting with symptoms persisting longer than a month presents greater challenge for diagnosis and treatment. Three basic goals have been identified for evaluating and managing nausea and vomiting:

(1) recognize and correct any consequences or complications, (2) identify and specify therapy for the primary cause, and (3) suppress and eliminate symptoms.[49] A thorough history and physical exam are essential first steps in the management of patients experiencing nausea and vomiting because they define the severity of the symptoms and provide clues to the underlying etiology. Once the most likely cause is determined, a clinician can discern the mechanism by which this etiology is triggering nausea and vomiting as well as specific transmitters and receptors involved in the process. Subsequently, management focuses on prescribing the appropriate pharmacologic antagonist to the implicated receptors.[48]

Nonpharmacological therapy such as avoiding strong smells or other nausea triggers, eating small, frequent meals, and limiting oral intake during periods of extreme emesis can help patients control their nausea and vomiting to certain degree. Psychological techniques, especially those that promote relaxation can help calm the condition also. Acupuncture and acupressure, especially in geriatric population, may provide some benefit in the setting of chemotherapy or surgery.[50,51] All potential underlying causes, such as constipation, opioids, and electrolyte abnormalities should be addressed simultaneously to provide the greatest chance of rapidly resolving nausea and vomiting.[48]

To date, no head-to-head comparison between mechanism-based and empirical therapy have been published.[48] However, a mechanism-based treatment scheme administering the most potent antagonist to the implicated receptors has been shown to be effective in up to 80% to 90% of patients near the end of life.[52] This management approach facilitates systematically caring for the patient, identifying all potential symptomatic contributors, directing therapy, and minimizing the risk of overmedicating a vulnerable population.[48]

Generally, opioid-induced nausea and vomiting occurs with initiation of opioids or with dose escalation and resolves within 3–5 days of continued use. In this situation, the antiemetic dose should not be prescribed on an as needed basis to prevent precipitating nausea. A dose reduction by 10–20% of daily opioid dose can alleviate nausea without loss of analgesia for patients with persistent nausea due to opioid use.[48] If symptoms are refractory despite adequate dosage and around-the-clock prophylactic administration, then empirical trial combining several therapies to block multiple emetic pathways should be attempted. A mechanism-based approach helps facilitate a step-wise introduction of medications that exert their effects at different receptor sites.[48] Often, refractory nausea and vomiting make oral administration of medication not feasible and alternate routes such as rectal suppositories, subcutaneous infusions, IV pushes, and orally dissolvable tablets need to be considered.[48]

Nontraditional agents may be utilized when nausea and vomiting persist despite a mechanism-based approach using several medications targeting multiple pathways, at appropriate doses taken around the clock. The nontraditional agents with limited evidence include mirtazapine (antidepressant) or dronabinol (cannabinoid).

Evidence Base Supporting Treatment Recommendations in Elderly Patients

Phenothiazines which have been used for many years to treat nausea and vomiting include promethazine, prochlorperazine, chlorpromazine, and trimethobenzamide. They are known to cause sedation, orthostatic hypotension and extrapyramidal symptoms (EPS). These adverse drug events (ADEs) render concerns for their use in older adults who are particularly vulnerable to suffer ill-effects from such problems. An ADEs study found geriatric status to be a significant risk factor for experiencing promethazine ADEs including sedation, delirium, and EPS.[53] Concomitant use of sedating drugs may further increase the risk for ADEs in the elderly. Promethazine has also been shown to slow the rate of recovery from opioid-induced respiratory depression.[53] This risk may be even greater in patients with renal insufficiency. Even though these ADEs are reversible upon discontinuation of the drug, the occurrence of delirium in the older patients can render long-term consequences including a 25–33% mortality rate, higher-level nursing care requirements, and great-

er health costs.[53] Trimethobenzamide carries high risk of extrapyramidal side effects at doses required for antiemetic effects, and is included on the Beer's criteria of potentially inappropriate medications among elderly patients.[54] Of these three agents, promethazine may be preferred if an inexpensive agent is required for occasional use, but in general their use should be minimized.

An alternative that may prove to be standard of care in the future are serotonin receptor antagonists. They have several advantages but the data at this time is lacking.

Metoclopramide, which can cause psychiatric symptoms as well as tardive dyskinesia and drug-induced Parkinsonism, is considered an inappropriate drug in the elderly, especially when used long-term or at doses higher than appropriate based on renal function.[55] Metoclopramide crosses blood brain barrier and has centrally-mediated adverse effects. Elderly are especially susceptible to these effects which include somnolence, reduced mental acuity, anxiety, depression, and EPS. Domperidone minimally crosses the blood brain barrier (BBB); it acts in the CTZ which lies outside of the BBB; less likely to cause the centrally-mediated adverse effects seen with metoclopramide, thus safer in elderly. However, domperidone is not available in the U.S. and has been associated with prolonged QT intervals, cardiac arrhythmias, and sudden death, thus it should not be used for patients with underlying long QT interval or for those on other medications that can prolong the QT interval.[52]

Droperidol, a centrally-acting anti-dopaminergic agent effective for preventing post-operative nausea and vomiting, and treating opioid-induced nausea and vomiting, can cause sedation, agitation, and restlessness.[52] Droperidol also carries the FDA black box warning for prolonging QT interval, cardiac arrhythmias that may result in torsades de pointes and sudden cardiac death. ECG is recommended prior to starting this agent, and treatment should be avoided in patients at risk for QT prolongation, which include elderly patients with arrhythmias and patients taking polypharmacy with potential to increase QT.[52]

Special Considerations Affecting Desired Clinical Outcomes

Nausea and vomiting can be caused by disturbances of the vestibular system in the inner ear, which can result from infection, traumatic injury, neoplasm and motion. Because the vestibular system is replete with muscarinic-type cholinergic and histamine (H_1) receptors, anticholinergics and antihistamines are the most commonly used therapeutic agents. Scopolamine, an anticholinergic used for motion sickness, is available as a transdermal patch delivery system, which may be helpful for patients who cannot tolerate oral medications or who require treatment for a prolonged period.[56] Drowsiness, reduced mental acuity, visual disturbances, dry mouth, and urinary retention can occur with antihistamine and anticholinergic use.[56] A 2007 Cochrane review summarized evidence from 14-randomised controlled studies evaluating the effectiveness and safety of scopolamine for motion sickness.[56] The review found scopolamine to be more effective than placebo for preventing motion sickness; however, scopolamine was not shown to be superior to antihistamines and combinations of scopolamine and ephedrine. Scopolamine was less likely to cause drowsiness, blurred vision or dizziness when compared to these other agents.[56] Therefore, scopolamine should be considered the first choice for treating nausea and vomiting due to motion sickness in the older population.

Dysphagia

Etiology, Epidemiology, and Clinical Presentation

Dysphagia, defined as difficulty swallowing, is a condition with a strong age-related bias. It is estimated to occur in up to 50% of patients in long-term care facilities, and said to be the most common esophageal disorder in the elderly.[57] Within the group of adults older than 65, estimated 10-30% have dysphagia, but true incidence and prevalence are unknown.[56] In general, the rate is lower in the community than in nursing home setting.[58] Overall, dysphagic patients have longer inpatient stay with higher incidence of complications, high-

er morbidity and increased need for inpatient rehabilitation and post-discharge institutionalized care compared to nondysphagic patients.[59]

Oropharyngeal dysphagia (OD) is defined as difficulty in initiating swallowing or transferring food from the oropharynx to the upper esophagus.[57] Whereas, esophageal dysphagia (ED) is difficulty in swallowing when ingested content cannot be transported from the hypopharynx through the esophagus into the stomach.[57] OD is more common in older adults with neurologic causes. Dementia is a major risk factor for both feeding problems and dysphagia. Post-stroke patients and those with dementia may not have the cognitive skills to recognize or understand the danger dysphagia presents regarding choking or aspiration.[59] Parkinson's disease is also a common cause of both OD and ED in the elderly.[60]

Additionally, medications can slow the passage of food and water through the esophagus into the stomach.[58] Drug-induced esophageal injury (e.g., ulcerations, circumferential lesions, strictures secondary to caustic injury) is a cause of ED, and conversely, ED may result in esophageal injury when certain drugs are temporarily lodged in the esophagus.[15] Healthcare providers should become familiar with the causes of higher risk for medication-induced esophageal injury in the elderly and recognize those agents considered to raise the risk in this vulnerable population.[60] One basic reason for increased risk is that the older patients often do not drink enough water when they take medications. Side effects of many commonly used medications can contribute to dysphagia as well, creating dry mouth, tardive dyskinesia, drowsiness, or suppressed gag or cough reflex.[61] Medications that commonly affect swallowing include the following[61]: neuroleptics (antidepressants, antipsychotics), sedatives (barbiturates), antihistamines, diuretics, mucosal anesthetics, and anticholinergics.

Common patient complaints of dysphagia include food sticking to the throat, coughing, choking, dyspnea, wet voice, and nasal or oral regurgitation. Patients may report the need to repetitively swallow or to clear throat progressively as well as pain on swallowing.[58] Lung crepitation and consolidation may be seen on the x-ray, and respiratory conditions need to be ruled out. Unexplained fever or low oxygen saturation should be evaluated for aspiration due to dysphagia.[58]

Standard Treatment and Management Strategies in General Adult Population

In a standardized bedside assessment, patient's level of consciousness, posture, voluntary cough, voice quality, and saliva control are examined. Then, a teaspoonful of water is given to drink followed by a small glass of water if the teaspoonful was cleared safely.[62] On the other hand, a recent article suggested Gugging swallowing screening (GU.S.S) method, in which after starting with a saliva swallow, patients are tested first on semi-solid thickened fluids, then thin fluids, then dry toast.[63] The initial diagnostic instrument for dysphagia is a barium swallow, along with videofluoroscopy (VFS), which uses continuous x-rays to view the barium as it passes through the pharynx, esophagus and stomach. VFS, which has been the accepted gold standard, can detect content entering the respiratory tract and how much, and whether pharyngeal or esophageal muscles are properly functioning.[63] Competitively, fiberoptic endoscopic evaluation of swallowing (FEES) is newer and has been established in differentiating the aspiration risk similar to VFS. The FEES involves passing an endoscope through the nose into level of the soft palate, and its advantages include no radiation exposure and possibility of frequent performance at bedside using normal meals.[64]

A multidisciplinary approach is necessary for effective diagnosis and treatment of dysphagia in older adults whether they are living in the community or in a long-term care facility. The multidisciplinary team may include the following members: physician, speech and language pathologist, dietitian, nursing staff, dentist, pharmacist, occupational therapist, social worker, and family or caregivers.[61] Treatment goals include identifying and maintaining safe swallowing techniques, avoiding aspiration, and ensuring adequate nutrition.[57] An early detection is the key to managing dysphagia and reducing morbidity. Evaluating and avoiding any medications that can aggravate

or trigger dysphagia can improve care for these patients, and pharmacists should be involved in this screening process. Main therapy for dysphagia is diet modification and swallowing rehabilitation. Many patients with dysphagia will have great difficulty with thin fluids but may safely take nectar-thick, pudding-thick, or honey-thick fluids.[58] Crushing medications and placing them in one of these thick fluids is often indicated when swallowing problems occur. A team of physician, pharmacist and nurse can work together to insure proper dosage forms (liquid formulations, or tablet or capsules that can be crushed or opened) are delivered to a dysphagic patient. It is also important to remember that certain formulations, such as sustained release products and enteric coated tablets, should not be crushed. Aggressive oral care should be part of the treatment plan to further reduce risk of pneumonia.[65] Both the patient and the caregiver should be educated on safe swallowing methods, including upright posture, chin tucking, and careful, slow swallowing.[58]

Evidence Base Supporting Treatment Recommendations in Elderly Patients

The treatment of dysphagia among geriatric patients is complicated by their cognitive decline, decreased immunity, malnutrition, and end-of-life decisions.[58] A large randomized controlled trial found differing effectiveness in eliminating aspiration among patients with Parkinson's disease and those with dementia.[66] Dietary consistency interventions were more effective in patients who had Parkinson's disease and not as effective in patients who had dementia. In the same trial, honey-thick fluids were more effective than nectar-thick fluids, and the least effective intervention was the chin-down swallowing posture.[66]

In a recent review, no randomized trials comparing tube feeding with oral feeding in dementia patients were identified.[67] There was also no data to suggest tube feeding for advanced dementia patients can prevent aspiration pneumonia, reduce infections, improve function or provide palliation.[67] Therefore, practice of tube feeding in elderly patients with dementia should be carefully reconsidered. Even though tube feeding [nasogastric (NG) or percutaneous (PEG)] may prevent malnutrition, it does not alter the risk of aspiration.[58] The Feed or Ordinary Diet (FOOD) trial aimed to evaluate commonly used feeding policies in hospitalized stroke patients.[68] The recommendation from this trial was to implement early NG tube feeding in the first few days following a stroke, with consideration of PEG tube feeding after several weeks if long-term nutritional supplementation is warranted.[68] Thus, if diet modification and swallowing training are ineffective, NG tube feeding may be a temporary option. Additionally, it is important to respect older adults' wishes regarding tube feeding. When a group of nursing home residents were asked about tube feeding as part of treatment of recurrent aspiration pneumonia, most refused tube feeding, via NG (69%) or PEG (71%), but wanted treatment for aspiration pneumonia (73%).[69]

Recent advances in the treatment of geriatric dysphagia have focused on rehabilitating swallowing function with active exercise. Evidence is emerging in support of resistance exercises that do not necessarily involve the act of swallowing itself but activities focused on tongue depressor, isometric lingual exercise, maximum expiratory training and head lifting, as effective interventions for specific dysphagic groups.[70] Ongoing clinical trials are being conducted for resistance exercises versus standard treatment and muscle exercise versus sensory postural therapy. Alternatively, a Cochrane Review reported the positive findings from randomized controlled trials supporting acupuncture in stroke patients with dysphagia.[71]

Special Considerations Affecting Desired Clinical Outcomes

The most common cause of death in patients with dysphagia due to neurologic disorders is aspiration pneumonia, which comprises 5% to 15% of the cases recorded as community-acquired pneumonia.[58] Forceful coughing, active ciliary transport, and normal immune response are presumed to be protective against acquiring aspiration pneumonia in healthy adults. There is a loss of muscular pharyngeal support and protective reflexes of coughing and swallowing in the older adults, which are thought to be results of age-related peripheral changes along with a decreased central nervous reflex activity.

Individuals with dysphagia will also often require alternative dosage formulations or crushed medications. Careful attention must be paid to extended release formulations or other medications that cannot be crushed. Liquid formulations may offer convenient alternatives, however these can be more expensive than tablet formulations and for individuals with complex medication regimens, doses of multiple liquid formulations can result in the need to swallow large or unpalatable volumes. Liquid formulations containing sorbitol or alcohol can also result in side effects caused by ingesting the larger quantities of drug vehicle. Therefore, when appropriate, it may often be preferable to crush oral formulations. If administering orally, crushed medication can be mixed into a small amount of jelly or similar substance. It is not recommended to stir or sprinkle medication into food or drink, as the entire portion must be consumed in order to assure the entire dose is administered. If medications are administered via feeding tube, the tube should be flushed with a small amount of water or saline before and after medication administration to prevent clogging.

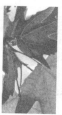

KEY POINT: Hospitalized older patients with no spontaneous complaints of dysphagia are still likely to have impaired swallowing function and an increased risk of aspiration.[72]

Brief assessment of swallowing function in all patients admitted to tertiary care geriatric wards can be useful. Dysphagic patients may be more prone to developing infections during long term hospital stays. A study associated the combination of dysphagia and hypoalbuminemia with increased risk of opportunistic microorganism colonization, including *Staphylococcus aureus*, *Pseudomonas aeruginosa*, *Streptococcus agalactiae*, and *Stenotrophomonas maltophilia*, in the oral cavity of geriatric patients hospitalized for longer than 3 months and bedridden.[73] Thus, the evaluation and management of dysphagia need to continue throughout a patient's long term hospital stay in order to prevent complications such as aspiration pneumonia.

Older dysphagic patients make up a heterogeneous mix of both healthy and disabled older adults who live across a wide spectrum of settings. It is important for clinicians to recognize this diversity in health, functional abilities, social supports, and resources among them and how these factors influence dysphagia care in different settings.

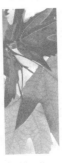

KEY POINT: Standard outcome measures of pneumonia, malnutrition, and mortality must be blended with other quality of life indices, and ultimately, patient and family decisions should dictate the interventions offered to older patients with dysphagia.[69]

Oral Health

Etiology, Epidemiology, and Clinical Presentation

Oral health is critical to systemic health and quality of life of the elderly. Oral health is also an integral component of overall nutritional health. Age is highly correlated with dental status. Physical and mental health of older adults influences access to services, including oral health care. Even though estimated 70% of the elderly population (23.3 million in the U.S.) who live in the community are independently functioning and are able to visit the dental office independently, loss of mobility increases with age, with the greatest decline in people aged 75 and older.[74] Multiple surveys report that compared to the younger adults, the older adults have worse oral hygiene, greater loss of teeth, poorer general oral functional capacity and higher level of dental caries and gingivitis.[75] Most common oral lesion in the elderly is denture stomatitis caused by poor denture hygiene and ill-fitting dentures,[76] which can also lead to problems with nutrition, communication and oral pain.

Microorganisms that cause dental caries and periodontal disease can spread from the oral cavity and have been linked to systemic disease, such as infective endocarditis, late prosthetic joint infections, and aspiration pneumonia.[77] The microflora present in the oral cavity because of poor oral hygiene has been associated with aspiration pneumonia, the leading cause of death and the second most common cause for hospitalization among nursing home residents. The risk for developing aspiration pneumonia increases as patients with poor oral health age and develop dysphagia. Typically, gram positive organisms, namely Streptococcus pneumonia and Staph aureus, are more commonly identified in residents of long-term care facilities compared to nonresidents, which is likely due to the differences in oral hygiene measures between these populations. Evidence shows that improved oral care can reduce risk of developing aspiration pneumonia in the elderly.[77]

A recent survey conducted among community-dwelling cognitively intact elderly with disabilities reported substantial oral health morbidities including dry mouth, jaw pain, and burning sensations.[75] Also, older adults are likely to develop several chronic diseases leading to polypharmacy use and are posed with adverse effects from the medications they take. Most common adverse effect to the oral mucosa is xerostomia.[74] Estimated 12–39% of non-institutionalized elderly patients present with xerostomia.[75] Most older patients use at least one drug with potential to cause dry mouth, particularly tricyclic antidepressants, certain antihypertensive agents (alpha blockers such as clonidine, beta adrenergic blockers, diuretics, and calcium channel blockers), cytotoxic drugs, anti-Parkinson's agents, antiepileptic drugs, and inhaled medications (beta-agonist, anticholinergic agent, corticosteroid, etc.).

Standard Treatment and Management Strategies in General Adult Population

Dental caries and gingivitis are detected by dental exam and confirmed by dental x-rays. Gingival bleeding and edema are signs of gingivitis. Oral hygiene, including brushing after meals with fluoride toothpaste and regular dental exam is the mainstay prevention. Powered toothbrushes with an oscillation-rotation action are found to be more effective in reducing plaque and improving gingival health than manual toothbrushes.[78] Antibiotics with mixed anaerobic and facultative bacteria coverage are needed for gingivitis. A review article noted that products containing triclosan/copolymer may reduce the progression of periodontitis in adults and high-risk individuals.[78] Advanced periodontal disease may require debridement to remove the inflammatory tissue and surgery to restore the normal gingival and bony architecture.

Evidence Base Supporting Treatment Recommendations in Elderly Patients

Overall, dental symptoms, signs, and diagnostic strategies are similar in elderly to younger adults. Wound healing after periodontal surgery is slower in the elderly, but the rates for long-term healing and regeneration are similar to younger adults.[74] Preventative oral hygiene is the first line of defense in this population. Development and maintenance of an individualized oral health care plan for the elderly in long term care facilities will enable early identification and prevention of known risk factors for aspiration pneumonia. There is a significant reduction in pneumonia among patients who regularly receive oral care and maintain good oral hygiene, and a trained nursing staff can minimize morbidity associated with poor oral hygiene.[79]

Oral mucosa hygiene using chlorhexidine mouth wash, bacteriocidal for gram-positive and gram-negative bacteria and fungicidal for candida, along with tooth brushing twice a day (after breakfast and dinner) is recommended in the elderly.[74] A 2004 review reported that the few studies that have been performed in older adults suggest using fluoride toothpaste and in the case of high caries risk individuals, the adjunctive use of other fluoride delivery systems to prevent dental caries. Some dentifrices containing triclosan have shown to improve plaque control and gingival health.[78] Older patients with impaired dexterity benefit from electric toothbrushes or manual toothbrushes with larger handles, and floss holders. Dentures need to be removed, brushed and cleansed as well.[74] There is a relationship between poor denture hygiene and denture stomatitis secondary to fungal infections.

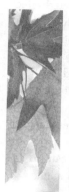

KEY POINT: Denture stomatitis can be reduced by proper hygiene measures, including brushing and soaking of the prosthesis using any of the over-the-counter cleansers available. Also, removable partial or full denture prosthetics should not be worn at night when saliva is reduced and bacterial counts rise.[76]

Patients with dementia and those with disorders that limit upper extremity mobility and dexterity (e.g., stroke, Parkinson's disease) may require tooth-brushing by others and professional cleaning more often than every 6 months.[74] Elderly residents of long-term nursing facilities often require continued professional oral care. There is a recommendation for dental hygiene sessions to be held at intervals of 1 week for 12 consecutive weeks and at intervals of 2 weeks for more than 20 weeks thereafter for this population. Alternatively, a recent study involving nurses who received hands-on instructions for oral cleaning in a geriatric institution found that the best outcome in both denture and dental hygiene occurred when the trained nurses provided daily dental care compared to every-3-week dental hygienist service or no intervention.[79]

Special Considerations Affecting Desired Clinical Outcomes

A recent collection of interviewer-administered questionnaires, to determine factors associated with oral health-related quality of life (OHQOL) in community-dwelling elderly, found that worse oral health, health, and disability status are related to poor OHQOL. However, less life satisfaction, low income, and living alone were not.[80] Nevertheless, low Medicaid reimbursements discourage dentists from accepting Medicaid patients and often older patients go without proper oral care. A randomized controlled trial concluded that implementing an oral health visit as part of a preventive health check within a primary care setting in patients 75 and older was feasible and effective in increasing the dental visits in this population.[81] Elderly patients have limited options when paying for dental care since Medicare does not generally cover routine dental work and Medicaid coverage varies widely between individual states.[82] The strategies needed to reduce the oral health disparities are complicated. This creates a setting with ample opportunities for investigators to test methods to improve delivery of oral care to the frail and functionally dependent older adults.

Malnutrition

Etiology, Epidemiology, and Clinical Presentation

Adequate nutrition promotes longevity and quality of life in geriatric population. Older adults have special nutritional needs due to processes of aging and disease. Increasingly being recognized is the importance of nutritional status of elderly patients having a variety of disease including cancer, heart disease, and dementia. Even though there is not a uniformly accepted definition of malnutrition in the elderly, common indicators such as decreased dietary intake, involuntary weight loss, abnormal body mass index (BMI), and specific vitamin deficiencies have been identified.[83] Within the large group of older adults, there are subgroups of the socially isolated, the economically challenged, and the institutionalized, who are more likely to consume imbalanced, low nutritional diet. Nutritional inadequacy has been shown to be more prevalent in the institutionalized elders compared to the community-dwelling elders.[83] Likewise, compared to the 11% of elderly living above the poverty level, 21% of the independent elderly living below the poverty level in the U.S. have poor diet.[83] A study on unhealthy lifestyle behaviors show that at age 70–75 years, low-quality diet, smoking, and physical inactivity together increased mortality risk in the participants.[84]

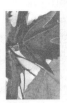 KEY POINT: Daily energy requirements decline as people age, even during healthy aging, due to decreased muscle mass and increased fat tissues.

This is because muscle mass is much more metabolically active than fat.[1] Elderly patient's caloric needs range from 1900 to 2400 calories a day, depending on their activity level.[85] 0.8 to 1.0 g/kg of protein, fat consumption of 30% of total calories, and 25–30 g of fiber can be set for healthy elders.[85] It is also important to include 6-8 glasses of water need into an older adult's daily nutritional plan. In addition to the change in proportion of muscle and fat tissues in the elderly, aging leads to decline in senses of taste and smell, negatively affecting appetite. Many elderly also have difficulty chewing and swallowing that interferes with eating. A study looking at characteristics of undernourished older medical patients in order to identify predictors for undernutrition revealed lower cognitive function, education less than 12 years and chewing problems as risk factors for malnutrition.[84] Having a lower dietary score which indicated low intake of vegetables, fruits and fluid, poor appetite, difficulties in eating (chewing problems, nausea and vomiting), and depression distinguished the malnourished group.[84]

Protein-energy malnutrition or undernutrition is common is older adults as unintended weight loss is found in up to 15% of community-dwelling elders and in 25–80% of nursing home residents.[1,85] The metabolic stress of insufficient protein intake combined with the effects of hepatic, renal or bowel disease can further impair an older patient's overall nutritional status. Acute illnesses can keep patients in a "nothing by mouth" status, which can contribute to anorexia after recovery. The body compensates for the low nutrition intake by reducing the metabolic rate and catabolizing the muscle mass, including heart and respiratory muscles. This can progress to a vicious cycle which ends in weakness and functional disability of the patient.

Common causes of weight loss in older adults are multifactorial and include social and psychological reasons such as isolation, depression, bereavement, loss of transportation to the market, poverty, and alcohol abuse. Physical causes include decreased mobility and functioning; neurological impairment such as stroke, dementia, and Parkinson's disease; GI disorders such as dysphagia, constipation, nausea, and reflux problems; and poor oral health including ill-fitting dentures.[1] Atrophic gastritis can lead to vitamin B12 deficiency by reducing absorption. Calcium is a risk nutrient in elderly who do not consume enough dairy in their diet. As a result of limited sunlight exposure in chronically-ill, homebound or frail elderly, vitamin D deficiencies have been noted. Medications that have been associated with poor food intake and failure to thrive in older adults include digoxin, cholinesterase inhibitors, antacids, laxative abuse, diuretics, NSAIDs, chemotherapy, anticonvulsants, antibiotics, certain antidepressants (e.g., fluoxetine, citalopram, bupropion, etc.), and any drug that can cause delirium.[1]

KEY POINT: Early signs and symptoms of malnutrition are nonspecific and mimic natural aging because the decline can take place very slowly.

Most common definition of weight loss that should be recognized is 5% in 1 month, 7% in 3 months, or 10% over 6 months; however, even more gradual weight loss such as 5% over 6–12 months is still associated with increased morbidity and mortality.[83] Multiple causes of weight loss in the elderly have been identified to include: alcohol and drug misuse, multiple comorbidities, dental problems, poor vision, dementia, adverse drug reactions, social isolation, functional dependencies, depression and other psychiatric disorders, poverty, limited access to food, food attitudes and cultural preferences, and elder abuse.[83] Body mass index (BMI) is used to describe weight in relation to height and categorize people to the following:

- Underweight = BMI <20 kg/m^2
- Healthy weight = BMI 20–25 kg/m^2
- Overweight = BMI 25–30 kg/m^2
- Obese = BMI >30 kg/m^2

The recommended BMI range in the elderly is 22–27 kg/m^2.[85] In BMI below 22–23 kg/m^2, there is steady increase in risk of death, particularly at BMI less than 18.5 kg/m^2 in women and 20.5 kg/m^2 in men.[86] Older patients who are smokers or have terminal illness or cancer may have BMI less than 20 kg/m^2 with poorer outcomes with respect to life expectancy than those with healthy or heavier weight. Available cross-sectional studies indicate that prevalence of obesity increases with age, up to about 60 years, remains steady for about 10 years until the age 70, then declines. Both weight gain and weight loss have been associated with adverse health outcomes to include decreased functional status, institutionalization, and increased mortality.[85] Nevertheless, BMI fails to recognize replacement of muscles with adipose tissue, and does not distinguish central obesity.

Recently in clinical practice, waist circumferences have been suggested as better measure of health consequences of obesity than BMI, especially in the case of identifying metabolic syndrome. Waist-to-hip ratio has also been positively correlated to mortality in women aged 55 to 69 years when corrected for smoking, alcohol, and estrogen use.[87] Yet, a study that looked at under- and overweight in relation to mortality in men in 7 countries showed that a large waist circumference was a better predictor of higher 5-year mortality than a waist-to-hip ratio or BMI.[87] But, low BMI was a better predictor of mortality than low waist circumference.[87] Overall, it can be summarized that increased fat tissue is better reflected by increased waist circumference, whereas low lean body mass is better reflected by a low BMI.

Standard Treatment and Management Strategies in General Adult Population

The initial laboratory assessment of weight loss should include a complete blood count, electrolytes and glucose, renal and liver function tests, thyroid panel, urinalysis and chest x-ray. Even though serum albumin less than 3.5 g/dL is associated with increased morbidity and mortality, it does not serve as an adequate clinical indicator of ongoing nutritional status due to its long half-life (approximately 3 weeks).[85] Conversely, prealbumin has shorter half-life of 2–3 days and can be used to confirm the clinical impression of poor nutritional status in the absence of inflammatory process.[85] Low prealbumin can verify malnutrition, whereas progressively rising prealbumin, along with clinical indicators such as wound healing and patient strengthening, can signify improving nutritional status. Sharp decline in cholesterol level can also indicate inadequate nutritional status.[85]

Several tools are available for use in clinical settings to determine patients' nutritional status such as the Subjective Global Assessment (SGA).[88] SGA collects a highly standardized medical history including weight change, changes in dietary intake, presence of GI symptoms, functional capacity, and knowledge of the metabolic demands of the patient's underlying disease state. Physical exam focuses on loss of subcutaneous fat, muscle wasting, edema in ankles, edema in sacral area, and ascites. Based on the features of history and physical exam a SGA rank is chosen by the clinician from the following: well nourished, moderate or suspected malnutrition, or severe malnutrition.[88]

Optimal treatment for malnutrition requires a multidimensional approach, starting with setting a realistic goal for the patient, recruiting family and social support, implementing an exercise regimen to increase appetite, providing pain management when needed, and incorporating the patient's food preferences and meal habits. Various liquid and powder supplements can be used when patients are unable to take enough oral foods, but they are most effective if consumed in between meals instead of replacing them. Supplements can be mixed in regular food if necessary, and targeted formulations are available for special populations such as renal failure patients and trauma patients.

A variety of medications have been used to stimulate appetite in order to promote weight gain. Megestrol acetate is often used in cancer patients and in immunocompromised as in AIDS patients. Other drugs with weight gaining properties that are used in clinical practice include Dronabinol (tetrahydrocannabinol), Cyproheptadine (antihistamine), and Testosterone (androgen). There are several drugs and alternative agents being studied for this purpose including omega-3 fatty acids. Malnourished patients with persistent anorexia can be tried on dexamethasone (steroid), mirtazapine (antidepressant), or a tricyclic antidepressant.

If a patient needs additional feeding in order to replenish or maintain their nutritional status and their GI tract is functioning, nutritional therapy utilizing the GI tract is preferred to parenteral feeding. Enteral nutrition (EN) is associated with lower infection rates than parenteral nutrition. Standard polymeric EN formulas are appropriate in most patients.[89] Therapeutic trial (2–4 weeks) with tube feeding may be utilized in a patient after their caloric goals are set. Head of the patient's bed should be kept elevated to 30 degrees to prevent aspiration, since all tube feedings, whether NG or PEG, are associated with aspiration and pneumonia. In bed-bound and post-operative patients with impaired bowel motility, metoclopramide can be given in low doses to promote bowel function along with the tube feeds. These patients should be monitored for adverse reactions and have a plan to discontinue the drug as soon as possible.

Parenteral nutrition (PN) is the intravenous administration of fluids, macronutrients, electrolytes, vitamins, and trace elements. PN is used if gut in not functioning or in conditions needing gut rest. PN is used to maintain or increase weight, preserve or replete lean body mass and visceral proteins, and support anabolism and nitrogen balance.[90] In patients whose liver and renal functions are normal, initial protein intake should not exceed 1.5 g/kg of the patient's weight. Weight gain greater than 1 kg/week denotes fluid retention and increasing heart rate indicates fluid overload status. PN is associated with many complications related to overfeeding including hyperglycemia, hypoglycemia, hyperlipidemia, hypercapnia, electrolyte disturbances, acid-base disturbances and refeeding syndrome. There are infectious and mechanical complications related to venous catheters as well.[90] Thus, patients on PN should be monitored closely for changes including vital signs, weight, electrolytes, and fluid status. A multidisciplinary nutrition team is a valuable service for initiating and monitoring this complicated, high-risk nutrition support.

Evidence Base Supporting Treatment Recommendations in Elderly Patients

Malnutrition is generally underdiagnosed in older adults. Careful and early detection facilitates development of comprehensive intervention of malnutrition in this population. There are several distinct screening tools validated for nutritional status in older adults, but no gold standard as assessed by a systemic review.[91] The Mini-Nutritional Assessment (MNA), shown in Figure 11-1, is one of the tools that is widely used.[92] In community-dwelling elderly patients, the MNA is designed to detect risk of malnutrition and lifestyle characteristics associated with nutritional risk, even when BMI and albumin are within the normal range. In outpatients and in hospitalized patients, the MNA predicts outcome and cost of care. Whereas, in home care and nursing home patients, the MNA targets living conditions, meal patterns, and chronic medical conditions allowing focused intervention.[92]

Another nutritional status screening tool validated for use in the elderly is the DETERMINE Nutrition Checklist, which lists a series of self-assessment statements for patients to check off regarding the following[93]:

- Disease—any disease, illness, or chronic condition that can change eating habits

- Eating poorly—eating too little or too much, or unbalanced meals

- Tooth loss/mouth pain—teeth, denture, mouth problems

- Economic hardship—having less or choosing to spend less than $25-30 per week for food

- Reduced social contact—living alone

- Multiple medicines—taking multiple medications or vitamins/minerals in high doses daily

- Involuntary weight loss or gain

- Need assistance in self care—trouble walking, shopping, buying or cooking food

- Elderly years above age 80

A score of 3–5 indicates moderate nutritional risk, whereas 6 or above warns high nutritional risk for a patient. The patient is directed to take the result to their provider for obtaining help to improve his or her nutritional health.

In frail elderly, combination of multinutrient supplementation (multivitamin + minerals) and micronutrient (enriched or fortified foods) can be used to enhance nutrition. The multinutrient dose should not exceed the recommended daily allowance to minimized adverse effects from high-dose vitamins. An interventional study, using approaches to increase food consumption including physical activity, improved meal ambiance, and flavor enhancement of the meal, increased nutritional status and quality of life in the frail elderly.[85] A Cochrane review examined the evidence from trials on nutritional status and clinical outcome improvements in elderly who received oral protein or energy supplementation.[94] They excluded patients who were in critical care and those recovering from cancer treatment. This review found that supplementation produced small but consistent weight gain in older adults, which may have beneficial effects on mortality.[94] While protein undernutrition has been associated with an increased risk of injury in older adults, protein supplementation has shown to reduce negative outcomes following injury in patients older than 65 years.[83]

Epidemiological studies on nutrition and aging show that guidelines for older adults are similar to those recommended for younger adults; however, the priorities are different. Recent reports have shown that applying screening protocols in long-term care institutions improved residents' nutritional status. The Modified MyPyramid for Older Adults, shown in Figure 11-2, is available to serve as a guide on diet, fluid needs, and physical activity for the older population.[95]

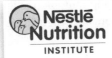

Mini Nutritional Assessment
MNA®

Last name: _____   First name: _____

Sex: _____ Age: _____ Weight, kg: _____ Height, cm: _____ Date: _____

Complete the screen by filling in the boxes with the appropriate numbers. Add the numbers for the screen. If score is 11 or less, continue with the assessment to gain a Malnutrition Indicator Score.

Screening

A Has food intake declined over the past 3 months due to loss of appetite, digestive problems, chewing or swallowing difficulties?
0 = severe decrease in food intake
1 = moderate decrease in food intake
2 = no decrease in food intake ☐

B Weight loss during the last 3 months
0 = weight loss greater than 3kg (6.6lbs)
1 = does not know
2 = weight loss between 1 and 3kg (2.2 and 6.6 lbs)
3 = no weight loss ☐

C Mobility
0 = bed or chair bound
1 = able to get out of bed / chair but does not go out
2 = goes out ☐

D Has suffered psychological stress or acute disease in the past 3 months?
0 = yes   2 = no ☐

E Neuropsychological problems
0 = severe dementia or depression
1 = mild dementia
2 = no psychological problems ☐

F Body Mass Index (BMI) (weight in kg) / (height in m²)
0 = BMI less than 19
1 = BMI 19 to less than 21
2 = BMI 21 to less than 23
3 = BMI 23 or greater ☐

Screening score
(subtotal max. 14 points) ☐☐

12 points or greater: Normal – not at risk – no need to complete assessment

11 points or below: Possible malnutrition – continue assessment

Assessment

G Lives independently (not in nursing home or hospital)
1 = yes   0 = no ☐

H Takes more than 3 prescription drugs per day
0 = yes   1 = no ☐

I Pressure sores or skin ulcers
0 = yes   1 = no ☐

J How many full meals does the patient eat daily?
0 = 1 meal
1 = 2 meals
2 = 3 meals ☐

K Selected consumption markers for protein intake
• At least one serving of dairy products (milk, cheese, yogurt) per day   yes ☐ no ☐
• Two or more servings of legumes or eggs per week   yes ☐ no ☐
• Meat, fish or poultry every day   yes ☐ no ☐
0.0 = if 0 or 1 yes
0.5 = if 2 yes
1.0 = if 3 yes ☐.☐

L Consumes two or more servings of fruit or vegetables per day?
0 = no   1 = yes ☐

M How much fluid (water, juice, coffee, tea, milk...) is consumed per day?
0.0 = less than 3 cups
0.5 = 3 to 5 cups
1.0 = more than 5 cups ☐.☐

N Mode of feeding
0 = unable to eat without assistance
1 = self-fed with some difficulty
2 = self-fed without any problem ☐

O Self view of nutritional status
0 = views self as being malnourished
1 = is uncertain of nutritional state
2 = views self as having no nutritional problem ☐

P In comparison with other people of the same age, how does the patient consider his / her health status?
0.0 = not as good
0.5 = does not know
1.0 = as good
2.0 = better ☐.☐

Q Mid-arm circumference (MAC) in cm
0.0 = MAC less than 21
0.5 = MAC 21 to 22
1.0 = MAC 22 or greater ☐.☐

R Calf circumference (CC) in cm
0 = CC less than 31
1 = CC 31 or greater ☐

Assessment (max. 16 points) ☐☐.☐

Screening score ☐☐.☐

Total Assessment (max. 30 points) ☐☐.☐

Malnutrition Indicator Score

17 to 23.5 points ☐ at risk of malnutrition

Less than 17 points ☐ malnourished

Ref. Vellas B, Villars H, Abellan G, et al. *Overview of MNA® - Its History and Challenges.* J Nut Health Aging 2006; 10: 456-465.
Rubenstein LZ, Harker JO, Salva A, Guigoz Y, Vellas B. Screening for Undernutrition in Geriatric Practice: *Developing the Short-Form Mini Nutritional Assessment (MNA-SF).* J. Geront 2001; 56A: M366-377.
Guigoz Y. The Mini-Nutritional Assessment (MNA®) *Review of the Literature – What does it tell us?* J Nutr Health Aging 2006; 10: 466-487.
© Nestlé, 1994, Revision 2006. N67200 12/99 10M
For more information: www.mna-elderly.com

Figure 11-1. The Mini-Nutritional Assessment (MNA).

Foods in the following categories, fluid, and physical activity are represented in the Modified MyPyramid for Older Adults[95] (Figure 11-2):

- Whole, enriched, and fortified grains and cereals such as brown rice and 100% whole wheat bread
- Bright-colored vegetables such as carrots and broccoli
- Deep-colored fruit such as berries and melon
- Low- and non-fat dairy products such as yogurt and low-lactose milk
- Dry beans and nuts, fish, poultry, lean meat and eggs
- Liquid vegetable oils and soft spreads low in saturated and *trans* fat

Added to the Modified MyPyramid is a foundation depicting physical activities characteristic of older adults such as walking, house work, yard work, and swimming.[95] This is an attempt to link regular physical activity with reduced risk of chronic disease, stable body weight, and improved quality of life. Emphasis is placed on the importance of consuming adequate amounts of fiber rich foods, which means choosing mainly whole grain products rather than highly refined forms, and whole fruits and vegetables rather than juices. Also included as an integral part of the Modified MyPyramid for Older Adults is a flag at the top suggesting that older adults may need certain supplemental nutrients. Calcium, vitamin D and vitamin B12 become difficult to obtain in adequate amounts from food alone and are depicted on the flag.[95]

Dietary calcium intake and vitamin D in older adults is largely important in prevention and treatment of osteoporosis, and is discussed in Chapter 15. It has also been reported that 5-20% of older adults have marginal or significant deficiency in vitamin B12. The most common clinical

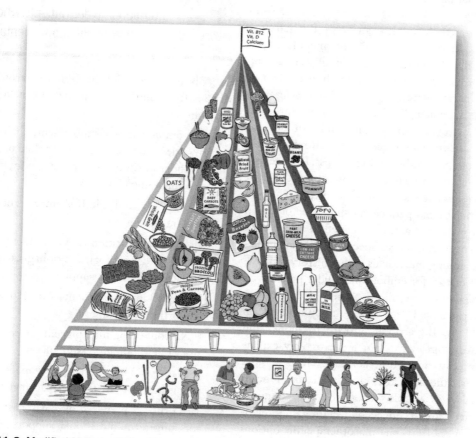

Figure 11-2. Modified MyPyramid for Older Adults. *Source:* Copyright 2007, Tufts University.

presentation of vitamin B12 deficiency in older adults include macrocytic anemia, subacute combined degeneration of the spinal cord, neuropathies, ataxia, glossitis and possibly dementia.[86] Recommendation for adults older than 50 years is to meet the recommended dietary allowance by taking vitamin B12 in the crystalline form, which does not require gastric acid or enzymes for digestion and absorption. A clinical trial identified that an oral dose of 500 mcg/d of crystalline vitamin B12 is required to reverse deficiency state in the elderly population.[96]

Medications used for appetite stimulation has many problems for elderly patients. Despite data from multiple trials among subjects with HIV wasting of cancer cachexia suggesting a benefit associated with daily doses of megestrol 400–800 mg, utility among elderly patients may be limited. Although a prospective study of 800 mg/day demonstrated modest weight gain among a population of long-term care residents, the weight gain was not significantly different from placebo at three months and only differed at 6 months, 3 months after active treatment had been discontinued.[97] Further, recent studies employing megestrol acetate found that weight gained tends to be in fat tissue rather than in muscles, and muscle mass actually decreased in patients who took the drug.[86] Such weight gain is not ideal for older patients who already lose lean muscle and gain fat as part of their aging process. If megestrol acetate is employed to combat unintended weight loss, parameters such as food intake, weight, and other nutritional parameters should be observed over 3–6 months and if no benefit is observed it should be discontinued. Special care should be exercised among individuals with a history of DVT or risk factors for embolism.[98] Older patients do not tolerate the dysphoria caused by dronabinol, and cyproheptadine has no efficacy evidence in the elderly. The anabolic growth hormones and insulin-like growth factor are extremely expensive and can cause intolerable side effects in older patients. Androgen therapy with testosterone or its analogues are also associated with frequent side effects and its effects on weight gain remains unknown.[86] Thus pharmacotherapeutic options are limited in this population for such indica-

tion. Older patients who are malnourished with persistent anorexia and have concurrent depression may be tried on mirtazapine therapy. There is actually no data evaluating the efficacy of mirtazapine among elderly patients with weight loss in the absence of depression, and it is not clear if any weight-gain that might be achieved is purely associated with the drug itself or with the alleviation of depression.[98] However as an acceptable antidepressant agent for elderly patients with depression, mirtazapine is a reasonable choice if weight loss is a concomitant symptom.[98]

The European Society for Parenteral and Enteral Nutrition (ESPEN) Guidelines provide recommendations for using enteral nutrition in geriatric population.[99]

KEY POINT: As in younger adult population, enteral nutrition is preferred over parenteral nutrition in older patients who need nutritional supplementation.

A brief summary of the Grade A recommendations from the ESPEN guidelines include the following[99]:

- Use oral nutritional supplementation (ONS) in patients who are undernourished or at risk of undernutrition to increase energy, protein and micronutrient intake

- Use ONS in frail elderly to improve or maintain nutritional status

- Use enteral nutrition (EN) in older patients with severe neurological dysphagia to ensure energy and nutrient supply

- Use ONS in older patients after hip fracture and orthopedic surgery

- ONS containing high protein can reduce the risk of developing pressure ulcers

- Initiate EN 3 hours after percutaneous endoscopic gastrostomy (PEG) placement

- PEG tube is preferred over nasogastric tube for long-term nutritional support in older patients with neurologic dysphagia; PEG is associated with less treatment failure and better nutritional status

- Use PEG tube if EN is anticipated to be longer than 4 weeks

- Use dietary fiber to normalize bowel function in tube-fed elderly

Ideally if parenteral nutrition is required and initiated, older patients should be closely monitored with daily assessment by a nutrition team. Overfeeding a frail patient can cause a potentially fatal refeeding syndrome. They are also subject to complications associated with parenteral nutrition described above.

Hospitalized older patients are at increased risk for malnutrition and need to be carefully assessed and aggressively managed. Reports show that up to 55% of the older patients admitted to hospital have pre-existing malnutrition.[83] Similarly, in the geriatric rehabilitation setting, the occurrence of protein undernutrition is estimated to be 57%.[100] The estimated mean resting energy intake in older hospitalized patients recovering from an acute illness have been reported to be 18.8 kcal/kg/day, which is just sufficient to cover the required energy expenditure.[84] Thus, the hospitalized elderly would most likely benefit from higher caloric intake. Additionally, malnutrition has been associated with skin breakdown, delayed wound healing, infection, longer hospital stay, readmission, and mortality.[83] Several randomized control trials have been conducted to demonstrate benefits of oral nutritional supplementation in the hospitalized elderly patients. For example, a Cochrane review of 22 trials found a reduction in relative risk of mortality in older patients who suffered hip fractures that received oral nutritional supplementation compared to those who did not receive the supplementation.[94] Nutritional support for older patients in hospitals and rehabilitation settings have improved nutritional status, reduce length of stay and mortality, and led to better functional outcomes as part of their recovery process.[83] Also, an early interdisciplinary intervention approach to managing nutrition in geriatric inpatients proved cost-effectiveness in reducing protein-energy malnutrition and related hospital-acquired infections.[100] At the time of hospital discharge, elderly patients at risk of malnutrition who received dietary counseling, and liquid and multivitamin supplementation maintained weight and improved activities of daily living functions compared to those who did not receive these interventions.[100]

Older patients who suffered a stroke possess a unique problem with eating and maintaining nutritional status. About half of all stroke patients have eating problems acutely after the stroke, and the problems can persist long-term. A variety of eating disabilities result as consequences of stroke, including functional decline related to arm or hand manipulation, posture, lip closure, chewing, swallowing, perception, sensation, and attention. According to a study assessing the needs of stroke patients at the time of hospital discharge, 67% of patients require support for eating and feeding. Of these, 42% of the patients had dysphagia and 60% poor food intake and appetite.[100] More than 80% of stroke patients in nursing home setting were assessed as having dependence in eating by the same study.[100] These results highlight the importance of making careful observation and evaluation, and consistent documentation regarding eating needs of the hospitalized elderly and the older stroke population to enable appropriate nutritional management.

Special Considerations Affecting Desired Clinical Outcomes

The presence of multiple diseases, polypharmacy, malnutrition, and altered metabolism, common in older patients, increases the risk of adverse events related to food-drug interactions. Pharmacists and nutritionist are integral part of the patient and provider education process in order to prevent such adverse events.

Examples of food-drug interactions commonly found in older adults are as follows[101]:

- Digoxin: decreased absorption with high-fiber products

- Fluoroquinolones and tetracyclines: decreased absorption with cations (calcium, iron, magnesium and zinc)

- Levodopa/carbidopa: decreased absorption with high protein diet

- Lithium: decreased level with high sodium diet; increased level with low sodium diet
- Monoamine oxidase inhibitors: thiamine-containing foods can precipitate hypertensive crisis or cardiovascular events
- Grapefruit juice: drug interactions with medications such as nifedipine, cyclosporin, simvastatin
- Warfarin: dietary vitamin K antagonizes effect

A recent study confirmed an independent association between nutritional deficit and depression in malnourished community-dwelling elderly population.[102] Findings emphasized the importance of early identification of depression among the older adults with nutritional disorders.

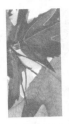

KEY POINT: Treating malnutrition in elderly population requires an Interdisciplinary approach to providing adequate nutrition across the spectrum of aging.

Furthermore, as the American Dietetic Association declared in their position paper, "National, state, local policies that promote coordination and integration of food and nutrition services into health and supportive systems are needed to maintain independence, functional ability, chronic disease management, and quality of life"[103] of the growing elderly population.

CASE 1: GERIATRIC PRIMARY CARE CLINIC

Subjective:
AM is a 69-year-old community dwelling woman who presents to a primary care clinic complaining of daily cough. No complaints of fever, chills, runny nose, increased sputum production, allergy or difficulty swallowing.

Past Medical History:
Hypertension, hyperlipidemia, transient ischemic attack and osteoarthritis

Medications:
Hydrochlorothiazide 25 mg daily, simvastatin 20 mg at bedtime, aspirin 81 mg daily and naproxen 250 mg twice daily as needed

Allergies:
Penicillin – Hives

Social History:
Cigarette smoking – half pack per day; 4–5 alcoholic drinks on weekends

Family History:
Mother died of breast cancer; father died when patient was young

Objective:
Height 5'2", Weight 174 pounds

Blood pressure 130/70; heart rate 68; respiratory rate 14; temperature 98.5 °F; BMI 31.8; pain 2/10 (on scale of 0–10)

Physical Exam:

Within normal limits

Laboratory/Radiology:

Complete metabolic panel and complete blood count within normal limits; lipid panel pending; chest x-ray negative

Assessment:

AM is a 69-year-old female with chronic cough without signs and symptoms of infection or allergy; possible GERD with several contributing factors including lifestyle and medication use.

Plan:

1. Lifestyle modification: Provide smoking cessation counseling; Educate on limiting alcohol use, eating small portions of low-fat diet, regular exercise for weight loss; provide other useful information such as elevating head of bed, not reclining after meals, etc.

2. Medication management: Discontinue naproxen use and avoid NSAIDs; take acetaminophen for arthritis pain; take aspirin after meal. Start omeprazole 20 mg daily; take 30 minutes before breakfast.

Rationale:

1. Once common causes of chronic cough are excluded and GERD is suspected for an elderly patient presenting with an atypical symptom, start lifestyle modification with intense education.

2. Medications that can irritate or potentiate GERD, such as NSAIDs, should be considered for discontinuation. Once-daily low-dose PPI therapy can be initiated for effective acid suppression in elderly patients when no alarm symptoms are present. Patients should be monitored for symptom control and progress of lifestyle modification.

CASE 2: NURSING HOME

Subjective:

TS is an 83-year-old male resident of a nursing home who has been living in the facility for past 11 months since suffering a right middle cerebral artery stroke. Since his admission to the nursing facility, TS has had difficulty eating due to trouble swallowing and decreased coordination required for feeding. He has lost 10kg. Also, he has developed a new coccyx ulcer.

Past Medical History:

Hypertension, stroke, osteoarthritis, and constipation

Medications:

Lisinopril 20 mg daily, clopidogrel 75 mg daily, acetaminophen 325 mg 2 tablets three times daily, docusate sodium 100 mg twice daily

Allergies:
Aspirin

Social History:
40-year history of cigarette smoking—quit 5 years ago; no alcoholic drinks

Family History:
Mother died of old age; father died of stroke at 70 years of age

Objective:
Height 5'9", weight 55 kg, BMI 17 kg/m^2
Blood pressure 122/62; heart rate 60; respiratory rate 14; temperature 98.6 °F; pain 1/10 (on scale of 0–10)

Physical Exam:
Slight edema in the ankles but otherwise within normal limits

Laboratory/Radiology:
Complete metabolic panel is within normal limits; complete blood count pending; albumin level pending but 2 months ago, it was 2.4 g/dL

Assessment:
TS is an 83-year-old male with severe malnutrition as evidenced by history of 15% weight loss over 11 months, underweight with BMI < 20 kg/m^2, MNA score of 14, and decreased dietary intake, declined physical function and mobility and possible dysphagia since suffering a stroke.

Plan:
1. Perform swallowing evaluation: Speech and language pathologist to provide bed-side swallowing assessment to determine the consistency of food that is appropriate for this patient.

2. Perform drug regimen review to evaluate all dosage formulations. Determine if this patient's medications need to be crushed or changed to liquid formulation if available. Consider whether all medications are absolutely needed and consider discontinuation if medication administration creates a hardship that outweighs any clinical benefit from drug therapy.

3. Provide occupational therapy: Occupational therapist to train TS on seating and positioning for successful eating, and offer assistive devices for meals.

4. Provide oral nutritional supplementation: High protein oral nutritional supplementation to be given in between regular meals as long as swallowing evaluation shows such consistency can be tolerated by the patient. Monitor prealbumin level weekly.

Rationale:
1. Dysphagia can also impair a patient's eating function greatly and place the patient at increased risk for malnutrition as well as aspiration. Speech and language pathologist should be a member of the team taking care of malnourished patients, providing swallowing evaluation and training to facilitate improved swallowing if necessary.

2. The patient may not be able to swallow medications or experience pain upon swallowing and refuse to take their medications. To insure adherence to necessary medications there must be an easy and reliable way to ingest each dose. Pharmacists can help with this need.

3. Seating and position are important requirements for successful eating and prevention of possible aspiration. Occupational therapists can train the patient and provide equipments such as special utensils, plates, or placemats to better facilitate self-feeding.

4. Oral nutritional supplementation, particularly high protein formula, can improve nutritional status of TS and promote healing of his pressure ulcer. TS's prealbumin level should be measured to objectively monitor nutritional treatment plan.

Clinical Pearls

- *Older patients are frequently prescribed a PPI in the hospital setting for stress ulcer prophylaxis, and continued on the medication after discharge inappropriately. Although a higher dose or chronic therapy may be indicated when the diagnosis of GERD is clearly established, the high prevalence of PPI continuation without true indication coupled with the possible risks of long term use underscore the need to critically evaluate the appropriateness of the PPI when performing drug regimen review.*

- *Although low fat, low sodium or other restrictive diets are often an integral part of disease management, the clinical outcomes of such diets are less clear in frail or institutionalized elderly. Restrictive diets may not be recommended, despite a history of heart disease, diabetes or other chronic diseases, among individuals with geriatric cachexia, swallowing problems, advanced dementia, palliative care directives, or in other situations in which enjoyment of food is prioritized above disease management.*

Chapter Summary

The prevalence and complications of GI disorders and nutritional deficiencies in older adults are widely known. Aging imparts various physiological changes and places the elderly patients at increased risk for GI problems such as gastroesophageal reflux disease, diverticular disease, constipation and fecal incontinence, *Clostridium difficile*-associated diarrhea, nausea and vomiting, dysphagia, and oral health needs. At the same time, decreased nutritional status increases their risk for becoming malnourished and frail. Among the available pharmacotherapies and management strategies for treating GI disorders and nutritional deficits, differing evidence exist between recommendations and treatment guidelines for older population as apposed to the younger patients. Becoming knowledgeable about these differences in evidence-based practices and being mindful of the special considerations specific to the older population can enrich the clinical service of a geriatric health care professional. In addition, Understanding the epidemiology of aging, associated with GI disorders and nutrition, can help eliminate disparities in health care and promote quality of life and longevity for our aging population.

Self-Assessment Questions

1. What physiologic changes related to aging affect GI disorders in the elderly?

2. How does the prevalence of protein-malnutrition compare between a community-dwelling elder with an elderly who is a nursing home resident?

3. What medical conditions can cause constipation in the elderly?

4. Which medications can negatively affect a patient's swallowing ability?

5. Compare and contrast the "step up" vs. "step down" therapy for treating GERD.

6. Which antibiotics are most commonly associated with developing *C. difficile*-associated diarrhea?

7. How does the treatment for nausea and vomiting differ for an elderly versus a younger patient?

8. What are the different components of the Modified MyPyramid for Older Adults that can be used to counsel a patient about their nutritional needs?

9. What are some strategies to maintaining optimal oral health and preventing stomatitis?

References

1. Ali MA, Lacy BE. Abdominal complaints and gastrointestinal disorders. In: Landefeld CS, Palmer RM, Johnson MA, et al., eds. *Current Geriatric Diagnosis and Treatment*. New York: McGraw-Hill Inc; 2004:220–238.

2. Greenwald DA. Aging, the gastrointestinal tract, and risk of acid-related disease. *Am J Med*. 2004;117 Suppl 5A:8S–13S.

3. Pathy MSJ, Sinclair A, Morely JE. Principles and practice of geriatric medicine. Available at: http://www3.interscience.wiley.com.ezproxy2.library.arizona.edu/cgi-bin/bookhome/112464097.

4. Pillotto A, Franceschi M, Leandro G, et al. Clinical features of reflux esophagitis in older people: a study of 840 consecutive patients. *J Am Geriatr Soc*. 2006;54(10):1537–1542.

5. De Vault KR, Castell DO. Updated guidelines for the diagnosis and treatment of gastroesophageal reflux disease. *A J Gastroenterol*. 2005;100:190–200.

6. Johnson DA. Gastroesophageal reflux disease in the elderly—a prevalent and severe disease. *Rev Gastroenterol Disord*. 2004;4 Suppl 4:S16–S24.

7. Pilotto A, Franceschi M, Paris F. Recent advances in the treatment of GERD in the elderly: focus on proton pump inhibitors. *J Clin Pract*. 2005;59(10):1204–1209.

8. Field SK. Gastroesophageal reflux and asthma: are they related? *J Asthma*. 1999; 36(8):631–644.

9. Laheij RJ, Sturkenboom MC, Hassing RJ, et al. Risk of community-acquired pneumonia and use of gastric acid-suppressive drugs. *JAMA*. 2004;292(16):1955–1960.

10. Yang YX, Lewis JD, Epstein S, et al. Long-term proton pump inhibitor therapy and risk of hip fracture. *JAMA*. 2006;296(24):2947–2953.

11. Leonard J, Marshall JK, Moayyedi P. Systematic review of the risk of enteric infection in patients taking acid suppression. *Am J Gastroenterol*. 2007;102(9):2047–2056.

12. Dial S, Delaney JA, Barkun AN, et al. Use of gastric acid-suppressive agents and the risk of community-acquired *Clostridium difficile*-associated disease. *JAMA*. 2005;294(23):2989–2995.

13. Gilard M, Arnaud B, Cornily JC, et al. Influence of omeprazole on the antiplatelet action of clopidogrel associated with aspirin: the randomized, double-blind OCLA (Omeprazole CLopidogrel Aspirin) study. *J Am Coll Cardiol*. 2008;51(3):261–163.

14. Food and Drug Adminstration. Public-health advisory: Updated safety information about a drug interaction between clopidogrel bisulfate (marketed as Plavix) and omeprazole (marketed as Prilosec and Prilosec OTC). November 17, 2009. http://www.fda.gov/Drugs/DrugSafety/PublicHealthAdvisories/ucm190825.htm. Accessed 11/19/09.

15. Comparato G, Pilotto A, Franze A, et al. Diverticular disease in the elderly. *Dig Dis*. 2007;25:151–159.

16. Farrell RJ, Farrell JJ, Morrin MM. Diverticular disease in the elderly. *Gastroenterology Clinics*. 2001;30(20). Available at : http://www.mdconsult.com/das/article/body/94936312-8.html. Accessed May 16, 2008.

17. Reisman Y, Ziv Y, Kravrovitc D, et al. Diverticulitis: the effect of age and location on the course of disease. *Int J Colorectal Dis*. 1999;14:250–254.

18. Standards Task Force of the American Society of Colon and Rectal Surgeons. Practice parameters for sigmoid diverticulitis: supporting documentation. *Dis Colon Rectum*. 1995;38:126–132.

19. Kockerling F, Schneider C, Reymond MA, et al. Laparoscopic resection of sigmoid diverticulitis: results of a multicenter study. *Surg Endosc*. 1999;13:567–571.

20. Aldoori WH, Giovannucci EL, Rockett HR, et al. A prospective study of dietary fiber types and symptomatic diverticular disease in men. *J Nutr*. 1998;128:714–719.

21. Schatzkin A, Lanza E, Corle D, et al. Lack of effect of a low-fat, high-fiber diet on the recurrence of colorectal

adenomas. Polyp Prevention Trial Study Group. *N Engl J Med.* 2000;342:1149–1155.

22. Aldoori WH, Giovannucci EL, Rimm EB, et al. Use of acetaminophen and non-steroidal anti-inflammatory drugs: a prospective study and the risk of symptomatic diverticular disease in men. *Arch Fam Med.* 1998;7:255–260.

23. Mitchell KL, Shaheen NJ. Preventive therapy in perforated colonic diverticular disease? Calcium channel blockers may hold the key. *Gastroenterology.* 2004;127:680–682.

24. Crane SJ, Talley NJ. Chronic gastrointestinal symptoms in the elderly. *Clin Geriatr Med.* 2007;23:721–734.

25. Ruby C, Fillenbaum G, Kuchibhatla M, et al. Laxative use in the community-dwelling elderly. *Am J Geriatr Pharmacother.* 2003;1(1):11–17.

26. Talley N, Fleming K, Evans J, et al. Constipation in an elderly community: a study of prevalence and potential risk factors. *Am J Gastroenterol.* 1996;91(1):19–25.

27. Bartz S. Gastrointestinal disorders in the elderly. *Ann Long-Term Care Clin Care Aging.* 2003;11(7):33–39.

28. Stern M. Neurogenic bowel and bladder in the older adult. *Clin Geriatr Med.* 2006;22:311–330.

29. Bharucha A, Zinsmeister A, Locke GR, et al. Prevalence and burden of fecal incontinence: a population-based study in women. *Gastroenterology.* 2005;129:42–49.

30. Goode P, Burgio K, Halli A, et al. Prevalence and correlates of fecal incontinence in community-dwelling older adults. *J Am Geriatr Soc.* 2005;53:629–635.

31. Lillo AR, Rose S. Functional bowel disorders in the geriatric patient: constipation, fecal impaction, and fecal incontinence. *Am J Gastroenterol.* 2000;95:901–905.

32. Coggrave M, Wiesel PH, Norton C, et al. Management of faecal incontinence and constipation in adults with central neurological disease. *Cochrane Database Syst Rev.* 2005;1:CD002115.

33. Johnson JF, Morton D, Geenen J, et al. Multicenter, 4-week, double-blind, randomized, placebo-controlled trial of lubiprostone, a locally-acting type-2 chloride channel activator, in patients with chronic constipation. *Am J Gastroenterol.* 2008;103:170–177.

34. Johnson AF, Ueno R. Lubiprostone, a locally acting chloride channel activator, in adult patients with chronic constipation: a double-blind, placebo-controlled, dose-ranging study to evaluate efficacy and safety. *Aliment Pharmacol Ther.* 2007;25:1351–1361.

35. Thomas J, Karver S, Cooney GA, et al. Methylnaltrexone for opioid-induced constipation in advanced illness. *N Engl J Med.* 2008;358:2332–2343.

36. Harari D, Norton C, Lockwood L, et al. Treatment of constipation and fecal incontinence in stroke patients: randomized controlled trial. *Stroke.* 2004;35:2549–2555.

37. Byrne CM, Solomon MJ, Young JM, et al. Biofeedback for fecal incontinence: short-term outcomes of 513 consecutive patients and predictors for successful treatment. *Dis Colon Rectum.* 2007;50(4):417–427.

38. Stenzelius K, Westergren A, Hallberg IR. Bowel function among people 75+ reporting fecal incontinence in relation to help seeking, dependency and quality of life. *J Clin Nursing.* 2007;16:458–469.

39. Prabhakar K. Diarrheal disease in the elderly. *Clin Geriatr Med.* 2007;23:833–856.

40. Crogan NL, Evans BC. *Clostridium difficile:* An Emerging Epidemic in Nursing Homes. *Geriatric Nursing.* 2007;28(3):161–164.

41. Simor AE, Bradley SF, Strausbaugh LJ, et al. *Clostridium difficile* in longer-term-care facilities for the elderly. *Infect Control Hosp Epidemiol.* 2002;23:696–703.

42. Bouza E, burillo A, Munoz P. Antimicrobial therapy of *Clostridium difficile*-associated diarrhea. *Med Clin N Am.* 2006;90:1141–1163.

43. Warny M, Pepin J, Fang A, et al. Toxin production by an emerging strain of *Clostridium difficile* associated with outbreaks of severe disease in North America and Europe. *Lancet.* 2005;366:1079–1084.

44. Tal S, Gurevich A, Guller V, et al. Risk factors for recurrence of *Clostridium difficile*-associated diarrhea in the elderly. *Scand J Infect Dis.* 2002;34:594–597.

45. Bobak DA. Rifaximin to Treat Recurrent *Clostridium difficile* Colitis. *Curr Infect Dis Rep.* 2008;10(2):90–91.

46. Cherifi S, Delmee M, Broeck JV, et al. Management of an outbreak of *Clostridium difficile*-associated disease among geriatric patients. *Infect Control Hosp Epidemiol.* 2006;27:1200–1205.

47. O'Connor KA, Kingston M, O'Donovan M, et al. Antibiotic prescribing policy and *Clostridium difficile* diarrhea. *Q J Med.* 2004;97:423–429.

48. Wood GJ, Shega JW, Lynch B, et al. Management of intractable nausea and vomiting in patients at the end of life. *JAMA.* 2007;298(10):1196–1207.

49. American Gastroenterological Association (AGA) Clinical Practice and Practice Economics Committee. AGA medical position statement: nausea and vomiting. *Gastroenterology.* 2001;120:261–262.

50. Vickers AJ. Can acupuncture have specific effects on health? A systematic review of acupuncture antiemesis trials. *J R Soc Med.* 1996;89(6):303–311.

51. Bertalanffy P, Hoerauf K, Fleischhackl R. Korean hand acupressure for motion sickness in prehospital trauma care: a perspective, randomized, double-blinded trial in a geriatric population. *Anesth Analg.* 2004;98:220–223.

52. Stephenson J, Davies A. An assessment of etiology-based guidelines for the management of nausea and vomiting in patients with advanced cancer. *Support Care Cancer.* 2006;14(4):348–353.

53. Sheth HS, Verrico MM, Skledar SJ, et al. Promethazine adverse events after implementation of a medication shortage interchange. *Ann Pharmacother.* 2005;39:255–261.

54. Fick DM, Cooper JW, Wade WE, Waller JL, Maclean JR, Beers MH. Updating the Beers Criteria for Potentially Inappropriate Medication Use in Older Adults. Results of a U.S. Consensus Panel of Experts. *Arch*

Intern Med. 2003;163:2716–2724

55. Esper CD, Factor SA. Failure of recognition of drug-induced Parkinsonism in the elderly. *Movement Disorders.* 2008;23(3):401–404.

56. Spinks AB,Wasiak J, Villanueva EV, Bernath V. Scopolamine (hyoscine) for preventing and treating motion sickness. *Cochrane Database of Syst Rev.* 2007;3:CD002851.

57. Beers MH, Jones TV, Berkwitz M, et al., eds. *The Merck Manual of Health & Aging. Whitehouse Station, NJ: Merck Research Laboratories*; 2004:735–743.

58. White GN, O'Rourke F, Ong BS, et al. Dysphagia: causes, assessment, treatment, and management. *Geriatrics.* 2008;63(5):15–20.

59. Runions S, Rodrigue N, White C. Practice on an acute stroke unit after implementation of a decision-making algorithm for dietary management of dysphagia. *J Neurosci Nurs.* 2004;36:200–207.

60. Robbins J, Barczi S. Disorders of swallowing. In: Hazzard WR, Blass JP, Halter JB, et al. *Principles of Geriatric Medicine and Gerontology.* 5th ed. New York: McGraw-Hill, Inc.; 2003:1193–1212.

61. Ashley J, Duggan M, Sutcliffe N. Speech, language, and swallowing disorders in the older adult. *Clin Geriatr Med.* 2006;22:291–310.

62. Westergren A. Detection of eating difficulties after stroke: a systematic review. *Int Nurs Rev.* 2006;53(2):143–149.

63. Trapl M, Enderie P, Nowotny M, et al. Dysphagia bedside screening for acute-stroke patients: the Gugging swallowing screen. *Stroke.* 2007;38(11):2948–2952.

64. Madden C, Fenton J, Hughes J, et al. Comparison between videofluoroscopy and milk-swallow endoscopic examination of swallowing (FEES) in determining the risk of aspiration in acute stroke patients. *Clin Otolaryngol Allied Sci.* 2000;25(6):504–506.

65. Marik PE, Kaplan D. Aspiration pneumonia and dysphagia in the elderly. *Chest.* 2003;124(1):328–336.

66. Logemann JA, Gensler G, Robbins J, et al. A randomized study of three interventions for aspiration of thin liquids in patients with dementia or Parkinson's disease. *J Speech Lang Hear Res.* 2008;51(1):173–183.

67. Finucane TE, Christmas C, Leff BA. Tube feeding in dementia: how incentives undermine health care quality and patient safety. *J Am Med Dir Assoc.* 2007;8(4):205–208.

68. Dennis MS, Lewis SC, Warlow C, for the FOOD Trial Collaboration. Effect of timing and method of enteral tube feeding for dysphagic stroke patients (FOOD): a multicenter randomized controlled trial. *Lancet.* 2005;365(9461):764–772.

69. Low JA, Chan DK, Hung WT, et al. Treatment of recurrent aspiration pneumonia in end-stage dementia: preferences and choices of a group of elderly nursing home residents. *Intern Med J.* 2003;33(8):345–349.

70. Kays S, Robbins J. Effects of sensorimotor exercise on swallowing outcomes relative to age and age-related disease. *Seminars in Speech and Language.* 2006;27(4):245–259.

71. Xie Y, Wang L, Zhao J, et al. Acupuncture for dysphagia in acute stroke (Protocol). *Cochrane Database Syst Rev.* 2006;(3):CD006076.

72. Okubo PD, Dantas RO, Troncon LE, et al. Clinical and scintigraphic assessment of swallowing of older patients admitted to a tertiary care geriatric ward. *Dysphagia.* 2008;23:1–6.

73. Tada A, Shiiba M, Yokoe H, et al. Relationship between oral motor dysfunction and oral bacteria in bedridden elderly. *Oral Surg oral Med oral Pathol Oral Radiol Endod.* 2004;98:184–188.

74. Ettinger RL. Oral health and the aging population. *JADA.* 2007;138:55–65.

75. Saunders R, Friedman B. Oral health conditions of community-dwelling cognitively intact elderly persons with disabilities. *Gerodontology.* 2007;24:67–76.

76. MacDonald DE. Principles of geriatric dentistry and their application to the older adult with a physical disability. *Clin Geriatr Med.* 2006;22:413–434.

77. Sarin J, Balasubramaniam, R, Corcoran A, et al. Reducing the risk of aspiration pneumonia among elderly patients in long-term care facilities through oral health interventions. *J Am Med Dir Assoc.* 2008;9:128–135.

78. Davies RM. The rational use of oral care products in the elderly. *Clin Oral Invest.* 2004;8:2–5.

79. Peltola P, Vehkalahti MM, Simoila R. Effects of 11-month interventions on oral cleanliness among the long-term hospitalized elderly. *Gerodontology.* 2007;24:14–21.

80. Jensen PM, Saunders RL, Thierer T, et al. Factors associated with oral health-related quality of life in community-dwelling elderly persons with disabilities. *J Am Geratr Soc.* 2008;56:711–717.

81. Lowe C, Blinkhorn AS, Worthington HV. Testing the effect of including oral health in general health checks for elderly patients in medical practice—a randomized controlled trial. *Community Dent Oral Epidemiol.* 2007;35:12–17.

82. Jablonski RA, Munro CL, Grap MJ, et al. The role of biobehavioral, environmental, and social forces on oral health disparities in frail and functionally dependent nursing home elders. *Biological Research for Nursing.* 2005;7(1):75–82.

83. Wells JL, Dumbrell AC. Nutrition and aging: assessment and treatment of compromised nutritional status in frail elderly patients. *Clin Interv Aging.* 2006;1(1):67–79.

84. Feldblum I, German L, Castel H, et al. Characteristics of undernourished older medical patients and the identification of predictors for undernutrition status. *Nutr J.* 2007;6:37–47.

85. Davis-Smith YM, Boltri JM. Nutrition and exercise in the elderly. In: Olsen CG, Tindall WN, Clasen ME, eds. *Geriatric Pharmacotherapy: A Guide for the Helping Professional.* Washington, DC: APhA; 2007:219–237.

86. Chapman IM. Nutritional disorders in the elderly. *Med Clin N Am.* 2006;90:887–907.

87. Visscher TLS, Seidell Jc, Menotti A et al. Under- and overweight in relation to mortality among men 40–59 and 50–69: the seven countries study. *Am J Epidemiol.* 2000;151:660–666.

88. Makhija S, Baker, J. The subjective global assessment: a review of its use in clinical practice. *Nutr Clin Pract.* 2008;23(4):405–409.

89. Miller S. Enteral Nutrition. In: Chisholm-Burns MA, Wells BG, Schwinghammer TL, et al., eds. *Pharmacotherapy: principles and practice.* New York: McGraw Hill, Inc; 2008:1511–1527.

90. Kraft MD, Btaiche IF. Parenteral nutrition. In: Chisholm-Burns MA, Wells BG, Schwinghammer TL, et al., eds. *Pharmacotherapy: principles and practice.* New York: McGraw Hill, Inc; 2008:1493–1510.

91. Donini LM, Savina C, Rosano A, et al. Systematic review of nutritional status evaluation and screening tools in the elderly. *J Nutr Health Aging.* 2007;11(5):421–432.

92. Guigoz Y, Lauque S, Vellas BJ. Identifying the elderly at risk for malnutrition—the mini nutritional assessment. *Clin Geriatr Med.* 2002;18:737–757.

93. Brunt AR. The ability of the DETERMINE checklist to predict continued community-dwelling in rural, white women. *J Nutr Elder.* 2006;25(3–4):41–59.

94. Avenell A, Handoll HH. Nutritional supplementation for hip fracture aftercare in older people. *Cochrane Database Syst Rev.* 2005;(2):CD001880.

95. Lichtenstein AH, Rasmussen H, Yu WW, Epstein SR, Russell RM. Modified MyPyramid for Older Adults. *J Nutr.* 2008; 138:78–82.

96. Park S, Johnson MA. What is an adequate dose of oral vitamin B12 in older people with poor vitamin B12 status? *Nutr Rev.* 2006;64(8):373–378.

97. Yeh S, Wu S, Lee T, et al. Improvement in quality-of-life measures and stimulation of weight gain after treatment with megestrol acetate oral suspension in geriatric cachexia: results of a double-blind, placebo-controlled study. *J Am Geriatr Soc.* 2000;48:485–492.

98. Fox CB, Treadway AK, Blaszczyk AT, Sleeper RB. Megestrol acetate and mirtazapine for the treatment of unplanned weight loss in the elderly. *Pharmacotherapy.* 2009 Apr;29(4):383–397.

99. Volkert D, Berner YN, Berry E, et al. ESPEN guidelines on enteral nutrition: geriatrics. *Clin Nutr.* 2006;25:330–360.

100. Persson M, Hytter-Landahl A, Brismar K et al. Nutritional supplementation and dietary advice in geriatric patients at risk of malnutrition. *Clinical Nutr.* 2007;26:216–224.

101. Akamine D, Filho MK, Peres CM. Drug-nutrient interactions in elderly people. *Curr Opin Clin Nutr Metab Care.* 2007;10:304–310.

102. Cabrera MAS, Mesas AE, Garcia ARL, et al. Malnutrition and depression among community-dwelling elderly people. *J Am Med Dir Assoc.* 2007;8:582–584.

103. American Dietetic Association. Position paper of the American Dietetic Association: nutrition across the spectrum of aging. *J Am Diet Assoc.* 2005;105:616–633.

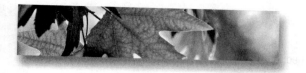

12

The Central Nervous System

AMIE TAGGART BLASZCZYK AND LISA C. HUTCHISON

Learning Objectives

1. Compare the prevalence of dementia across different age groups.

2. Contrast the different etiologies, symptoms and therapies for mild cognitive impairment, Alzheimer's dementia, vascular dementia, dementia with Lewy bodies, and frontotemporal dementia.

3. Design a treatment plan for behavioral symptoms associated with dementia.

4. Distinguish the epidemiology and features of dementia and delirium in an elderly patient.

5. Devise a prevention and treatment plan for an elderly patient with delirium.

6. Recognize the impact of Parkinson's disease and its treatment on the quality of life of patients and caregivers.

7. Recommend appropriate therapy for a senior individual with Parkinson's disease throughout the course of the disease.

8. Recommend nonpharmacologic and pharmacologic interventions for a person with Parkinson's experiencing depression and constipation.

9. Recognize the different etiologies and clinical presentation of seizures in the senior population versus the younger population with seizures.

10. Recommend appropriate therapy for a senior individual diagnosed with epilepsy adjusting for pharmacokinetic and pharmacodynamic problems.

11. Recommend an appropriate titration schedule for a senior to switch anti-epileptic drugs.

Key Terms

BETA-AMYLOID: Peptide of 39-43 amino acids formed after cleavage of the amyloid precursor protein. Beta-amyloid is insoluble in the brain and forms plaques associated with AD.

CHEMICAL RESTRAINT: Use of psychoactive medications as a matter of convenience in order to prevent a patient from moving about or to control behavior. No medical indication or safety issue which would require treatment for the patient's best interest is present for use of a psychoactive medication to be considered inappropriate.

DYSKINESIAS: Uncontrollable, automatic, dance-like movements, commonly occurring when levodopa doses are peaking or "peak-dose dyskinesias."

EPILEPSY: Chronic neurologic condition characterized by recurrent unprovoked seizures.

HYPODERMOCLYSIS: Infusion of isotonic fluids into the subcutaneous tissue. This avoids the potential safety issues of an intravenous infusion therefore requiring less monitoring by nursing staff. However, the solution is limited to normal saline or 5% dextrose with 0.45% sodium chloride without additives.

LEWY BODY: Abnormal collection of proteins, usually alpha-synuclein, ubiquitin, and others, that forms inside nerve cells. In PD, they are initially found in the substantia nigra while in DLB they are found in the hippocampus. However, as disease progresses, Lewy bodies will extend to many other parts of the brain, as observed at autopsy.

MOTOR COMPLICATIONS: Wearing off or dyskinesias.

MOTOR SYMPTOMS: Commonly include tremor, bradykinesia, rigidity and postural instability.

NEUROLEPTIC SENSITIVITY: Excess sensitivity to the dopamine effects of agents with dopamine effects resulting in increased extrapyramidal effects. This is most often described as an attribute of patients with DLB seen when treated with antipsychotic agents.

NEUROPSYCHIATRIC SYMPTOMS: Refers to non-cognitive symptoms secondary to moderate-severe dementia including psychosis, agitation, aggression, wandering, crying out, hostility, suspiciousness, anxiety, or depression.

NON-MOTOR SYMPTOMS/COMPLICATIONS: Commonly include swallowing difficulties, constipation and other GI transit slowing, autonomic dysfunction, shuffling gait, masked facies, depression, dementia, and anosmia, among others.

OFF: State in which medications are not working and the patient feels symptoms of PD.

ON: Symptom-free state; when medication for PD is working.

REFRACTORY EPILEPSY: While the definition is controversial, the generally accepted definition is the failure of two or more drugs and occurrence of one or more seizures per month over 18 months.[96]

WEARING OFF: Feeling of medications for PD, typically levodopa, diminishing; typically felt in between doses of levodopa, and occurs with disease progression.

Introduction

The workings of the brain remain a mystery in many respects. Some elderly patients maintain a quick wit, enthusiasm for learning and wisdom to share with the younger generations. Yet others are plagued with neurologic abnormalities that are not normal with aging. Dementia, delirium, Parkinson's disease and **epilepsy** are more common in older adults, and their exact causes and cures are yet to be identified. This chapter reviews these neurologic conditions in the elderly patient, focusing upon the optimal use of medications in this population.

Dementia

Etiology, Epidemiology, and Clinical Presentation Specific to Geriatrics

Dementia is a disease of the white matter of the brain with various etiologies. It is defined by the DSM-IV-TR as presence of a memory disorder with at least one of the following: aphasia, apraxia, agnosia, or executive dysfunction.[1] In addition, the cognitive deficits must interfere with social or work activities for the diagnosis to be applied. Mild cognitive impairment (MCI) is a term used when the patient has memory or cognitive problems which do not qualify for the definition of dementia. Pharmacists may be one of the first to recognize that a patient may have MCI or dementia when problems with medication management are identified. Table 12-1 provides information related to the various subtypes of dementia and related disorders. Dementia is estimated to occur in 6–10% of individuals over 65 years of age however, prevalence increases from 1–2% of the young-old (age 65–74 years), to 30% of those over 85 years of age and crests at 58% of individuals older than 94 years.[2]

When a patient presents with complaints of memory impairment, reversible causes should be identified and treated. These include hypothyroidism, depression, electrolyte disturbances, hepatic insufficiency, anemia, and vitamin B-12 deficiency. In addition, if patient history indicates, serologic testing for neurosyphilis is performed.

Many medications can cloud mentation as part of their pharmacologic effect. The most commonly associated medications are benzodiazepines, medications with anticholinergic properties, opioid analgesics and anticonvulsants; however, amiodarone, digoxin, corticosteroids, NSAIDs, H-2 blockers and many other medications have been reported to cause delirium. Dosage reduction or drug discontinuation is desirable to eliminate iatrogenic memory loss.

Vitamin B-12 deficiency is associated with increasing age, atrophic gastritis, and acid-suppression therapy. Anemia may occur with vitamin B-12 deficiency, but this effect may be masked with the current level of folic acid supplementation in cereals and breads consumed in the U.S.[3] The typically normal range (150–900 pg/mL) for vitamin B-12 serum concentrations, also named cobalamin, is not a good marker of tissue vitamin B-12 levels; measurement of folic acid and methylmalonic acid are required to clearly document vitamin B-12 deficiency when vitamin B-12 serum concentrations are in the low normal range.[4] In many cases it is easier and less expensive to replace vitamin B-12 in individuals to bring serum concentrations above 300–500 pg/mL.

KEY POINT: Reversible causes of memory loss must be addressed, including medication-related issues, before a diagnosis of dementia can be applied.

Alzheimer's Disease

Alzheimer's disease (AD) is the most common type of dementia, occurring in 60-80% of dementia diagnoses. Definite risk factors identified for AD are age, family history, head trauma, identified apolipoprotein ε-4 mutations/polymorphisms, and Down syndrome. Early onset cases of AD are usually attributed to inherited genetic mutations, or in the case of Down syndrome, an additional copy of chromosome 21. Late-onset AD is associated with polymorphism of the apolipoprotein ε-4. Protective factors, such

Table 12-1. **Some Diseases of Cognition**

Disease	Prevalence	Characteristics	Risk Factors
Mild cognitive impairment	5.4 million U.S. citizens (10–22% of older adults); 12% progress to dementia annually 8% mortality rate	Varied, including prodromal AD, medical conditions, vascular disease, depression, or neurologic conditions	• Age • Low educational attainment
Alzheimer's disease	2.5–4.5 million U.S. citizens (10% of individuals > 71 years old); 70% of dementias	Early symptoms include difficulty remembering names and recent events, apathy and depression; later symptoms of impaired judgment, confusion and behavior change	• Age • APO ε–4 alleles
Vascular dementia	(2.4% of individuals >71 years old); 17% of dementias	Symptoms overlap with AD, but progression occurs in a stairstep fashion with lower plateaus of functional impairment and focal neurological deficits	• Hypertension • Diabetes • Age • Atherosclerosis • Male sex • Atrial fibrillation • Myocardial infarction • Heart disease • Smoking • History of stroke
Dementia with **Lewy bodies**	15–20% of dementias; (0.7% of individuals > 65 years old)	Symptoms overlap with AD, but alertness and cognition fluctuate day to day; visual hallucinations, muscle rigidity and tremors occur	Duplicate or triplicate copies of α-synuclein gene (familial cases only)
Frontotemporal dementia	5–10% of dementias	Personality and behavior changes; difficulty with language and self-care; onset at younger age (average 58 years old); rarely occurs after age 75	• Family history • Tau protein genetic mutation
Creutzfeldt-Jakob disease	1 case per million per year worldwide; Increased 30–100 fold where familial cases cluster	Rapidly progressive memory impairment, incoordination and behavior changes; mortality within 1–2 years	• Prion protein gene on chromosome 20 (familial cases) • Medical history of psychosis • Multiple surgeries • Live 10+ years on a farm
Normal pressure hydrocephalus	2–20 cases per million per year worldwide	Symptoms include memory loss, difficulty walking, and incontinence	
Dementia of advanced Parkinson's disease		In later stages of PD, dementia may develop	

Source: Compiled from references 2, 10, and 93–95.

as increased educational attainment or dietary antioxidant consumption, may exist but have yet to be proved.

Multiple pathophysiologic theories are proposed and guide investigational drug development in AD. The cholinergic hypothesis involves the loss of cholinergic neuronal activity in the hippocampus and cortex. Currently available drug therapy with acetylcholinesterase inhibitors (CIs) supports this hypothesis. Another hypothesis is the **beta-amyloid** hypothesis which has developed because the location of beta-amyloid plaques, one of the hallmark features of AD at autopsy, corresponds to cognitive deficits. Researchers have outlined the process by which beta-amyloid proteins join to form plaques, and drugs to decrease production or increase clearance of the toxic protein are under investigation. Cytokines and inflammatory mediators are elevated in the brains of individuals with AD giving rise to the inflammation hypothesis. It is based upon evidence that neuronal injury gives rise to interleukin-1 production, which in turn triggers a host of immune-mediated responses and beta-amyloid protein deposition.

A definitive diagnosis of AD is only given with autopsy where beta-amyloid plaques and neurofibrillary tangles are found in the brain. More useful in practice are the National Institute of Neurologic and Communicative Disorders–developed criteria for clinical diagnosis of probable AD:

- Dementia established by clinical examination and objective testing (e.g., MMSE, 7MS)

- Deficits in two or more areas of cognition (memory impairment, deterioration of language, or visuospatial defects)

- Progressive worsening of memory and other cognitive functions

- No disturbance of consciousness

- Onset between ages 40–90 years

- No other explainable cause of symptoms[5]

However, the differentiation of AD from other dementias through objective tests is becoming accepted, including MRI findings of loss of volume in the area of the hippocampus, entorhinal cortex and amygdala; alterations of amyloid beta 1-42 or tau protein concentrations in the cerebrospinal fluid; reduced glucose metabolism in bilateral temporal parietal regions on PET scanning; and detection of homozygous apolipoprotein ε-4 genotype. These newer objective measures are being evaluated as possible additions or replacements for the criteria for diagnosis of probable AD. The hope is that an objective biomarker which will identify individuals at risk for developing AD can be found, and the biomarker will test positive early on in the disease process, allowing for the use of effective interventions for prevention or cure while the disease is in a preclinical stage.[6]

Frequently, a patient may have symptoms of AD for several years prior to diagnosis, but family, co-workers and friends begin to take on duties and responsibilities which the patient can no longer handle. For example, the spouse may take over paying bills and balancing the checkbook if the patient starts to make mistakes or forgets to pay bills on time. The timeline after diagnosis varies but survival can range from 3 to 20 years with a median of 4.2 years for men and 5.7 years for women.[7] Some patients have a rapid decline, losing 5 points or more on the Mini-Mental State Examination (MMSE) each year, while others lose fewer than 2 points per year. Whatever the initial progression rate, patients tend to continue with that rate throughout the course of the disease. AD is the fifth leading cause of death in the U.S., and the disease is probably a significant contributor to deaths attributed to pneumonia, sepsis, and trauma.

Vascular Dementia or Vascular Cognitive Impairment

Multiple names are applied to patients with cognitive impairment related to vascular disease in the brain including vascular dementia, multi-infarct dementia, Binswanger's disease, lacunar state or vascular cognitive impairment.[8,9] Vascular dementia is diagnosed when new-onset dementia occurs within 3 months of a cerebrovascular accident. In many cases, the course of vascular dementia follows a stair-step decline, with specific cognitive or functional deficits occurring that place the patient on a lower plateau. However, silent infarctions may occur and build until cognitive impairment is the first symptom of disease. Because the location and amount of tissue damage influence the cognitive deficits, patients with vascular dementia have differing clinical presentations. Small cerebrovascular infarcts less than 15 mm, called lacunar infarcts, may or may not precipitate cognitive changes dependent upon where they occur in the brain. AD can co-exist with vascular dementia as 77% of brain autopsies meeting criteria for vascular dementia also had AD in the Florida Brain Bank study.[10] The pathology of vascular dementia involves evidence of cerebrovascular disease and infarction in the white matter of the brain. Diagnosis is frequently supported with MRI or CT scan which shows infarction coupled with evaluation of vascular risk factors. Risk factors for vascular dementia mirror those for stroke, heart disease and atherosclerosis.

Dementia with Lewy Bodies

Dementia with Lewy bodies (DLB) was originally felt to be a rare disease, but with newer staining techniques for recognition of cortical Lewy bodies (at autopsy) it is now known to be the second or third most common type of dementia, depending upon the study. It usually occurs in patients age 75–80 years and has many overlapping features with AD. In addition to dementia, to be diagnosed with DLB the patient must have at least two of three features:

- fluctuating cognition with pronounced variations in attention and alertness,
- recurrent detailed visual hallucinations, and/or
- spontaneous features of parkinsonism.[11]

To differentiate DLB from dementia of advanced Parkinson's disease , the timing of dementia and parkinsonian symptoms must be considered. In DLB, the onset of dementia should occur concurrently with the onset of parkinsonism (within 12 months) while in dementia of advanced Parkinson's disease the dementia occurs late in the course after Parkinson's disease has been well-established in the individual.

Neuroleptic sensitivity is a secondary feature that is suggestive of DLB and particularly important in considering drug therapy because antipsychotic therapy may be considered for a patient with visual hallucinations. Excessive sensitivity to D2 receptor blocking agents is seen and causes an increased morbidity and mortality in about half of patients with DLB treated with these agents. Patients with DLB exposed to neuroleptics had significantly more sedation, confusion, rigidity, and immobility. Mortality in one retrospective study was 2.7 times that of control patients.[12] The atypical antipsychotics have been tried as an alternative with mixed results. Case reports indicate enhanced sensitivity to adverse effects with clozapine, risperidone, olanzapine and quetiapine although some small studies indicate a modest therapeutic response to olanzapine and quetiapine.[12] Small doses and close monitoring is indicated if an atypical antipsychotic is prescribed for a patient with DLB. In many cases, clinicians can educate caregivers and patients that hallucinations can remain untreated as long as they do not cause unnecessary fear or safety concerns, thereby preventing exposure to antipsychotic agents in a patient with DLB.

 KEY POINT: Sensitivity to dopamine antagonists in patients with DLB occurs within 2 weeks of initiation or dose increase.

Frontotemporal Dementia

Frontotemporal dementia, also known as Pick's Disease, is supported by atrophy of the prefrontal or anterior temporal areas of the brain on MRI. Patients will present with dementia and decline in interpersonal conduct with socially inappropriate behaviors such as rude, caustic, or sexually explicit remarks; loss of empathy and emotional blunting; and decline in personal hygiene. A subset of FTD, progressive aphasia, is diagnosed when a patient presents with nonfluent spontaneous speech with at least one of the following: agrammatism, phonemic paraphasias, or anomia. Patients who are early in progressive aphasia will preserve social skills, but these break down similar to FTD at later disease stages as they progress to mutism. The incidence of FTD is highest in the youngest old and does not increase in the higher age groups.

Other Types of Dementia

Normal pressure hydrocephalus (NPH) is a reversible dementia caused by increased pressure in the ventricles of the brain, although upon spinal tap, the opening pressure is normal. Diagnosis is based upon a classic triad of dementia, gait disturbance and urinary incontinence. This etiology is important to identify because surgical placement of a ventriculoperitoneal shunt can potentially reverse the progression of the disorder.

Creutzfeldt-Jakob disease is a rare cause of dementia that develops over weeks to months with rapid progression to death over 1–2 years. Characteristic findings on the EEG and in the CSF support it as a diagnosis, whether inherited or infectious in etiology. Neurosyphilis is another infectious cause of dementia. It occurs 10–20 years after a primary syphilis infection manifesting as dementia, anxiety, paranoia and mania. A positive reactive plasma reagin (RPR) or fluorescent treponemal antibody absorption (FTA-Abs) test indicate prior syphilis infection and raise the possibility of neurosyphilis in a patient with dementia. Positive testing of the cerebrospinal fluid is required for definitive diagnosis. Because of its rare occurrence, current guidelines for dementia assessment do not recommend these tests in every patient presenting with dementia. However, if a patient presents with a new episode of psychosis along with dementia, screening with FTA-Abs followed with lumbar puncture is indicated in order to identify a potentially reversible cause of dementia.

Summary of Standard Treatment of Dementias

When mild cognitive impairment or dementia is diagnosed, comorbid conditions should be addressed early in the course of disease to limit their contribution to functional declines. Elimination of unnecessary medications should occur first, especially those with any anticholinergic properties. Retrospective studies have shown an increase in progression of dementia when patients with AD receive anticholinergic medications. In addition

the patient should be assessed for depression, and treated if it is present. Depression causes apathy and difficulty with concentration, which can augment cognitive impairment.

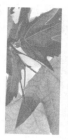

KEY POINT: Up to one third of patients with AD will have concurrent depression, plus patients with depression may present with memory loss. These overlaps complicate the clinical picture.

Cardiovascular risk factors should be addressed, particularly for patients with AD or vascular dementia as several observational studies indicate a more rapid decline may occur when hypertension and hyperlipidemia are not controlled. Vision and hearing should be assessed to assure that communication can be optimized for as long as possible. Finally, exercise programs for both physical and cognitive activities are recommended.[7]

Social issues should be tackled with family, friends and caregivers. Patients should be encouraged to draw up advanced care directives and durable power of attorney documents. Wishes for long-term care may be discussed, as the disease course is expected to reduce the patient's functional abilities over time until she will require 24 hour care, 7 days a week.

Currently the mainstays of pharmacotherapy for dementia are the CIs and memantine, an NMDA receptor antagonist. Tacrine was the first CI on the market in the U.S., but due to risk for hepatotoxicity, it is no longer used. The pharmacokinetic comparisons of other agents are shown in Table 12-2. These agents have a FDA-labeled indication for treatment of AD, but are frequently used off-label for other types of dementia, some with evidence and some without.

AD is the most studied of the dementias and current treatment algorithms from the American College of Physicians and the American Academy of Family Physicians distinguish a pathway for patients with mild-to-moderate as compared

Table 12-2. **Pharmacology of Medications for Alzheimer's Disease**

Generic Drug (Trade Name)	Mechanism of Action	Serum Half-life	Protein Binding	Food Delays Absorption	Metabolism	Renal Elimination
Acetylcholinesterase (ACH) Inhibitors						
Donepezil (Aricept)	Reversible and non-competitive inhibition of ACH	70–80 hours	96%	No	CYP2D6, 3A4	17% as unchanged drug
Galantamine (Razadyne)	Reversible and competitive inhibition of ACH; modulates nicotinic acetylcholine receptors	5–7 hours	10–20%	Yes	CYP2D6, 3A4	20–32% as unchanged drug
Rivastigmine (Exelon)	Reversible inhibition of both acetyl- and butyl-cholinesterases	2 hours	40%	Yes	Hydrolysis in brain; D-methylation or sulfation in liver	Insignificant
NMDA Receptor Antagonist						
Memantine (Namenda)	Prevents over-stimulation of glutamate receptors to prevent excitotoxicity of neurons	60–80 hours	45%	No	Glucuronidation Reduction Hydrolysis	52–80% as unchanged drug

to moderate-to-severe AD. For mild-to-moderate AD, first line therapy is a CI to be titrated to maximally tolerated dose in the therapeutic range. (See Table 12-3.) No clinical data places one CI above the other as an initial choice. If ineffective or not tolerated, a switch to another CI is suggested. If poor clinical response is noted, addition or substitution of memantine in patients with moderate AD is the next step. In moderate-to-severe AD, the pathway allows for a CI or memantine first-line, followed by combination therapy. Intolerance or loss of clinical benefit is addressed by switching from one CI to another, just as in the mild-to-moderate pathway. If there is a treatment failure, loss of benefit or intolerance after all three CIs and memantine have been tried, withdrawal of either or both medications is recommended for both algorithms. In essence, the current pathways are equivalent except that memantine can be tried first line as monotherapy or as dual therapy with a CI in moderate-to-severe disease.[13]

Monitoring of Therapy

Monitoring for effectiveness of both CIs and memantine involves assessment from the patient, caregiver and physician. Generally, effectiveness can be assessed after treatment for 3 months using standard instruments such as the MMSE, Clinician's Interview-Based Impression of Change-Plus Caregiver Input, Activities of Daily Living, and/or the Neuropsychiatric Inventory-Questionnaire, as described in Chapter 4.[13]

Most commonly, CIs cause gastrointestinal adverse effects including nausea, vomiting, diarrhea and anorexia in 5–20% of patients due to the increased peripheral cholinergic stimulation. This pharmacologic effect can also cause incontinence and bradycardia. Dizziness and insomnia have been reported frequently. Once daily CIs are generally started at bedtime to reduce patient complaints of gastrointestinal side effects, however, if insomnia occurs, doses can be given in the

Table 12-3. Initiation and Titration of Drugs Used in Dementia

Drug	Initial Dose	Titration Schedule Every	Recommended Dose	Minimum Therapeutic Dose	Renal Adjustment	Formulations
Donepezil	5 mg daily	4 weeks	10 mg daily	5 mg daily	No	5 and 10 mg tablets; 5 and 10 mg orally disintegrating tablets
Galantamine IR	4 mg 2×/day	4 weeks	12 mg 2×/day	8 mg 2×/day	Yes	4, 8, 12 mg tablets; 4 mg/mL solution
Galantamine ER	8 mg daily	4 weeks	24 mg daily	16 mg daily	Yes	8, 12, 24 mg capsules
Rivastigmine	1.5 mg 2×/day	4 weeks	6 mg 2×/day	3 mg 2×/day	No	1.5, 3, 4.5, 6 mg capsules; 2 mg/mL solution
Rivastigmine transdermal	4.6 mg daily	4 weeks	9.5 mg/day	9.5 mg daily	No	4.6, 9.5 mg patches
Memantine	5 mg daily	1 week	10 mg 2×/day	10 mg daily	Yes	5 and 10 mg; 2 mg/mL solution

morning. If more than 2–3 days therapy of a CI is missed, the drug should be re-titrated from the initial dose to avoid increased adverse effects.

Memantine is generally well-tolerated with dizziness, headache, constipation and somnolence reported more frequently than in placebo-treated subjects.[14] Other reported adverse effects such as agitation, falls and accidental injuries did not occur more often in the memantine-treated patients, although important issues in this patient group.

Pharmacotherapy of Other Dementias

Less is known about optimal pharmacotherapy of other dementias. Generally the medications used to treat AD may be tried, and patients are assessed for clinical response within a similar timeframe as with AD.

Review of Evidence Base Supporting Treatment Recommendations for Elderly Patients

As dementia is a syndrome found primarily in older adults, all studies have included geriatric

patients. Several reviews and meta-analyses have been published to summarize the evidence for effectiveness and safety of the CIs and memantine in treatment of dementia and mild cognitive impairment.[15-17] For AD, effectiveness data agree across most studies and all meta-analyses that cognition, function and behavior are improved with CIs, although debate continues as to whether the statistical significance translates to clinically important differences. At least 26 well-controlled studies of CIs in AD were evaluated by one author and 59 studies including over 16,000 subjects in CIs and/or memantine for dementia or MCI by another.[15,17] The beneficial effect is modest at best, and a subgroup of individuals appears to have clinical benefit. Similar conclusions were drawn in the evidence review that included AD along with other dementias, although the numbers of subjects were much smaller in the non-AD studies. Although some pharmacologic differences are seen in the CIs, no clinical differences are seen with therapeutic or adverse effects when the agents are compared; therefore, no currently available CI is preferred for initial treatment over another.

Similarly, evidence for the effectiveness of memantine in dementia shows statistically significant improvement in cognition, function, and reduction in caregiver burden although clinical significance is not as clear. Withdrawal rates are similar for both treatment and placebo groups at 7–13%. However, only case studies have been published on use of memantine in DLB and they report mixed results. Of note, delusions, hallucinations, agitation and parkinsonism worsened in some patients.[12] Randomized, controlled trials are needed.

The combination of a CI and memantine is recommended in clinical practice guidelines for moderate to severe AD and is frequently tried for patients who continue to deteriorate. Few studies have been done with the combination; donepezil in combination with memantine has shown statistically significant improvements in measures designed for severe dementia assessment.[18,19] A trial which allowed any CI for maintenance did not show significant change when memantine was added.[20]

Three randomized, controlled trials evaluated over 3500 subjects with MCI for the effect of CIs on progression to dementia.[16] Dropout rates were high: 40% in treatment groups and 29% in placebo groups, but the risk for progression to dementia or AD was reduced 25% in treated subjects compared to control subjects. One study noted this positive effect to occur predominantly in subjects who were carriers of the apolipoprotein ε-4 genotype.

Only one controlled study with a CI in DLB has been performed and indicates benefit with reduction of apathy, anxiety, delusions and hallucinations.[21] No evidence supports the use of CIs in FTD, although a trial in an individual patient may be warranted because a definitive diagnosis may not be possible and mixed dementias are common.

Common Problems Encountered When Treating Elderly Patients with this Condition

Neuropsychiatric Symptoms

While cognitive decline is the hallmark feature of dementia, neuropsychiatric (NP) symptoms typically cause the most anxiety and stress for patients and caregivers. They include delusions, hallucinations, repetitive activities, sleep disturbances and mood changes. These symptoms are frequently called behavior problems in that they precipitate agitation, physical aggression, psychosis and wandering; behaviors that cause problems with caregiving. However, the better term refers to them as symptoms because they frequently result from an undiagnosed underlying problem which the patient with dementia cannot communicate effectively to caregivers in order to achieve a resolution.[22]

NP symptoms generally manifest as the disease progresses into a moderate to severe stage when the patient is partially functional, but has begun to lose the ability to perceive and communicate effectively. Nursing home admission becomes likely as caregivers are unable to provide the amount of care that is needed. When the dementia progresses to the end stage, the patient's functional status will have diminished such that he is unable to interact with others or the environment and becomes bedbound. NP symptoms are no longer discernible.

When new NP symptoms develop, the first step is to assess the patient for a medical or environmental precipitant that can be corrected. For example, a patient with moderate stage AD who starts wandering at night should be evaluated for changes in caffeine intake, new medications, excess heat in the bedroom or strange noises at night. Any of these items could cause the patient to have sleep problems which he could not communicate effectively to caregivers and may begin wandering. Pain is a common medical precipitant to NP symptoms and should always be considered.

Evidence supports the use of nonpharmacologic treatments for NP symptoms although the treatments are widely varied. Person-centered bathing where the patient was kept covered at all times during the bath showed significant reduction in agitation compared to standard bathing procedures. Use of lavender oil, lemon balm, pet therapy, and music therapy has likewise shown reduction in agitation. Exercise training coupled with caregiver education reduced depression and improved functional status in a randomized controlled trial.[7,22]

Medications are frequently used when non-pharmacologic interventions fail or are impractical. Generally a patient should be evaluated to determine if only acute, as-needed medication is required, or if chronic/maintenance treatments are necessary. Benzodiazepines and antipsychotics are most commonly used when acute rescue medication is needed and CIs, memantine, selective serotonin re-uptake inhibitors or atypical antipsychotic agents are more often prescribed for maintenance medications as described below.

CIs and/or memantine may be tried if the patient is not already being treated with these agents. However, evidence to support their effectiveness is meager. In DLB, it is especially useful to try CIs first, as increased sensitivity to adverse effects of other agents is likely. Selective serotonin re-uptake inhibitors may be effective if anxiety is present, although it may be difficult to objectively assess the presence of anxiety, making their use off-label. However, withdrawal may be attempted after 3–6 months as these symptoms do not persist as the disease progresses. Valproic acid at a dose of 125–500 mg daily may be tried for symptoms of agitation and aggression, sleep-wake disruption and disinhibition (manic-like behaviors) although evidence of effectiveness is also sparse.

Antipsychotics are frequently the drugs of choice for psychosis, psychomotor agitation and aggression in patients with dementia. Evidence of effectiveness is not strong, and concerns over an increased risk for mortality in elderly patients with dementia when these medications are used have forced manufacturers to include a black box warning on both typical and atypical antipsychotics. A multi-center randomized controlled clinical trial compared risperidone, olanzapine and quetiapine to placebo in treatment of psychosis, aggression and agitation in nursing home residents with AD. The primary outcome of interest was time until discontinuation of treatment for either lack of effectiveness or adverse effects. No difference was seen with discontinuation occurring from 5–8 weeks after initiation of the antipsychotic or placebo, although the reason for discontinuation was lack of effectiveness for the placebo group compared to presence of significant adverse events in the antipsychotic groups. Improvement was seen in 21% of placebo-treated subjects and 26–32% of antipsychotic-treated subjects.[23]

The Agency for Healthcare Research and Quality has published a summary on the use of atypical antipsychotic agents for off-label indications. It states that no strong evidence supports the use of these agents in elderly patients with dementia. It lists the risk of death to increase from 23 deaths per 1,000 elderly people on placebo to 35 deaths per 1,000 elderly people on an atypical antipsychotic. Specifically, risperidone and olanzapine are noted to increase the risk of stroke.[24]

Delirium

Etiology, Epidemiology and Clinical Presentation Specific to Geriatrics

Definition

Just as dementia is a memory disorder, so is delirium. However, delirium is seen in patients with an altered state of consciousness which must be ruled out for a diagnosis of dementia. The patient with delirium may develop confusion, distractibility, disorientation, disordered thinking, hallucinations and agitation all within hours or days. The hyperactive, agitated subtype of delirium is most recognized and concerning to the clinician, as frequently the patient is pulling out catheters, intravenous lines or other tubes and may be a danger to themselves or others. However, patients experiencing a hypoactive delirium are subdued and quiet, unable to interact with their surroundings. A third type of delirium is mixed, with the patient switching between hyperactive and hypoactive states.[25]

The DSM IV TR states that delirium is a disturbance in consciousness, developing over hours to days, with fluctuation over the course of the day. In delirium, the patient is inattentive and unaware of the environment. Memory impairment and disorientation are identified when the patient is questioned. Sensory impairment is also seen as the patient may confuse loud noises with gunshots, misinterpret television programs as a party occurring in the room, or have the inability to interact appropriately with objects at the bedside.[1]

Delirium has a highly variable course. Studies indicate from 20–69% of patients recover from delirium within one day; however, as many as 15% may have symptoms lasting 10 days or more.[26] Individuals with advanced age or pre-existing dementia are likely to have a more prolonged course, as will those with multiple contributing causes. Therefore, delirium is considered a syndrome of the elderly.

Epidemiology and Pathophysiology

Delirium has been reported in 10–40% of hospital admissions, with an incidence of 10–15% of patients on medical surgical hospital wards.[27] One study of post-operative patients identified delirium occurring within seven days after surgery in 44% of subjects.[28] Within the geriatric nursing home population, the prevalence of delirium is as high as 60%.[25] Recognizing delirium is important because it is associated with an increase in mortality at 30 days and 6 months, reportedly as high as 76% in one study. Morbidity is also higher in patients with delirium, evidenced by longer hospital stays, increased time in the intensive care unit, pneumonias and pressure sores. Finally, costs increase when delirium is present.

Several pathophysiologic theories have been proposed, however, cholinergic deficiency likely plays a role. The cholinergic deficit may develop as a result of impaired synthesis of acetylcholine, increased anticholinergic burden at the neuronal synapse or imbalance of dopaminergic/serotonergic activity with the cholinergic activity.[29]

Numerous risk factors for delirium have been identified. Many medical and surgical conditions can precipitate delirium, but increased age and the presence of dementia are clearly associated with an increase in the risk for delirium. Postoperative delirium increases from 22% for age 50–59 years to 92% in patients over the age of 80.[28] Individuals with pre-existing brain pathology lack sufficient cognitive reserve to balance a sudden cholinergic decrease.

Medications have been implicated as a cause in 30% of delirium cases. Any medication that has central nervous system effects can cause delirium and confusion, especially anticholinergic agents, analgesics, sedative/hypnotics, antimicrobial agents, muscle relaxants, corticosteroids, anticonvulsants, antidiabetic drugs, and gastrointestinal agents. In addition, abrupt discontinuation of alcohol or depressant medications may cause delirium as part of the withdrawal syndrome.

Clinical Presentation

Delirium is frequently overlooked by clinicians, especially if the patient exhibits hypoactive symptoms. The criteria for diagnosis from the DSM-IV TR have been adapted into several screening tools. The Confusion Assessment Method is one simple tool that has been validated in multiple populations and can be applied by any healthcare provider to identify the patient likely to have delirium. (See Table 12-4.)[30] Generally features are assessed by asking a series of questions to a family member, friend or nurse who has spent time with the patient and knows the patient's baseline cognitive status. For delirium to be present, the patient must have features 1 and 2 and either feature 3 or 4.

Delirium should be distinguished from dementia or depression, as all of these may cause a patient to be unable to correctly answer questions about orientation; however, delirium has the contrasting features of inattention, acute onset, and fluctuation in alertness or consciousness. Patients with dementia will have a slow onset of symptoms and are alert. Patients with depression have a slow onset; they will display apathy and provide few (if any) answers to orientation questions because of this rather than because of cognitive loss.

Summary of Standard Treatment of Delirium

Preventive Strategies

Interventions have been proven to reduce the incidence of delirium in elderly hospitalized patients. In a multi-component model for hospitalized elderly patients, delirium episodes occurred in 9.9% of the intervention group compared to 15% of the control group.[31] Interventions included an orientation protocol, cognitive stimulation, environment control, nonpharmacologic sleep

Table 12-4. Confusion Assessment Method

Feature	Description Ask family member or nurse the following questions:	Requirement
1. Acute onset and fluctuating course	1. Is there evidence of an acute change in mental status from the patient's baseline? 2. Did the abnormal behavior fluctuate during the day, that is tend to come and go, or increase and decrease in severity?	Must be present
2. Inattention	Did the patient have difficulty focusing attention? For example: Was the patient easily distractible? Did the patient have difficulty keeping track of what was being said?	Must be present
3. Disorganized thinking	Was the patient's thinking disorganized or incoherent, such as rambling or irrelevant conversation, unclear or illogical flow of ideas, or unpredictable switching from subject to subject?	If absent, Feature 4 must be present
4. Altered level of consciousness	How would you rate this patient's level of consciousness? Alert (normal) Vigilant (hyperalert) Lethargic (drowsy, easily aroused) Stupor (difficult to arouse) Coma (unarousable)	If absent, Feature 3 must be present

Source: Adapted from reference 30.

aids, early mobilization, minimization of physical restraints, visual and hearing aids for those with impairment, dentures for those without teeth, other personal affects and early volume repletion for patients with dehydration. This intervention has been successfully replicated in other institutions.[32-33] Similar interventions can be adapted for use in nursing home and home care patients to reduce the risk of delirium. Volunteers may be recruited to provide added nonpharmacologic support when friends, family or nursing staff are not available.

Treat or Remove Underlying Cause

Early identification and treatment of delirium is expected to improve outcomes, but data to support this is lacking. However, not every case of delirium can be prevented. Once delirium is identified, the first step is to conduct an assessment for the underlying cause(s). The history, physical examination, and basic laboratory testing to identify infection, myocardial infarction, electrolyte abnormalities, pain or a change in medications is necessary.[25] Serum drug levels and/or a urine drug screen may provide valuable information. Medical or surgical treatment to correct the underlying cause is imperative for the patient to regain previous cognitive function.

Supportive Measures

Supportive measures should be instituted simultaneously with treatment of the underlying cause. Having a friend or family member present to re-assure and re-direct the patient can help avoid the need to apply restraints, which usually make delirium worsen. In addition, patients may injure themselves as they attempt to get out of bed while in restraints. But if the patient is at risk for injuring themselves or others, restraints may be required. The re-direction by a caregiver at the bedside distracts the patient from pulling out a parenteral line or catheter. It is useful to remind the patient of the time and place; a clock, calendar and family pictures may help with this task. In communicating with the patient in delirium, it is best to use clear language, little medical terminology, a tranquil voice and few abstractions.

The environment should be kept at a comfortable temperature, with controlled excesses of noise. A radio or television can be soothing if tuned into appropriate programming. Lighting should be adequate during the daytime and a nightlight may be helpful at night. If the patient wears glasses, hearing aids or dentures, have them in place as much as possible to reduce sensory deficits and possible misperceptions. Both over- and under-stimulation should be avoided.

A nonpharmacologic approach to improving sleep in patients with insomnia may improve delirium. Use of warm drinks (non-caffeinated tea or milk), soothing music, and back massage have been used. Hospital or nursing home noises and interruptions should be minimized during the night to prevent waking patients and residents.

Inadequate hydration was identified as a risk factor for delirium in nursing home residents. Frail elderly patients frequently reduce intake of nutrition and fluids in response to infection, pain or other insult, quickly resulting in dehydration given that elderly persons already have lower total body water compared to younger patients. Quick attention to providing maintenance fluids either orally, intravenously or through **hypodermoclysis** may prevent severe dehydration and its related morbidity or risk for delirium.[34]

Pharmacologic Management

Once nonpharmacologic measures are in place and steps to address the underlying cause of delirium are implemented, the patient should be re-evaluated. If the behaviors associated with delirium are not problematic, no further therapy is necessary. However, in some cases agitation and combative behavior must be managed pharmacologically to prevent danger to the patient or others and to allow evaluation and treatment by the medical team. This should be a small minority of patients. Pharmacologic measures for delirium management can be considered **chemical restraints** when used to control behavior that is undesirable but innocuous, especially if administered for extended periods of time.

Review of Evidence Base Supporting Treatment Recommendations for Elderly Patients

Little published data is available to guide the use of medications in this situation and no medications have FDA approval for use in delirium. One study in hip fracture patients found that low-dose haloperidol administered prophylactically reduced the severity and duration, but not the incidence, of delirium.[35] Clinical practice has moved away from the typical antipsychotics like haloperidol and quetiapine, olanzapine and risperidone appear to work as well as haloperidol with a lower risk for extrapyramidal side effects. No double-blind, randomized, placebo-controlled trials support the efficacy and safety of these medications, but small uncontrolled studies provide limited evidence that low-dose, short-term use of antipsychotics reduce delirium severity by 43–70%.[36] Doses recommended for elderly patients with delirium are significantly lower than for younger adults as shown in Table 12-5. In an elderly patient, haloperidol 0.5-1mg is the preferred drug and dose to be used as needed. Patients should be re-evaluated no sooner than 30-60 minutes after the dose for effect. The dose may be repeated after this time until the patient is manageable or until a maximum of haloperidol 5mg is reached. If longer term therapy is needed, atypical antipsychotic agents should be considered.

Benzodiazepines have been used as second-line treatment when antipsychotic agents were not effective. Again, their use in delirium is not well studied and as CNS depressants, they may worsen confusion and sedation. Furthermore, benzodiazepines are associated with increasing incidence of delirium. Lorazepam is most frequently used as it is more water-soluble than other benzodiazepines, has an intermediate elimination half-life and is available in oral, intramuscular and intravenous formulations.

Parkinson's Disease
Etiology, Epidemiology, and Clinical Presentation of Parkinson's Disease

Parkinson's disease (PD) affects approximately 1% of the population over the age of 60 and 4–5%

Table 12-5. Antipsychotic Agents Used in Delirium with Older Adults

Medication	Initial Recommended Dose	Maximum Daily Dose	Comments
Aripiprazole	5 mg PO	15 mg	Case series and reports in young and older adults
Haloperidol	0.25–0.5 mg PO or IV	2–5 mg	IV route is off-label and associated with QTc prolongation
Olanzapine	2.5–5 mg PO	10 mg	Anticholinergic side effects
Quetiapine	12.5–25 mg PO	150 mg	Postural hypotension
Risperidone	0.25–0.5 mg PO	4 mg	EPS with higher doses
Ziprasidone	20 mg IM	100 mg	Case reports in young, critically ill patients; Significant risk for dose-related QTc prolongation

over the age of 85.[37,38] Next to Alzheimer's disease, it is the second most common neurodegenerative disease.

The primary cause of PD is believed to be the depletion of the dopamine-producing neurons in the substantia nigra pars compacta. Symptoms of the disease are believed to become present when ~80% of these neurons have been destroyed. The decrease in dopamine is the primary target of symptomatic treatment, as currently there is no cure or disease-modifying therapy available. The disease is slowly progressive, which makes follow-up absolutely necessary.

Clinically, patients with PD present with one or more of the following **motor symptoms**: resting tremor, bradykinesia, stiffness and postural instability. Typically, a person presents asymmetrically, with symptoms being worse or only present on one side of the body. As the disease progresses, there is bilateral involvement. There are also many non-motor complications of the disease which may be present at initial presentation or may occur as the disease progresses. The non-motor symptoms include micrographia, a masked appearance of the face, anosmia, urinary incontinence, depression, dementia, orthostatic hypotension, constipation, sialorrhea, increased sweating and oily skin, as well as sexual dysfunction. It is important to know these non-motor symptoms will not occur in all patients and complaints of these problems may occur at any point in the disease process. The initial presentation is not different in an elderly

patient, compared to a younger cohort, however the reasons for presentation may be different. The stiffness and slowness experienced with PD may be attributed to other disease states in older adults, such as osteoarthritis. The elderly patient may also present later in the disease course secondary to their ability to manipulate their routine around deficits versus a younger individual who may have a job, and thus the inability to avoid the tasks which are becoming more difficult with the PD. Attributing symptoms of PD to "getting old" may be another reason elderly patients do not present as early in the disease course as younger patients.

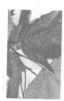

KEY POINT: Elderly patients may attribute symptoms of PD, such as slowing of movement and rigidity to other disease states or "getting old."

As the disease progresses, motor complications may arise. These can include **wearing off** between doses and **dyskinesias**, which are involuntary, repetitive movements typically seen when a person with PD is in the "on," or treated, state. Dyskinesias occur in approximately 40% of patients with PD at some point in their disease process.

PD has a significant impact on both the lives of those patients affected with PD, as well as their caregivers. People with PD lose their ability to function independently as the disease progresses, and early in the disease process they commonly lose their fine-motor skills. And, approximately 50% of PD patients will experience depression.[39]

As the disease progresses and functional deficits increase, so does caregiver strain. The caregiver's quality of life is typically impacted negatively as care demands increase.[40] Some of the factors which can increase the risk of nursing home placement include impairment of function of the person with PD, decreased ability to complete activities of daily living, dementia and hallucinations.[41]

Summary of Standard Treatment

The American Academy of Neurology (AAN) produces guidelines for the initially presenting patient , as well as the patient experiencing motor complications which may occur as the disease progresses and dopaminergic therapy is continued.[42,43] The gold-standard of symptomatic treatment, levodopa/carbidopa, is an available option for treating the initially presenting patient. (See Table 12-6.) However, due to the risk of dyskinesias seen with long-term use of levodopa, clinicians will typically elect to delay starting levodopa in younger patients and utilize alternative agents as first line therapy unless symptoms of PD are overly bothersome and impact quality of life. Other initial options available for the patient with mildly bothersome symptoms include the monoamine oxidase type B inhibitors, selegiline and rasagiline, as well the dopamine agonists, bromocriptine, pramipexole and ropinirole.[42] Selegiline has shown to decrease the rate of decline in motor scores of the UPDRS[42,44,45] and rasagiline has shown improvement of the ADL and motor subscales.[46] Dopamine agonists, are typically not the first choice in those experiencing PD symptoms which are having a significant impact on function and quality of life. Practitioners typically employ levodopa/carbidopa in these patients.[42,47,48]

Over time, wearing off and dyskinesias are seen with long-term use of levodopa/carbidopa. The AAN offers guidance on managing these complications.[43] The addition of entacapone or rasagiline are both level A evidence interventions in those individuals experiencing wearing off be-tween doses of levodopa/carbidopa. The addition of ropinirole or pramipexole is also an option in the patient experiencing wearing off. It is important to remember that the dose of levodopa should be empirically decreased, as add-on therapies can worsen dyskinesias by increasing the peak level of levodopa. Apomorphine has class C evidence for use in wearing off, and clinically is used for episodes of sudden "off" or freezing. Apomorphine, however, is only appropriate for as needed use and should not be used as a scheduled medication unless freezing is occurring at consistent times. Although not supported by evidence, the practice of decreasing the dosing interval (increasing the number of daily doses) is also a viable option for wearing off. Changing from immediate-release to sustained-release levodopa/carbidopa for relief of wearing off is not supported by evidence, and clinically is not effective for this problem.[43]

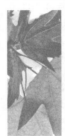

KEY POINT: Doses of levodopa/carbidopa should be empirically decreased when a dopamine agonist, COMT inhibitor or MAO-B inhibitor is added to a regimen to decrease the incidence of peak-dose dyskinesias.

Dyskinesias, resulting from levodopa/carbidopa doses, can be extremely bothersome, and the addition of amantadine has level C evidence to support its use.[43] Although evidence is not available to support the practice, decreasing the dose of levodopa/carbidopa and decreasing the dosing interval at the same time is used clinically to assuage dyskinesias.

Review of Evidence Supporting Treatment Recommendations in the Elderly

Upon initial presentation, the clinician treating the elderly patient is faced with the challenge of balancing good symptom control and improved quality of life with the side effect burden of currently available treatment options. The clinician must also ensure drug interactions are avoided

Table 12-6. Drugs, Common Dosages, and Required Dose Adjustments

| Drug | Daily Dose (mg) | Adjustment Required | | |
		Mild-Moderate Renal Impairment	Moderate-Severe Renal Impairment	Hepatic Impairment
Levodopa	200–1000+	No	No	No
Carbidopa	25–75	No	No	No
Amantadine	200–400	Yes	Yes	No
Dopamine Agonists				
Bromocriptine	15–90	No	No	Use with caution
Pramipexole	1.5–4.5	Yes	Yes	No
Ropinirole IR	1.5–24	No	Use with caution*	Use with caution*
Ropinirole CR	2–24	No	Use with caution*	Use with caution*
Apomorphine	3–6	Yes	Use with caution*	Use with caution
COMT inhibitors				
Entacapone	400–1600	No	No	Use with caution*
Tolcapone	300–600	No	Use with caution	Do not use
MAO-B inhibitors				
Selegiline	5–10	No	No	No
Selegiline ODT	1.25–2.5	No	No	No
Rasagiline	0.5–1	No	Use with caution	Yes
Anticholinergics				
Benztropine	0.5–4	No	No	No
Trihexyphenidyl	1–6	No	No	No

*Not studied in this specific subset of patients.

and make certain to not exacerbate other disease-states with the therapy. These tenets continue to be important as the disease progresses and motor complications develop, as well as when electing to treat the non-motor symptoms responsive to drug therapy.

The American Academy of Neurology does not currently have a guideline for treating the elderly patient specifically with Parkinson's disease. However, keeping the patient's concomitant diseases and agent characteristics in mind will help circumvent major problems in treatment.

Due to the increased incidence of the disease with age, virtually all clinical trials of agents for the treatment of PD do not have a maximum age at which individuals are excluded. However, most trials of agents include the common, broad and loosely-defined exclusion criteria of individuals with severe systemic disease, dementia, depression or other psychiatric illnesses. This has a great impact on the inclusion of a more aged cohort into these trials and the typical average age seen in these trials is between 60 and 65.

Currently, there are no clinical trials which specifically target the safety and efficacy of agents for elderly PD patients in a randomized fashion. A retrospective analysis of the dopamine agonists in a small cohort of patients 80 years old and older showed >50% of patients were unable to tolerate dopamine agonists, or did not see efficacy with the use of the agents.[49] Hallucinations were seen in 21% and 25% of patients receiving pramipexole and ropinirole, respectively. Orthostasis was also seen in 5–6% of patients receiving a non-ergot alkaloid dopamine agonist. A subgroup analysis of rasagiline trials showed individuals greater than age 70 were no more likely to experience adverse effects of rasagiline than those patients under 70, however there was no analysis of efficacy.[50]

Common Problems Encountered in the Senior Population with Parkinson's Disease

Agent-related

Levodopa/carbidopa will likely become a part of any PD regimen at some point during the disease course, and in geriatric individuals many times will be the starting point of therapy. Individuals taking levodopa/carbidopa typically commence with three times daily dosing. However, as the disease progresses this dosing interval typically decreases, with some patients taking upwards of 8 doses of levodopa/carbidopa per day. This can be difficult for patients to manage, especially in those with other concomitant disease states for which medications are taken. The ability to adhere to such a regimen should always be considered. Levodopa/carbidopa is also a medication for which timely medication administration is important, and for those patients residing in long-term care facilities, this can prove difficult. The dietary considerations with levodopa/carbidopa also make it a difficult medication to administer. Preferably, the medication should be taken on an empty stomach, and dietary protein should be avoided close to medication administration. This is due to the body's preferred uptake of dietary protein when compared to levodopa/carbidopa and can result in a decreased blood level, as well as a delay in "on."

The dopamine agonists are still considered by many to be first line therapy, in order to delay use of levodopa/carbidopa. However, the elderly patient is more likely to experience the hallucinations and confusion which can be seen with the dopamine agonists.[51] "Sleep attacks," the experience of suddenly and unexpectedly falling asleep, are a problem with increasing dopamine by any means, but are seen with increased incidence in those receiving dopamine agonists. Case reports of repetitive, compulsive behaviors, such as gambling, eating, drinking and sexual behaviors, are

becoming more common. And while the elderly are not more prone to these behaviors specifically when compared to a younger cohort, this has become an important counseling point for patients and caregivers. Currently, the non-ergot alkaloid dopamine agonists, pramipexole and ropinirole controlled-release are not available generically, and can be cost-prohibitive for those patients with limited income. Ropinirole immediate-release is, however, now available generically. Pergolide, an ergot-derived dopamine agonist, was withdrawn from the market secondary to valvular heart defects associated with its use.[52,53] The use of bromocriptine was associated with multivalvular heart disease in a patient with no pre-existing valvular disease[54] and attempts should be made to limit its use.

The monoamine oxidase type B inhibitor, selegiline, has an amphetamine-like metabolite, which can be a problem in a person with concomitant hypertension or cardiovascular disease. This metabolite may decrease appetite and therefore has the potential to cause weight loss. Insomnia is also believed to be a side effect of selegiline, and typically the last dose of the day is given no later than noon. Rasagiline is without an amphetamine-like metabolite, and could potentially be a less bothersome agent. Again, a small sub-group analysis showed no age-related effect on experiencing an adverse event with the use of rasagiline.[50] The drug interaction profile of the MAO-B inhibitors is quite extensive, making their use in the elderly difficult, given the extensive polypharmacy seen within the population. Rasagiline trials, however, included participants on a number of drugs and drug classes stated to be contraindicated within the package insert. Fluoxetine and fluvoxamine, however, were not used likely secondary to their long half-lives. Clinically, many times PD patients are on concomitant SSRIs without incident. However, those clinical trials did not look at the risk of adverse effects specifically in the group receiving rasagiline and one of these medications. Because of this, close monitoring of blood pressure specifically, and other symptoms of serotonin syndrome, is warranted if these agents are used concomitantly.

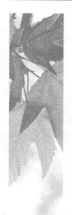

KEY POINT: Concomitant use of rasagiline with SSRIs is common, and selected SSRIs have been used in combination with rasagiline in clinical trials. However, close monitoring of blood pressure and other symptoms of serotonin syndrome is extremely important in the first few weeks of concomitant therapy.

The COMT inhibitor, tolcapone, has significant monitoring associated with its use due to reports of hepatotoxicity, and is therefore rarely used clinically. Entacapone is typically well tolerated overall, and is available in a combination tablet with levodopa/carbidopa for ease of dosing. The cost of the combination product is typically similar to buying each agent separately, however this fixed dose combination does not allow for easy tailoring of levodopa doses.

The anticholinergics, benztropine and trihexyphenidyl, are many times used for treating bothersome tremor. However, these agents are a poor choice in an elderly patient secondary to their cadre of side effects. The side effects include constipation, urinary retention, dry mucous membranes, tachycardia and, most disturbing in an elderly cohort, confusion. Another agent with anticholinergic activity in addition to its other effects is amantadine. It is used most often to treat dyskinesias and has an increased risk of CNS side effects in the elderly patient, such as confusion and psychosis.[55,56] Of particular note for the elderly patient, amantadine requires dose adjustment for renal impairment.

Apomorphine, an agent available for relief of freezing episodes, is a subcutaneously delivered dopamine agonist. The most distressing side effect of this medication is the extreme hypotension which can be seen shortly after a dose is given. So much so, that the manufacturer requires the first dose to be given in the care provider's office or under their care. This hypotension can increase the risk of falls and subsequent fracture. This agent can also cause nausea and vomiting, which typically requires scheduled dosing with an anti-emetic, such as trimethobenzamide. However, the 5HT3 receptor antagonists (e.g., ondansetron) are absolutely contraindicated due to additive hypotension.

Disease-related

Autonomic dysfunction is a common occurrence in PD, manifesting as one or more of the following: constipation, urge urinary incontinence, orthostatic hypotension, sexual dysfunction, seborrheic dermatitis and thermal dysregulation. While no clinical trials exist to address these autonomic abnormalities specifically in the elderly with PD, general treatment principles outlined elsewhere in this text are prudent management of these conditions. Avoidance of medications which may exacerbate these conditions is especially important, when practical. An interesting clinical dilemma is the patient with orthostatic hypotension and concomitant hypertension. Usually these individuals are on antihypertensive medications, as their blood pressures can be significantly elevated when in the supine position. If the patient can safely be taken off the antihypertensive, every effort should be made to do so. However, if this is not possible, the addition of fludrocortisone or midodrine may help the patient with hypotension feel better. The patient should be educated to avoid lying in the supine position when one of these medications is given in order to avoid extremely high blood pressure.

PD may cause drowsiness or a feeling of lethargy, and many of the medications used to treat the symptoms of PD may cause drowsiness. Sleep patterns are often disrupted in PD. Insomnia may also occur as a result of uncontrolled PD symptoms or restless legs syndrome, a common concomitant syndrome with PD. Many times maximizing PD therapy around bedtime can ameliorate this, as well as education on proper sleep hygiene. Chapter 13 provides information on treatment of insomnia which can be applied to patients with PD.

Anosmia or hyposmia can be a presenting symptom of the disease. This inability to smell, and thereby taste, is especially concerning in the elder who has stopped eating or decreased eating because they are no longer able to taste, and thereby enjoy, their food. This can lead to weight loss, which in a nursing home elder is monitored closely, but is truly a concern in any senior individual.

Depression, dementia and psychosis occur in the PD population with increased frequency over age-matched counterparts. While the disease process can be implicated in these psychiatric non-motor complications, medications must always be reviewed to ascertain whether these psychiatric manifestations may be an untoward side effect. Depression can be seen in approximately 50% of patients with PD at some point in their disease course and although there is no specific literature existing for the elderly with PD, SSRIs are typically employed in clinical practice with good results.[39] The AAN notes in their 2006 practice parameter that level C evidence exists for amitriptyline, however, they also note amitriptyline is not a first line agent.[57] They go on to state that the lack of literature showing efficacy of other agents is not the same as the absence of efficacy.[57] This implies using agents other than TCAs, while not supported in the literature, is an acceptable intervention for the depressed patient with PD. Dementia in PD is also experienced with increased frequency as the disease progresses. The acetylcholinesterase inhibitors rivastigmine and donepezil both have level B evidence to support their use in dementia associated with PD, however rivastigmine is the only product FDA-approved for this indication.[57] Psychosis, typically resulting from medications, is especially burdensome, and is a common reason for nursing home placement.[41] Hence, dopamine agonists are used cautiously in the elderly with PD. When symptoms are controlled on a PD medication regimen and psychosis is experienced, the clinician may elect to treat the psychosis, rather than change the regimen. The atypical antipsychotics quetiapine and clozapine are the first and second line agents, respectively, for treating this side effect.[58,59] And while the dopamine antagonism of the antipsychotic medications as a class would seem to contribute to disease exacerbation, these two agents do not. When quetiapine is not effective or side effects to this agent prevent its use, clozapine is employed. However, the agranulocytosis seen with this agent requires significant monitoring, which can be burdensome to patients, caregivers and providers.

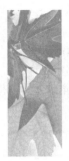

KEY POINT: Quetiapine and clozapine are appropriate choices for the treatment of psychosis which may be experienced secondary to PD therapies, as they decrease psychotic symptoms yet do not exacerbate PD symptoms.

The slowness of movement is not limited to the extremities, and many patients with PD experience slowing of the GI tract, which may manifest as swallowing difficulties, delayed gastric emptying and constipation. Swallowing difficulties in PD must always be at the forefront of any care plan for the elderly. This includes both the therapies used to treat PD, as well as other disease states. Crushing medications to help with administration is common when swallowing problems occur. However it is prudent to consider a medication regimen review when crushing medications is employed, as long-acting or enteric-coated formulations may need to be changed. Non-oral routes may also be considered when swallowing becomes difficult.

Seizures

Etiology, Epidemiology, and Clinical Presentation of Seizures

A seizure is defined as abnormal electrical activity in the brain manifesting with or without convulsions. Elderly patients may experience a single seizure as a result of electrolyte abnormalities or other acute illness. Instead, epilepsy is a disease manifested by multiple seizures. Status epilepticus is typically defined as continuous seizure activity of 30 minutes or more, or multiple seizures without full recovery of consciousness between seizures.[60]

Cerebrovascular disease is the most common cause of new onset seizures in the senior population, with post-stroke seizures accounting for ~55% of new onset seizures in this population.[61] Those who experience a stroke in the cortical region of the brain are more likely to have seizures than those with a stroke in subcortical regions. Brain tumors, trauma and dementias are other causes of new onset seizures in this population.[62,63] Iatrogenic causes must always be ruled out, with offending agents removed as quickly as possible. Status epilepticus occurs at a higher incidence in the elderly, with almost twice the incidence of the general population, and a much higher mortality rate.[60,64,65] Status epilepticus which occurs along with an ischemic stroke has been shown to increase the risk of mortality by 3 times, compared to ischemic stroke alone.[66]

Seizures typically fall into one of two categories: partial or generalized.[67,68] Partial seizures start in one hemisphere of the brain and manifest as unilateral motor symptoms. If consciousness is not lost, these are deemed simple partial seizures, however with loss of consciousness, these are categorized as complex partial seizures. Generalized seizures involve both hemispheres of the brain and manifest as bilateral motor involvement. The tonic-clonic seizure is an example of a generalized seizure. If a seizure starts as a partial seizure, but becomes generalized, these seizures are deemed secondary generalized and are typically treated as partial seizures. Generalized absence seizures are typically manifested without motor symptoms, but with a sudden "interruption of ongoing activities, a blank stare and possible a brief upward rotation of the eyes."[69] In general, absence seizures occur in a much younger population and will not be addressed in this chapter.

The clinical presentation of seizures in the elderly may differ from the presentation in a younger cohort. For instance, seniors are less likely to have auras associated with their seizures.[70] Seizures in a senior population may also be confused with an acute confusional state, or syncope, which makes the diagnosis of a seizure in an elderly person quite difficult.[70] Generalized seizures are also less common in the elderly, than in a younger cohort,

with partial seizures being a much more common type of seizure experienced.[70,71] And, although clinical presentation may be different, seizures can have a significant impact on quality of life in an elderly cohort, just as they do in the younger population with seizures.[72]

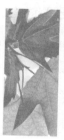

KEY POINT: The cholinesterase inhibitors and memantine have the potential to decrease seizure threshold, and should therefore be used with caution in those with a prior history of seizure disorder.

Summary of Standard Treatment

The goal of any treatment for epilepsy, is to acutely stop the clinical and electrical seizure activity, and to prevent future seizures. A single seizure may not require chronic therapy especially if an underlying illnesses is corrected. Despite many studies of seizure medications having an endpoint of "reduction in seizure frequency by 50%," the goal number of seizures in an individual is always zero. Minimizing side effects, maximizing quality of life and retaining independence and confidence are goals of treatment in all patients.

Standard treatment of seizures depends on the type of seizure being treated. Status epilepticus typically is treated with an intravenous benzodiazepine first line, followed by either intravenous phenytoin or intravenous fosphenytoin.

Table 12-7 identifies the agents recommended for monotherapy of newly diagnosed epilepsy, for refractory partial epilepsy and as add-on therapy by the American Academy of Neurology (AAN) and the American Epilepsy Society (AES).[73,74] Initial choice of an agent should be individualized, however all agents listed have efficacy data to support their use. Forty to fifty percent of adults who are refractory to the first anti-epileptic drug (AED) they are tried on, will have adequate seizure control on another AED as monotherapy.[75] However, if two agents as monotherapy at maxi-

Table 12-7. Seizure Medications: Indications and Common Dosages[95]

Agent	Seizure-related Indications[a]	Common Daily Dosages[b]
Carbamazepine	Partial seizures with complex symptomatology Generalized tonic-clonic Mixed seizure patterns Monotherapy for newly diagnosed	800–1200 mg/daily[c]
Felbamate	Monotherapy or adjunctive therapy for partial seizures ± secondary generalization[d]	2400–3000 mg/day[c]
Fosphenytoin	Control of generalized status epilepticus (SE) Prevention and treatment of seizures during neurosurgery	SE: Loading dose: 15–20 mg PE/kg with a rate of: 100–150 mg PE/min Non-emergent: Loading dose: 10–20 mg PE/kg IV or IM Maintenance dose: 4–6 mg PE/kg/day IV or IM[c]
Gabapentin	Adjunct for partial seizures ± secondary generalization Monotherapy for newly diagnosed Add-on for **refractory epilepsy**	900–2400 mg/day[c] Adjust dose for renal insufficiency
Lacosamide	Adjunctive therapy for partial onset seizures	200–400 mg/day[c] Adjust dose for renal insufficiency
Lamotrigine	Adjunctive for primary generalized tonic-clonic Adjunctive for partial seizures Monotherapy for newly diagnosed Mono- or add-on therapy for refractory epilepsy (although evidence for monotherapy in this setting is weaker)	225–375 mg/daily[c] Regimens with valproic acid: 100–400 mg/daily[c] Regimens with an enzyme-inducing AED: 300–500 mg/daily[c] Adjust dose for renal insufficiency
Levetiracetam	Adjunctive therapy for partial seizures Adjunctive therapy for myoclonic and/or primary generalized tonic-clonic Add-on for refractory epilepsy	2000–3000 mg/daily[c] Adjust dose for renal insufficiency
Oxcarbazepine	Monotherapy or adjunctive therapy for partial seizures Monotherapy for newly diagnosed Mono- or add-on therapy for refractory epilepsy	1200–2400 mg/daily[c]
Phenytoin	Management of generalized tonic-clonic Management of complex partial seizures Seizure prevention in head trauma/neurosurgery Monotherapy for newly diagnosed	300–1200 mg/daily[c]
Phenobarbital	Management of generalized tonic-clonic seizures Management of partial seizures Monotherapy for newly diagnosed	100–300 mg/day[c]
Pregabalin	Adjunctive therapy for partial seizures	150–600 mg/day[c] Adjust dose for renal insufficiency
Primidone	Management of grand mal, psychomotor, or focal seizures	750–1500 mg/day[c]

(continued)

Table 12-7. Seizure Medications: Indications and Common Dosages[95] (cont'd)

Agent	Seizure-related Indications[a]	Common Daily Dosages[b]
Rufinamide	(No adult indications at present)	1600–3200 mg/day[c]
Topiramate	Monotherapy or adjunctive therapy for partial seizures Monotherapy or adjunctive therapy for tonic-clonic seizures Monotherapy for newly diagnosed Mono- or add-on therapy for refractory epilepsy	Monotherapy: 100–400 mg/day[c] Adjunctive partial: 100–200 mg BID Adjunctive tonic-clonic: 200 mg BID
Tiagabine	Adjunctive therapy for partial seizures Add-on for refractory epilepsy	Regimens with enzyme-inducing AEDs: 32–56 mg/day[c]
Valproic acid	Monotherapy or adjunctive therapy for complex partial seizures Monotherapy for newly diagnosed	15–60 mg/kg/day[c]
Zonisamide	Adjunctive therapy for partial seizures Add-on for refractory epilepsy	100–400 mg/day[c]

[a]Indications applicable to older adults.
[b]Indicates common total daily dosages.
[c]In divided doses.
[d]Not indicated for first-line therapy.
PE, phenytoin equivalents

mum dosages are ineffective, adjunctive therapy should be considered.[72] Valproate is the supported treatment of first choice for generalized seizures, and, for generalized tonic-clonic seizures refractory to treatment, adjunctive therapy with topiramate is recommended based on safety and efficacy data.[74]

The SANAD Study Group trials were large, open-label trials designed to best reflect clinical practice in that providers were able to change agents if it was deemed there was treatment failure or intolerability.[76,77] There were two arms of the study: one for the treatment of partial epilepsy and another for the treatment of generalized or otherwise unclassified epilepsy.[76,77] In the first arm, investigators studied carbamazepine, gabapentin, lamotrigine, oxcarbazepine and topiramate as monotherapy for the treatment of new onset partial epilepsy. The majority of the individuals randomized had never received a prior therapy. The median age was 38.3 years old and the time to treatment failure (defined as stopping of the medication because of either intolerable side effects or inadequate seizure control) was statisti-

cally significantly better in the group receiving lamotrigine, with carbamazepine and oxcarbazepine both having statistically significant results as well. In the time to 12-month remission, another primary endpoint, lamotrigine was found to be non-inferior to carbamazepine.[77] In the second arm of SANAD, individuals with generalized or otherwise unclassified epilepsy were randomized to either valproate, lamotrigine or topiramate. Valproate showed superiority in both primary endpoints of time to treatment failure (defined as above) and time to 12-month remission.[77] However, the median age in the B arm of SANAD was 22.5 years old.

In December 2008, the FDA completed an analysis of trials in which AEDs were compared to placebo for a variety of conditions (e.g., epilepsy, psychiatric disorders, migraines) and determined an increased risk of suicidal thoughts and behaviors existed on treatment with an AED. Warnings are now included in the package labeling to this end, and a MedGuide is required to be given with each dispensation of an AED, for any indication.

Review of Evidence Supporting Treatment Recommendations in the Elderly

The goals of therapy for a senior patient are no different than that of the younger cohort, with an additional goal of minimizing drug interactions, secondary to the increased number of medications seniors typically take. The senior population, as is the case with many disease states, is typically excluded from trials of AEDs, despite the fact that those over age 60 account for 25% of new cases of epilepsy.[78] Seniors are typically excluded from trials because of their high number of co-morbid conditions, and thus medications taken, as well as the increased risk of side effects seen in this population which could impact safety data presented. Even when they are included in trials of seizure medications, exclusion criteria often eliminate those with severe chronic disease (which is typically ill-defined in the literature), those with psychiatric disease, those with other neurological illnesses, and even those individuals who are receiving medications known to interact with the agent being researched. A prime example is a study done to assess the tolerability and safety of oxcarbazepine which utilized the pharmaceutical company's database.[79] Of 1626 patients in oxcarbazepine trials, 52 (3.2%) were older than 65, and 18 (1.1%) were older than 75. Trials involving the senior population often are small, open-label, prospective, single-center trials, limiting the validity of the results, as well as limiting the ability to apply the results to the general population of seniors. The few agents which have looked at efficacy, safety and quality of life measures specifically in the elderly include: lamotrigine, carbamazepine, topiramate, oxcarbazepine, and levetiracetam.

By far, the most widely researched AED in the elderly is lamotrigine. It has shown efficacy as both monotherapy and in combination with other therapies, as well as better tolerability when compared to other therapies, most notably carbamazepine.[80-84] Most trials are in elderly patients with any type of seizure, but lamotrigine was studied specifically in those who had an ischemic stroke and developed seizures, and although it was a small study, there was no differ-ence in seizure frequency with lamotrigine versus carbamazepine.[84] However, there was increased tolerability with lamotrigine. Carbamazepine in these trials, although less tolerable than lamotrigine in this population, was noted to be an efficacious therapy for seizures in the elderly. A small, open-label study of patients aged 60 and older who wished to change AED, either secondary to intolerable side effects or continuing seizures, were given a trial of lamotrigine first as add-on therapy and then as monotherapy if they wished.[82] In those patients who chose to convert to lamotrigine monotherapy, 64% achieved seizure freedom.

Topiramate has some data to support its use as monotherapy in the elderly in a small trial and a subgroup analysis of a larger seizure trial.[85,86] Both showed similar efficacy to trials in younger patients, with seizure freedom ranging from 63% at 7 months and 44% at 12 months.[85,86] Adverse effects experienced by individuals in the trials were dizziness, nausea, loss of appetite and paresthesias. Of note, there was a statistically significant decrease in weight from baseline in one of the trials.[86]

A small subgroup of elderly patients within a larger clinical trial of oxcarbazepine as monotherapy for partial seizures showed good response in the 12-month remission rates among the seniors in the cohort (n = 19).[87] There was no breakdown within the subgroup in regards to adverse events. However, a retrospective analysis of the elderly patients within a large database of trials of oxcarbazepine as monotherapy showed similar safety and tolerability with oxcarbazepine compared to the remainder of the cohort, although the number of seniors in this cohort were small.[79] Hyponatremia, vertigo, nausea and abnormal vision were more common in the elderly drop-outs than in the younger drop-outs. This analysis did not assess efficacy.

A small study of levetiracetam monotherapy in post-stroke patients with at least two seizures showed seizure freedom at 4 months in 85% of the patients. One person discontinued treatment due to intolerable somnolence.[88] A retrospective chart review of elderly patients with partial epilepsy receiving levetiracetam noted good response and relatively good tolerability.[89] In an observational study of Alzheimer's patients with new onset seizures, a trial of levetiracetam was given after removal of all medications which could increase risk of seizures, including their cholinesterase inhibitor and any neuroleptic they were receiving.[90] At a dose of 1000-1500 mg/day, levetiracetam was associated with seizure freedom in 18 of the 25 patients; 4 patients discontinued the drug because of intolerable side effects, including somnolence, gait disturbance, agitation and increased confusion. However, it is unclear whether discontinuation of other therapies could have confounded these adverse events.

Many trials of AEDs look specifically at tolerability in the elderly population, relying on efficacy data from the younger cohort. However, given the differing etiologies of seizures in the senior population, this extrapolation of data should be done with caution. Elderly patients also tend to achieve seizure control with lower doses of AEDs and at lower AED serum levels than in a younger cohort.[91] This begs the question of whether serum monitoring should be done in an elderly patient if lower AED serum levels are effective. Most experts would agree that monitoring is appropriate when one is adjusting phenytoin doses specifically or if assessing adherence or toxicity of any AED.

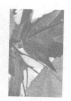

KEY POINT: Therapeutic drug monitoring with AEDs is most appropriate when one is adjusting phenytoin doses or if assessing adherence or toxicity of an AED.

The treatment of status epilepticus in the elderly typically follows that of the general population. No specific evidence supporting or refuting current guidelines in the elderly subpopulation exists.

There is currently no evidence to suggest an increase in suicidal behaviors or thoughts specifically in the elderly, and given the low numbers of elderly in trials of these agents, conclusions are not likely to be drawn. However, the FDAs new warnings and the receipt of a MedGuide with each AED prescription include those dispensed to seniors.

Common Problems Encountered in the Senior Population with Seizure Disorder

Seniors, by their very nature of being high consumers of healthcare, can be more prone to the drug interactions and untoward side effects of the AEDs. The pharmacokinetic and pharmacodynamic changes associated with aging also make the choice of AED somewhat difficult. (See Table 12-8.) While many newer generation AEDs tend to be better tolerated, the cost associated with the agents themselves can be a limiting factor to their use in the senior population.

Agent-related

Despite being used frequently in the elderly with seizure disorder, phenytoin has many issues associated with its use, especially long-term. It induces many CYP450 isoenzymes, making it highly likely to interact with many common medications used in the elderly population. When given concomitantly with tube feedings, its bioavailability is significantly reduced, putting patients at risk for lower blood levels and also an increased risk for seizures. Tube feedings should be stopped for 2 hours prior to phenytoin administration and should be held for at least 1 hour after phenytoin administration. This can be very difficult in someone receiving twice daily administration of phenytoin on continuous tube feeds, and in most cases if this cannot be done easily, switching to another AED is often employed. However, in those whom phenytoin is unable to be stopped, doses may be increased to compensate for this interaction. However, it is of the utmost importance to be consistent with dosing, and to remember dosage adjustments have been made should the tube feeding be stopped for any length of time or discontinued. Phenytoin can increase the risk for falls by both inducing vitamin D metabolism, as well as the potential to cause cerebellar atrophy with long-term use. In order to assess true steady state, levels should be drawn 2–3 weeks after starting phenytoin in the elderly secondary to an increased half-life in this population. And, due to

Table 12-8. **Antiepileptic Drug-Disease Interactions**[72]

Selected Conditions[a]	Precaution	Contraindication
Anorexia, weight loss	Felbamate, topiramate, carbamazepine (anorexia), rufinamide, zonisamide (anorexia)	
Cardiac conduction abnormalities, ventricular arrhythmia	Carbamazepine, fosphenytoin, lacosamide, lamotrigine, phenytoin (parenteral), oxcarbazepine	Phenytoin if sinus bradycardia, sinoatrial block, 2nd-or 3rd-degree AV block, Adams-Stokes block Rufinamide if familial short QT syndrome
Cognitive impairment	Barbiturates,[b] benzodiazepines, topiramate, tiagabine, zonisamide	
Gait unsteadiness, dizziness	Barbiturates, carbamazepine,[c] felbamate, gabapentin, lacosamide, lamotrigine, levetiracetam, oxcarbazepine, phenytoin, pregabalin, rufinamide, tiagabine, topiramate, valproate,[c] zonisamide	
Hepatic disease, impairment	Carbamazepine, felbamate, lacosamide, rufinamide, tiagabine, valproate, zonisamide, oxcarbazepine, phenytoin	Felbamate, Phenobarbital, Valproate
Hyponatremia	Carbamazepine, oxcarbazepine	
Narrow-angle glaucoma	Topiramate	Gabapentin
Osteomalacia, osteoporosis[d]	Carbamazepine, oxcarbazepine, phenobarbital, phenytoin, primidone, valproate	
Respiratory disease (obstructive, dyspnea)	Benzodiazepines, phenytoin (IV, IM)	Phenobarbital
Tremor (familial, Parkinson's disease)	Gabapentin, lacosamide, lamotrigine, pregabalin, rufinamide, tiagabine, topiramate, valproate	
Renal impairment	Gabapentin, lacosamide, levetiracetam, phenobarbital, pregabalin, topiramate, zonisamide	
Sedation	Barbiturates, benzodiazepines, carbamazepine, felbamate, gabapentin, lacosamide, lamotrigine, pregabalin, oxcarbazepine, rufinamide, tiagabine, topiramate, valproate	Rufinamide if familial short QT syndrome
Urinary incontinencee	Carbamazepine, clonazepam, gabapentin, lamotrigine, oxcarbazepine, phenobarbital, phenytoin, tiagabine, topiramate, valproate	
Nephrolithiasis	Topiramate, zonisamide	

AV block = atrioventricular nodal block.
[a]Hypersensitivity to the antiepileptic drug, its ingredients, or related class of drugs is a contraindication.
[b]Phenobarbital is commonly believed to impair cognition; however, at equivalent serum drug concentrations, this effect was no different than antiepileptic drugs with an uncertain effect (phenytoin, carbamazepine, oxcarbazepine, valproate).
[c]Carbamazepine and valproate may pose a lower risk of gait disturbance than other antiepileptic drugs.
[d]The risk of osteoporosis with the newer antiepileptic drugs is not established.
[e]Urinary incontinence is a potential untoward effect of some antiepileptic drugs.
Source: Adapted from reference 72 with permission.

its being highly protein bound, a free phenytoin level should be drawn in a frail elderly patient who is likely to have hypoalbuminemia, rather than a total phenytoin assay.

Phenytoin can block alpha-receptors and thereby may decrease internal bladder sphincter tone, which can exacerbate stress urinary incontinence. The gingival hyperplasia seen in a younger cohort is not typically seen in the elderly population. Fosphenytoin has very little research specifically in the elderly, however its ability to induce many P450 isoenzymes makes it use in the elderly difficult. But it is typically only used short-term in emergent situations, or when the oral route of administration is not available in a patient receiving phenytoin.

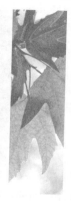

KEY POINT: If phenytoin doses are increased to compensate for decreased absorption secondary to tube feedings, it is of utmost importance to be consistent with dosing, and to remember doses have been adjusted if tube feedings are stopped for any length of time or discontinued.

Hyponatremia, rash and SIADH are side effects which can occur with carbamazepine, however they can be seen with increased frequency in the elderly population.[72] Due to its induction of many CYP450 isoenzymes, carbamazepine is highly likely to interact with many medications found commonly on the profiles of elderly patients. Carbamazepine also induces its own metabolism. Carbamazepine binds to alpha-glycoprotein which is known to increase in the elderly, which can make total carbamazepine levels look therapeutic, but not really be so. Carbamazepine can induce vitamin D metabolism, potentially leading to an increased risk of osteoporosis and falls. Overflow incontinence, secondary to increased parasympathetic stimulation of the detrusor, is also an untoward consequence of car-

bamazepine use which is commonly overlooked.[72] Similar to carbamazepine, oxcarbazepine has an increased risk of hyponatremia in the elderly and can decrease the efficacy of estrogen, something to note in an individual receiving estrogen-replacement therapy.

Valproic acid is commonly used in elderly patients. Its time to steady state may be doubled in an elderly cohort, so this should be taken into consideration for drug monitoring. Platelet count and ammonia levels should be monitored and, in those with hypoalbuminemia, the unbound concentration should be tested. Weight gain and a fine hand tremor may also be seen in the elderly receiving valproic acid.

Phenobarbital, another older agent, should be used in the elderly with extreme caution, if at all, due to its long half-life and ability to cause cognitive disturbances. It can also interfere with vitamin D metabolism and is highly protein bound, which can be an issue in an elderly patient with decreased albumin. Due to additive respiratory depression, phenobarbital is contraindicated with the concomitant use of an opioid. It is noted as a drug to be avoided in the elderly and is associated with dependence. Primidone, the parent drug of phenobarbital, has the same issues and warnings. When discontinuing these agents, doses should be tapered slowly to avoid withdrawal reactions.

Gabapentin's ability to cause weight gain is well documented in the literature in the younger cohort, and is also seen in the elderly in clinical practice. Elderly are much more prone to the effects of ataxia and somnolence, however. Gabapentin has the potential to cause edema, yet is commonly overlooked when iatrogenic causes are being investigated. Pregabalin has a similar side effect profile.

Lamotrigine is well known for the potential to cause a rash which can occur at any time during its use, but most often is seen in the titration phase. A Stevens-Johnson Syndrome-type rash may also occur in patients taking lamotrigine, therefore any complaint of rash needs to be quickly addressed, given the life-threatening nature of this particular syndrome. This risk for rash is increased in those receiving concomitant valproic acid. However, with slow titration, over more than 8 weeks, this adverse effect can be minimized. This need for slow titration limits its use to those who do not need immediate therapeutic doses of their seizure medication.

Levetiracetam is gaining in popularity, despite lack of significant literature support in the elderly. This is likely because it lacks CYP450 interactions and has a fairly mild side effect profile when compared to other agents.

Topiramate's most common side effect in the elderly is weight loss. On average, in small clinical trials in the elderly, patients lost ~5 pounds, with a subgroup analysis noting those with an increased BMI losing the most weight.[85,86] Cognitive disturbance and word-finding difficulties can be experienced in the elderly on topiramate. In the younger population, topiramate has an increased risk of kidney stones, which should be monitored for in the elderly, especially those with decreased water intake or on water restriction due to other disease states, such as CHF.

Zonisamide is rarely used in the elderly for several reasons. It should be used with caution in those with a creatinine clearance less than 50 mL/min and in those allergic to sulfonamides. Zonisamide may also increase the risk of renal stones, so like topiramate it should be used with caution in those with low water intake. Zonisamide has also been implicated in causing cognitive impairment and psychosis, as well as increasing the chance of metabolic acidosis.

Two new AEDs have not been evaluated in older adults. Lacosamide should be used with caution in those with conduction disorders as it has the potential to prolong the PR interval. It should be avoided in those with CHF, and in those who are taking other medications which prolong this interval. Rufinamide is indicated only as adjuvant therapy for generalized seizures secondary to Lennox-Gastaut, a type of epilepsy seen in children. It can shorten the QT interval and must be used with caution in those patients with pre-existing conduction disorders, and in those on concomitant QT interval shortening medications.

Disease-related

Many medications and herbal products commonly used by the geriatric population may lower seizure threshold (see Table 12-9). It is important to avoid the use of these medications whenever possible in a patient with seizure disorder. If a patient should have a new onset of a seizure disorder, a thorough medication review should take place, ensuring the patient is asked about over-the-counter product use, as well as herbals.

Certain AEDs are excreted by the kidneys. Dose adjustments are frequently required in elderly patients due to renal insufficiency. Table 12-7 notes the agents which necessitate this modification.

AEDs which may cause or worsen osteoporosis should be looked at critically and ascertained whether another agent which doesn't cause osteoporosis might be a better option, taking risk versus benefit into account. Osteoporosis should be treated. However, the choice of agent should be based on patient- and agent-related variables, given there are no agents currently approved for AED-induced osteoporosis. For patients using an AED known to induce vitamin D metabolism, it is a prudent recommendation to follow 25-OH vitamin D levels regularly and supplement if necessary.

Patients with seizures should be screened on a regular basis for depression and anxiety, as these conditions can be seen with increased incidence in those with seizure disorder.[92] Again, the choice of agent should be chosen with the patient- and agent-related variables in mind.

Table 12-9. Medications that Can Decrease Seizure Threshold[72]

Bupropion	Lithium
Cephalosporins	Ma huang
Cholinesterase inhibitors	Maprotiline
	Memantine
Duloxetine	Meperidine
Ephedrine	Metoclopramide
Fluoroquinolones	Penicillins
Fluvoxamine	Phenothiazines
Ginkgo biloba	St. John's Wort
Ginseng	Theophylline
Insulin	Tramadol
Isoniazid	Tricyclic antidepressants
Kava kava	Venlafaxine

CASE 1: DELIRIUM

Setting:
Hospital

Subjective:
GM is a 74-year-old man who presents with a chief complaint of confusion and incontinence. His wife says he became confused about 2 days ago. The confusion at first was minor, but worsened until he tried getting into the car and going to work at 5:00 a.m., although he has been retired for 9 years. Today he was incontinent and she brought him to the hospital for evaluation.

PMH:
Mild cognitive impairment for 2 years, hypertension, benign prostatic hypertrophy. Medications prior to admission: lisinopril 10 mg daily, doxazosin 4 mg at bedtime, aspirin 81mg daily.

Social History:
Retired schoolteacher, lives at home with his wife.

Physical Examination:
Well developed, well nourished older gentleman. Oriented × 2. Otherwise unremarkable except for pain with palpation at the costo-vertebral angles.

Laboratory:
BUN 48 mg/dL; serum creatinine 1.8 mg/dL; CBC: WBC 13,000; urinalysis: positive leukocyte esterase, positive nitrites; CK-MB WNL, Tropinins WNL, ECG: no change from previous.

Assessment:
Urinary tract infection and delirium secondary to infection.

Plan:
1. Start oral levofloxacin dosed per creatinine clearance.
2. Avoid intravenous lines, urinary catheter and other tethers.
3. Non-pharmacologic measures for reduction of delirium including music, massage, redirection and stimulation during the day/quiet at night.

Rationale:
1. Infections and myocardial infarctions frequently do not present with the same symptoms in elderly patients as they do in younger adults. Individuals with cognitive impairment from any source may become delirious as a result of the insult. When a patient presents in delirium, work-up must include evaluation for the common precipitants. As this patient did not have any medication changes, focus upon infection or cardiac conditions is appropriate.
2. Levofloxacin is an appropriate antibiotic to choose in a complicated urinary tract infection, however, it has been associated with causing delirium. Appropriate dosing in renal insufficiency will help minimize this effect.
3. Avoiding intravenous lines and urinary catheters when they are not needed will eliminate the risk of the delirious patient pulling them out, causing more damage. Nonpharmacologic measures such as music therapy, massage, aromatherapy, and behavior techniques have been shown to reduce the risk for delirium and may aid in recovery once delirium has developed. Using these early in the hospitalization will help prevent the need for pharmacologic treatment of delirium and hopefully speed recovery.

CASE 2: PARKINSON'S DISEASE

Setting:
Assisted living facility

Subjective:
PG is an 86-year-old female patient with a past medical history positive for Parkinson's disease for 3 years. Her PD symptoms have been controlled on levodopa/carbidopa 200/25 mg 3 times daily for the past 2 years. However, she is currently experiencing "wearing off" before her next dose of levodopa/carbidopa is due, as well as problems "getting moving" when she wakes up in the morning around 7:00 a.m.

PMH:
PD × 3 years, osteoporosis × 17 years, s/p hip fracture 12 years ago, episodic hypotension, & glaucoma. Her concurrent medications include: calcium/vitamin D3 500 mg/200 I.U. three times daily; alendronate 70 mg once weekly; dorzolamide/timolol 1 drop both eyes twice daily; travoprost 1 drop both eyes at bedtime, aspirin 81 mg once daily, acetaminophen 650 mg as needed for headache

Objective:
Ht: 5'0" Wt: 96 pounds
Blood pressure: 131/89 (sitting), 113/79 (standing); pulse: 79 (sitting), 90 (standing)
Temperature: 98.2, respiratory rate: 17
Pertinent physical examination findings: resting tremor present R>L, shuffling gait, slight stooped posture

Assessment:
86-year old Parkinson's patient experiencing wearing off and morning bradykinesia

Plan:
1. Change dosing interval of levodopa/carbidopa 200/25 mg to four times daily 7:00 a.m., 1:00 p.m. and 7:00 p.m. and 11:00 p.m.
2. Counsel patient to take levodopa/carbidopa in the morning before rising from bed and to wait 30 minutes or more for it to take effect.
3. Review medication for issues with administration.
4. Return to clinic in 4 weeks to assess improvement in wearing off and possible dyskinesias.

Rationale:
1. The wearing off PG is experiencing can be attributed to disease progression, and while there are other options other than decreasing the dosing interval, PG appears to be tolerating the levodopa/carbidopa well. If possible, it is best to stay with the single drug, levodopa/carbidopa, to avoid additional exposure and risk for adverse effects. Other options are available should this one not be optimal. A dopamine agonist could be added, however, PG is of advanced age, and may be more prone to the psychiatric adverse effects of this medication. A COMT inhibitor could also be added with each dose of levodopa/carbidopa, however these are expensive agents and would add to pill burden (unless the combination product, another expensive product, was used). Another option is addition of selegiline or rasagiline. Selegiline is the least expensive option, except for the orally disintegrating tablet although it offers an important dosing option for the early morning. Rasagiline has been shown effective in this situation, and is dosed conveniently at once a day, but is a more expensive alternative.
2. Due to the swallowing difficulties and slowed GI transit seen with PD, the alendronate has the potential to cause ulceration if it gets caught in the esophagus. And the question must be

asked, can she administer her eye drops correctly secondary to possible tremor and rigidity? All medications require reassessment due to the motor and non-motor deficits seen with PD.

Summary:

Wearing off between levodopa doses and dyskinesias are common occurrences as PD progresses. Knowing how to manage these occurrences are important concepts. While there is little data to support specific interventions in the elderly when these occur, keeping the tenets of geriatrics at the heart of the plan is key to success. These include making one intervention at a time in order to best assess efficacy and tolerability, as well as starting low with doses and going slow in titration. Timely reassessment of interventions and continued follow-up are similarly important. Interventions may result in symptom improvement, but with concomitant bothersome dyskinesias. And, as the disease process progresses and symptoms worsen, additional intervention may be required.

Clinical Pearls

- *The appropriate duration of therapy with CIs or memantine has not been fully investigated. Patients who experience adverse effects, perceive little benefit, have rapid worsening or are concerned about medication costs may elect to discontinue treatment based upon risk/benefit assessment. In some studies, rapid deterioration occurred when the CIs were discontinued and some patients never regained this loss. However, patients should be evaluated annually, upon entry into long-term care or when the patient becomes bedbound with advanced disease to determine continued need for CI or memantine therapy.*

- *Switching AEDs, especially when one is intolerable or due to patient preference, should be done slowly with the dose of the new agent maximized prior to the older agent being titrated off. Once the new agent is at the minimally effective dose, a 20% reduction in dose of the older agent should occur every 1–2 weeks until discontinued. The new agent can have further increases in dose as needed for seizure control and as tolerated.*

Chapter Summary

One of the most dreaded diseases associated with aging is dementia, as no preventive treatment has been identified, therapies do not alter its course substantially and over time the patient must rely upon around-the-clock care without a clear sense of self. Dementia may occur due to vascular causes, but the most common etiology is AD. CIs are the mainstays of therapy, particularly for mild-to-moderate AD with memantine an option for those who are intolerant or progress to severe disease. NP symptoms also remain a challenge for treatment as medications have little evidence that efficacy outweighs the risk for side effects in this population.

Delirium, most common in patients with neurologic compromise, is a syndrome of the elderly that complicates therapy of other disease states and can lead to significant morbidity and mortality. Preventive measures have been successful in hospitalized patients. Once a diagnosis of delirium is established, nonpharmacologic measures should be instituted with pharmacologic therapy reserved for patients who pose safety problems for themselves or others.

As another progressive neurologic disease without cure, PD requires timely re-evaluation of interventions. Levodopa/carbidopa remains the gold-standard of symptomatic treatment and rasagiline has some literature supporting its tolerability in those greater than 70 years old. Dopamine agonists are likely not the best first choice in an elderly patient, and if used should be titrated slowly and monitored closely for adverse effects. In patients experiencing wearing off or dyskinesias, one must keep the tenets of geriatrics at the center of the plan, avoiding anticholinergics as much as possible due to their myriad side effects.

Seizures, the final neurologic condition covered in this chapter, are common among the elderly, especially amongst those with a history of stroke, tumors, trauma and dementia. There is a paucity of good quality trials of AEDs specifically in the elderly population, which makes the choice of an AED even more confusing. Lamotrigine, carbamazepine, topiramate, oxcarbazepine and levetiracetam have been studied specifically in the elderly population for safety, efficacy and tolerability, with lamotrigine having the most data in this population. However, given the quality of these trials, additional research is desperately needed to help clinicians make an evidence-based decision.

Self-Assessment Questions

1. Why are serum vitamin B-12 concentrations measured in the work-up of dementia?

2. What are the important counseling points for a patient who is started on a CI?

3. When would antipsychotics be appropriate in treating a patient with dementia?

4. What are the risk factors for developing delirium?

5. What nonpharmacologic treatments for delirium are useful?

6. What are the pros and cons of starting levodopa/carbidopa versus a dopamine agonist in an elderly patient newly diagnosed with Parkinson's disease?

7. What are the options available to treat the patient who is experiencing wearing off?

8. How do dyskinesias contrast with wearing off?

9. How do the non-motor complications of PD impact the quality of life in a community-dwelling senior?

10. Which AEDs should have the free concentration measured when conducting therapeutic drug monitoring? Why?

11. Which AEDs should be renally dose adjusted in an elderly person?

12. What precautions should be undertaken when adding lamotrigine to a valproate-based regimen?

13. What are the advantages and disadvantages of using the newer AEDs for the treatment of partial seizures in the elderly?

14. Why might the diagnosis of a seizure disorder in an elderly person be difficult?

References

1. *American Psychiatric Association Diagnostic and Statistical Manual.* 4th ed. Washington, DC: APA Press; 1994.

2. Chapman DP, Williams SM, Strine TW, Anda RF, Moore MJ. Dementia and its implications for public health. *Prev Chronic Dis.* 2006;3(2):A34.

3. Selhub J, Morris MS, Jacques PF, Rosenberg IH. Folate-vitamin B-12 interaction in relation to cognitive impairment, anemia, and biochemical indicators of vitamin B-12 deficiency. *Am J Clin Nutr.* 2009;89(2):702S–706S.

4. Smith AD, Refsum H. Vitamin B-12 and cognition in the elderly. *Am J Clin Nutr.* 2009;89(2):707S–711S.

5. McKhann G, Drachman D, Folstein M, Katzman R, Price D, Stadlan EM. Clinical diagnosis of Alzheimer's disease: report of the NINCDS-ADRDA Work Group under the auspices of Department of Health and Human Services Task Force on Alzheimer's Disease. *Neurology.* 1984;34(7):939–944.

6. Cummings JL, Doody R, Clark C. Disease-modifying therapies for Alzheimer disease: challenges to early intervention. *Neurology.* 2007;69(16):1622–1634.

7. Rubin CD. The primary care of Alzheimer disease. *Am J Med Sci.* 2006;332(6):314–333.

8. Rojas-Fernandez CH, Moorhouse P. Current concepts in vascular cognitive impairment and pharmacotherapeutic implications. *Ann Pharmacother.* 2009;43:1310–23.

9. Kirshner HS. Vascular dementia: a review of recent evidence for prevention and treatment. *Curr Neur Neuroscience Rep.* 2009;9:437–42.

10. Barker WW, Luis CA, Kashuba A, et al. Relative frequencies of Alzheimer disease, Lewy body, vascular and frontotemporal dementia, and hippocampal sclerosis in the State of Florida Brain Bank. *Alzheimer Dis Assoc Disord.* 2002;16(4):203–212.

11. McKeith IG, Dickson DW, Lowe J, et al. Diagnosis and management of dementia with Lewy bodies: third report of the DLB Consortium. *Neurology.* 2005;65(12):1863–1872.

12. Henriksen AL, St Dennis C, Setter SM, Tran JT. Dementia with Lewy bodies: therapeutic opportunities and pitfalls. *Consult Pharm.* 2006;21(7):563–575.

13. Farlow MR, Cummings JL. Effective pharmacologic management of Alzheimer's disease. *Am J Med.* 2007;120(5):388–397.

14. Robinson DM, Keating GM. Memantine: a review of its use in Alzheimer's disease. *Drugs.* 2006;66(11):1515–1534.

15. Raina P, Santaguida P, Ismaila A, et al. Effectiveness of cholinesterase inhibitors and memantine for treating dementia: evidence review for a clinical practice guideline. *Ann Intern Med.* 2008;148(5):379–397.

16. Diniz BS, Pinto JA, Jr., Gonzaga ML, Guimaraes FM, Gattaz WF, Forlenza OV. To treat or not to treat? A meta-analysis of the use of cholinesterase inhibitors in mild cognitive impairment for delaying progression to Alzheimer's disease. *Eur Arch Psychiatry Clin Neurosci.* 2009;259(4):248–256.

17. Hansen RA, Gartlehner G, Webb AP, Morgan LC, Moore CG, Jonas DE. Efficacy and safety of donepezil, galantamine, and rivastigmine for the treatment of Alzheimer's disease: a systematic review and meta-analysis. *Clin Interv Aging.* 2008;3(2):211–225.

18. Tariot PN, Farlow MR, Grossberg GT, Graham SM, McDonald S, Gergel I. Memantine treatment in patients with moderate to severe Alzheimer disease already receiving donepezil: a randomized controlled trial. *JAMA.* 2004;291(3):317–324.

19. van Dyck CH, Schmitt FA, Olin JT. A responder analysis of memantine treatment in patients with Alzheimer disease maintained on donepezil. *Am J Geriatr Psychiatry.* 2006;14(5):428–437.

20. Porsteinsson AP, Grossberg GT, Mintzer J, Olin JT. Memantine treatment in patients with mild to moderate Alzheimer's disease already receiving a cholinesterase inhibitor: a randomized, double-blind, placebo-controlled trial. *Curr Alzheimer Res.* 2008;5(1):83–89.

21. McKeith I, Del Ser T, Spano P, et al. Efficacy of rivastigmine in dementia with Lewy bodies: a randomised, double-blind, placebo-controlled international study. *Lancet.* 2000;356(9247):2031–2036.

22. Sutor B, Rummans TA, Smith GE. Assessment and management of behavioral disturbances in nursing home patients with dementia. *Mayo Clin Proc.* May 2001;76(5):540–550.

23. Schneider LS, Tariot PN, Dagerman KS, et al. Effectiveness of atypical antipsychotic drugs in patients with Alzheimer's disease. *N Engl J Med.* 2006;355(15):1525–1538.

24. Agency for Heath Care Research and Quality. Available at: http://effectivehealthcare.ahrq.gov/repFiles/Atypical_Antipsychotics_Off_Label_Use.pdf

25. Gleason OC. Delirium. *Am Fam Physician.* 2003;67(5):1027–1034.

26. van Zyl LT, Seitz DP. Delirium concisely: condition is associated with increased morbidity, mortality, and length of hospitalization. *Geriatrics.* Mar 2006;61(3):18–21.

27. Dharmarajan TS, Norman RA, eds. *Clinical Geriatrics.* New York: Parthenon Publishing; 2003.

28. Robinson TN, Raeburn CD, Tran ZV, Angles EM, Brenner LA, Moss M. Postoperative delirium in the elderly: risk factors and outcomes. *Ann Surg.* Jan 2009;249(1):173–178.

29. Hshieh TT, Fong TG, Marcantonio ER, Inouye SK. Cholinergic deficiency hypothesis in delirium: a synthesis of current evidence. *J Gerontol A Biol Sci Med Sci.* Jul 2008;63(7):764–772.

30. Inouye SK, van Dyck CH, Alessi CA, Balkin S, Siegal AP, Horwitz RI. Clarifying confusion: the confusion assessment method. A new method for detection of delirium. *Ann Intern Med.* Dec 15 1990;113(12):941–948.

31. Inouye SK, Bogardus ST, Jr., Charpentier PA, et al. A multicomponent intervention to prevent delirium in hospitalized older patients. *N Engl J Med.* Mar 4 1999;340(9):669–676.

32. Inouye SK, Baker DI, Fugal P, Bradley EH. Dissemination of the hospital elder life program: implementation, adaptation, and successes. *J Am Geriatr Soc.* Oct 2006;54(10):1492–1499.

33. Marcantonio ER, Flacker JM, Wright RJ, Resnick NM. Reducing delirium after hip fracture: a randomized trial. *J Am Geriatr Soc.* May 2001;49(5):516–522.

34. Mei A, Auerhahn D. Hypodermoclysis: maintaining hydration in the frail older adult. *Ann Long-Term Care.* 2009; 17:28–30.

35. Kalisvaart KJ, de Jonghe JF, Bogaards MJ, et al. Haloperidol prophylaxis for elderly hip-surgery patients at risk for delirium: a randomized placebo-controlled study. *J Am Geriatr Soc.* Oct 2005;53(10):1658–1666.

36. Seitz DP, Gill SS, van Zyl LT. Antipsychotics in the treatment of delirium: a systematic review. *J Clin Psychiatry.* Jan 2007;68(1):11–21.

37. de Rijk MC, Launer LJ, Berger K, et al. Prevalence of Parkinson's disease in Europe: a collaborative study of population-based cohorts. *Neurology.* 2000;54(Suppl 5): S21–S23.

38. de Laul M, Giesbergen PC, de Rijk MC, et al. Incidence of parkinsonism and Parkinson's disease in

a general population: the Rotterdam study. *Neurology.* 2004;63:1240–1244.

39. McDonald WM, Richard IH, DeLong MR. Prevalence, etiology and treatment of depression in Parkinson's disease. *Biol Psychiatry.* 2003;54:363–375.

40. Carter JH, Stewart BJ, Archbold PG, et al. Living with the person who has Parkinson's disease: the spouse's perspective by stage of disease. *Mov Disord.* 1998;13:20–28.

41. Aarsland D, Larsen JP, Tandberg E, et al. Predictors of nursing home placement in Parkinson's disease: a population-based, prospective study. *J Am Geriatr Soc.* 2000;48:938–942.

42. Miyasaki JM, Martin W, Suchowersky OK, et al. Practice parameter: Initiation of treatment for Parkinson's disease: An evidence-based review: Report of the Quality Standards Subcommittee of the American Academy of Neurology. *Neurology.* 2002;58:11–17.

43. Pahwa R, Factor SA, Lyons KE, et al. Practice Parameter: Treatment of Parkinson disease with motor fluctuations and dyskinesia (an evidence-based review): report of the quality standards subcommittee of the American Academy of Neurology. *Neurology.* 2006;66:983–995.

44. Parkinson Study Group. Effect of deprenyl on the progression of disability in early Parkinson's disease. *N Engl J Med.* 1993;328:176–183.

45. Palhagen S, Heinonen EH, Hagglung K, et al. Selegiline delays the onset of disability in de novo parkinsonian patients. *Neurology.* 1998;51:520–525.

46. Parkinson Study Group. A controlled trial of rasagiline in early Parkinson disease: the TEMPO study. *Arch Neurol.* 2002;59:1937–1943.

47. Rascol O, Brooks DJ, Korczyn AD, et al. A five-year study of the incidence of dyskinesia in patients with early Parkinson's disease who were treated with ropinirole or levodopa. *N Engl J Med.* 2000;342:1484–1491.

48. Parkinson Study Group. Pramipexole versus levodopa as initial treatment for Parkinson's disease: a 4-year randomized, controlled trial. *Arch Neurol.* 2004;61:1044–1053.

49. Shulman LM, Minagar A, Rabinstein A, et al. The use of dopamine agonists in very elderly patients with Parkinson's disease. *Mov Disord.* 2000;15:664–668.

50. Goetz CG, Schwid SR, Eberly SW, et al. Safety of rasagiline in elderly patients with Parkinson disease. *Neurology.* 2006;66:1427–1429.

51. Hristova AH, Koller WC. Early Parkinson's disease: What is the best approach to treatment. *Drugs Aging.* 2000;17:165–181.

52. Schade R, Andersohn F, Suissa S, et al. Dopamine agonists and the risk of cardiac-valve regurgitation. *N Engl J Med.* 2007;356:29–38.

53. Zanettini R, Antonini A, Gatto G, et al. Valvular heart disease and the use of dopamine agonists for Parkinson's disease. *N Engl J Med.* 2007;356:39–46.

54. Serratrice J, Disdier P, Habib G, et al. Fibrotic valvular heart disease subsequent to bromocriptine treatment. *Cardiol Rev.* 2002;10:334–336.

55. Clane SM, Kumar A. Nursing care of patients with late-stage Parkinson's disease. *J Neurosci Nurs.* 2003;35:242–251.

56. Lees A. Alternatives to levodopa in the initial treatment of early Parkinson's disease. *Drugs Aging.* 2005;22:731–740.

57. Miyasaki JM, Shannon K, Voon V, et al. Practice parameter: evaluation and treatment of depression, psychosis, and dementia in Parkinson disease (and evidence-based review): report of the quality standards subcommittee of the American Academy of Neurology. *Neurology.* 2006;66:996–1002.

58. Parkinson Study Group. Low-dose clozapine for the treatment of drug-induced psychosis in Parkinson's disease. *N Engl J Med.* 1999;340:757–763.

59. French Clozapine Parkinson Study Group. Clozapine in drug-induced psychosis in Parkinson's disease. *Lancet.* 1999;353:2041–2042.

60. Waterhouse EJ, DeLorenzo RJ. Status epilepticus in older patients: Epidemiology and treatment options. *Drugs Aging.* 2001;18(2):133–142.

61. Herman ST. Epilepsy after brain insult. *Neurology.* 2002;59(Suppl):21–26.

62. Hauser WA, Annegers JF. Risk factors for epilepsy. *Epilepsy Res.* 1991;4(Suppl):45–52.

63. Sriven JI, Ozuna J. Diagnosing epilepsy in older adults: what does it mean for the primary care physician? *Geriatrics.* 2005;60:30–35.

64. Pryor FM, Ramsay RE, Rowan AJ. Epilepsy in older adults: update from VA Cooperative Study #428. *Epilepsia.* 2002;43(Suppl 7):165–166.

65. DeLorenzo RJ, Hauser WA, Towne AR, et al. A prospective, population-based epidemiologic study of status epilepticus in Richmond, Virginia. *Neurology.* 1996;46:1029–1035.

66. Waterhouse EJ, Vaughan JK, Barnes TY, et al. Synergistic effect of status epilepticus and ischemic brain injury on mortality. *Epilepsy Res.* 1998;29:175–183.

67. Commission on Classification and Terminology of the International League Against Epilepsy. Proposal for revised clinical and electroencephalographic classification of epileptic seizures. *Epilepsia.* 1981;22:489–501.

68. Commission on Classification and Terminology of the International League Against Epilepsy. Proposal for revised classification of epilepsies and epileptic syndromes. *Epilepsia.* 1989;30:389–399.

69. Gidal BE, Garnett WR. Epilepsy. In: DiPiro JT, ed. *Pharmacotherapy: A Pathophysiology Approach, 6th edition.* New York: McGraw-Hill; 2005:1023–1048.

70. Poza JJ. Management of epilepsy in the elderly. *Neuropsychiatr Dis Treat.* 2007;3:723–728.

71. Hiyoshi T, Yagi K. Epilepsy in the elderly. *Epilepsia.* 2000;41(Suppl 9):31–35.

72. Lackner TE. Strategies for optimizing antiepileptic drug therapy in elderly people. *Pharmacotherapy.* 2002;22:329–364.

73. French JA, Kanner AM, Bautista J, et al. Efficacy and tolerability of the new antiepileptic drugs I: Treat-

ment of new onset epilepsy: Report of the therapeutics and technology assessment subcommittee and quality standards subcommittee of the American Academy of Neurology and the American Epilepsy Society. *Neurology*. 2004;62:1252–1260.

74. French JA, Kanner AM, Bautista J, et al. Efficacy and tolerability of the new antiepileptic drugs II: Treatment of refractory epilepsy: Report of the therapeutics and technology assessment subcommittee and quality standards subcommittee of the American Academy of Neurology and the American Epilepsy Society. *Neurology*. 2004;62:1261–1273.

75. Lammers MW, Hekster YA, Keyser A, et al. Monotherapy or polytherapy for epilepsy revisited: a quantitative assessment. *Epilepsia*. 1995;36:440–446.

76. Marson AG, Al-Kharusi AM, Alwaidh M, et al. The SANAD study of effectiveness of carbamazepine, gabapentin, lamotrigine, oxcarbazepine, or topiramate for treatment of partial epilepsy: an unblinded, randomized controlled trial. *Lancet*. 2007;369:1000–1015.

77. Marson AG, Al-Kharusi AM, Alwaidh M, et al. The SANAD study of effectiveness of valproate, lamotrigine, or topiramate for generalised and unclassifiable epilepsy: an unblinded randomised controlled trial. *Lancet*. 2007;369:1016–1026.

78. Sander JWAS, Shorvon SD. Epidemiology of the epilepsies. *J Neurol Neurosurg Psychiatr*. 1996;61:433–443.

79. Kutluay E, McCague K, D'Souza J, Beydoun A. Safety and tolerability of oxcarbazepine in elderly patients with epilepsy. *Epilepsy Behav*. 2003;4:175–180.

80. Rowan AJ, Ramsay RE, Collins JF, et al. New onset geriatric epilepsy: a randomized study of gabapentin, lamotrigine and carbamazepine. *Neurology*. 2005;64:1868–1873.

81. Brodie MJ, Overstall PW, Giorgi L, the UK Lamotrigine Elderly Study Group. Multicentre, double-blind, randomised comparison between lamotrigine and carbamazepine in elderly patients with newly diagnosed epilepsy. *Epilepsy Res*. 1999;37:81–97.

82. Evans BK, Kustra RP, Hammer AE. Assessment of tolerability in elderly patients: changing to lamotrigine therapy. *Am J Geriatr Pharmacother*. 2007;5:112–119.

83. Saetre E, Perucca E, Isojarvi J, Gjerstad L, on behalf of the LAM 40089 Study Group. An international multicenter randomized double-blind controlled trial of lamotrigine and sustained-release carbamazepine in the treatment of newly diagnosed epilepsy in the elderly. *Epilepsia*. 2007;48:1292–1302.

84. Gilad R, Sadeh M, Rapoport A, Dabby R, Boaz M, Lampl Y. Monotherapy of lamotrigine versus carbamazepine in patients with poststroke seizure. *Clin Neuropharmacol*. 2007;30:189–195.

85. Stefan H, Hubbertz L, Peglau I, et al. Epilepsy outcomes in elderly treated with topiramate. *Acta Neurol Scand*. 2008;118:164–174.

86. Groselj J, Guerrini R, Van Oene J, et al. Experience with topiramate monotherapy in elderly patients with recent-onset epilepsy. *Acta Neurol Scand*. 2005;112:14–150.

87. Dogan EA, Usta BE, Bilgen R, et al. Efficacy, tolerability, and side effects of oxcarbazepine monotherapy: a prospective study in adult and elderly patients with newly diagnosed partial epilepsy. *Epilepsy Behav*. 2008;13:156–161.

88. Kutlu G, Gomceli YB, Unal Y, Inan LE. Levetiracetam monotherapy for late poststroke seizures in the elderly. *Epilepsy Behav*. 2008;13:542–544.

89. Alsaadi TM, Koopmans S, Apperson M, Farias S. Levetiracetam monotherapy for elderly patients with epilepsy. *Seizure*. 2004;13:58–60.

90. Belcastro V, Costa C, Galletti F, et al. Levetiracetam monotherapy in Alzheimer's patients with late-onset seizures: a prospective observational study. *Euro J Neurol*. 2007;14:1176–1178.

91. Ramsay R, Rowan A, Slater J, et al. Effects of age on epilepsy and its treatment: results of the VA Cooperative Study. *Epilepsia*. 2004;35(Suppl 8):91.

92. Baker GA, Jacoby A, Buck D, et al. The quality of life of older people with epilepsy: findings from a UK community study. *Seizure*. 2001;10:92–99.

93. Plassman BL, Langa KM, Fisher GG, et al. Prevalence of cognitive impairment without dementia in the United States. *Ann Intern Med*. 2008;148(6):427–434.

94. Plassman BL, Langa KM, Fisher GG, et al. Prevalence of dementia in the United States: the aging, demographics, and memory study. *Neuroepidemiology*. 2007;29(1–2):125–132.

95. Lexi-Comp Online™, Lexi-Drugs Online™, Hudson, Ohio: Lexi-Comp, Inc.; 2009; June 19, 2009.

96. Berg AT, Vickrey BG, Testa FM, et al. How long does it take for epilepsy to become intractable? A prospective investigation. *Ann Neurol*. 2006;60:73–79.

13

Psychiatric Disorders

MONICA MATHYS AND MYRA T. BELGERI

Learning Objectives

1. Recognize the DSM-IV criteria for major depressive disorder, generalized anxiety disorder and panic disorder and features commonly observed in late-life depression and anxiety.

2. Recommend an appropriate treatment plan for a geriatric patient suffering from depression and/or anxiety.

3. Recognize the changes in sleep that occur with normal aging and the impact of insomnia on an elderly patient's health and quality of life.

4. Recommend appropriate therapy for insomnia based upon published evidence in the elderly patient.

5. Describe the limitations of the DSM-IV criteria for substance abuse and dependence when used to diagnose elderly patients with substance use disorders.

6. List the alcohol drinking limits for geriatric patients and discuss the reasons why guidelines suggest lower limits compared to younger adults.

7. Recommend an appropriate treatment plan for alcohol withdrawal and long-term abstinence for a geriatric patient.

Key Terms

CLINICAL GLOBAL IMPRESSION OF IMPROVEMENT (CGI-I): Seven-point scale which measures how much a patient's symptoms have improved or worsened compared to baseline.

COGNITIVE BEHAVIORAL THERAPY: Therapy focused to help patients correct negative thoughts associated with depression and to cope with anxiety disorders. The therapy includes breathing retraining, muscle relaxation, cognitive restructuring to focus on the consistent worrying, and graded exposure so the patient can learn how to cope in stressful/phobic situations.

EARLY-ONSET ALCOHOLISM/ABUSE/DEPENDENCE: Alcohol abuse/dependence in which onset occurs before the age of 50.

HAMILTON RATING SCALE FOR ANXIETY (HAM-A): Fourteen-item assessment tool appropriate for measuring symptom severity and treatment response for GAD.

INTERPERSONAL PSYCHOTHERAPY: Therapy focused on finding and dealing with interpersonal causes of depression.

LATE-LIFE ANXIETY: Anxiety episode which occurs when a patient is an older adult.

LATE-LIFE DEPRESSION: Depressive episode which occurs when a patient is an older adult.

LATE-LIFE SUBSTANCE ABUSE/DEPENDENCE: Substance abuse or dependence in an older adult.

LATE-ONSET ALCOHOLISM/ABUSE/DEPENDENCE: Alcohol abuse/dependence in which onset occurs at or after the age of 50.

LATE-ONSET DEPRESSION: Major depression in which the first depressive episode occurs when the patient is an older adult. He/she has never had a depressive episode as a younger adult.

PARTIAL RESPONSE: Less than 50% reduction in symptoms.

PROBLEM-SOLVING THERAPY: Therapy which focuses on helping the patients learn strategies for solving everyday problems associated with their depression.

RECURRENCE: New episode of depression 6 months or longer after achieving remission.

RELAPSE: Increase in depressive symptoms within 6 months from remission.

REMISSION: Asymptomatic state.

RESPONSE: 50% reduction in symptoms.

SLEEP LATENCY: Amount of time required to initiate sleep.

SUPPORTIVE THERAPY: Therapy which focuses on providing an environment in which patients can discuss and be open about their symptoms and causes of depression.

Introduction

Psychiatric disorders discussed in this chapter include depression, anxiety, insomnia and substance abuse. Although diagnostic criteria are the same as for younger adults for these disorders, it is sometimes difficult to elicit clear symptoms of depression or anxiety from older patients, especially if they have underlying dementia. Luckily, newer pharmacologic agents add options that are better tolerated in individuals with co-morbidities, multiple medications and altered pharmacodynamics.

Sleep architecture changes with aging; co-morbidities and the environment contribute to insomnia in the elderly patient. If underlying factors cannot be corrected and non-pharmacologic therapy is not effective, medications may help the patient achieve sleep goals. However, it is important to choose drug therapy that will minimize adverse events and for the patient to understand how these agents work to set proper expectations.

Finally, substance and alcohol abuse should not be dismissed as a possible health issue in older adults. Alcohol withdrawal can be life-threatening in any age group and is even more of a risk for individuals with heart or lung disease. Psychosocial interventions appropriate to older age groups may be coupled with pharmacologic treatment to maintain sobriety.

Depression
Etiology, Epidemiology, and Clinical Presentation Specific To Geriatrics

Epidemiology

Depression is the most common psychiatric disorder diagnosed in the elderly with approximately 5% to 15% of community-based elderly individuals meeting criteria for major depressive disorder rising to 6% to 32% in the nursing home population.[1,2] Often times, a depressive episode witnessed in older adults is a **recurrence** of the disorder that was diagnosed as a young adult. However, 30% of cases are noted to be purely late-onset depression.[2]

Common late-life diseases such as cerebral vascular disease, cardiovascular disease, and dementia often coexist or precipitate late-onset depression.[3,4] For patients who have suffered a stroke, major depression is noted to develop in 15–25% of individuals.[4] Left-sided stroke is associated with early onset of symptoms (≤ 3 months) while right-sided stroke is more likely to result in later-onset depression.[5] Approximately 25% of patients who experience a myocardial infarction or undergo cardiac catheterization develop major depression.[3] The prevalence of depression in patients with Alzheimer's dementia is approximately 17% and noted to be higher in those with subcortical dementias.[3]

Physiologic Changes Associated with Late-Life Depression

Physiologic factors that may predispose individuals to **late-life depression** include abnormalities in the frontostriatal region, amygdala, and hippocampus. These abnormalities may be a result of one or both of the following factors: (1) age-related changes such as a decline in neurons and receptors within the central nervous system and (2) disease-related changes such as increased cortisol levels (often observed in those with chronic illnesses), inflammation, and ischemia.[3]

Research has shown that executive dysfunction and inattention are caused by frontostriatal abnormalities. Executive dysfunction and inattention are often observed in late-onset depression and continue to be present even after treatment of the depressive symptoms. Other depressive symptoms possibly associated with frontostriatal deficits include psychomotor retardation and apathy.[2,3] The most likely cause of frontostriatal impairment is cerebrovascular disease, therefore, this type of late-onset depression is labeled "vascular depression."[2]

Abnormalities of the amygdala also predispose patients to depression. Larger amygdala volumes are observed in older adults experiencing a first episode of depression compared to nondepressed patients or those with recurring depression. Increased output from the amygdala leads to increased cortisol levels which over time can lead to depression and negative emotion.[3]

It is also theorized that abnormal hippocampal activity may be associated with late-life depression although the mechanism is not clearly defined. Studies have shown hippocampal volume to decline with depressive episodes and the degree of decline appears to correlate with the duration of depression over a person's lifetime.[2-3]

Diagnostic Criteria

While many clinicians screen for depression using the Geriatric Depression Scale as discussed in Chapter 4, diagnosis is made using criteria from the *Diagnostics and Statistical Manual of Mental Disorders*, 4th edition (DSM-IV).[6] A patient meets the criteria for major depressive disorder if he/she experiences either depressed mood or decreased interest or pleasure in usual activities and meets at least four of the following criteria: significant appetite and weight changes, increased agitation or motor retardation, loss of energy, changes in sleep (insomnia or hypersomnia), feelings of guilt or worthlessness, problems with memory or concentration, or thoughts of suicide. According to the DSM-IV, symptoms must exist almost daily for at least 2 weeks, lead to functional impairment, and not be the result of substance abuse, medical conditions, or bereavement.[6] Normal bereavement usually does not lead to depression, but patients who have experienced a major loss within the last 6–8 weeks with functional impairment should be assessed for depressive symptoms. If present, then treatment is often recommended.[7]

Other mood disorders such as dysthymia or minor depression are frequently assessed in the geriatric population and about 25% of these cases will develop into major depression within 2 years.[3] Minor depressive disorder is defined as having at least two but fewer than five of the symptoms listed under major depressive disorder for 2 weeks or longer. Dysthymia is described as a sad mood on most days with two other symptoms listed under major depressive disorder lasting for 2 years or more. To meet the criteria for depressive disorders, patients cannot have a history of mania or psychotic disorders.[6]

Assessment and Presentation

Issues often coexisting with late-life depression include multiple comorbidities, chronic pain, disability, and cognitive impairment. Common social stressors include loss of spouse, forced relocation (e.g., being forced to move in with family, assisted-living, or nursing home placement), and retirement which may lead to decreased self-worth, boredom, and loss of income.[3,7]

Elderly depressed patients often complain of decreased concentration and show deficits in mental processing speed and executive function. These deficits often improve after treatment of depression (therefore sometimes referred to as pseudodementia) but evidence suggests mild cognitive dysfunction does not always resolve completely. In fact, individuals who develop late-life depression and cognitive impairment have a higher risk of developing true dementia.[3,8] Elderly patients with depression are more likely to present to their health provider complaining of somatic complaints such as vague aches and pains and may not realize or mention anything about depressed mood. This leads to a delayed diagnosis and treatment since providers are often focused on treating the physical complaints of the patient.[9]

If depression is left untreated, symptoms may persist for years and result in decreased daily function, poor quality of life, and increased rates of suicide and nonsuicidal mortality.[9-14] One of the more recent large epidemiologic studies found that depressed elderly patients had a significantly increased relative risk of 1.67 for impairment of activities of daily living and 1.73 for mobility impairment compared to non-depressed elderly.[14] Over the last two decades, there have been several studies showing a correlation with depression and increased cardiovascular mortality.[9,11,13]

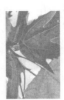

KEY POINT: When cognitive impairment is observed with a late-life depressive episode, the patient may be at higher risk for dementia later in life.

Suicide Risk

Age is a major risk factor for suicide. Suicidal ideation appears to occur more frequently in younger adults but completed suicides are highest among older men.[7] The use of a firearm is the most common method of death for elderly suicide patients.[15] Risk factors for suicidal behavior in older adults include (1) a coexisting psychiatric disorder, (2) substance abuse, (3) a coexisting personality disorder, (4) chronic medical illness, (5) poor coping mechanisms, (6) loneliness/isolation, and (7) functional impairment.[5,7,15]

Recent data suggest antidepressant medications may increase the risk of suicidal ideation in adolescents and young adults. However, this risk has not been observed in older adults. In fact, data suggest antidepressants may have a protective effect against suicidal ideation in the older population.[16]

Summary of Standard Treatment in the Adult Population

When depression is suspected, the duration and severity of symptoms should be assessed and a treatment history addressing current and past therapies (nonpharmacologic and pharmacologic) should be performed. A physical examination, laboratory tests, and a thorough medical history should be obtained in order to assess whether medical conditions or medications may be worsening depressive symptoms (Table 13-1).[7]

Symptom **remission** rather than just **response** should be the optimal goal for clinicians and their patients. The large, multicenter STAR-D (Sequenced Treatment Alternatives to Relieve Depression) study showed patients who achieved remission were more likely to have increased daily function and less risk of **relapse** in the long-term compared to those who only achieved a response with treatment.[17]

Psychotherapy should be discussed as a treatment option and patients should also be aware that it can often be used without drug therapy for

Table 13-1. Medical Conditions and Medications Associated with Depression, Anxiety, and Insomnia[3,5,54,57,71,74,76,85,142]

Medical Conditions	Medications
Depression	
Thyroid disorders	Benzodiazepines
Malignant Disease	Beta Blockers
Cerebrovascular Disease	Steroids
Myocardial Infarction	Cimetidine
B12 deficiency	Clonidine
Malnutrition	Hydralazine
Diabetes Mellitus	Tamoxifen
Parkinson's Disease	Opioid analgesics
Multiple Sclerosis	Anticonvulsants
Chronic Pain	
HIV/AIDS	
Anxiety	
Hyperthyroidism	Theophylline
Heart Failure	Alcohol withdrawal
Pulmonary Embolism	Benzodiazepine withdrawal
Angina	Caffeine
Arrhythmias	Sympathomimetics
Chronic Obstructive Pulmonary Disease	Steroids
Parkinson's Disease	Thyroid hormones
Stroke	Anticholinergics
	Antidepressants (initiation of therapy)
Insomnia	
Benign prostatic hyperplasia	Alcohol
Cardiovascular disease	Anticholinergics
Chronic kidney disease	Antidepressants
Congestive heart failure	Antihistamines,
Chronic obstructive pulmonary disease	Benzodiazepines
Chronic pain	Beta agonists
Dementia	Corticosteroids
Depression	Decongestants,
Malignancy	Diuretics
Nasal problems	Nicotine
Nocturnal wheezing	Xanthines
Parkinson's disease	
Restless Leg Syndrome	
Sleep apnea	
Stroke	
Thyroid disease	

mild depression. According to recent treatment guidelines,[18] any second generation antidepressant (SSRI, SNRI, bupropion, or mirtazapine) can be used as a first-line agent when drug treatment is needed. If a response is seen after 4 to 6 weeks of therapy and the patient is tolerating the medication, then therapy should be continued. If only a **partial response** is observed then the current antidepressant dose should be increased further or an additional agent can be added with the current therapy for augmentation. Recommended agents for augmentation include another second generation antidepressant that has a different mechanism of action, liothyronine (T3), or buspirone. In cases where no response is seen with the first-line agent, then the patient should switch to another antidepressant preferably one from a different drug class. When switching agents, cross-tapering is recommended. TCAs, monoamine oxidase inhibitors, lithium and atypical antipsychotic augmentation are recommended as third and fourth line treatments after patients have failed at least two trials with second generation antidepressants.

Using the results from the STAR-D study[17] as reference, clinicians can assume 30% of patients are likely to achieve remission (~ 50% will have a response) after taking one antidepressant for 12 weeks. For patients who move on to a level 2 treatment (augmentation agent or switching antidepressants), approximately 20% more will obtain remission. For resistant patients, third and fourth round treatments can be beneficial but achieving remission continues to be difficult.[17]

Once remission has been achieved, treatment should continue for at least 6 to 9 months. Long-term therapy is recommended for patients who have had multiple episodes of depression in order to decrease the chance for recurrence.[18]

Review of Evidence Supporting Treatment Recommendations for Geriatric Patients

Evidence-based treatment options for depression in elderly patients also include psychotherapy and antidepressant medications. Medications are frequently prescribed in both the outpatient and institutionalized setting. However, psychotherapy

has been shown to have equivalent efficacy compared to antidepressants in older adults with 45 to 70% having clinical improvement.[19] Combination therapy including both psychotherapy and antidepressant therapy has shown to be most efficacious for severe or chronic depression.[20-21]

For mild depression, either psychotherapy alone or medication therapy alone can be used for treatment. Methods of psychotherapy which have shown clinical efficacy in late-life depression include **cognitive behavioral therapy, interpersonal psychotherapy, supportive therapy** and problem-solving therapy. Therapy is usually provided for at least 6 to 12 treatments and is highly recommended for patients refusing pharmacologic treatment or for those who have not responded or only partially responded to drug therapy.[22]

When depression is assessed as moderate, medication treatment is strongly recommended with or without psychotherapy. Combination therapy of psychotherapy and antidepressant is recommended for severe or chronic depression.[23]

To date there have been several positive studies[24-30] supporting SSRI therapy for treatment of late-life depression. The mean age of patients in these studies ranged from 67–75 years, and rates ranged from 35–89% for response, 19-72% for remission and 9–32% for recurrence.

These agents appear to be as efficacious in the elderly as first generation agents such as tricyclic antidepressants[5] but they are associated with fewer adverse effects and are safer in overdose situations.[9,31,32] SSRI and SNRI antidepressants are recommended as first-line agents for elderly patients due to adequate efficacy data and their low risk for serious adverse effects.[5,23] When initiating antidepressant treatment, a low dose should be started but therapy should continue to be titrated to a moderate dose to receive an adequate response. A recent meta-analysis addressing antidepressant efficacy showed medication response is most likely to be observed after 10 to 12 weeks of therapy (versus 6 weeks in younger adults).[32] However, literature also suggests approximately two thirds of patients who do respond to antidepressants are likely to report partial improvement after 4 weeks of therapy.[33]

If only a partial response is observed after 12 weeks of an appropriate treatment dose of the initial antidepressant treatment, then augmentation with an additional agent is recommended.[23] Although studies which focus on dual pharmacotherapy in late-life depression are lacking there is one recent study which supports augmentation in older patients.[34] During this study, patients 70 years and older who had an inadequate response after 12 weeks of paroxetine were augmented with either bupropion sustained-release, lithium, or nortriptyline. Fifty percent of these patients achieved a full response after 28 weeks of augmentation.

Consensus guidelines state the augmenting agent should be another antidepressant in a different drug class than the initial medication.[23] Low-dose lithium is also mentioned in the guidelines as a possible choice for augmentation. However, this medication must be used cautiously due to risk of toxicity mainly caused by age-related decline in glomerular filtration. Studies have suggested that older adults are more likely to relapse or have a recurrence of depression sooner after adequate treatment compared to younger adults.[35] Therefore, maintenance therapy should continue for at least one year after remission is achieved. Maintenance therapy for 1 to 3 years is suggested for patients with more than one depressive episode.[23]

Electroconvulsive Therapy

A number of studies have shown electroconvulsive therapy (ECT) to be effective in late-life depression with efficacy rates ranging from 60 to 80 percent.[36-38] This treatment is indicated for treatment-resistant depression or for patients at high risk of serious harm because of psychotic depression or suicidal ideation. ECT is usually administered three times weekly for 2 to 6 weeks (total of 6–12 treatments) in an inpatient psychiatric setting, which limits its utilization. Common adverse effects include headache, temporary amnesia and cognitive impairment. Permanent memory loss of the events surrounding the ECT treatments is a rare event but can occur.[7] After ECT treatment is completed, maintenance therapy with an antidepressant medication is recommended to decrease the risk of relapse.[39]

Common Problems Encountered When Treating Elderly Patients

Selective Serotonin Reuptake Inhibitors (SSRIs)

Overall, SSRIs do not antagonize muscarinic, histaminic, or adrenergic receptors. Therefore, the common adverse effects observed with tricyclic antidepressants and monoamine oxidase inhibitors are not usually a concern with most SSRI agents.[9] The exception is paroxetine. Paroxetine has moderate antimuscarinic activity and this is one reason it is not recommended as a first-line SSRI for the elderly.[9] Case reports of prolonged QT interval associated with SSRI use are reported, however, cardiotoxicity is rare with this drug class. Common adverse effects associated with SSRIs are due to increased activity at serotonin receptors. Gastrointestinal symptoms such as nausea, vomiting, and diarrhea are frequently noted. SSRIs are also associated with sexual dysfunction, appetite suppression, and sleep changes (both hypersomnia and insomnia).[9,31] Fluoxetine is associated with more anxiety and agitation compared to other SSRIs. Because of these adverse effects and its long half-life, fluoxetine is not considered a first-line SSRI for older adults.[40]

There are particular SSRI adverse effects more prevalent in the elderly population compared to younger adults. These include hyponatremia, extrapyramidal adverse effects, and increased bleeding. SSRI-induced hyponatremia occurs in 10–15% of older adults and is more common in women. Paroxetine appears to have the highest incidence within this class. The hyponatremia is likely the result of increased secretion of antidiuretic hormone. Extrapyramidal side effects such as parkinsonism, dystonia, and akathisia are observed in 10% of older adults taking SSRI therapy. These effects are possibly due to decreased nigrostriatal dopaminergic transmission indirectly caused by increase serotonin activity. Bleeding risk appears to be higher in elderly patients who take SSRIs compared to younger adults. Gastrointestinal bleed risk is increased when these agents are taken concurrently with nonsteroidal anti-inflammatory drugs. Bleeding risk is possibly due to SSRIs preventing platelet reuptake of serotonin and resulting in decreased platelet action.[9,31] Bleeding risk should be seriously assessed and monitored closely especially for patients taking antiplatelets and anticoagulants concurrently with SSRI therapy.

All SSRIs are metabolized by cytochrome P450 enzymes. Paroxetine significantly inhibits 2D6 isoenzymes while fluoxetine inhibits 2D6, 3A4 and 1A2 making these two agents more likely to interact with other medications. Sertraline weakly inhibits 2D6 at higher doses and citalopram and escitalopram have very little inhibition activity, often making these three agents the preferred ones for elderly patients taking multiple medications.[31]

Serotonin and Norepinephrine Reuptake Inhibitors

Venlafaxine and duloxetine result in increased levels of serotonin and norepinephrine in the synaptic cleft by inhibiting the reuptake of these neurotransmitters back into the presynaptic neuron. Patients who fail to respond to SSRIs may find efficacy with SNRIs due to the dual neurotransmitter effect. These agents may also be beneficial for patients with concurrent neuropathic pain or fibromyalgias.[7] Studies[41-44] have shown venlafaxine and duloxetine to be efficacious and well-tolerated in the elderly although one trial did suggest that venlafaxine may be less well tolerated in the frail elderly compared to SSRIs.[45]

Serotonergic adverse effects such as gastrointestinal upset, sexual dysfunction, and sleep changes are commonly observed with SNRIs. Cases of hyponatremia have also been noted with venlafaxine use. Typically SNRIs should be given in the morning because of the risk of insomnia if given at bedtime. These agents are also associated with elevated blood pressure at high doses (risk is greater for venlafaxine vs. duloxetine); therefore, blood pressure should be monitored regularly with therapy.[9]

Both venlafaxine and duloxetine are metabolized by the cytochrome P-450 isoenzymes. Venlafaxine has very weak inhibition and duloxetine has moderate inhibition at the 2D6 pathway. However, these effects have not been shown to be clinically significant in most cases. Overall, venlafaxine and duloxetine can be used in older patients taking multiple medications without cause

of concern, though dosage recommendations should follow the standard recommendation in older adults to, "Start low and go slow, but go."[31]

Bupropion and Mirtazapine

Bupropion inhibits the reuptake of dopamine and norepinephrine in the CNS causing an increase in these neurotransmitters in the neuronal synaptic cleft. Because of bupropion's mechanism of action, it is the most activating agent compared to other antidepressants. Doses should not be taken at night because of the risk of insomnia. Due to limited data in the elderly,[46] it is difficult to label bupropion's role in late-life depression. However, it may be useful for depression associated with apathy, lack of motivation, and hypersomnia.[3,7] Recent data suggests bupropion may have a role in augmentation therapy when used in treatment-resistant depression.[34]

Common adverse effects of bupropion include tremors, nervousness, and elevated blood pressure and pulse. Bupropion is contraindicated in patients with a history of seizures and should not be used in patients with anxiety disorders. Compared to other antidepressants, bupropion is most likely to cause appetite suppression and weight loss and therefore should be used cautiously in elderly patients who have decreased oral intake. When using the medication, blood pressure and pulse should be monitored regularly.[3,5,7]

Mirtazapine acts as a central alpha antagonist resulting in increased release of serotonin and norepinephrine in the CNS. This agent is also a potent antagonist of histamine receptors and therefore causes sedation and increased appetite. Compared to the quantity of SSRIs and SNRIs data, there is significantly less published information regarding the efficacy of mirtazapine in late-life depression. However, small studies do suggest mirtazapine is as effective as all other antidepressants in first-line therapy and may be useful for depressed elderly who also have decreased oral intake or insomnia.[47,48]

Tricyclic Antidepressants

In general, tricyclic antidepressants work similarly to SNRIs by inhibiting the reuptake of both serotonin and norepinephrine. However, each tricyclic agent has varying degrees of potency on the reuptake transporters making some agents more serotonergic and others more noradrenergic in action. Tricyclic antidepressants are effective but are less well tolerated in older adults compared to SSRIs and SNRIs.[9,49] These agents also inhibit cardiac Na/K ATPase pump and act as antagonists at alpha, muscarinic, and histaminic receptors which can lead to significant adverse effects. Tricyclic antidepressants can worsen symptoms of chronic conditions such as benign prostate hyperplasia, urinary retention, constipation, cognitive impairment, glaucoma, orthostatic hypotension, cardiac disease, and arrhythmias.[7,9]

Secondary amines such as nortriptyline and desipramine are associated with less anticholinergic, antihistaminic, and orthostatic hypotension compared to the tertiary amines. However, cardiac toxicity is equal among both groups of drugs.[9,31] Compared to the other classes of antidepressants, tricyclic antidepressants are more likely to be fatal in overdose situations. Even though tricyclic antidepressants have been proven to be efficacious for late-life depression, they should not be used as first line therapy due to the high risk of adverse effects.[5,40] If tricyclic therapy is necessary then nortriptyline is usually recommended.[46] Nortriptyline has data to support its efficacy as monotherapy[25,43] and as an augmentation agent[34,50] for patients who fail SSRI therapy. Drug levels should be obtained and monitored. A concentration of 80–120 ng/L is the goal range for efficacy and safety.[50]

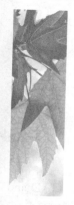

KEY POINT: The benefits of using SSRI therapy as a first line agent for late-life depression outweigh the risks. However, geriatric patients are at higher risk of developing hyponatremia, extrapyramidal adverse effects, and gastrointestinal bleeding with SSRI therapy compared to younger adults.

Anxiety

Etiology, Epidemiology, and Clinical Presentation Specific to Geriatrics

Compared to late-life depression, fewer studies exist and less is known about the presentation, treatment, and prognosis of **late-life anxiety** disorders.[51] The most recent epidemiologic data[52,53] found the prevalence rates of anxiety disorders ranged from 10% to 15% in older adults. This recent data suggests the prevalence of anxiety is higher than what is observed in younger adults. However, the majority of older adults with anxiety did not have pure anxiety but also suffered from depression with anxiety symptoms.

Comorbid anxiety and depression are observed three times more often than pure anxiety.[51,54] The prevalence of older adults with depression who also suffer from an anxiety disorder is approximately 35%.[55] Elderly patients with both depression and generalized anxiety disorder are more likely to have severe depressive symptoms and suicidal ideation compared to those only suffering from depression.[55] In addition, older adults suffering from any anxiety disorder with depression suffer from lower social functioning and increased health services compared to elderly patients with pure anxiety.[56]

Anxiety disorders is a broad term which includes multiple individual disorders such as generalized anxiety disorder (GAD), panic disorder, specific phobias, social anxiety disorder, obsessive-compulsive disorder (OCD), acute stress disorder, and post-traumatic stress disorder (PTSD).[6] Two of the most common anxiety diagnoses observed in the elderly in which pharmacotherapy plays a major role in treatment are generalized anxiety disorder and panic disorder. Therefore, these two disorders will be the focus of this chapter section.

Diagnostic Criteria and Presentation Specific to Geriatric Patients

Generalized Anxiety Disorder

According to the DSM-IV, an individual meets criteria for generalized anxiety disorder (GAD) if he/she continues to have excessive worry over 6 months about a number of situations and continues to experience at least 3 of the following symptoms: (1) restlessness, (2) fatigue, (3) trouble concentrating, (4) irritability, (5) muscle tension, or (6) sleep disturbance. An individual with GAD also finds it difficult to control worry and experiences significant distress and impairment of daily function.[6]

The Amsterdam Longitudinal Aging Study[2] reported 7.3 % of older adults met DSM-IV criteria for GAD with approximately 1% having pure GAD without other psychiatric diagnoses. Episodes of late-life GAD are found to be an even combination of chronic patients who report having anxiety symptoms since early adulthood and patients whose symptoms started in late-life.[51,54] Older adults with late-onset GAD often present to their primary care provider complaining of unexplained physical symptoms such as fatigue, aches, pains, gastrointestinal symptoms, or trouble sleeping which may result in a delay of the correct diagnosis.[54]

Panic Disorder

For an individual to be diagnosed with panic disorder, he/she must have a history of experiencing a panic attack. A panic attack is defined as a specific period of intense fear or discomfort in which at least four of the following symptoms develop: (1) heart palpitations, (2) sweating, (3) trembling/shaking, (4) chills or hot flashes, (5) shortness of breath or sensation of being smothered, (6) feeling of choking, (7) chest pain, (8) gastrointestinal distress, (9) paresthesias, (10) dizziness or lightheadedness, (11) depersonalization, (12) fear of losing control, or (13) fear of dying. An attack will generally peak within 10 minutes and last 20-30 minutes.[6]

Patients with a history of panic attacks often worry about future attacks and the outcome if an attack were to happen in public. Panic disorder can lead to agoraphobia in which an individual becomes anxious and fearful of places in which he/she cannot escape easily if a panic attack were to occur. This can make the individual fearful of leaving the house and going to public places, resulting in social isolation.[57]

Panic disorder without comorbid psychiatric diagnoses is found to be prevalent in 0.1 to 1% of

the elderly population and is diagnosed more frequently in women.[52,53,57] However, a more recent study noted 9.3 % of depressed elderly also met criteria for panic disorder.[55] Most older adults diagnosed with panic disorder have had symptoms since early adulthood and many have not had adequate treatment through the years. New onset of panic disorder in late-life is rare.[51,57] Studies have shown panic attacks in older adults tend to be less frequent and the severity of symptoms and avoidant behavior is less compared to younger adults with the disorder.[58-60]

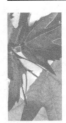 KEY POINT: There is a high prevalence of comorbid depression with late-life anxiety. Patients who meet diagnostic criteria for anxiety should also be screened for major depressive disorder.

Summary of Standard Treatment in the Adult Population

Goals of treatment for all patients with anxiety disorders include decreasing anxiety severity, improving level of function, and obtaining remission. For patients with panic disorder, goals also include decreasing the frequency of panic attacks and treating phobic avoidance.[61,62]

For acute treatment, benzodiazepines are the only pharmacologic treatment available with a quick onset of action. Benzodiazepines may also need to be used for chronic treatment for patients who obtain only a partial response with antidepressants. Guidelines recommend SSRIs and SNRIs as first-line agents for the chronic treatment of GAD and primarily SSRIs for the treatment of panic disorder. If first-line agents are ineffective then tricyclic antidepressants can be tried. Buspirone can also be considered as a second or third-line agent for chronic treatment of GAD. Once an adequate response is achieved, treatment should continue for 3–10 months for GAD and 12–24 months for panic disorder. Long-term therapy is recommended for patients with multiple episodes of anxiety.[61-62]

Cognitive-behavioral therapy (CBT) has been shown to be equally efficacious for treatment of anxiety disorders compared to pharmacotherapy for younger adults and if available, patients may choose this option over drug therapy. Combination therapy can be useful for those with severe agoraphobia or for those who only partially respond to either treatment alone.[61,62]

Review of Evidence Supporting Treatment Recommendations for Geriatric Patients

Psychotherapy

Although drug therapy is often recommended for late-life anxiety, psychotherapy may also be efficacious and be preferred for older adults who are sensitive to medication adverse effects or trying to avoid polypharmacy. Cognitive-behavioral therapy (CBT) is the most studied psychotherapy in older adults with anxiety and may include breathing retraining, muscle relaxation, cognitive restructuring to focus on the consistent worrying, and graded exposure so the patient can learn how to cope in stressful/phobic situations.[54]

Study results regarding the efficacy of CBT for anxious elderly patients are conflicting. Several small studies have found CBT to be no more or even less useful than supportive therapy. Past research has also suggested that CBT therapy may be less efficacious for older adults than younger adults with GAD.[54] However a recent meta-analysis[63] which included these small studies found CBT significantly reduced anxiety symptoms compared to the active control groups.

Antidepressants

Many of the SSRIs and SNRIs are FDA labeled for anxiety disorders and considered first-line treatment for chronic management of anxiety in the adult population. There is limited data addressing these antidepressants and their efficacy in late-life anxiety, but they are still commonly prescribed by geriatric clinicians because of their low risk of serious adverse effects.[51] Agents which have clinical data supporting their use in the elderly with anxiety disorders include citalopram and venlafaxine, although sertraline, escitalopram, paroxetine, mirtazapine, and duloxetine have proven effective in younger adult populations.

Katz and colleagues[64] investigated the efficacy and tolerability of venlafaxine extended-release for treatment of GAD in elderly patients. The researchers performed a retrospective review of data from five randomized placebo-controlled trials. Data pertaining to the older adults (≥ 60 years of age) enrolled in the studies was collected. All five studies were at least 8 weeks in duration and two of them continued through 24 weeks. Overall, the researchers found that assessment score changes from baseline to follow-up for the intention-to-treat group were not significantly different compared to placebo. One assessment score, the **Clinical Global Impression of Improvement (CGI-I)**, was the only score that significantly improved among the venlafaxine group compared to placebo. Remission and response rates were noted as secondary objectives. For the intention-to-treat group, response rates were significantly higher according to the CGI-I scale for patients taking venlafaxine at both weeks 8 and 24. When the researchers looked at the **Hamilton Rating Scale for Anxiety (HAM-A)** scores, response rates were only noted to be significantly higher at week 24. Remission rates were not found to be significantly different at either follow-up point. Venlafaxine was found to cause more gastrointestinal adverse effects compared to the placebo group but the overall discontinuation rates were not significantly different.[64]

The authors also noted the outcomes for the younger population (< 60 years of age). Interestingly, patients taking venlafaxine had more improvement compared to the placebo group according to all assessment reports. Also, the younger patients taking venlafaxine continued to have significantly higher response and remission rates through week 8 and 24. These results suggest that a better response to venlafaxine is observed in younger adults compared to older adults. However, one should keep in mind the number of geriatric patients may not have been high enough to meet the power requirement of the study.[64]

Lenze and colleagues lead a randomized, placebo-controlled study of citalopram for the treatment of anxiety disorders in the elderly.[65] Diagnoses of the patients included GAD, panic disorder, and post-traumatic stress disorder, although, a great majority of the patients were diagnosed with GAD. Sixty-five percent of patients assigned to citalopram treatment (dose = 20–30 mg/day) achieved a response by 8 weeks while only 24% in the placebo responded.

After 8 weeks of treatment were completed, the study patients were eligible to continue an open label study of citalopram for 24 more weeks. Patients who responded to citalopram during the first 8 weeks continued to take citalopram and those who were non-responders taking placebo were switched to citalopram for the rest of the long-term study. Those who were taking citalopram and did not respond during the first 8 weeks were omitted from the long-term study. Blank and colleagues[66] published the results of the long-term study and found anxiety rating scale scores continued to improve throughout the study and 60% were responders at the end of the study.

Antidepressants need be taken at a therapeutic dose for 6 weeks before a response will be seen. Initially, these agents may appear to worsen anxiety symptoms by causing jitteriness and activation. Counseling the patient on these transient adverse effects ahead of time is recommended along with frequent follow-up during the first 2 months of therapy. Also, initiating therapy at a low dose and titrating carefully can decrease the severity of adverse effects.[51,54] Additional information regarding which SSRIs are better in the elderly and common adverse effects are discussed above in the depression section of the chapter.

Benzodiazepines

Benzodiazepines have a rapid onset of action and are currently the only option for acute treatment of GAD and panic disorder. These agents are efficacious but can cause significant adverse effects such as excessive sedation, depressed mood, cognitive impairment, tolerance and dependence, amnesia, unstable gait, increase risk for falls, and respiratory depression. Severe withdrawal symptoms such as seizures and exacerbation of anxiety can occur if these agents are suddenly stopped or tapered too quickly. Since the risk of benzodiazepines often outweighs their benefit in the elderly population, they are generally not recommended for long-term use.[51,40] However, a recent study found that over 50% of older adults with anxiety disorders were using a benzodiazepine at baseline and use did not decline over a nine year period suggesting this drug class is still overused.[67]

If a benzodiazepine is needed, lorazepam and oxazepam are the preferred agents due to their short half-life, no active metabolite, and lack of CYP 450 involvement.[51,54] Patients who have been on benzodiazepine therapy for many years may find it difficult to taper off therapy due to worsening anxiety symptoms. In this case, if the medication is not causing significant adverse effects, it may be better for the patient to continue therapy while trying to use the lowest dose possible to control symptoms.[54]

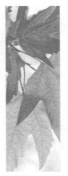

KEY POINT: Generally, the risks of chronic benzodiazepine use outweigh the benefits. However, older patients who have been taking therapy for years find it difficult to discontinue therapy (even with gradual tapering) without anxiety symptoms recurring.

Buspirone

Buspirone works as a partial agonist at the 5-HT_{1A} receptors. Although the medication is efficacious for GAD, it does not work well for panic disorder. Buspirone is not associated with dependence, sedation, depressed respiratory rate, or psychomotor impairment as seen with benzodiazepine therapy. Older studies have shown buspirone to be effective and well-tolerated in the geriatric population. However, buspirone's therapeutic response is less predictable compared to the antidepressants and benzodiazepines. Clinicians must remember buspirone is not quick acting and can take up to 2 to 3 weeks before an effect is observed. The twice to three times a day dosing schedule can often times be burdensome for elderly who have multiple medications to organize.[51,54] Also, buspirone has been shown to be less efficacious for those who have chronically used benzodiazepines in the past.[68] For treatment of GAD, buspirone is considered a second or third line agent for chronic management falling behind antidepressants. If used, the recommended starting dose in older adults is 5 mg twice daily. The dose can be increased by 5 mg every 4–5 days to a target dose of 20–30 mg/day given in divided doses.[54]

Common Problems Encountered When Treating Elderly Patients

Due to the lack of data in older adults, much of the treatment guidelines are extrapolated from data obtained from younger adults.[54,57] When anxiety is suspected, a thorough history of the illness should be obtained and include current symptoms, past symptoms, history of medications used, family history of mental illness and history of substance abuse. Along with a mental status examination, a physical examination with laboratory values should be performed. A full medical history will help decide whether physical factors or medications are contributing to a patient's anxiety (Table 13-1).[51,54]

Because of the high prevalence of psychiatric comorbidity, elderly patients who screen positive for GAD or panic disorder, should also be assessed for depression.[54,57] For patients who meet diagnostic criteria for both major depressive disorder and GAD, a separate diagnosis of GAD is not needed unless it is clear the patient has experienced GAD symptoms outside the depressive episodes.[54]

Due to the conflicting results of CBT in older adults, pharmacotherapy is recommended over psychotherapy for treatment of anxiety.[54] However, CBT can be used as adjunctive treatment or for patients who do not tolerate medications. SSRIs and SNRIs should be considered first-line therapy for long-term treatment of GAD. There is limited efficacy data addressing the use of these agents for anxiety in the elderly. However, the agents have been proven effective in younger adults and there are trials to support that these medications are safe and well-tolerated in the older adults.[51] Doses of the agents should be started low but continue to be titrated to therapeutic doses. If a patient does not respond to the

first-line agent after 6 weeks of therapy, switching to a different class of antidepressant (i.e., switch from an SSRI to a SNRI or vice versa) is recommended.[54] For treatment of panic disorder, SSRIs are first-line for the elderly. Dosing initiation and titration are the same as described above. If a response is not observed after 6 weeks of using a therapeutic dose then a further dose increase is recommended. Once the patient has failed high dose therapy then he/she should be switched to another SSRI.[57]

Because antidepressants take several weeks to induce a response, short-term benzodiazepine use is indicated if the patient needs acute treatment. An antidepressant should be started with the benzodiazepine, and the purpose of each, along with expected outcome should be translated to the patient. After 6 weeks of combination therapy, a tapering schedule for the benzodiazepine should be initiated and eventually discontinued if possible.[51,54] For patients who do not receive adequate anxiety relief with an antidepressants alone, long-term treatment with benzodiazepines may be necessary. In this case, the lowest dose possible to treat symptoms should be used. Agents of choice for older adults include lorazepam (0.5–2 mg/day) and oxazepam (10–30 mg/day).[54]

Once an adequate response is achieved, therapy should be continued for at least one year for late-onset GAD and 12 to 18 months for panic disorder. Elderly with chronic recurrence of anxiety should continue treatment long-term. If anxiety presents with major depressive disorder then treatment duration should be decided by the patient's depression history.[54,57]

Insomnia

Etiology, Epidemiology, and Clinical Presentation Specific to Geriatrics

Insomnia is a condition that can affect patients at any age during their lifetime. It is often assumed that older patients require less sleep, especially since sleep complaints are common in the elderly population. However, insomnia is not a normal characteristic of aging and should be evaluated and treated appropriately.

Many epidemiologic studies have described the prevalence of sleep complaints in elderly patients. Of those residing in the community, about 60% of elderly patients reported some form of disruption of sleep, with nocturnal waking, insomnia, and difficulty falling asleep being the most common.[69] When compared to the younger population (<60 years of age), older patients (>80 years of age) have more complaints regarding waking repeatedly during sleep and having a difficult time getting back to sleep after waking up in the middle of the night.[70] These sleep complaints, if left undiagnosed and untreated, can significantly impact a patient's quality of life.[69-72]

Sleep Changes in the Elderly

On polysomnography, several changes are present in an elderly patient. **Sleep latency**, the amount of time spent in sleep stages 1 and 2, and the number of awakenings after sleep onset increase as the patient ages. On the other hand, total sleep time, sleep efficiency, the amount of time spent in sleep stages 3, 4, and REM, and REM sleep latency decrease.[73] Some risk factors for excessive sleepiness in elderly patients have been associated with decreased time spent in REM sleep and REM sleep latency.[74]

It is unknown whether elderly patients actually require less sleep as compared to when they were younger. The average adult patient requires 7 to 8 hours of sleep, which may remain true for an average elderly patient; however, elderly patients have difficulty sleeping uninterrupted in this 7 to 8 hour period. The amount of time spent in nocturnal sleep diminishes, which may be offset by an increase in naps during the normal waking hours.[75] From midlife until the ninth decade, total sleep time may decrease by an average of 27 minutes per decade.[76]

Sleep initiation and sleep maintenance become problematic as a patient ages: total sleep time diminishes despite more time spent lying in bed, sleep efficiency decreases, the number of nocturnal awakenings and arousal increase, and the ability to sleep continuously over an 8-hour period decreases.[73] Almost 50% of elderly patients have sleep maintenance problems, from waking during the night to waking too early, as compared to only 20% that just had difficulty falling asleep.[69] Contributing to the problem of sleep maintenance is the increase in nocturnal awakenings in an elderly patient. Though brief (<30 seconds) nocturnal awakenings occur in patients of any age, elderly patients exhibit an increased frequency and increase duration (5 minutes) of nocturnal awakenings.[77]

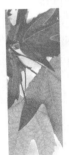

KEY POINT: Elderly patients should be told that it is normal to wake up several times during the night. This wakening should not seriously interfere with daytime functioning as long as they can get back to sleep within a reasonable time frame.

Age-related shifts in the circadian rhythm may explain why elderly patients go to bed earlier and wake up earlier as compared to when they were younger. Several studies have demonstrated that these changes are associated with poor sleep quality, altered sleep architecture, increased awakenings during sleep, early morning awakenings, and increased daytime sleepiness.[73,76]

Growth hormone and cortisol levels have been associated with sleep quality in healthy, older men. In one study, growth hormone levels decreased by nearly 75% from young adulthood to midlife (fifth decade) and continued to decreased into late adulthood. Reduced amounts of shortwave/deep sleep were associated with reduced amounts of growth hormone secretion. Cortisol levels, specifically the evening nadir levels, were significantly increased from midlife to late life as compared to younger counterparts. This was associated with decreased amounts of REM sleep and increased amount of wake time.[78]

Changes in sleep patterns in an elderly patient may also be exacerbated by the patient's environment. Residing in a long-term care facility is not conducive to promoting quality sleep due to reasons such as night-time noise or light and room-sharing. Long-term care residents are often in poor physical health as compared to their counterparts residing in the community, which may impact their sleep quality.[79,80]

Assessment of Insomnia in the Elderly

Since there is no standard or guideline on what is normal in the elderly, the assessment of daytime functioning is an appropriate clinical measure to evaluate the significance of insomnia on an individual patient. Negative impact on daytime functioning is stressed in the DSM-IV TR diagnostic criteria for primary insomnia.[6] Sleep disturbances in an elderly patient may adversely affect daytime functioning, including complaints of napping and not feeling well-rested upon awakening.[69] Daytime sleepiness in elderly patients has been associated with increased mortality rate and increased cardiovascular disease, especially in women.[72]

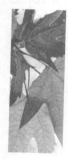

KEY POINT: It is important to ask the patient how sleep difficulties are affecting overall daytime functioning. Assessing daytime functioning will help the clinician select appropriate therapy, thereby, positively impacting an elderly patient's quality of life.

Chronic insomnia has been shown to impact cognitive function. One study found that elderly patients with chronic insomnia had impaired cognitive functioning (which included memory, executive functioning, and attention) as compared to elderly patients without insomnia.[81] There was no difference between these groups as far as hypnotic medication use; however, the investigators did not analyze the use of alcohol or other psychiatric medications that may affect cognitive functioning. Older patients with insomnia performed poorly on tests for attention/concentration as compared to older patients without sleep problems. This was true whether or not the older patient with insomnia took a benzodiazepine to aid in sleep.[82]

Insomnia is often assessed with the use of sleep diaries or questionnaires, which can be difficult to obtain or complete in an elderly patient.

Some questions that may be helpful include asking the patient what time they fall asleep at night and wake up in the morning, if they feel excessively drowsy during the day, if they have difficulties falling asleep, how long it takes them to fall asleep, how many hours per night are they asleep, how many times they wake up during the night, and if other symptoms are present while sleeping (such as snoring, leg discomfort, breathing difficulty, movements).[71,83,84] Asking the spouse or caregiver these questions may also provide some insight for the clinician.

When assessing an elderly patient's complaint of insomnia, it is important to perform a thorough evaluation of the patient's overall physical and psychological health status and medication use. Multiple conditions may affect the quality and quantity of sleep by impacting a patient's pain/discomfort level, ability to breathe, ability to urinate, or general mental condition. Almost all diseases that are common in the elderly population can adversely affect sleep (see Table 13-1).[71,74,85] When identifying these comorbid conditions, the clinician should consider if these diseases are appropriately treated or controlled before initiating therapy for the insomnia complaint.

Medications that cause stimulation, anxiety, increased urination, excessive drowsiness, or mental status changes should be evaluated. Some examples of medications that may cause these symptoms are found in Table 13-1. Many of these medications also have specific negative effects on sleep staging and quality.[71,76]

Summary of Standard Treatment in the Adult Population

When the average adult patient complains of insomnia, they are often initially educated on proper sleep hygiene or provided cognitive behavioral therapy. When this nonpharmacologic therapy is ineffective, a short course of a hypnotic agent, typically a benzodiazepine receptor agonist is added. Other choices include sedating antihistamines, benzodiazepines or ramelteon. Chronic use of these agents may be warranted after adequate assessment of the patient's underlying medical conditions that could contribute to the sleep disturbances.[86]

Review of Evidence Supporting Treatment Recommendations for Geriatric Patients

As with any patient with insomnia, good sleep hygiene (addressing healthy lifestyle habits and environmental factors that influence sleep) should be instituted. However, sleep hygiene alone is often not sufficient to treat insomnia in an elderly patient. A variety of other nonpharmacologic therapies, such as relaxation, stimulus control, sleep restriction, and cognitive behavioral therapy can be beneficial for an elderly patient.[76,87] Cognitive behavioral therapy and pharmacologic therapy, in combination, is more effective in the treatment of insomnia than either treatment approach alone. The use of cognitive behavioral therapy when drug therapy is discontinued maintains remission of insomnia; and is preferred and perceived by patients to be an effective therapy option.[88,89]

Several studies have demonstrated that Tai Chi is effective in improving sleep quality and daytime sleepiness in elderly patients.[90,91] Moderate exercise, consisting of 30–40 minutes of low-impact aerobics or brisk walking performed four times per week, has been shown to improve sleep quality, sleep latency, and sleep duration in patients between 50–76 years of age.[92] However, exercise should not be performed within an hour of bedtime so the body and mind will have time to relax. Decreasing or eliminating daytime napping may not be as beneficial as initially thought, as one study revealed that day or evening naps were not correlated with poor sleep characteristics (sleep latency, awakenings after sleep onset, sleep efficiency) in older patients.[93]

The benzodiazepine receptor agonists include zolpidem, zaleplon, and eszopiclone. These agents have all been studied in the elderly population and have been shown to be effective for the treatment for insomnia. Their effects on improving sleep onset and sleep maintenance enable these agents to target the common sleep disturbances in an elderly insomniac. As compared to the benzodiazepines, the benzodiazepine receptor agonists have their advantages by causing minimal effects on tolerance, rebound insomnia, and residual daytime sleepiness.

Zolpidem has been shown to be as effective as triazolam in the short-term treatment of insom-nia by increasing total sleep time, decreasing the number of nocturnal awakenings, and decreasing sleep latency in elderly patients.[94] The extended release formulation, at a dosage of 6.25 mg, has demonstrated similar efficacy in these parameters as well.[95] Sleep parameters in which zaleplon has been effective in elderly patients include decreasing the number of nocturnal awakenings, self-reported sleep latency and sleep quality, and total sleep time.[96,97] Eszopiclone, at a dosage of 2 mg, has been proven to be efficacious in improving sleep latency, decreasing the number of nocturnal awakenings, improving sleep quality, and decreasing the duration of daytime naps in elderly subjects.[98,99] Additionally, patients who took eszopiclone reported improved daytime alertness and sense of well-being.

Benzodiazepine receptor agonists have the potential to cause complex sleep-related behaviors, such as sleep-driving, making phone calls, and preparing and eating food (while asleep), with subsequent amnesia of these behaviors. Patients should be counseled to take the medication immediately before going to bed and to alert the bed partner to watch for these behaviors so alternative treatment can be tried. These agents may also cause anaphylaxis and angioedema. As a result of post-marketing surveillance, these products are now required to state the potential of these effects in their labeling.[100]

The hypnotic benzodiazepines (flurazepam, estazolam, temazepam, triazolam, quazepam) are effective in treating insomnia and can be used in short courses (<14 days). Several epidemiologic studies have shown that benzodiazepines are commonly prescribed in the elderly population.[80,101] These agents reduce sleep latency, reduce the number of awakenings, and increase total sleep time. Though benzodiazepines have little or no effect on REM sleep, the duration of sleep stages 1 and 4 is decreased whereas the duration of sleep stage 2 is increased. Due to the high frequency of adverse effects that can typically occur in an elderly patient with the use of these agents, they should be avoided as treatment for chronic insomnia. Benzodiazepines have been associated with increased falls, excessive daytime sleepiness, increased fractures, and motor vehicle crashes in elderly patients.[36,71,102-104]

In melatonin-deficient elderly patients, replacement with melatonin is beneficial in improving sleep latency and sleep efficiency.[105] In contrast, using melatonin in patients who are not specifically deficient in this hormone is ineffective in treating primary insomnia.[106] The melatonin receptor agonist, ramelteon, has been proven to be effective in elderly patients with insomnia as well. Ramelteon improves self-reported sleep latency and total sleep time.[107,108] Ramelteon carries the revised warning labeling regarding possible anaphylaxis and angioedema but in general is much safer in elderly patients than the benzodiazepine receptor agonists.[100]

Common Problems Encountered When Treating Elderly Patients

Hangover symptoms during the next morning after taking a dose of most sedative-hypnotics for sleep induction or latency is a common phenomenon for geriatric patients due to the pharmacokinetic alterations in renal function, hepatic function and volume of distribution which occur with aging. For this reason, the lowest doses are recommended even for agents that are short acting. Extended release agents may not be an optimal choice due to slowed motility of the gastrointestinal tract in addition to the other altered pharmacokinetic parameters.

Because of their availability, over-the-counter (OTC) products are frequently chosen in younger adults for the treatment of sleep disturbances. However, these medications typically contain diphenhydramine or doxylamine which are listed as potentially inappropriate medications for use in the elderly patient. Due to the high potential of anticholinergic effects, possible mental status changes, and residual daytime drowsiness/excessive somnolence, OTC sleep products should be avoided in the elderly population.[84,101]

The use of antidepressants, such as trazodone and mirtazapine, for the treatment of insomnia should be reserved for elderly patients who have depression. Trazodone was commonly recommended by many experts as a safe medication for sleep before the availability of the benzodiazepine receptor agonists, however, there is no data to support this assertion. Additionally, antipsychotics with sedating adverse effects should be reserved for elderly patients with psychotic symptoms because of the multitude of adverse effects associated with their use.[80,84]

Substance Abuse
Etiology, Epidemiology, and Clinical Presentation Specific to Geriatrics

Substance abuse is one of the leading causes of disability. With the elderly population increasing and with the "baby boomers" now entering their sixties, it is predicted the prevalence of late-life substance abuse and dependence will also continue to increase.[109] Alcohol abuse is noted to be a significant health issue for the elderly population and over the last 15 years, more data has become available addressing the epidemiology, assessment, and treatment of late-life alcoholism.

Non-alcohol substance disorders include illicit and prescription drug abuse. Clinicians are more likely to encounter prescription abuse than illicit drug use in older adults.[110] Currently, the prevalence of illicit drug use is very low in the elderly population even though the numbers will most likely increase as the geriatric population continues to grow.[111] Due to the higher prevalence[110] and moderate amount of data available, late-life alcohol and prescription drug abuse disorders will be the primary focus of this chapter section.

Recent reports note the majority of older adults (50–60%) are reported to abstain (no alcohol within the previous year) from alcohol compared to 30–40% of younger adults.[109] The prevalence of alcohol dependence within community dwelling elderly is reported to be low at 1.5–2%[112] but prevalence of unhealthy or at-risk drinking is higher at 6–16%.[113] Based on results of alcohol screening programs within the primary care setting, 10–15% of elderly patients screened positive for at-risk or problem drinking.[114,115] In the nursing home setting, 29–49% of patients met criteria for alcohol dependence or abuse during their lifetime with 10–18% having met criteria within 1 year of admission to the home.[116,117]

Two thirds of older alcoholics developed alcoholism earlier in life and continued to drink through their elder years. These individuals are considered to have **early-onset alcoholism**. Late-onset abusers, who encompass the remaining one-third, include individuals who did not drink heavily until late in life. There are many differences between these groups in regards to epidemiology and social history.[113]

Early-onset alcoholics are more likely to have a family history of alcoholism, socioeconomic decline due to their alcohol use, and antisocial behavior. Due to their many years of use, these patients will often have significant medical history such as cirrhosis, cognitive decline, and other psychiatric disorders. Late-onset alcoholics usually do not report any alcohol-related problems until after 50 years of age. These individuals are often times well educated and have maintained a high socioeconomic status through their working life. Alcohol-related illnesses are less frequent in this population. A stressful life event is usually what precipitates the excessive drinking. Late-onset alcoholics are noted to be more agreeable to treatment and recover easier compared to early-onset patients. However, late-onset abuse and dependence are often missed by health care providers.[113,118]

Alcohol and drug abuse are often associated with other psychiatric illnesses in younger adults. The few epidemiology studies published addressing comorbidity in older adults have shown 20–50% of elderly who abuse alcohol also suffer from a mood disorder such as depression or dysthymia.[119,120] It has also been found that approximately 20% of elderly patients who are referred for alcohol treatment show cognitive impairment due to their alcohol use.[121]

Risk Factors for Alcohol Abuse and Comorbidities

Major risk factors identified for elderly alcohol abuse include male gender, major life changes or stressors, and recent loss. Overall, elderly women were found to be less likely to drink heavily, however they are more likely than men to develop late-onset alcohol abuse.[113]

Although moderate consumption of alcohol has shown to decrease risk of cardiovascular disease, cancer risk, and dementia; alcohol dependence is associated with increased morbidity and mortality. Morbidities associated with chronic alcohol use include pancreatitis, peptic ulcer disease, cirrhosis, thrombocytopenia, cardiomyopathy, hypertension, and increased trauma from falls or motor vehicle accidents.[109] Chronic alcohol use results in cognitive impairment with cerebral atrophy and cerebellar degeneration. Cerebrovascular accidents are more common in alcoholics which also result in significant cognitive and functional decline.[113] Sleep disturbances are frequently reported by individuals who drink heavily including those who use alcohol to help initiate sleep. Alcohol has been proven to decrease sleep maintenance, rapid eye movement (REM) sleep, and delta sleep. For elderly alcoholics, the negative effects of sleep are in addition to the reduced REM and deep sleep that accompany normal aging.[113]

Alcoholics are often deficient in several essential vitamins due to altered absorption and decreased intake. Vitamin B12 and folate deficiencies are common and can lead to macrocytic and hemolytic anemias, peripheral neuropathy, paresthesias, and weakness in the lower extremities if not supplemented.[118] Thiamine deficiency results in both Wernicke's encephalopathy and Korsakoff's syndrome. Wernicke's encephalopathy presents as acute confusion, ataxia, and abnormal eye movements while Korsakoff's presents as memory impairment.[113]

Diagnostic Criteria

According to the DSM-IV, one meets criteria for substance abuse if he/she has persistent abuse of a substance that leads to significant impairment defined by one or more of the following and occurs within a 12-month period: (1) recurrent abuse resulting in not being able to meet obligations at work, home, or school, (2) recurrent abuse in situations which are dangerous (e.g. driving while intoxicated), (3) legal problems as a result of substance abuse, and (4) continued abuse despite experiencing social and personal problems as a result of substance use.[6]

Substance dependence is defined as persistent use of a substance which leads to significant impairment defined by three or more of the following and occurring within a 12-month period: (1) development of tolerance, (2) experiencing withdrawal when not using the substance, (3) using larger amounts of the substance at one time than what was intended, (4) continuing efforts or unsuccessful attempts to decrease use, (5) a significant amount of time is spent seeking, using, and recovering from the substance, (6) normal social and work related activities decrease due substance use, and (7) substance use continues despite the patient knowing concurrent illnesses and psychiatric disorders are related to the use.[6]

Presentation Specific to Geriatric Patients

Due to age related physical changes, older adults have an increased sensitivity to alcohol and other mood altering medications. As people age, lean body mass and total body water decreases which leads to decreased distribution and higher serum concentrations of these substances.[109] Impaired hepatic blood flow and enzyme activity can lead to reduced metabolism of alcohol. It and other abused substances can easily penetrate the CNS making older adults more sensitive to the effects of these substances compared to younger adults. The interaction between alcohol and prescription medications, especially psychotropic medications, is a major concern in this age group.[113]

Because of these age related factors, the recommended appropriate intake of alcohol for older adults is lower than the standards established for young to middle age adults. The National Institute on Alcohol Abuse and Alcoholism (NIAAA)[122] and the Substance Abuse and Mental Health Services Administration/Center for Substance Abuse Treatment (SAMSHA/CSTAT) Improvement Protocol on Older Adults[111] recommends no more than one standard drink per day and no more than two standard drinks on any occasion for adults older than 65 years of age. A standard drink is defined as 5 ounces of wine, 12 ounces of beer, or a mixed drink containing 1.5 ounces of hard liquor. Use beyond these recommendations is considered hazardous or at-risk drinking.[111]

Many geriatric and substance abuse specialists agree there are limitations with using the DSM-IV criteria to diagnose substance abuse and dependence in the elderly.[111] Because of these limitations, it is suspected there is low reporting of substance disorders in older adults. As mentioned in the previous section, one of the criteria for substance dependence is developing tolerance which is usually shown by increased use of the substance to receive the same level of effect. For older adults, substance use may appear to decrease or stay the same due to increased sensitivity and higher blood levels at lower amounts. Lower quantities used may also make it difficult for older users to meet the criterion of spending a great deal of time in activities related to substance use. The criterion of withdrawal may not be applicable for patients who develop late-onset substance dependence and have not yet experienced a period of withdrawal. To meet criteria for substance abuse, patients often fail to meet daily obligations because of their use. Again, this criterion is less likely to apply for older users because they are often retired or isolated from social situations.[113]

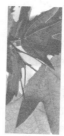

KEY POINT: Limitations exist when trying to use the DSM-IV criteria for substance abuse and dependence to diagnose geriatric patients. These limitations result in under diagnosing of late-life substance abuse.

Screening for Alcohol Dependence or Hazardous Drinking

Alcohol abuse/dependence screening should be part of a patient's regular physical examination.[111] Common screening tools used in older adults include the Short Michigan Alcoholism Screening Test–Geriatric version (SMAST-G), the CAGE questionnaire, and the Alcohol Use Disorders Identification Test (AUDIT). Out of the three screening tools, the SMAST-G was developed specifically for older adults. The CAGE questionnaire is considered the easiest tool to use in a clinic setting and has high specificity for detecting alcohol abuse. However, it has low sensitivity for detecting alcohol dependence and at-risk drinking.[109,113] Patient self-reporting continues to be the primary method of obtaining history of alcohol use, although any collateral information from the patient's spouse and family is helpful.[109] If a patient states he abstains from alcohol, clinicians should continue to question the reasons for abstaining. Some individuals currently abstain from alcohol because of abuse problems in the past.[109]

Common Problems Encountered When Treating Elderly Patients

Ethanol Withdrawal and Acute Treatment

Older age has not been shown to increase risk of drug and alcohol withdrawal. However, older adults may experience longer duration of withdrawal symptoms and are more likely to have complications due to longer history of alcohol abuse, medical comorbidities, baseline cognitive impairment, and sensitivity to drug treatments.[109,123] Older age has also been noted to be associated with longer hospital stays for treatment and greater risk of being discharged to an extended care facility.[124]

Patients experiencing alcohol withdrawal typically present with autonomic hyperactivity including increased pulse and blood pressure, increased temperature, restlessness, anxiety, tremor and insomnia. These symptoms usually present within the first 12–48 hours after the last drink consumed. Severe symptoms such as hallucinations, delirium tremens, seizures, and coma can develop as late as 2–10 days after withdrawal. Because alcohol withdrawal can be severe and fatal, careful evaluation and benzodiazepine regimens should be made available as recommended using the Clinical Institute Withdrawal Assessment (CIWA) tool (Table 13-2).[113,123,125]

Patients who are predicted to have minimal to moderate withdrawal symptoms, no history of complicated withdrawal, no significant comorbidities, and who have a caregiver available to monitor closely, may complete the detoxification process as an outpatient. The patient and caregiv-

Table 13-2. Clinical Institute Withdrawal Assessment for Alcohol[125]

Symptom	Range of Scores
Agitation	0 = normal activity 7 = constantly moving
Anxiety	0 = calm, at ease 7 = acute panic symptoms
Auditory hallucinations	0 = no hallucinations 7 = continuous hallucinations
Disorientation	0 = oriented, no cognitive impairment 4 = disoriented to time, place, and person
Headache	0 = no pain 7 = extremely severe
Nausea/ vomiting	0 = no GI symptoms 7 = constant nausea/vomiting/ dry heaves
Sweating	0 = no sweating 7 = drenching sweats
Tactile hallucinations	0 = no hallucinations 7 = continuous hallucinations
Tremor	0 = no tremor present 7 = severe tremor
Visual hallucinations	0 = no hallucinations 7 = continuous hallucinations

Maximum score is 67. Minimal-mild withdrawal symptoms < 8, moderate withdrawal symptoms = 8–15, severe withdrawal symptoms > 15.

er should be educated on how to use the CIWA (Table 13-2) to assess the severity of withdrawal symptoms. If the patient experiences moderate withdrawal (CIWA score between 8 and 15) then a benzodiazepine can be administered to help relieve symptoms. The CIWA should be used every 4 hours and a clinician should follow-up with the patient daily during the withdrawal period.[123]

Patients should be admitted for inpatient detoxification if he/she has a history of withdrawal delirium or seizures, complex medical or psychiatric illnesses, has suicidal thoughts, does not have a strong support system, or has a CIWA score greater than 15. Hospitalization can also provide further treatment benefits such as lack of access to alcohol and removing the patient out of his/her usual environment.[123]

For relief and prevention of alcohol withdrawal symptoms, benzodiazepines are first line therapy for all patients including older adults. Benzodiazepines act on the GABA A-type receptor similar to alcohol and augment the inhibition effect of GABA. Much data exist showing that benzodiazepines reduce the risk of delirium and seizures during the withdrawal period.[123] However, the choice of benzodiazepine (long-acting versus short-acting) to treat elderly patients is not as clear. As discussed in the anxiety section of this chapter, long-acting benzodiazepines with active metabolites may be less tolerated in the elderly due to age-related pharmacokinetic and pharmacodynamic changes. Adverse effects of these benzodiazepines may be one of the reasons more complications and longer hospital stays have been observed in elderly patients undergoing detoxification versus younger adults.[124,126-128]

Based on the possible risk of adverse effects with long-acting benzodiazepines, clinicians may wish to use short-acting agents such as lorazepam or oxazepam for withdrawal treatment in the elderly. However, one should also keep in mind the risk of using these agents. It is possible a patient may not be provided adequate coverage of withdrawal symptoms with short-acting agents.[123]

In regards to dosing schedules, unless a patient has a seizure disorder, history of alcohol withdrawal seizures, or history of delirium tremens, scheduled benzodiazepine regimens are not recommended for older adults. For most cases of detoxification, a symptom-triggered approach such as a CIWA protocol should be used to prevent unneeded benzodiazepine use.[123]

In addition to treating withdrawal symptoms, electrolytes and vitamins should be supplemented if needed. Thiamine supplementation (100 mg daily) should be provided in all cases of alcoholism. Vitamin B12 and folate are also recommended if serum levels are low or macrocytic anemia is present. Electrolytes including magnesium should be checked and corrected if abnormal.[113]

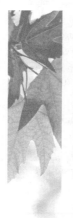

KEY POINT: Although short-acting benzodiazepines are usually recommended over long-acting agents for elderly patients, long-acting benzodiazepines are more likely to ensure adequate coverage during the withdrawal period without increasing risk of seizures. Careful dosing and diligent monitoring of therapeutic and adverse effects are required to balance the risk-benefit of these agents.

Long-term Treatment for Alcohol Dependence

Treatment research for late-life substance abuse/dependence is lacking but published data has slowly emerged over the last 15 years especially for alcohol treatment. Studies have shown psychosocial and pharmacological treatments to be effective for older adults and result in increased quality of life.[109] Community programs for older adults assisting with alcohol abstinence have shown to be just as or more beneficial in improving quality of life compared to middle-aged adults.[128-130]

Brief advice interventions during clinic visits have been shown to significantly decrease drinking in the elderly. Two studies which included 158 and 452 elderly patients, demonstrated that brief 10–15 minutes of counseling regarding alcohol use at clinic visits can significantly reduce drinking compared to usual care patients.[109,130,131]

Psychosocial intervention is considered the cornerstone of therapy when treating substance abuse and maintaining sobriety. This intervention has also shown to be beneficial for older adults and interestingly, the best results are observed when older patients are involved in age-specific programs versus mixed-age groups. Studies have shown older adults to have higher program completion rates, higher group attendance, and higher abstinence rates at 6 months and 1 year after completing a program when placed in age-specific versus those placed in mixed-age programs.[132-134] Age-specific programs should include the following: (1) group therapy with other older adults that is supportive and helps build self-esteem, (2) a focus on coping with common psychosocial issues in the elderly such as depression, loneliness, and loss of spouse, (3) a focus on increasing social support for the patient, (4) clinicians who are experienced in working with the elderly, and (5) being able to refer patients to a case manager and other outside services for older adults.[111]

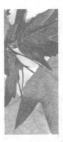

KEY POINT: Psychosocial intervention is considered the cornerstone of therapy when treating substance abuse and maintaining sobriety. Age-specific programs have been shown to work best for older adults.

Three agents (disulfiram, naltrexone, and acamprosate) are currently FDA approved to help maintain abstinence from alcohol. All agents have been shown to be most efficacious when used along with psychosocial therapy. Patients should understand that pharmacotherapy is prescribed as an adjunct and not as a replacement for individual or group therapy.

Disulfiram is the oldest agent available for treatment of alcohol dependence Patients use disulfiram as a deterrent from drinking in order to avoid the symptoms associated with the alcohol-disulfiram interaction. This medication is not recommended for elderly patients due to the adverse effects of acetaldehyde and the risk of exacerbating concurrent illnesses.[109]

Naltrexone is an opioid antagonist with a recommended dosing of 50 mg daily orally or 380 mg monthly if given intramuscularly. The most common adverse effects reported are gastrointestinal symptoms (nausea, stomach pain, anorexia) and injection site reactions with the parenteral product. Elevation in liver transaminases and hepatotoxicity are reported for both the oral and injectable drug. Therefore, baseline liver function tests should be obtained and monitored periodically with therapy. Naltrexone should not be used in patients with history of liver impairment or those taking opioid therapy.[135]

There is data to support the efficacy and safety of naltrexone in older adults. Oslin and colleagues lead a double-blind, randomized placebo-controlled study in 50–70 year old veterans. The treatment group was assigned naltrexone 50 mg daily. Naltrexone did not significantly improve complete abstinence but those taking naltrexone were less likely to relapse to heavy drinking.[136] Another study comparing compliance among older and younger patients found adherence to naltrexone and psychosocial therapy was better among older adults.[137] In this study, a higher naltrexone dose of 100 mg daily was used and there was no difference in tolerability of the medication in the older versus younger group.

Acamprosate is the newest agent approved for maintenance of alcohol abstinence. It is recommended that acamprosate be initiated after detoxification and the patient has been sober for at least seven days. A dose of 666 mg three times a day is normally prescribed. Although food has no significant effect on absorption of acamprosate, patients may be encouraged to take with meals to increase compliance. The medication is renally cleared; therefore, dose adjustments should be made for decreased renal function. Patients with a creatinine clearance between 30-50 ml/min should start with 333 mg three times daily and acamprosate should not be used in patients with creatinine clearance less than 30 ml/min. Acamprosate is usually well tolerated with diarrhea being the most common adverse effects.[138] To date, there have been no trials published addressing the efficacy of acamprosate in the elderly population. It is suspected the medication should be well tolerated in older adults without exacerbating any chronic diseases. However, many elderly should be dosed the lower dose of 333 mg three times daily due to age-related renal impairment.

Prescription Drug Abuse

The overall prevalence of prescription drug abuse in the elderly has not been directly reported.

However, it should be noted that abuse appears to be uncommon among elderly especially if they do not have a history of other types of substance abuse. According to a recent study involving older adults, female gender, depression, social isolation, and history of alcohol and other substance abuse appear to be risk factors for prescription medication abuse.[139,140] Late-life abusers usually do not have to use illegal methods to obtain controlled substances. Unsafe amounts of medications are often obtained by using multiple physicians, borrowing medication from family and friends, or by keeping and collecting prescriptions over time.[139]

Benzodiazepines are a drug class that may be of concern for abuse due to their addiction potential and they continue to be one of the most prescribed medications in the elderly.[111,141] Benzodiazepines are used for many psychiatric symptoms such as agitation, anxiety, and insomnia. As discussed in the anxiety section of this chapter, chronic use of benzodiazepines should be avoided in the elderly if possible due to their high risk of adverse effects in this population. If the use of benzodiazepines outweighs the risks then shorter acting agents such as lorazepam and oxazepam are recommended. For patients who are at risk for abuse, highly lipophilic agents such as diazepam and alprazolam should be avoided.[111]

Benzodiazepine withdrawal symptoms are more likely to present as confusion and disorientation in older adults rather than increased anxiety and insomnia which is often witnessed in younger adults.[113] Treatment of benzodiazepine abuse is gradual tapering of the medication. Patients addicted to short-acting benzodiazepines such as alprazolam, should be switched to a longer-acting agent first (clonazepam is often a popular choice). The longer-acting benzodiazepine can then be slowly tapered.[113]

Opioid prescribing has increased over the recent years for all age groups in order to meet national guidelines for adequate pain control. Hydrocodone/acetaminophen is noted to be the most prescribed medication for outpatient use and at least eight other opioid analgesics are listed in the top 200 medications dispensed. Despite these recent statistics, opioid abuse is noted to be rare in the elderly population especially for patients who do not already have a history of substance abuse.[139] Clinicians should be aware that drug-seeking behavior is often times the result of inadequate pain control. Chronic opioid users will develop physical dependence and can experience uncomfortable withdrawal symptoms such as diarrhea, nausea, rhinorrhea, shivering, anxiety, and agitation if therapy is discontinued abruptly. Whether abuse is suspected or the patient wishes to simply discontinue therapy, opioids should be gradually tapered to prevent withdrawal.[139] This is true for opioids of lower abuse potential also, such as tramadol and propoxyphene. Physical and psychological dependence to these agents can occur, even if addiction is not present.

CASE 1: PRIMARY CARE CLINIC

Subjective:

TM is a 72-year-old male patient who presents to his primary care provider for the first time in 5 years with complaints of stomach and joint pain, trouble sleeping, increased anxiety, impaired concentration and short-term memory, and lack of energy. TM is worried he has something seriously wrong with him such as cancer to be causing all his symptoms.

After interviewing the patient, it is also discovered the patient is no longer exercising or visiting the community senior center like he was in the past. TM mentions that he is getting old and his joint pain has worsened over the last year to where he has trouble walking. TM states, "I'm not sure why I'm still alive. I wish I would just pass in my sleep." TM becomes tearful when he talks about his deceased wife.

Medications:
No prescription medications, has been using OTC omeprazole 20 mg daily for stomach pain and uses occasional acetaminophen for joint pain

Past Medical History:
Obstructive sleep apnea (uses CPAP as prescribed), osteoarthritis

Allergies:
NKA

Family History:
Both parents are dead, but neither parent had a history of mental illness.

Social History:
Patient's wife died unexpectedly a year ago while hospitalized for pneumonia, TM has 3 children and 6 grandchildren but they all live out of state, denies alcohol, tobacco, or illicit drug use.

Objective: Height = 70 inches, weight = 265 lb, BP = 138/89 mmHg, P = 65 BPM, pain = 7/10

Labs:
Basic metabolic panel and complete blood count are normal, TSH 3.5mIU/L; vitamin B-12 450 mg/mL.

Assessment:
TM meets the diagnostic criteria for major depressive disorder—moderate to severe. He has decreased interest in his daily activities, trouble sleeping, decreased energy, memory complaints, and passive suicidal ideation. In addition, he has symptoms of generalized anxiety with trouble sleeping, decreased energy, impaired concentration and anxiety. He also complains of joint and stomach pain which may be associated with his depression.

Plan:
1. Sertraline 25 mg can be offered to the patient as a first-line agent. Begin 25 mg daily × 1 week then titrate to 50 mg daily.
2. Refer patient to the neuropsychologist for psychotherapy, if patient agrees.
3. Begin schedule acetaminophen 1000 mg every 8 hours for joint pain.
4. Return to clinic in 1 week.

Rationale:
Psychotherapy and medication therapy should be offered to the patient for optimal treatment. Sertraline or citalopram are appropriate choices for a first-line SSRI as they have a favorable pharmacokinetic profile for older adults and are available as generic medications. Because TM has several risk factors for suicide (age, white male, chronic pain, immobility, isolation) he should be followed frequently in the beginning of therapy (every week or every other week). Further work-up for stomach and joint complaints may be required but symptoms may improve as depression is treated. This can be addressed at his return appointment.

Case Summary:
TM is a 72-year-old man who suffered the loss of his wife 1 year ago and now presents with late-onset depression and anxiety. He also has somatic complaints of stomach and joint pains. Some

thoughts of death are evident which increase concern that he may consider suicide. He is not on medications which are associated with depression. The stomach and joint pain may be separate diagnoses or may be associated with his depression. Treatment with an SSRI is appropriate to begin, as is more effective management of his pain symptoms with acetaminophen.

CASE 2: PCP OFFICE

Subjective:

SB is an 81-year-old male who presents to his primary care physician for routine physical exam. Upon questioning, SB states that he concerned that he is not getting a full 8 hours of sleep at night. He complains of bothersome nocturia and is getting up 4–5 times during the night to urinate. He denies fevers, chills, or dysuria. SB wakes up well-rested and is able to perform his usual ADLs and IADLs without drowsiness.

Social History:

Negative for tobacco use, occasional alcohol use during special occasions

Objective:

PMH: Benign prostatic hypertrophy, hypertension, congestive heart failure; medications: terazosin 1 mg at bedtime, finasteride 5 mg daily, furosemide 20 mg every morning, lisinopril 20 mg every morning, aspirin 81 mg daily; blood pressure: 152/78, pulse 76 sitting; 148/78, pulse 78 standing

Physical Exam:

Within normal limits except trace pitting edema in ankles bilaterally and a slightly enlarged prostate

Labs:

Urinalysis negative

Assessment:

SB is an 81-year-old man with concerns about his total sleep time and presents with uncontrolled lower urinary tract symptoms likely due to his BPH.

Plan:

1. Titrate dose of terazosin to 2 mg at bedtime to maximize pt's BPH therapy. Monitor blood pressure and symptoms of dizziness.
2. Educate patient regarding his sleep pattern–as long as his interrupted sleep is not adversely affecting his daytime functioning, pharmacologic treatment is not necessary. Caution patient on self-treating with OTC sleep aids which contain diphenhydramine or doxylamine, as these agents may worsen his comorbid conditions. Educate patient on proper sleep hygiene.

Rationale:

Because his comorbidity of BPH causes him to wake up at night, SB is concerned about his sleep efficacy and is a "worried well" geriatric patient. Reassurance and counseling about normal sleep patterns and that OTC sleep aids are not appropriate for him given his comorbidity are important.

Case Summary:

SB has concerns about his sleeping pattern, although he wakes up well-rested and without functional issues. More effective treatment of his BPH may provide him with an uninterrupted night of sleep. Counseling about normal sleep patterns, the effect of BPH on sleep and the problems associated with OTC sleep aids are indicated.

Clinical Pearls

- *Insomnia is an especially difficult problem in long-term care settings. Routines include turning bed-bound residents every 2 hours, checking incontinent residents periodically at night, early morning vital sign measurements or other standard practices which do not lend themselves to good sleep. In addition, most residents have a roommate, doubling the occurrence of these activities. Efforts to reduce interruptions and noise in this setting would help reduce the use of sedatives in the older, frail adult who is most prone to experience adverse effects.*

- *Current federal regulations require periodic dose reductions for all psychoactive medications for nursing home residents. Antidepressants, benzodiazepines and benzodiazepine receptor agonists must be tapered to lower doses within 6 months to meet this regulation. This is repeated until the medication is discontinued or until the resident demonstrates symptoms of disease recurrence. This is problematic with the use of antidepressants, which are recommended for use a minimum of 9 months with late-life depression, and sometimes needed for life-long therapy. Clear documentation of medication need is necessary to ensure optimal pharmaceutical care and prevent placing the nursing home at risk for regulatory non-compliance.*

Chapter Summary

Depression and GAD are the most common psychiatric disorders observed in geriatric patients and if left untreated, lead to decreased daily function and increased morbidity and mortality. SSRI and SNRI therapy are recommended as first-line when medications are needed. Doses should be started at the lower end of the range but eventually titrated to a moderate dose to provide an adequate response. Frequent follow-up, monitoring, and support should be provided once therapy is initiated to increase chances of remission, compliance, and quality of life.

Benzodiazepines can be used if acute treatment of GAD or panic disorder is needed. Short-acting agents such as lorazepam and oxazepam are the preferred agents to use in the elderly. Generally, chronic benzodiazepine use is discouraged due to the risk of adverse effects and should be gradually tapered after a patient has had time to respond to antidepressant therapy.

Insomnia is a common complaint among elderly patients. If left undiagnosed and untreated, insomnia may have detrimental effects on the patient's overall health status and quality of life. When an older patient complaints of insomnia, it is important to evaluate the patient "as a whole," which includes assessing comorbid conditions, medication use, and where they reside. Additionally, assessing the elderly patient's daytime functioning can help the clinician in selecting the appropriate therapy. Nonpharmacologic therapy is beneficial for the elderly patient. However, if non pharmacologic strategies are ineffective, the use of drug therapy, specifically a benzodiazepine receptor agonist or melatonin receptor agonist, may be warranted. The prevalence of substance abuse and dependence in older adults is less than observed in young to middle age adults. However, as the geriatric population continues to grow and the "baby boomers" begin to enter into their sixties, the prevalence of late-life abuse is expected to increase. Currently, alcohol abuse is noted to be more concerning in the elderly population compared to prescription drug or illicit substance abuse.

Self-Assessment Questions

1. What are the criteria for diagnosing major depressive disorder, GAD and panic disorder according to the DSM-IV?

2. What other complaints are associated more with late-life depression and late-life anxiety compared to young adult depression and anxiety?

3. Which therapies are considered first-line for treatment of late-life depression and late-life anxiety?

4. What is the overall consensus regarding the efficacy versus the risks of using benzodiazepines for late-life anxiety?

5. Which benzodiazepines are considered "safer" for older adults? When and how should benzodiazepines be discontinued?

6. What physiologic changes on sleep architecture and circadian rhythm occur as a patient gets older? How do chronic diseases and medication use contribute to sleep disturbances in elderly patients?

7. What types of nonpharmacologic therapies can be beneficial for insomnia in an elderly patient?

8. Of the available pharmacologic therapies indicated for insomnia, which are preferred in the elderly population and why?

9. What are the limitations of using the DSM-IV criteria to diagnose a geriatric patient with substance abuse and dependence?

10. Why are older adults more sensitive to alcohol and other psychotropic substances?

11. What is the CIWA tool and why is it recommended for detoxification treatment protocols?

12. What are the pros and cons of using short-acting and long-acting benzodiazepines for prevention and treatment of alcohol withdrawal symptoms in the elderly?

13. What benefits have been observed when age-specific psychosocial therapy is used for treatment of late-life substance abuse/dependence?

14. Which pharmacologic agents can be considered as adjunct therapy for older adults trying to abstain from alcohol?

References

1. Snowden M, Steinman L, Frederick J. Treating depression in older adults: challenges to implementing the recommendations of an expert panel. *Prev Chronic Dis.* 2008;5:1–7.

2. Rapp MA, Dahlman K, Sano M, Grossman HT, Haroutunian V, Gorman JM. Neuropsychological

differences between late-onset and recurrent geriatric major depression. *Am J Psychiatry.* 2005;162:691–8.

3. Alexopoulos GS. Depression in the elderly. *Lancet.* 2005;365:1961–70.

4. Robinson RG. *The Clinical Neuropsychiatry of Stroke: Cognitive, Behavioral, and Emotional Disorders Following Vascular Brain Injury.* 2nd ed. Cambridge: Cambridge University Press; 2006.

5. Shanmugham B, Karp J, Drayer R, Reynolds CF, Alexopoulos G. Evidence-based pharmacologic interventions for geriatric depression. *Psychiatr Clin N Am.* 2005;28:821–35.

6. American Psychiatric Association. *Diagnostic and Statistical Manual of Mental Disorders.* 4th ed., Text Revision. Washington, DC: American Psychiatric Association; 2000.

7. Unutzer J. Late-life depression. *N Engl J Med.* 2007;357:2269–76.

8. Alexopoulos GS. The course of geriatric depression with "reversible dementia": a controlled study. *Am J Psychiatry.* 1993;150:1693–99.

9. Berra C, Torta R. Therapeutic rationale of antidepressant use in the elderly. *Arch Gerontol Geriatr.* 2007;1:83–90.

10. Wells KB, Stewart A, Hays RD, et al. The functioning and well being of depressed patients. Results from the Medical Outcomes Study. *JAMA.* 1989;262:914–9.

11. Frasure-Smith N, Lesperance F, Talajic M. Depression following myocardial infarction. Impact on 6-month survival. *JAMA.* 1993;270:1819–25.

12. Whooley MA, Browner WS. Association between depressive symptoms and mortality in older women. *Arch Intern Med.* 1998;158:2129–35.

13. Wassertheil-Smoller S, Shumaker S, Ockene J, et al. Depression and cardiovascular sequelae in postmenopausal women. *Arch Intern Med.* 2004;164:289–98.

14. Pennix BW, Leveille S, Ferrucci L, Van Eijk JT, Guralnik JM. Exploring the effect of depression on physical disability: longitudinal evidence from the Established Populations for Epidemiologic Studies of the Elderly. *Am J Public Health.* 1999;89:1346–52.

15. Heisel MJ. Suicide and its prevention among older adults. *Can J Psychiatry.* 2006;51:143–54.

16. Kuehn BM. FDA panel seeks to balance risks in warnings for antidepressants. *JAMA.* 2007;297:573–4.

17. Gaynes BN, Rush AJ, Trivedi MH, Wisniewski SR, Spencer D, Fava M. The STAR-D study: treating depression in the real world. *Cleveland Clinic J Med.* 2008;75:57–66.

18. Texas Implementation of Medication Algorithms. Major depressive disorder algorithms. Available at: www.dshs.state.tx.us/mhprograms/tima.shtml. Accessed 10/31/08.

19. Pinquart M, Duberstein PR, Lyness JM. Treatments for later-life depressive conditions: a meta-analytic comparison of pharmacotherapy and psychotherapy. *Am J Psychiatry.* 2006;163:1493–501.

20. Keller MB, McCullough JP, Klein DN, et al. A comparison of nefazodone, the cognitive behavioral-analysis system of psychotherapy, and their combination for the treatment of chronic depression. *N Engl J Med.* 2000;342:1462–70.

21. Reynolds CF III, Frank E, Perel JM, et al. Nortriptyline and interpersonal psychotherapy as maintenance therapies for recurrent major depression: a randomized controlled trial in patients older than 59 years. *JAMA.* 1999;281:39–45.

22. Cuijpers P, van Straten A, Smit F. Psychological treatment of late-life depression: a meta-analysis of randomized controlled trials. *Int J Geriatr Psychiatry.* 2006;21:1139–49.

23. Alexopoulos GS, Katz IR, Reynolds CF III, Carpenter D, Docherty JP, Ross RW. Pharmacotherapy of depression in older patients: a summary of the expert consensus guidelines. *J Psychiatr Pract.* 2001;7:361–76.

24. Tollefson GD, Bosomworth JC, Heiligentstein JH, Potvin JH, Holman S. Fluoxetine Collaborative Group: a double-blind, placebo-controlled clinical trial of fluoxetine in geriatric patients with major depression. *Int Psychogeriatrics.* 1995;7:89–104.

25. Bondareff W, Alpert M, Friedhoff AJ, Richter EM, Clary CM, Batzar E. Comparison of sertraline and nortriptyline in the treatment of major depressive disorder in late life. *Am J Psychiatry.* 2000;157:729–36.

26. Schneider LS, Nelson JC, Clary CM, et al. An 8-week multicenter, parallel-group, double-blind, placebo-controlled study of sertraline in elderly outpatients with major depression. *Am J Psychiatry.* 2003;160:1277–85.

27. Rapaport MH, Schneider LS, Dunner DL, Davies JT, Pitts CD. Efficacy of controlled-release paroxetine in the treatment of late-life depression. *J Clin Psychiatry.* 2003;64:1065–74.

28. Karlsson I, Godderis J, Augusto De Mendonca LC, et al. A ramdomised, double-blind comparison of the efficacy and safety of citalopram compared to mianserin in elderly, depressed patients with or without mild to moderate dementia. *Int J Geriatr Psychiatry.* 2000;15:295–305.

29. Klysner R, Bent-Hansen J, Hansen HL, Lunde M, Pleidrup E, Poulsen DL. Efficacy of citalopram in the prevention of recurrent depression in elderly patients: placebo-controlled study of maintenance therapy. *Br J Psychiatry.* 2002;181:29–35.

30. Gorwood P, Weiller E, Lemming O, Katona C. Escitalopram prevents relapse in older patients with major depressive disorder. *Am J Geriatr Psychiatry.* 2007;15:581–93.

31. Lotrich FE, Pollock BG. Aging and clinical pharmacology: implications for antidepressants. *J Clin Pharmacol.* 2005;45:1106–22.

32. Nelson JC, Delucchi K, Schneider LS. Efficacy of second generation antidepressants in late-life depression: a meta-analysis of the evidence. *Am J Geriatr Psychiatry.* 2008;16:558–67.

33. Mulsant BH, Houck PR, Gildengers AG, et al. What

is the optimal duration of a short-term antidepressant trial when treating geriatric depression? *J Clin Psychopharmacol.* 2006;26:113–20.

34. Dew MA, Whyte EM, Lenze EJ, et al. Recovery from major depression in older adults receiving augmentation of antidepressant pharmacotherapy. *Am J Psychiatry.* 2007;164:892–99.

35. Mitchell AJ, Subramaniam H. Prognosis of depression in old age compared to middle age: a systematic review of comparative studies. *Am J Psychiatry.* 2005;162:1588–1601.

36. Van de Wurff FB, Stek ML, Hoogendijk WJ, Beekman AT. The efficacy and safety of ECT in depressed older adults: a literature review. *Int J Geriatr Psychiatry.* 2003;18:894–904.

37. Kujala I, Rosenvinge B, Bekkelund SI. Clinical outcome and adverse effects of electroconvulsive therapy in elderly psychiatric patients. *J Geriatr Psychiatry Neurol.* 2002;15:73–6.

38. Dombrovski AY, Mulsant BH. The evidence for electroconvulsive therapy (ECT) in the treatment of severe late-life depression: ECT, the preferred treatment for severe depression in late life. *Int Psychogeriatr.* 2007;19:10–14, 24–35.

39. Sackeim HA, Haskett RF, Mulsant BH, et al. Continuation pharmacotherapy in the prevention of relapse following electroconvulsive therapy: a randomized controlled trial. *JAMA.* 2001;285:1299–307.

40. Fick DM, Cooper JW, Wade WE, Waller JL, Maclean R, Beers MH. Updating the Beers criteria for potentially inappropriate medication use in older adults. *Arch Intern Med.* 2003;163:2716–24.

41. Wohlreich M, Mallinckrodt CH, Watkin JG, Hay DP. Duloxetine for the long-term treatment of major depressive disorder in patients aged 65 and older: an open-label study. *BMC Geriatrics.* 2004;4:11.

42. Raskin J, Wiltse CG, Siegal A, et al. Efficacy of duloxetine on cognition, depression, and pain in elderly patients with major depressive disorder: an 8-week, double-blind, placebo-controlled trial. *Am J Psychiatry.* 2007;164:900–9.

43. Gasto C, Navarro V, Marcos T, et al. Single-blind comparison of venlafaxine and nortriptyline in elderly major depression. *J Clin Psychopharmacol.* 2003;23:21–6.

44. Allard P, Gram L, Timdahl K, et al. Efficacy and tolerability of venlafaxine in geriatric outpatients with major depression: a double-blind, randomised 6-month comparative trial with citalopram. *Int J Geriatr Psychiatry.* 2004;19:1123–30.

45. Oslin DW, Ten Have TR, Streim JE, et al. Probing the safety of medications in the frail elderly: evidence from a randomized clinical trial of sertraline and venlafaxine in depressed nursing home residents. *J Clin Psychiatry.* 2003;64:875–82.

46. Weihs KL, Settle EC, Batey SR, et al. Bupropion sustained release versus paroxetine for the treatment of depression in the elderly. *J Clin Psychiatry.* 2000;61:196–202.

47. Roose SP, Nelson JC, Salzman C, Hollander SB, Rodrigues H. Open-label study of mirtazapine orally disintegrating tablets in depressed patients in the nursing home. *Curr Med Res Opin.* 2003;19:737–46.

48. Schatzberg AF, Kremer C, Rodrigues HE, Murphy GM. Double-blind, randomized comparison of mirtazapine and paroxetine in elderly depressed patients. *Am J Geriatr Psychiatry.* 2002;10:541–50.

49. Wilson K, Mottram P. A comparison of side effects of selective serotonin reuptake inhibitors and tricyclic antidepressants in older depressed patients: a meta-analysis. *Int J Geriatr Psychiatry.* 2004;19:754–62.

50. Whyte EM, Basinski J, Farhi P, et al. Geriatric depression treatment in nonresponders to selective serotonin reuptake inhibitors. *J Clin Psychiatry.* 2004;65:1634–41.

51. Lauderdale SA. Sheikh JI. Anxiety disorders in older adults. *Clin Geriatr Med.* 2003;19:721–41.

52. Beekman ATF, Bremmer MA, Deeg DJH, et al. Anxiety disorders in later life: a report from the longitudinal aging study Amsterdam. *Int J Geriatr Psychiatry.* 1998;13:717–26.

53. Manela M, Katona C, Livingston G. How common are the anxiety disorders in old age? *Int J Geriatr Psychiatry.* 1996;11:65–70.

54. Flint AJ. Generalised anxiety disorder in elderly patients: epidemiology, diagnosis, and treatment options. *Drugs Aging.* 2005;22:101–14.

55. Lenz EJ, Mulsant BH, Shear MK, et al. Comorbid anxiety disorders in depressed elderly patients. *Am J Psychiatry.* 2000;157:722–28.

56. De Beurs E, Beekman ATF, Van Balkom AJLM, Deeg DJH, Van Dyck R, Van Tildburg W. Consequences of anxiety in older persons: its effect on disability, well-being and use of health services. *Psychological Med.* 1999;29:583–93.

57. Flint AJ, Gagnon N. Diagnosis and management of panic disorder in older patients. *Drugs Aging.* 2003;20:881–91.

58. Sheikh JI, Swales PJ, Carlson EB, Lindley SE. Aging and panic disorder: phenomenology, comorbidity, and risk factors. *Am J Geriatr Psychiatry.* 2004;12:102–109.

59. Katerndahl DA, Talamantes M. A comparison of persons with early versus late-onset panic attacks. *J Clin Psychiatry.* 2000;61:422–7.

60. Segui J, Salvador-Carulla L, Marquez M, et al. Differential clinical features of late-onset panic disorder. *J Affect Disord.* 2000;57:115–24.

61. Kirkwood CK, Melton ST. Anxiety disorders I: generalized anxiety, panic, and social anxiety disorders. In: DiPiro JT, Talbert RL, Yee GC, Matzke GR, Wells BG, Posey LM, eds. *Pharmacotherapy: A Pathophysiologic Approach.* 6th ed. McGraw-Hill Companies, Inc., 2005:1289–95.

62. Treatment of Patients with Panic Disorder. American Psychiatric Association. Available at: www.psychiatryonline.com/pracGuide/pracGuideTopic_9.aspx.

63. Hendriks GJ, Oude Voshaar RC, Keijsers GPJ,

Hoogduin CAL, Van Balkom AJLM. Cognitive-behavioural therapy for late-life anxiety disorders: a systematic review and meta-analysis. *Acta Psychiatr Scand.* 2008;117:403–11.

64. Katz IR, Reynolds III CF, Alexopoulos GS, Hackett D. Venlafaxine ER as a treatment for generalized anxiety disorder in older adults: pooled analysis of five randomized placebo-controlled clinical trials. *J Am Geriatr Soc.* 2002;50:18–25.

65. Lenze EJ, Mulsant BH, Shear MK, et al. Efficacy and tolerability of citalopram in the treatment of late-life anxiety disorders: results from an 8-week randomized, placebo-controlled trial. *Am J Psychiatry.* 2005;162:146–50.

66. Blank S, Lenze EJ, Benoit H, et al. Outcomes of late-life anxiety disorders during 32 weeks of citalopram treatment. *J Clin Psychiatry.* 2006;67:468–72.

67. Benitez CIP, Smith K, Vasile RG, Rende R, Edelen MO, Keller MB. Use of benzodiazepines and selective serotonin reuptake inhibitors in middle-aged and older adults with anxiety disorders. *Am J Geriatr Psychiatry.* 2008;16:5–13.

68. DeMartinis N, Rynn M, Rickels K, et al. Prior benzodiazepine use and buspirone response in the treatment of generalized anxiety disorder. *J Clin Psychiatry.* 2000;61:91–4.

69. Foley DJ, Monjan AA, Brown SL, et al. Sleep complaints among elderly persons: an epidemiologic studies of three communities. *Sleep.* 1995;18:425–432.

70. Schubert CR, Cruickshanks KJ, Dalton DS, et al. Prevalence of sleep problems and quality of life in an older population. *Sleep.* 2002;25(8):889–893.

71. McCall WV. Sleep in the elderly: burden, diagnosis, and treatment. *Prim Care Companion J Clin Psychiatry.* 2004;6:9–20.

72. Newman AB, Spiekerman CF, Enright P, et al. Daytime sleepiness predicts mortality and cardiovascular disease in older adults. The cardiovascular health study research group. *J Am Geriatr Soc.* 2000;48(2):115–123.

73. Espiritu JRD. Aging-related sleep changes. *Clin Geriatr Med.* 2008;24:1–14.

74. Pack AI, Dinges DF, Gehrman PR, et al. Risk factors for excessive sleepiness in older adults. *Ann Neurol.* 2006;59:893–904.

75. Roth T. Characteristics and determinants of normal sleep. *J Clin Psychiatry.* 2004;65[suppl 16]:8–11.

76. Phillips B, Ancoli-Israel S. Sleep disorders in the elderly. *Sleep Med.* 2001;2:99–114.

77. Webb WB. Age-related changes in sleep. *Clin Geriatr Med.* 1989;5(2):275–287.

78. Van Cauter E, Leproult R, Plat L. Age-related changes in slow wave sleep and REM sleep and relationship with growth hormone and cortisol levels in healthy men. *JAMA.* 2000;284:861–868.

79. Martin JL, Ancoli-Israel S. Sleep disturbances in long-term care. *Clin Geriatr Med.* 2008;24:39–50.

80. Conn DK, Madan R. Use of sleep-promoting medications in nursing home residents. *Drugs Aging.* 2006;23(4):271–287.

81. Haimov I, Hanuka E, Horowitz Y. Chronic insomnia and cognitive functioning among older adults. *Behav Sleep Med.* 2008;6(1):32–54.

82. Vignola A, Lamoureux C, Bastien CH, et al. Effects of chronic insomnia and use of benzodiazepines on daytime performance in older adults. *J Gerontol B Psychol Sci Soc Sci.* 2000;55(1):P54–P62.

83. Misra S, Malow BA. Evaluation of sleep disturbances in older adults. *Clin Geriatr Med.* 2008;24:15–26.

84. Bloom HG, Ahmed I, Alessi CA, et al. Evidence-based recommendations for the assessment and management of sleep disorders in older persons. *J Am Geriatr Soc.* 2009;57:761–789.

85. Garcia AD. The effect of chronic disorders on sleep in the elderly. *Clin Geriatr Med.* 2008;24:27–38.

86. Dopp JM, Phillips BG. Sleep Disorders. In: Dipiro JT, Talbert RL, Yee GC, et al, eds. *Pharmacotherapy: A Pathophysiologic Approach.* 7th ed. New York: McGraw Hill; 2008:1193–1195.

87. Joshi S. Nonpharmacologic therapy for insomnia in the elderly. *Clin Geriatr Med.* 2008;24:107–119.

88. Morin CM, Colecchi C, Stone J, et al. Behavioral and pharmacological therapies for late-life insomnia: a randomized controlled trial. *JAMA.* 1999;281(11):991–999.

89. Morin CM, Vallieres A, Guay B, et al. Cognitive behavioral therapy, singly and combined with medication, for persistent insomnia: a randomized controlled trial. *JAMA.* 2009;301(19):2005–2015.

99. Li F, Fisher KJ, Harmer P, et al. Tai chi and self-rated quality of sleep and daytime sleepiness in older adults: a randomized controlled trial. *J Am Geriatr Soc.* 2004;52(6):892–900.

91. Irwin MR, Olmstead R, Motivala SJ. Improving sleep quality in older adults with moderate sleep complaints: a randomized controlled trial of Tai Chi Chih. *Sleep.* 2008;31(7):1001–1008.

92. King AC, Oman RF, Brassington GS, et al. Moderate-intensity exercise and self-rated quality of sleep in older adults. A randomized controlled trial. *JAMA.* 1997;277(1):32–37.

93. Dautovich ND, McCrae CS, Rowe M. Subjective and objective napping and sleep in older adults: are evening naps "bad" for nighttime sleep? *J Am Geriatr Soc.* 2008;56:1681–1686.

94. Roger M, Attalie P, Coquelin JP. Multicenter, double-blind, controlled comparison of zolpidem and triazolam in elderly patients with insomnia. *Clin Ther.* 1993;15(1):127–136.

95. Walsh JK, Soubrane C, Roth T. Efficacy and safety of zolpidem extended release in elderly primary insomnia patients. *Am J Geriatr Psychiatry.* 2008;16(1):44–57.

96. Hedner J, Yaeche R, Emilien G, et al. Zaleplon shortens subjective sleep latency and improves subjective

sleep quality in elderly patients with insomnia. *Int J Geriatr Psychiatry.* 2000;15:704–712.

97. Ancoli-Israel S, Walsh JK, Mangano RM, et al. Zaleplon, a novel nonbenzodiazepine hypnotic, effectively treats insomnia in elderly patients without causing rebound effects. *Prim Care Companion J Clin Psychiatry.* 1999;1:114–120.

98. Scharf M, Erman M, Rosenberg R, et al. A 2-week efficacy and safety stuffy of eszopiclone in elderly patients with primary insomnia. *Sleep.* 2005;28(6):720–727.

99. McCall WV, Erman M, Krystal AD, et al. A polysomnography study of eszopiclone in elderly patients with insomnia. *Curr Med Res Opin.* 2006;22(9):1633–1642.

100. FDA.gov. FDA requests label change for all sleep disorder drug products. [Internet] Rockville (MD). Available from: http://www.fda.gov/bbs/topics/NEWS/2007/NEW01587.html

101. Basu R, Dodge H, Stoehr GP, et al. Sedative-hypnotic use of diphenhydramine in a rural, older adult, community-based cohort. *Geriatr Psychiatry.* 2003;11:205–213.

102. Ray WA, Griffin MR, Schaffner W, et al. Psychotropic drug use and the risk of hip fracture. *N Engl J Med.* 1987;316:363–369.

103. Sorock GS, Shimkin EE. Benzodiazepine sedatives and the risk of falling in a community-dwelling elderly cohort. *Arch Intern Med.* 1988;148:2441–2444.

104. Hemmelgarn B, Suissa S, Huang A, et al. Benzodiazepine use and the risk of motor vehicle crash in the elderly. *JAMA.* 1997;278:27–31.

105. Haimov I, Lavie P, Laudon M, et al. Melatonin replacement therapy for elderly insomniacs. *Sleep.* 1995;18(7):598–603.

106. Almeida Montes LG, Ontiveros Uribe MP, Sotres JC, et al. Treatment of primary insomnia with melatonin: a double-blind, placebo-controlled, crossover study. *J Psychiatry Neurosci.* 2003;28(3):191–196.

107. Roth T, Stubbs C, Walsh JK. Ramelteon (TAK-375), a selective MT1/MT2 receptor agonist reduces latency to persistent sleep in a model of transient insomnia related to a novel environment. *Sleep.* 2005;28:303–307.

108. Roth T, Seiden D, Zee P, et al. Phase III trial of ramelteon for the treatment of chronic insomnia in elderly patients. *J Am Geriatr Soc.* 2005;53:S25.

109. Oslin DW. Late-life alcoholism. Issues relevant to the geriatric psychiatrist. *Am J Geriatr Psychiatry.* 2004;12:571–83.

110. Substance Abuse among Older Adults. SAMHSA/CSAT Treatment Improvement Protocols. Available at: www.ncbi.nlm.nih.gov/books/bv.fcgi?rid=hstat5.chapter.48302. Accessed December 30, 2008.

111. Colliver JD, Compton WM, Gfroerer JC, Condon T. Projecting drug use among aging baby boomers in 2020. *Ann Epidemiol.* 2006;16:257–65.

112. Kandel D, Chen K, Warner LA, Kessler RC, Grant B. Prevalence and demographic correlates of symptoms of last-year dependence on alcohol, nicotine, marijuana, and cocaine in the U.S. population. *Drug Alcohol Depend.* 1997;44:11–29.

113. Menninger JA. Assessment and treatment of alcoholism and substance-related disorders in the elderly. *Bull Menninger Clinic.* 2002;66:166–83.

114. Barry KL, Blow FC, Walton MA, et al. Elder-specific brief alcohol intervention:3-month outcomes. *Alcohol Clin Exp Res.* 1998;22:30A.

115. Callahan CM, Tierney WM. Health services use and mortality among older primary care patients with alcoholism. *J Am Geriatr Soc.* 1995;43:1378–83.

116. Joseph CL, Ganzini L, Atkinson RM. Screening for alcohol use disorders in the nursing home. *J Am Geriatr Soc.* 1995;43:368–73.

117. Oslin DW, Streim JE, Parmelee P, Boyce AA, Katz IR. Alcohol abuse: a source of reversible functional disability among residents of a VA nursing home. *Int J Geriatr Psychiatry.* 1997;12:825–32.

118. Culberson JW. Alcohol use in the elderly: beyond the CAGE. Part 1 of 2:prevalence and patterns of problem drinking. *Geriatrics.* 2006;61:23–7.

119. Blow F, Cook CA, Booth BM, Falcon SP, Friedman MJ. Age-related psychiatric comorbidities and level of functioning in alcoholic veterans seeking outpatient treatment. *Hosp Community Psychiatry.* 1992;43:990–5.

120. Blazer DG, Hughes DC, George LK. The epidemiology of depression in an elderly community population. *Gerontologist.* 1987;27:281–7.

121. Finlayson RE, Hurt RD, Davis LJ Jr, Morse RM. Alcoholism in elderly persons: a study of the psychiatric and psychosocial features of 216 inpatients. *Mayo Clin Proc.* 1988;63:761–8.

122. Alcohol and Aging. Alcohol Alert (updated April 1998). Available at: www.pubs.niaaaa.nih.gov/publications/aa40.htm. Accessed December 29, 2008.

123. Kraemer KL, Conigliaro J, Saitz R. Managing alcohol withdrawal in the elderly. *Drugs Aging.* 1999;14:409–25.

124. Kraemer KL, Mayo-Smith MF, Calkins DR. Impact of age on the severity, course, and complications of alcohol withdrawal. *Arch Intern Med.* 1997;157:2234–41.

125. Kosten TR, O'Conner PG. Management of drug and alcohol withdrawal. *N Engl J Med.* 2003;348:1786–95.

126. Brower KJ, Mudd S, Blow FC, Young JP, Hill EM. Severity and treatment of alcohol withdrawal in elderly versus younger patients. *Alcohol Clin Exp Res.* 1994;18:196–201.

127. Foy A, Kay J, Taylor A. The course of alcohol withdrawal in a general hospital. *Q J Med.* 1997;90:253–61.

128. Lemke S, Moos RH. Outcomes at 1 and 5 years for older patients with alcohol use disorders. *J Subst Abuse Treat.* 2003;24:43–50.

129. Oslin DW, Slaymaker VJ, Blow FC, Owen PL, Colleran C. Treatment outcomes for alcohol dependence among middle-aged and older adults. *Addict Behav.* 2005;30:1431–6.

130. Lemke S, Moos RH. Treatment and outcomes of older patients with alcohol use disorders in community residential programs. *J Stud Alcohol.* 2003;65:219–26.

131. Fleming MF, Manwell LB, Barry KL, Adams W, Stauffacher EA. Brief physician advice for alcohol problems in older adults: a randomized, community-based trial. *J Fam Pract.* 1999;48:378–84.

132. Kofoed LL, Tolson RL, Atkinson RM, Toth RL, Turner JA. Treatment compliance of older alcoholics: an elder-specific approach is superior to "mainstreaming." *J Stud Alcohol.* 1987;48:47–51.

133. Atkinson RM, Tolson RL, Turner JA. Factors affecting outpatient treatment compliance of older male problem drinkers. *J Stud Alcohol.* 1993;54:102–6.

134. Kashner TM, Rodell DE, Ogden SR, Guggenheim FG, Karson CN. Outcomes and costs of two VA inpatient treatment programs for older alcoholic patients. *Hosp Community Psychiatry.* 1992;43:985–9.

135. Naltrexone. In: Lacy CF, Armstrong LL, Goldman MP, Lance LL, eds. Lexi-Comp's Drug Information Handbook, 17th ed. Hudson, OH: Lexi-Comp, Inc., 2008:1084–5.

136. Oslin D, Liberto JG, O'Brien J, Krois S, Norbeck J. Naltrexone as an adjunctive treatment for older patients with alcohol dependence. *Am J Geriatr Psychiatry.* 1997;5:324–32.

137. Oslin DW, Pettinati H, Volpicelli JR. Alcoholism treatment adherence: older age predicts better adherence and drinking outcomes. *Am J Geriatr Psychiatry.* 2002;10:740–7.

138. Acamprosate. In: Lacy CF, Armstrong LL, Goldman MP, Lance LL, eds. *Lexi-Comp's Drug Information Handbook.* 17th ed. Hudson, OH: Lexi-Comp, Inc., 2008:19–20.

139. Culberson JW, Ziska M. Prescription drug misuse/abuse in the elderly. *Geriatrics.* 2008;63:22–6, 31.

140. Simoni-Wastila L, Yang HK. Psychoactive drug abuse in older adults. *Am J Geriatr Pharmacother.* 2006;4:380–94.

141. Benitez CIP, Smith K, Vasile RG, Rende R, Edelen MO, Keller MB. Use of benzodiazepines and selective serotonin reuptake inhibitors in middle-aged and older adults with anxiety disorders. *Am J Geriatr Psychiatry.* 2008;16:5–13.

142. Kotlyar M, Dysken M, Adson DE. Update on drug-induced depression in the elderly. *Am J Geriatr Pharmacother.* 2005;3:288–300.

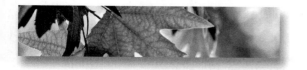

14

Sensory Disorders

MERI HIX

Learning Objectives

1. Discuss the risk factors and etiology of cataract, glaucoma, macular degeneration, dry eye, and diabetic retinopathy.

2. Evaluate the evidence supporting treatment guidelines in elderly patients.

3. Assess a therapeutic regimen for appropriateness, efficacy, and adverse effects.

4. Describe strategies for improving communication with patients with vision and hearing impairment.

5. Describe the presentation of persistent pain in elderly patients.

6. Explain the challenges in assessing pain in elderly patients with or without cognitive impairment.

7. List the classes of medications commonly used to treat nociceptive and neuropathic pain.

8. Recommend a safe treatment strategy for an elderly patient with pain.

Key Terms

BREAKTHROUGH PAIN: Acute pain that occurs despite consistent treatment with long-acting analgesia.

DERMATOME: Localized region of skin that is innervated by a single nerve root.

DRUSEN: Yellow or white deposits on the retina that are more common in older patients; correlated with the risk of developing macular degeneration.

MACULAR DEGENERATION: Eye disease of the macular retina affecting central vision; classified as either exudative/neovascular or nonexudative.

NOCICEPTORS: Receptors preferentially sensitive to a noxious stimulus or to a stimulus which would become noxious if prolonged.

NEUROPATHIC PAIN: Pain initiated or caused by a primary lesion or dysfunction in the nervous system.

PRESBYCUSIS: Bilateral, high frequency hearing loss that is the most common hearing disorder in older patients.

PRESBYOPIA: Inability to focus near vision due to decreased lens accommodation.

Introduction

Sensory deficits in the elderly individual are a chief contributor to decreased quality of life. As vision, taste, smell, and hearing diminish, simple daily pleasures are reduced. Loss of vision or hearing is especially difficult and contributes to increased dependence upon others for activities of daily living. In addition, the sense of touch may become altered with neuropathy from a variety of etiologic sources. Pain management is especially problematic in older adults due to the effects of analgesic medications on the senses and the major organ systems. This chapter focuses upon vision and hearing loss, pain management and the pharmacotherapy associated with these disorders.

Vision and Hearing Impairment

Etiology, Epidemiology, and Clinical Presentation Specific to Geriatrics

Visual impairment in geriatric patients is largely due to age-related changes in the eye that may be either structural or functional in nature (Table 14-1). **Presbyopia,** a functional change, and increased intraocular pressure, a structural change, are common age-related changes. Increased intraocular pressure is a risk factor for glaucoma. Dry eye results from reduced tear production, a functional change, but may also have an inflammatory component.[2] Other etiologies of visual impairment include cataract, **macular degeneration**, and diabetic retinopathy.

Visual impairment affects an estimated 3.3 million people in the United States over the age of 40 and is projected to increase to 5.5 million (3.6% of the population) in the year 2020.[3] Race, ethnic group, and age account for differences in prevalence of low vision and blindness. Cataract is the most common cause of low vision across ethnic groups; whereas, in black persons, cataract is also the leading cause of blindness.[3,4] Macular degeneration and glaucoma are the leading causes of blindness in white and Hispanic persons, respectively. The prevalence of visual impairment increases with age. Depending on ethnic group, blindness and low vision has been estimated to increase two- to eight-fold after the age of 80 years old.

Table 14-1. Age-related Eye Changes

Functional	• Presbyopia
	• Decreased refractive power
	• Decreased dark adaptation
	• Decreased contrast sensitivity
	• Visual field constriction
	• Decreased tear production, resulting in dry eyes
	• Increased difficulty with upward gaze, convergence
Structural	• Lens enlargement, resulting in narrowing of the anterior chamber angle
	• Decreased lens translucency resulting in decreased retinal illumination
	• Increased lens stiffness and decreased curvature
	• Rod cell loss
	• Liquefaction of vitreous gel
	• Loss of eyelid tone, resulting in entropion or ectropion
	• Rising intraocular pressure

Source: Lewis T, Warshaw G. *Current Geriatric Diagnosis and Treatment.* ©2004. McGraw-Hill. Reproduced with permission from the McGraw-Hill Companies.

The etiology of hearing loss falls into two categories: conductive and sensorineural. Cerumen impaction, excessive noise, cerebrovascular accident, trauma, tumors, ototoxic medications, and **presbycusis** are common causes.[1] The prevalence of hearing loss increases with age. Close to 17% of adults in the United States report hearing loss. This number almost doubles in people ages 65 to 74 and almost triples in people ages 75 and above.[5] Hearing loss is common and may go undetected because of its gradual onset or apprehension on the part of the patient when admitting impairment.[6]

Elderly patients may experience visual and hearing impairments because of natural age-related declines, but drug-induced causes may also be present, either due to chronic toxicities or due to increased sensitivity to adverse effects. For instance, antipsychotic medications have been associated with cataracts. Corticosteroid use can cause cataract and open-angle glaucoma, whereas, anticholinergics and adrenergics have both caused acute closed-angle glaucoma.[7] Aminoglycoside antibiotics and nonsteroidal anti-inflammatory drugs are common causes of ototoxicity.

Comorbidities also increase risk for visual and hearing issues in older patients. Sjogren's syndrome, an autoimmune disease that affects exocrine glands, increases the risk for dry eye. Diabetes is the most common cause of retinopathy.[1]

Functional losses and emotional problems are consequences of visual and hearing impairment. Both activities of daily living and self-administration of medication can become limited.[8] Depression, social isolation, and cognitive impairment are reported consequences of declining hearing and vision.[4,8,9]

 KEY POINT: Vision and hearing loss affect cognitive and psychosocial function of older adults.

Summary of Standard Treatment in General Adult Population

Management of glaucoma is targeted at decreasing intraocular pressure and preventing angle closure. First-line pharmacotherapy for primary open-angle glaucoma includes topical beta-blockers or prostaglandin analog eye drops.[10] Other pharmacotherapeutic options include topical alpha-2 adrenergic agonists, topical or oral carbonic anhydrase inhibitors, and topical cholinergic agents.

Decreasing intraocular pressure is accomplished by either decreasing aqueous production or increasing its outflow. Beta-adrenergic blockers and carbonic anhydrase inhibitors decrease aqueous humor production (Table 14-2). Prostaglandin analogs and cholinergic agents increase outflow of aqueous humor.[11] Alpha-adrenergic agonists perform both of these actions. It is recommended that if one agent is effective but a target intraocular pressure has not been reached, then combination therapy should be used. However, if one agent is ineffective, an alternative drug class should be used.[10]

The common management of dry eyes includes lubricant and anti-inflammatory eye drops. Lubricant eye drops are effective in both mild and severe disease.[12] The efficacy of lubricants is limited by short contact time with the eye. Hypotonic solutions, tear stabilizing molecules, and lipid formulations have enhanced contact time with the eye, viscosity, and stability of the tear film.[2]

Cyclosporine and corticosteroid eye drops inhibit inflammation and increase the health of the ocular surface.[2] With both of these agents, little systemic absorption occurs, although prolonged use of topical corticosteroids is not recommended because of the increased risk of cataract development and elevated intraocular pressure.[2] Other methods to treat dry eyes have been examined. A diet of omega-3 fatty acids, topical or oral secretagogues, and hormone replacement have been studied or used off-label for dry eye.[2,12]

The treatment for cataract is primarily surgical with very few non-surgical options that may reduce some symptoms of cataract. Although

Table 14-2. Common Treatments that Decrease Intraocular Pressure in Open-angle Glaucoma

Class	Medication Examples	General Adult Treatment Principles	Geriatric Considerations
Beta-blockers	Timolol Betaxolol	First-line therapy. Possible systemic absorption. Available in combination with other agents.	May be difficult to administer. Once or twice daily dosing improves compliance. Cautious use with concomitant disease states such as heart failure, bradycardia, asthma, and chronic obstructive pulmonary disease.
Prostaglandin analogs	Latanoprost Travoprost Bimatoprost	First-line therapy. Available in combination with other agents.	May be difficult to administer. Once-daily dosing improves compliance. Fewer adverse effects than beta-blockers. Long-term use may lead to macular edema.
Alpha adrenergic agonists	Brimonidine Apraclonidine	Alternative or add-on therapy. Possible systemic absorption.	May be difficult to administer. Frequent dosing will decrease compliance. Additive effects on the cardiovascular system may be more pronounced.
Carbonic anhydrase inhibitors	Dorzolamide Acetazolamide	Alternative or add-on therapy. Available in combination with other agents.	May be difficult to administer. Frequent dosing will decrease compliance. Acetazolamide given orally is an easier-to-administer alternative. Age-related declines in renal and hepatic function may lead to increased adverse effects.
Cholinergic agents	Pilocarpine Carbachol	Alternative or add-on therapy. Possible systemic absorption.	May be difficult to administer. Frequent dosing will decrease compliance. Long-term use may lead to cataract. Cautious use in patients with Parkinson's disease.

many studies have examined nutritional supplementation, such as beta-carotene, to reduce the incidence of cataract, they have been largely unsuccessful.[13] Reducing the risk of developing cataract, such as smoking cessation, avoidance of certain medications that may cause cataract, and reduction of sun exposure, is recommended.

For age-related macular degeneration (AMD), treatment depends on the type of AMD, either wet or dry. Initial treatment of dry, or atrophic, AMD is reserved until there is intermediate macular degeneration, evidenced by the presence of **drusen** in both eyes, or advanced disease in one eye, evidenced by drusen accompanied by blurred vision.[14] Oral antioxidant vitamin and mineral supplements which include vitamin C, vitamin E, beta-carotene and zinc are the treatments of choice in advanced dry macular degeneration, as determined by a group of studies undertaken by the Age-Related Eye Disease Research Group.[15] Copper has been added to prevent copper deficiency associated with zinc intake. A smoker's formulation which does not include beta-carotene because it has been associated with increased risk for lung cancer in this group is also used.

KEY POINT: Prophylactic treatment of AMD with eye formulations of vitamins and minerals is not currently recommended.

Photodynamic therapy with verteporfin, which destroys abnormal blood vessels, may be used with more advanced disease with neovascularization, or wet AMD. Vascular endothelial growth factor is a target for therapy aimed at reducing angiogenesis in macular degeneration. These agents include pegaptanib, ranibizumab, and bevacizumab administered periodically as intravitreal injections.[14]

Treatment of hearing loss depends on the etiology. If the cause is treatable, then hearing may be restored. However, in cases where the cause is irreversible, management of the hearing loss with hearing aids, assistive listening devices, or cochlear implants may be necessary.[1] The decision as to what kind of aid is most beneficial is the specialty practice of audiologists.

Review of Evidence Supporting Treatment Recommendations for Elderly Patients

The presence of visual impairment increases with age, emphasizing the importance of follow-up eye examinations, even in the oldest patients. It has been shown that nursing home records often lack reports of eye examinations even when known visual impairment exists.[1] These patients are at the greatest risk of psychosocial impairment as a result of sensory impairment and should be evaluated.

Although glaucoma studies do not specifically study the effects of therapy in the geriatric population, there is still a large proportion of participants who are at least 60 years old.

Monotherapy with beta-adrenergic blockers or prostaglandin analogs is recommended by glaucoma guidelines.[10] Bimatoprost, a prostaglandin analog, was compared to twice daily timolol in patients with an average age of 60 years old, ranging up to 90 years old.[17] Bimatoprost given once daily, significantly reduced intraocular pressure compared with timolol. Twice-daily dosing of bimatoprost was not more beneficial than once-daily dosing. Once-daily latanoprost lowered intraocular pressure more than twice-daily timolol in chronic closed-angle glaucoma.[18] The average age of participants was 63 years old, ranging up to 82 years old. Aside from ocular hypotensive effects, latanoprost showed a significant improvement in contrast sensitivity compared with timolol in a study of patients with an average age of 61 years old, ranging up to 69 years old.[19]

Combination therapy is commonly studied because of the additive efficacy of two classes of medications versus monotherapy. Studies enrolled patients with an average age less than 65 but included patients up to 93 years old. A combination of brimonidine, an alpha-adrenergic agonist, and timolol demonstrated significantly greater reductions in intraocular pressure compared with either agent alone.[20] A combination of timolol with either latanoprost or dorzolamide, a topical carbonic anhydrase inhibitor, is feasible under current glaucoma guidelines. A study of over 200 patients randomized to either group demonstrated that the combination with latanoprost significantly lowered intraocular pressure when compared with the dorzolamide combination.[21] Timolol combined with either dorzolamide or brimonidine, an alpha-adrenergic agonist showed that both combinations were effective and comparable at lowering intraocular pressure.

Trials in the management of dry eye disease are not specific for older patients. One study of topical cyclosporine demonstrated significant symptomatic improvement of mild to moderate dry eye and objective improvement in severe dry eye.[22] These patients ranged in age from 23 to 88 years old, with an average age of 63 years old. Blurred vision, grittiness, itchiness, and dryness were significantly decreased from baseline in cyclosporine treatment groups compared to a placebo vehicle in another study.[23] The patients in this study were an average of 60 years old but ranged up to 73 years old. Objective measures were also significantly improved. Two strengths of cyclosporine solution were compared but no dose effects were seen. Newer therapies for chronic dry eye are commonly studied in younger populations or in those patients receiving corrective eye surgery.

Larger trials of at least 1,000 patients evaluating dietary supplements in cataracts have included a fair number of patients over the age of 65 years old. The Age Related Eye Disease Study (AREDS)[24], the Clinical Trial of Nutritional Supplements (CTNS),[25] and the Carotenoids in the Age-Related Eye Disease Study (CAREDS)[26] have studied antioxidants and multivitamins in relation to incidence or progression of lens opacities. Investigators in the largest study, AREDS[24], reported no effect with high doses of vitamin C, vitamin E, and beta carotene on the development of any type of lens opacity. Results of a later study, CTNS,[25] demonstrated an 18% reduction of the development or progression of lens opacities with intake of a multivitamin supplement. There is some evidence to suggest higher dietary lutein and zeaxanthin may reduce the risk of developing nuclear cataract.[26] With conflicting results, pharmacotherapy is not recommended.

Large studies have demonstrated a reduced occurrence of age-related macular degeneration with concurrent intake of vitamins E and C, beta carotene, and zinc. The Age-Related Eye Disease Studies (AREDS),[15,27] Blue Mountains Eye Disease Study,[28] and other similar studies of age-related macular degeneration included 2,400 to 4,170 patients with either double-blind,[15] case-control,[27] or prospective cohort designs.[28,29] The average age of participants in these trials was at least 65 years old.

Higher dietary or supplemental intake of zinc, lutein and zeaxanthin, and zinc combined with other vitamins or antioxidants reduced incidence of AMD and a synergistic effect was seen with combination of vitamins C and E, zinc, and beta carotene.[15,29] One study concluded that beta-carotene or vitamin E alone may increase the incidence of AMD and another that high dietary intake of omega-3 long-chain polyunsaturated fatty acids decreases the incidence of AMD.[27,28] Although current guidelines recommend treatment with supplements after signs of AMD are evident, there is some evidence that supports the use of antioxidants for primary prevention in elderly patients.[29]

Treatment with vascular endothelial growth factor inhibitors has been studied for more advanced macular degeneration. Ranibizumab in patients with an average age of 77 years old increased or maintained visual acuity in over 90% of patients compared to 62% or less in the control group.[30] Ranibizumab also decreased neovascularization. Preservation of visual acuity has also been reported in patients with mean ages of 75 to 77 years old treated with pegaptanib.[31] These studies both show lasting effect with continued treatment over a 2-year period of time.

Common Problems Encountered When Treating Elderly Patients with This Condition

Eye drop containers may be difficult to handle for an elderly person trying to administer the solution. Older patients, especially those with lower visual acuity, have greater difficulty opening and administering eye drops than younger patients.[32] The pharmacist should instruct patients on proper administration technique, which includes pulling down the lower eye lid with one hand and steadying the other hand that is holding the bottle against the forehead. To prevent some systemic absorption, the patient should apply pressure on the tear duct in the corner of the eye after administration of eye drops. Mobility impairments, such as tremor, arthritis, or paralysis, also make it difficult for patients to administer these medications. There are aids to help with squeezing and holding bottles so that placement of eye drops is accurate for individuals with these problems. The pharmacist has a unique opportunity in the community setting to assess a patient's ability to self-administer eye drops. In settings where eye drops are administered by a health professional, such as a long term care facility, the pharmacist should periodically observe administration technique by the patient and/or nursing staff.

 KEY POINT: Instillation of eye drops is a difficult task for older patients that requires aids and innovative techniques for sufficient administration.

Eye drops for the treatment of glaucoma range in the frequency of dosing. Some require only once-daily dosing, like latanoprost, while others require three-times daily dosing, like brimonidine monotherapy. If dual therapy is required, the patient is required to wait between the administrations of two separate agents. The option of using fixed-dose combination products is convenient for patients who could benefit from more than one class of medication.

Elderly patients with visual impairment may rely on caregivers to perform or communicate tasks required for daily living and medical care. However, many patients want to maintain independence. Strategies for effective communication with patients with vision loss include the use of corrective lenses, magnifying aids, large print on written material, and adequate lighting.[33]

Communication can be difficult with someone who has hearing loss. Someone with presbycusis needs extra time to process what has been said. Speech should be clear and louder than normal but not necessarily slower.[34] Any communication should occur in a quiet place, free from extraneous background noise, and in close proximity, directly face-to-face with the patient.[1] Rephrasing to less complicated and shorter sentences, pausing between sentences, and using written communication are all strategies to better communicate if the first attempt is unsuccessful.[1,34]

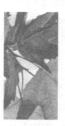 KEY POINT: Many patients with hearing impairment rely on lip reading and facial gestures, and exaggerated enunciation or slowed speech impairs this process.

Pain

Etiology, Epidemiology, and Clinical Presentation Specific to Geriatrics

Pain is a subjective sensation that often serves as a signal of damage or potential damage to nerve fibers. Pain is classified by its onset, duration, or etiology. Acute injury or sudden onset of pain defines acute pain. Chronic, or persistent, pain may be initiated by an acute injury but has lasted beyond the normal healing time. Persistent pain may also arise from chronic diseases, cancer, or unknown causes and include both nociceptive and neuropathic features.

Nociceptive pain is initiated by thermal, electrical, or mechanical impulses that stimulate nerve fibers, called **nociceptors**. This type of pain may be less severe in older patients because of age-related changes in nerve fibers, but modulation of persistent pain may be impaired due to age-related declines in neurotransmitter production.[35] **Neuropathic pain** is often associated with conditions like diabetic peripheral neuropathy, postherpetic neuralgia, phantom limb pain after amputation, and central post-stroke pain. It also arises from persistent, nociceptive pain.

Regardless of etiology, neuropathic pain is often characterized by a burning, buzzing, stinging, shock-like, or deep aching pain or discomfort. The location of symptoms may vary. Peripheral diabetic neuropathic pain is bilateral and symmetrical, usually affecting the lower limbs.[36] Postherpetic neuralgia occurs asymmetrically along a **dermatome**, typically weeks to months after onset of rash.[37]

Despite adequately treated pain, incidents of acute pain, or **breakthrough pain**, may occur.

Causes of breakthrough pain include end-of-dose failure, when analgesia wanes before the next dose is scheduled; incident pain, when movement provokes pain; and spontaneous pain.[38]

In residents of long-term care facilities, prevalence of pain ranges from about 50 to 80 percent.[39] The most common type of pain reported in older patients is musculoskeletal. Neuropathic pain represents 10% of all pain, but prevalence increases with age.[40] Peripheral diabetic neuropathic pain affects close to 25% of all patients with diabetes.[41] Post-stroke pain affects 21% of patients after first stroke.[42] Inadequately treated pain in the elderly population leads to depression, anxiety, sleep disturbance, decreased quality of life, and reduced independence in daily living.[38,43]

Assessment of the presence and severity of pain can be difficult in elderly patients. Reluctance to admit pain may be for cultural or social reasons. The most common methods of assessment are visual analog scales; numerical rating scales; verbal descriptor scales; or faces scales comprised of simple drawings of faces depicting varying levels of discomfort. These scales may be used reliably in patients who are cognitively intact. The faces scale has demonstrated utility in patients with cognitive impairment. However, patients with advanced dementia may not express pain and will instead display behaviors like aggression, irritability, groaning, rigidity, altered facial expressions, changes in eating patterns, or social withdrawal.[35,38]

Summary of Standard Treatment in the General Adult Population

The experience of pain is subjective, and a systematic approach to assessment is needed to create a successful treatment plan. Pain level, quality of life, mood, and sleep quality is evaluated in patients with persistent pain. Nociceptive pain can be successfully treated with typical analgesics, like acetaminophen, non-steroidal anti-inflammatory drugs, and opioids. Neuropathic pain is less predictably responsive to these analgesics. Alternative classes, or adjuvant drugs, like antidepressants, antiepileptic drugs, and topical agents, have demonstrated efficacy in neuropathic pain.

The World Health Organization describes a step-wise approach to the management of cancer pain which is often extended to other types of pain.[44] This approach uses non-opioid analgesics in mild pain. As pain persists, the addition of an opioid analgesic is recommended. Scheduling doses or using long-acting agents will provide more consistent pain relief. Short-acting opioids with a fast onset should be added for breakthrough pain as needed. Titration to higher doses of long-acting agents should be based on the usage of as-needed doses. At any pain level, skeletal muscle relaxants, benzodiazepines, or other adjuvant drugs used for neuropathic pain are recommended.

KEY POINT: Opioids have similar efficacy and adverse effects when used in equipotent doses.

Consensus guidelines and literature reviews for the treatment of diabetic peripheral neuropathic pain and postherpetic neuralgia describe the general approach for management of neuropathic pain.[45,46] Pharmacologic treatment includes the use of tricyclic antidepressants, serotonin-norepinephrine reuptake inhibitors, antiepileptic drugs, long-acting opioids, and topical lidocaine or capsaicin (Table 14-3). General approaches to therapy include initiating at low doses; slow titration to an effective dose to avoid excessive adverse effects; switching to a different class if monotherapy fails; and addition of a different class if monotherapy demonstrates suboptimal efficacy. Efficacy of these treatments may take several weeks, and a change in therapy should not be considered until an adequate amount of time has passed.

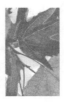

KEY POINT: Combination therapy with analgesics and adjuvant drugs may be necessary to effectively manage persistent pain.

Table 14-3. **Common Treatments for Neuropathic Pain**

Class	Medication Examples	General Adult Treatment Principles	Geriatric Considerations
Tricyclic antide-pressants	Amitriptyline Desipramine Nortriptyline	First-line treatment. Effective doses lower than those used for depression.	Potential for anticholinergic adverse effects; sedating.
Anticonvulsants	Pregabalin Gabapentin Carbamazepine	A first-line treatment for neuropathic pain. Pregabalin has FDA-approved indication for DPNP and PHN.	Requires lower starting doses and slower titration. Pregabalin and gabapentin are renally eliminated and may require dose adjustments.
Serotonin-norepinephrine reuptake inhibitors	Duloxetine Venlafaxine	A first-line treatment for neuropathic pain. Duloxetine has FDA-approved indication for DPNP.	Duloxetine not recommended in hepatic impairment or CrCl < 30 mL/min. Venlafaxine may need dose reduction in hepatic or renal impairment.
Opioids	Oxycodone Methadone Tramadol	May be used as initial monotherapy or add-on therapy. Methadone also has NMDA antagonist activity. Tramadol also has weak serotonin reuptake activity.	Adverse effects such as dizziness, sedation, constipation, and respiratory suppression are more common in the elderly. Methadone has long half-life that requires careful dose titration. Tramadol may increase risk of serotonin syndrome when given with antidepressants.
Topical	Lidocaine Capsaicin	May be used as initial therapy or as add-on therapy. Useful in localized pain.	Ease of use in elderly (lidocaine), especially if in patch form. Capsaicin causes increased burning during initial use. Capsaicin should not be used in acute herpes zoster due to risk of mucosal contact.

CrCl = creatinine clearance; DPNP = diabetic peripheral neuropathic pain; NMDA = N-methyl-D-aspartate; PHN = postherpetic neuropathy.

Review of Evidence Supporting Treatment Recommendations for Elderly Patients

The American Geriatrics Society provides guidelines for the assessment and treatment of persistent pain in the geriatric population.[38] Two follow-up guidelines specifically address pharmacologic management outlining use of non-opioid and opioid analgesics.[47,48] Few studies of chronic or persistent pain syndromes using typical analgesics have been conducted, with almost none in the elderly, and recommendations are made based on expert opinion.

Initial treatment of musculoskeletal pain with acetaminophen is recommended.[47] Non-steroidal anti-inflammatory drugs should not routinely be used in elderly patients due to a high risk of causing gastrointestinal bleeding, renal dysfunction, hypertension, and heart failure. Two studies providing evidence for the treatment of chronic pain with acetaminophen in older adults with osteoarthritis used 3.9–4 grams for periods as long as 12 months. The mean age of subjects was around 60 years, but ranged as high as 90 in one study. Patients in both studies reported significant improvement in pain scores, but in one study, 1.9% of patients had clinically significant elevations in hepatic transaminases in the treatment arm.[49,50]

Opioids are recommended for moderate-severe pain, and doses should be scheduled around-the-clock for frequent or persistent pain.[38,47,48] These recommendations are based on expert opinion, pharmacokinetic and pharmacodynamic data, and extrapolation of results from adult patients.[48] A weakness of many studies is that efficacy and safety data specific to elderly participants is lacking. One placebo-controlled study evaluated controlled-release oxycodone in 133 subjects with osteoarthritis (average age 62 years with 43% of patients ≥65).[51] Although this was only a 2-week trial, a clinically meaningful pain reduction (20%) from baseline was achieved within 1 day for the 10-mg arm and 2 days for the 20-mg arm and statistically significant improvements in mood, enjoyment of life, and sleep when compared with placebo were evident in the 20-mg arm. However, over one half of the patients withdrew participation, primarily due to adverse effects and dose-related ineffectiveness.

The use of adjuvant drugs in the treatment of neuropathic pain is recommended in guidelines for elderly patients.[47] A caution against the use of the tricyclic antidepressants amitriptyline, imipramine, and doxepin is detailed in the guidelines, owing to adverse effects. Other common oral adjuvant drugs are not mentioned specifically, but the evidence for their use comes from studies of disease states that are more common in the elderly population. These studies do not specifically include elderly patients and rarely include more than a few patients over 75. Results should be extrapolated with caution because patients with conditions common in the elderly, such as renal, hepatic, and cardiac diseases, are excluded from the studies. A summary of representative trials using adjuvant drugs for neuropathic pain is included in Table 14-4.

Topical agents are recommended for well-localized neuropathic pain.[47] They have the advantage of few systemic adverse effects or drug interactions. Lidocaine is most commonly recommended and has demonstrated efficacy in small studies of patients with a wide range of ages.[63,64]

Common Problems Encountered When Treating Elderly Patients with This Condition

There are often discrepancies in prevalence studies of pain in older patients because of the failure to recognize, report, or treat pain in these patients.[39] Pain in the older population in general is not adequately treated, whether or not the patient is cognitively impaired or the pain is acute or persistent.[65-67]

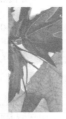

KEY POINT: Pain is often under-recognized and undertreated in elderly patients. Close monitoring and proactive approaches to dose titration will provide better management.

Patients with cognitive impairment may not be able to recall pain over a period of time, but the ability to report current pain often remains intact.[68] Rating scales to assess pain in non-verbal or cognitively impaired patients are available but not always reliable. Observing facial gestures, for example, during painful movements (e.g., during transfers) provides useful clues to how a patient behaves when in pain.[68] Similarly, administering a test dose of an analgesic when pain is suspected and then observing for a decrease in pain-related behaviors may provide helpful information. Family or caregivers who closely observe these patients may be called upon to report the presence of pain with relative accuracy.

Table 14-4. **Summary of Trials of the Management of Neuropathic Pain**

	Tricyclic antidepressants[52-55]	Serotonin-norepinephrine reuptake inhibitors[56,57]	Antiepileptic drugs[58-60]	Opioids[52,55,61,62]
Study drug(s)	Amitriptyline, desipramine, nortriptyline	Duloxetine	Pregabalin, gabapentin	Oxycodone, morphine
Etiology of pain	Postherpetic neuralgia, diabetic peripheral neuropathic pain	Diabetic peripheral neuropathic pain	Postherpetic neuralgia, diabetic peripheral neuropathic pain	Postherpetic neuralgia, diabetic peripheral neuropathic pain
Average ages (years)	60–71	59–61	62–73	60–71
Size of individual trials (n)	Less than 50	Over 300	81–217	Less than 65
Average pain reduction from baseline (%)	32–66	45	33–40	38–63
Patients with significant pain reduction (%)	34–67	39–69	43–61	38–58
Limitations	Small study size, oldest demographic not represented	Younger patient population, studies supported by drug manufacturer, many concomitant disease states excluded	Pregabalin studies supported by drug manufacturer, many concomitant disease states excluded	Most studies used opioid in combination with an adjuvant or as a comparator arm

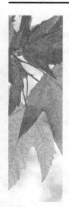

KEY POINT: Non-verbal behaviors suggestive of pain can be observed to assist in pain management of patients with an inability to communicate. In patients with cognitive impairment, close family members or caretakers are reliable sources for assessing pain and the efficacy of pain management.

Most adverse effects of analgesics and adjuvant drugs are transient, and tolerance develops when they are used consistently. Initially, adverse effects like sedation, dizziness, and orthostatic hypotension caused by antidepressants, antiepileptic drugs, and opioids can be made less bothersome by administering these drugs at bedtime.

Tolerance to opioid-induced constipation does not typically occur. The goal to managing constipation is prevention. Older patients are at greater risk for developing constipation because of decreased mobility or increased likelihood of taking concomitant drugs that cause constipation. A bowel regimen containing a stimulant laxative like senna should be used in all patients receiving opioids, starting with an "as needed" schedule. The dose can be titrated upward to assure bowel movements occur every 3 days. A stool softener may be added to improve consistency of the stool and comfort for the patient.

Renal and hepatic impairment, whether age-related or due to other causes, predisposes patients to toxicities caused by analgesic and adjuvant drugs. Non-steroidal anti-inflammatory drugs can worsen renal function by causing vasoconstriction of renal arterioles. Neurotoxicity caused by opioids may rarely occur and is due to accumulation of renally eliminated active metabolites or rapid escalation of dose. Signs and symptoms of neurotoxicity include hyperalgesia, seizures, confusion, and twitching. Pregabalin, gabapentin, and duloxetine are renally eliminated and should be dosed accordingly in older patients. Duloxetine, tricyclic antidepressants, and most opioids are hepatically metabolized. Age-related hepatic impairment partially contributes to the increased sensitivity of elderly patients to the effects of these drugs. Longer intervals between doses and smaller doses of these agents are recommended for initial therapy with careful titration to achieve pain control in order to avoid drug-related problems.[48]

 KEY POINT: First doses of adjuvant drugs should be given at bedtime because adverse effects like sedation and dizziness will be less bothersome.

Acetaminophen is usually the first agent of choice in the older adult because it has a good safety profile. Although it undergoes hepatic metabolism, the primary route is through sulfation and glucuronidation, which generally remain intact as a person ages. However, with excess amounts of acetaminophen the mixed function oxidase system is used for metabolism. It requires adequate glutathione to metabolize acetaminophen to an inactive compound. If glutathione is not available, a toxic metabolite is produced which causes hepatic cell necrosis. A maximum dose of 4 g per day of acetaminophen is recommended to reduce the risk of hepatoxicity. Individuals who consume alcohol are at an increased risk. An additional cause of concern is the multitude of combination analgesics which contain acetaminophen increasing the potential for unintentional overdose. The FDA updated the requirements for labeling of over-the-counter products containing acetaminophen in an attempt to better educate consumers.[69]

Increased adipose tissue in the body composition of older patients is also a concern with certain drugs. Fentanyl is highly lipophilic and may unpredictably release into circulation after depositing in adipose tissue. In addition, absorption of transdermal fentanyl is highly variable, may be affected by normal changes in older skin and is temperature dependent. Transdermal fentanyl should always be started at 25 mcg or less for opiate-naïve patients, and this is particularly important in the geriatric population.

Methadone, meperidine and propoxyphene are not recommended for use in the elderly. Methadone is complicated to dose, making an already dangerous class of drugs in the elderly even more complicated. It may be of some benefit in neuropathic pain. Meperidine and propoxyphene are opioids that are hepatically metabolized to active, and toxic, metabolites with a longer half-life than the parent drug. The metabolites are renally eliminated, interact with other drugs, and accumulate in older patients. Normeperidine, the active metabolite of meperidine, can precipitate anxiety, tremors and seizures. The adverse effects of propoxyphene become disproportionate to the analgesia conferred to the patient. Propoxyphene is no longer available in Europe due to its risk/benefit profile and the FDA has also considered removing it from the U.S. market. Nonsteroidal anti-inflammatory drugs cause gastrointestinal ulceration, hypertension, and renal failure and are not routinely recommended for older patients. Pregabalin and gabapentin cause edema, often dose-related and troubling in patients with heart failure. Tricyclic antidepressants and serotonin norepinephrine reuptake inhibitors cause cardiac rhythm abnormalities. In patients with comorbid conditions that predispose them to these effects, these agents should be used cautiously, if at all.

Patients cite fear of adverse effects, concerns for overdosing, and addiction as reasons for inadequate analgesia.[70] An understanding of the etiology of pain syndromes, increased sensitivity to analgesics in older patients, and measures to prevent adverse effects will promote safer pain management. Although addiction may occur in older patients, the fear is often unfounded. Educating the patient that daily use of opioids to treat pain is not addiction and that it is similar to treating high blood pressure with an antihypertensive drug will help to allay this concern.

CASE 1: OUTPATIENT OPHTHALMOLOGY CLINIC

Subjective:

TP is a 67-year-old Hispanic woman who presents with a progressive loss of field vision and no headache or pain.

PMH:

Hypertension, chronic atrial fibrillation, and arthritis in the hands

Medications:

hydrochlorothiazide 25 mg daily
metoprolol tartrate XL 50 mg daily
acetaminophen 650 mg every 4 to 6 hours prn
asa 81 mg daily

Objective:

BP 134/64 mm Hg HR 58
IOP 28 mmHg (normal: 10–22 mmHg)

Assessment:

TP has open-angle glaucoma with elevated IOP with vision loss

Plan:

Initiate therapy with latanoprost eye drops for open-angle glaucoma.

Rationale:

Prostaglandin analogs are a first-line treatment for open-angle glaucoma as well as beta-blockers. Topical beta-blockers would not be a first choice in this patient because she has a low heart rate due to the beta blocker therapy for atrial fibrillation.

Case Summary:

TP is at risk for glaucoma secondary to age and Hispanic ethnicity. She presents with symptoms of open-angle glaucoma (loss of field vision). Closed-angle glaucoma is uncommon and typically presents as an acute worsening of vision with associated eye pain or headache. Since there are two first-line agents for open-angle glaucoma, concomitant diseases and ease of use must be carefully considered in an elderly patient. Although administered topically, beta-blockers may have some systemic absorption which would be additive to an oral beta blocker. Latanoprost is dosed once daily in the evening, which improves compliance.

CASE 2: OUTPATIENT PAIN CLINIC

Subjective:

LM is a 77-year-old man with chronic non-malignant back pain presenting with worsening pain that he describes as dull and aching. Until recently his pain had been very well managed (3/10 visual analog score) with hydrocodone/acetaminophen and occasional ibuprofen, but now requires more frequent doses (up to maximum prescribed) with little added benefit.

Past Medical History:

Hypertension, obesity, obstructive sleep apnea, back pain

Past Surgical History:

Back surgery 8 years ago to fix a bulging disc

Allergies:

NKDA

Medications:

hydrochlorothiazide 25 mg daily
hydrocodone/acetaminophen 10/500, 2 tabs five to six times daily
ibuprofen 600 mg three to four times daily
docusate 200 mg twice daily

Social/Work History:

Used to raise cattle on a farm. Lives with wife of 45 years.

Objective:

height 5'8"
weight 265 lb
visual analog score: 7/10
blood pressure: 154/70 mmHg
heart rate: 87
BUN 25 mg/dL
serum creatinine 1.4 mg/dL

Assessment:

LM is experiencing worsening pain that may have components of neuropathic pain and is not controlled with his current regimen. His daily dose of acetaminophen exceeds maximum recommendations.

Plan:

1. Start morphine sulfate extended release 30 mg every 12 hours, change hydrocodone/acetaminophen to 1–2 tablets every 6 hours as needed dosing (maximum daily acetaminophen limited to 4 g), discontinue ibuprofen, and add gabapentin 200 mg at bedtime for 3 days, then increase to 200 mg twice daily.

2. Add senna as needed for opioid-induced constipation. Consider docusate in addition to senna according to patient needs.

3. Counsel patient and spouse to observe for worsening sleep apnea with addition of long-acting opioid and gabapentin.

Rationale:

LM has a history of a bulging disc and surgery on his back, has persistent pain that is worsening, and has neuropathic features. LM should be placed on a consistent opioid regimen and an adjuvant drug for his neuropathic pain. There is ample evidence to suggest how much opioid he requires, and an equivalent regimen of a long-acting opioid can be created using an equipotent dose, adjusted for possible cross tolerance and renal function. The combination of hydrocodone/acetaminophen is appropriate for moderate breakthrough pain as long as the patient does not take excessive amounts of acetaminophen. Ibuprofen should be discontinued due to its adverse effect on blood pressure and renal function. Gabapentin is a reasonable choice for the neuropathic symptoms as long as the dose is adjusted based on renal function. Although LM has not complained of constipation, a stimulant laxative should be made available with the initiation of scheduled opiate therapy to be proactive. Finally, older patients frequently have co-morbidities that require more intense monitoring or careful titration. Patients with obstructive sleep apnea are at an increased risk for respiratory depression from sedatives and pain medications.

Case Summary:

This patient requires multiple interventions because pain is not sufficiently responding to increased doses of analgesics. The analgesic drugs LM currently takes could potentially lead to renal and hepatic toxicity, as well as increasing blood pressure, if they are continued at a higher frequency. Other classes of analgesics and adjuvant drugs should be considered for better management of this pain syndrome.

Clinical Pearls

- *Patients with hearing loss may be mistakenly labeled with cognitive impairment because it may require more time for them to process information or it may appear that they do not understand the conversation. Patients whose hearing loss has not been officially diagnosed may be particularly vulnerable to this inappropriate diagnosis.*

- *The effective dose of tricyclic antidepressants for neuropathic pain is often less than the dose used for depression. Desipramine and nortriptyline have less anticholinergic activity than other tricyclic antidepressants and are preferred over amitriptyline in the elderly patient.*

Chapter Summary

Visual and hearing impairment are commonly linked with aging. Patient age is a risk factor for many causes of decreased visual acuity. Guidelines for treatments are developed from studies that contain many elderly patients. In elderly patients, however, maintenance of quality of life is just as important as managing the disease state. The pharmacist should consider quality of life when recommending therapy and ensure adequate communication techniques when interacting with patients.

Pain management recommendations in the elderly are largely based on expert opinion and based on knowledge of pain syndromes and the altered pharmacokinetics and pharmacodynamics of drugs in elderly patients. Pain is a subjective disease in which patients will direct therapeutic decisions by rating their pain and pain reduction. However, in elderly patients, therapeutic choices must be more conservative.

Treatments for neuropathic and nociceptive pain have a high rate of adverse effects like sedation, dizziness, confusion, respiratory suppression, and constipation. Many effects are transient, but older patients should begin treatment at lower doses or with longer intervals between doses in order to lessen these effects. A balance must be achieved between conservative dosing and sufficient pain management in elderly patients.

Self-Assessment Questions

1. Why does the prevalence of glaucoma increase in patients over the age of 65?

2. What age-related changes contribute to the development of dry eyes?

3. What are the two general mechanisms of action in the pharmacotherapy of open-angle glaucoma?

4. Which common drug classes in the elderly increase the risk for developing cataract?

5. Which types of visual impairment have pharmacologic prevention strategies?

6. Why are elderly patients more at risk for developing drug-related causes of hearing impairment?

7. What common disorders in elderly patients makes administration of eye drops more difficult?

8. What behavior should be avoided when communicating with a patient with presbycusis?

9. What are the most common causes of pain in elderly patients?

10. What methods can be used to assess pain in patients with cognitive impairment?

11. Which drugs would not be considered first-line choices in the treatment of neuropathic pain in elderly patients?

12. How do pain management guidelines for adult and elderly patients differ?

13. What physiologic age-related changes should be considered when designing a pain regimen for an elderly patient?

14. What points of education are important when counseling a patient and caregivers about the treatment of pain?

15. Which adverse effect of opioids should be managed with another class of drugs?

16. In what disease states should pregabalin and gabapentin be used with caution?

References

1. Lewis T, Warshaw G. Visual and hearing impairment. In: Landefeld CS, Palmer RM, Johnson MA, Johnston CB, Lyons WL, eds. *Current Geriatric Diagnosis and Treatment.* 1st ed. New York: McGraw Hill; 2004:122.

2. Foulks GN. Pharmacological management of dry eye in the elderly patient. *Drugs Aging.* 2008;25:105–118.

3. The eye diseases prevalence research group. Causes and prevalence of visual impairment among adults in the United States. *Arch Ophthalmol.* 2004;122:477–485.

4. Johnston CB. Geriatric assessment. In: Landefeld CS, Palmer RM, Johnson MA, Johnston CB, Lyons WL, eds. *Current Geriatric Diagnosis and Treatment.* 1st ed. New York: McGraw Hill; 2004:16.

5. Quick Statistics Page. National Institute on Deafness and Other Communication Disorders. Available at: http://www.nidcd.nih.gov/health/statistics/quick.htm. Accessed September 29, 2008.

6. Gates GA, Murphy M, Rees TS, Fraher A. Screening for handicapping hearing loss in the elderly. *J Fam Pract.* 2003;52:56–62.

7. Li J, Tripathi RC, Tripathi BJ. Drug-induced ocular disorders. *Drug Saf.* 2008;31:127–141.

8. Sloan FA, Ostermann J, Brown DS, Lee PP. Effects of changes in self-reported vision on cognitive, affective, and functional status and living arrangements among the elderly. *Am J Ophthalmol.* 2005;140:618–627.

9. Age-related eye disease study research group. Cognitive impairment in the age-related eye disease study. *Arch Ophthalmol.* 2006;124:537–543.

10. Primary open-angle glaucoma. Glaucoma panel, preferred practice patterns committee. San Francisco:

American Academy of Ophthalmology; 2005. Available at: http://one.aao.org/CE/PracticeGuidelines/PPP_Content.aspx. Accessed October 1, 2008.

11. Weinreb RN, Khaw PT. Primary open-angle glaucoma. *Lancet.* 2004;363:1711–1720.

12. Lemp MA. Management of dry eye disease. *Am J Manag Care.* 2008;14:S88–S101.

13. Cataract in the adult eye. Cataract and anterior segment panel, preferred practice patterns committee. 2006. Available at: http://one.aao.org/CE/PracticeGuidelines. Accessed October 1, 2008.

14. Age-related macular degeneration. Retina panel, preferred practice patterns committee. 2006. Available at: http://one.aao.org/CE/PracticeGuidelines. Accessed October 1, 2008.

15. Age-related eye disease study group. A randomized, placebo-controlled, clinical trial of high-dose supplementation with vitamins C and E, beta carotene, and zinc for age-related macular degeneration and vision loss. *Arch Ophthalmol.* 2001;119:1417–1436.

16. Owsley C, McGwin G, Scilley K, Meek GC, Dyer A, Seker D. The visual status of older persons residing in nursing homes. *Arch Ophthalmol.* 2007;124:925–930.

17. Whitcup SM, Cantor LB, VanDenburgh AM, Chen K. A randomized, double masked, multicentre clinical trial comparing bimatoprost and timolol for the treatment of glaucoma and ocular hypertension. *Br J Ophthalmol.* 2003;87:57–62.

18. Chew P, Aung T, Aquino MV, Rojanapongpun P. Intraocular pressure-reducing effects and safety of latanoprost versus timolol in patients with chronic angle-closure glaucoma. *Ophthalmology.* 2004;111:427–434.

19. Evans DW, Bartlett JD, Houde B, Than TP, Shaikh A. *J Pharmacol Ther.* 2008;24: 224–229.

20. Sherwood MB, Craven ER, Chou C, DuBiner HB, Batoosingh AL, Schiffman RM, et al. Twice-daily 0.2% brimonidine-0.5% timolol fixed-combination therapy vs monotherapy with timolol or brimonidine in patients with glaucoma or ocular hypertension. *Arch Ophthalmol.* 2006;124:1230–1238.

21. Shin DH, Feldman RM, Sheu WP. Efficacy and safety of the fixed combinations latanoprost/timolol versus dorzolamide/timolol in patients with elevated intraocular pressure. *Ophthalmology.* 2004;111:276–282.

22. Perry HD, Solomon R, Donnenfeld ED, Perry AR, Wittpenn JR, Greenman HE, et al. Evaluation of topical cyclosporine for the treatment of dry eye disease. *Arch Ophthalmol.* 2008;126:1046–1050.

23. Sall K, Stevenson OD, Mundorf TK, Reis BL. Two multicenter, randomized studies of the efficacy and safety of cyclosporine ophthalmic emulsion in moderate to severe dry eye disease. *Ophthalmology.* 2000;107:631–639.

24. Age-related eye disease study research group. A randomized, placebo-controlled, clinical trial of high-dose supplementation with vitamins C and E and beta carotene for age-related cataract and vision loss: AREDS report no. 9. *Arch Ophthalmol.* 2001;119:1439–1452.

25. A randomized, double-masked, placebo-controlled clinical trial of multivitamin supplementation for age-related lens opacities. Clinical trial of nutritional supplements and age-related cataract study group. *Ophthalmology.* 2008;115:599–607.

26. Moeller SM, Voland R, Tinker L, Blodi BA, Klein ML, Gehrs KM, et al. Associations between age-related nuclear cataract and lutein and zeaxanthin in the diet and serum in the carotenoids in the age-related eye disease study (CAREDS), and ancillary study of the women's health initiative. *Arch Ophthalmol.* 2008;126:354–364.

27. Age-related eye disease study research group. The relationship of dietary lipid intake and age-related macular degeneration in a case-control study. *Arch Ophthalmol.* 2007;125:671–679.

28. Tan JSL, Wang JJ, Flood V, Rochtchina E, Smith W, Mitchell P. Dietary antioxidants and the long-term incidence of age-related macular degeneration. *Ophthalmology.* 2008;115:334–341.

29. Van Leeuwen R, Boekhoorn S, Vingerling JR, Witteman JCM, Klaver CW, Hofman A, et al. Dietary intake of antioxidants and risk of age-related macular degeneration. *JAMA.* 2005;294:3101–3107.

30. Rosenfeld PJ, Brown DM, Heier JS, Boyer DS, Kaiser PK, Chung CY, et al. Ranibizumab for neovascular age-related macular degeneration. *N Engl J Med.* 2006;355:1419–1431.

31. VEGF inhibition study in ocular neovascularization clinical trial group. Year 2 efficacy results of 2 randomized controlled clinical trials of pegaptanib for neovascular age-related macular degeneration. *Ophthalmology.* 2006;113:1508–1521.

32. Dietlein TS, Jordan JF, Luke C, Schild A, Dinslage S, Krieglstein GK. Self-application of single-use eye drop containers in an elderly population: comparisons with standard eye drop bottle and with younger patients. *Acta Ophthalmol.* 2008;86(8):856–859.

33. Rosenberg EA, Sperazza LC. The visually impaired patient. *Am Fam Physician.* 2008;77:1431–1436.

34. Morgan DE. Assessment and treatment of hearing loss among elders. In: Osterweil D, Brummel-Smith, K, Beck JC, eds. *Comprehensive Geriatric Assessment.* 1st ed. New York: McGraw-Hill; 2000:253.

35. Karp JF, Shega JW, Morone NE, Weiner DK. Advances in understanding the mechanisms and management of persistent pain in older adults. *Br J Anaesth.* 2008;101:111–120.

36. Argoff CE, Cole BE, Fishbain DA, Irving GA. Diabetic peripheral neuropathic pain: clinical and quality-of-life issues. *Mayo Clin Proc.* 2006;81:S3–S11.

37. Niv D, Maltsman-Tseikhin A. Postherpetic neuralgia: the never-ending challenge. *Pain Practice.* 2005;5:327–340.

38. AGS Panel on Persistent Pain in Older Persons. The management of persistent pain in older persons. *J Am Geriatr Soc.* 2002;50:S205–S224.

39. Fox PL, Raina P, Jadad AR. Prevalence and treatment of pain in older adults in nursing homes and other

long-term care institutions: a systematic review. *CMAJ.* 1999;160:329–333.

40. Torrance N, Smith BH, Bennett MI, Lee AJ. The epidemiology of chronic pain of predominantly neuropathic origin. *J Pain.* 2006;7:281–289.

41. Davies M, Brophy S, Williams R, Taylor A. The prevalence, severity, and impact of painful diabetic peripheral neuropathy in type 2 diabetes. *Diabetes Care.* 2006;29:1518–1522.

42. Lundstrom E, Smits A, Terent A, Borg J. Risk factors for stroke-related pain 1 year after first-ever stroke. *Eur J Neurol.* 2009;16:188–193.

43. Weiner DK, Rudy TE, Morrow L, Slaboda J, Lieber S. The relationship between pain, neuropsychological performance, and physical function in community-dwelling older adults with chronic low back pain. *Pain Med.* 2006;7:60–70.

44. WHO's Pain Ladder. World Health Organization Web site. Available at: http://www.who.int/cancer/palliative/painladder/en/. Accessed October 1, 2008.

45. Christo PJ, Hobelmann G, Maine DN. Post-herpetic neuralgia in older adults. *Drugs Aging.* 2007;24:1–19.

46. Argoff CE, Backonja MM, Belgrade MJ, Bennett GJ, Clark MR, Cole BE, et al. Consensus guidelines: treatment planning and options. *Mayo Clin Proc.* 2006;81:S12–S25.

47. Pharmacological management of persistent pain in older persons. AGS Panel on pharmacological management of persistent pain in older persons. Available at: http://www.americangeriatrics.org/education/final_recommendations.pdf Accessed May, 14, 2009.

48. Pergolizzi J, Boger RH, Budd K, Dahan A, Erdine S, Hans G, et al. Opioids and the management of chronic severe pain in the elderly: consensus statement of an international panel with focus on the six clinically most often used World Health Organization step III opioids. *Pain Practice.* 2008;8:287–313.

49. Temple AR, Benson GD, Zinsenheim JR, Schweinle JE. Multicenter, randomized, double-blind, active-controlled, parallel-group trial of the long-term (6–12 months) safety of acetaminophen in adult patients with osteoarthritis. *Clin Ther.* 2006;28:222–235.

50. Altman RD, Zinsenheim JR, Temple AR, Schweinle JE. Three-month efficacy and safety of acetaminophen extended-release for osteoarthritis pain of the hip or knee: a randomized, double-blind, placebo-controlled study. *Osteoarthr Cartil.* 2007;15:454–461.

51. Roth SH, Fleischmann RM, Burch FX, Dietz F, Bockow B, Rapoport RJ, et al. Around-the-clock, controlled-release oxycodone therapy for osteoarthritis-related pain. *Arch Intern Med.* 2000;160:853–860.

52. Raja SN, Haythornthwaite JA, Pappagallo M, Clark MD, Travison TG, Sabeen S, et al. Opioids versus antidepressants in postherpetic neuralgia. *Neurology.* 2002;59:1015–1021.

53. Morello CM, Leckband SG, Stoner CP, Moorhouse DF, Sahagian GA. Randomized double-blind study comparing the efficacy of gabapentin with amitriptyline

on diabetic peripheral neuropathy pain. *Arch Intern Med.* 1999;159:1931–1937.

54. Dallocchi C, Buffa C, Mazzarello P, Chiroli S. Gabapentin vs. amitriptyline in painful diabetic neuropathy: an open-label pilot study. *J Pain Symptom Manage.* 2000;20:280–285.

55. Watson CP, Vernich L, Chipman M, Reed K. Nortriptyline versus amitriptyline in postherpetic neuralgia: a randomized trial. *Neurology.* 1998;51:1166–1171.

56. Raskin J, Pritchett YL, Wang F, D'Souza DN, Waninger AL, Iyengar S, et al. A double-blind, randomized multicenter trial comparing duloxetine with placebo in the management of diabetic peripheral neuropathic pain. *Pain Med.* 2005;6:346–356.

57. Wernicke JF, Pritchett YL, D'Souza DN, Waninger A, Tran MD, Iyengar S, et al. A randomized controlled trial of duloxetine in diabetic peripheral neuropathic pain. *Neurology.* 2006;67:1411–1420.

58. Rowbotham M, Harden N, Stacey B, Bernstein P, Magnus-Miller L. Gabapentin for the treatment of postherpetic neuralgia: a randomized controlled trial. *JAMA.* 1998;280:1837–1842.

59. Stacey BR, Dworkin RH, Murphy K, Sharma U, Emir B, Griesing T. Pregabalin in the treatment of refractory neuropathic pain: results of a 15-month open-label trial. *Pain Med.* 2008;9(8):1202–1208.

60. Baron R, Brunnmuller U, Brasser M, May M, Binder A. Efficacy and safety of pregabalin in patients with diabetic peripheral neuropathy or postherpetic neuralgia: open-label, non-comparative, flexible-dose study. *Eur J Pain.* 2008;12:850–858.

61. Gilron I, Bailey JM, Tu D, Holden RR, Weaver DF, Houlden RL. Morphine, gabapentin, or their combination for neuropathic pain. *N Engl J Med.* 2005;352:1324–1334.

62. Watson CPN, Moulin D, Watt-Watson J, Gordon A, Eisenhoffer J. Controlled-release oxycodone relieves neuropathic pain: a randomized controlled trial in painful diabetic neuropathy. *Pain.* 2003;105:71–78.

63. Lin PL, Fan, SZ, Huang CH, Huang HH, Tsai MC, Lin CJ, et al. Analgesic effect of lidocaine patch 5% in the treatment of acute herpes zoster: a double-blind and vehicle-controlled study. *Reg Anesth Pain Med.* 2008;33:320–325.

64. White WT, Patel N, Drass M, Nalamachu S. Lidocaine patch 5% with systemic analgesics such as gabapentin: a rational polypharmacy approach for the treatment of chronic pain. *Pain Med.* 2003;4:321–330.

65. Morrison RS, Siu AL. A comparison of pain and its treatment in advanced dementia and cognitively intact patients with hip fracture. *J Pain Symptom Manage.* 2000;19:240–248.

66. Nygaard HA, Jarland M. Are nursing home patients with dementia diagnosis at increased risk for inadequate pain treatment? *Int J Geriatr Psychiatry.* 2005;20:730–737.

67. Reynolds KS, Hanson LC, DeVellis RF, Henderson M, Stenihauser KE. Disparities in pain management

between cognitively intact and cognitively impaired nursing home residents. *J Pain Symptom Manage.* 2008;35:388–396.

68. Herr K, Bjoro K, Decker S. Tools for assessment of pain in nonverbal older adults with dementia: a state-of-the-science review. *J Pain Symptom Manage.* 2006;31:170–192.

69. Food and Drug Administration. Acetaminophen information. Available at: http://www.fda.gov/Drugs/ DrugSafety/InformationbyDrugClass/ucm165107. htm. Accessed 09/22/2009.

70. Zeppetella G. Opioids for cancer breakthrough pain: a pilot study reporting patient assessment of time to meaningful pain relief. *J Pain Symptom Manage.* 2008;35:563–567.

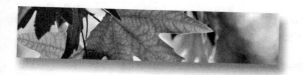

15

Musculoskeletal and Connective Tissue

MARY BETH O'CONNELL AND MICHELLE A. FRITSCH

Learning Objectives

1. Identify differences in the presentation and risk factors of common musculoskeletal disorders including falls, arthritis conditions, osteoporosis, and related pain syndromes; and pressure ulcers in seniors.

2. Apply evidence to support age adjusted therapies for common musculoskeletal disorders and pressure ulcers.

3. Recommend appropriate nonpharmacologic and medication therapy to achieve treatment goals for common musculoskeletal disorders and pressure ulcers.

4. Resolve pharmacotherapy related problems unique to seniors with musculoskeletal disorders.

Key Terms

BRM: Biologic response modifiers. Products that modulate the activity of immunologic substances such as monoclonal antibodies, cytokines, or colony stimulating factors.

DEBRIDEMENT: Removal of nonliving tissue from pressure ulcers, burns and other wounds. "Sharp" debridement is a form of selective debridement where surgical instruments are used to remove specific areas of necrotic tissue. "Wet to dry" and "enzymatic" debridement are non-selective techniques that employ the use of saline-soaked gauze or enzyme gels placed into the wound.

DMARD: Disease modifying antirheumatic drug. Refers to medications with the ability to modify the course of disease, as opposed to simply treating symptoms such as pain or inflammation.

FRAX QUESTIONNAIRE: A tool developed by the World Health Organization to evaluate 10-year fracture risk using a combination of clinical risk factors; can be done with or without femoral neck bone mineral density data.

FRICTION: Force resisting the relative parallel motion of solid surfaces. As a risk factor for pressure ulcers, this refers to stress on the skin surface caused by sliding a patient across bed sheets.

NUTRACEUTICALS: A term referring to a nutritional product that claims to have, in addition to nutritional benefits, medicinal effects.

PRESSURE: the force per unit area applied in a direction perpendicular to the surface of an object. As a risk factor for pressure ulcers, this refers to the downward pressure of the body against the surface of a bed or chair.

SHEAR: the stress applied in a direction parallel to the surface of an object. A little different from friction, this refers to the stress on the internal layers of skin and soft tissue caused by shifts of internal structures. For example, when raising the head of a bed without providing assistance in repositioning, the skin of the back is pulled slightly upward while gravity pulls the ribcage and internal structures downward.

Introduction

Mobility is very important to seniors, sometimes meaning the difference between independent and residential living. Aging is associated with changes in muscle, joint, and bone function that ultimately lead to musculoskeletal diseases such as osteoarthritis, osteoporosis, and polymyalgia rheumatica, all of which have higher incidences in seniors. Prevention can help eliminate or delay the onset of these conditions. For many seniors, these conditions require treatment, however, this treatment usually provides only symptom relief or slowing of disease progression without disease cure. Health care providers have an important role in educating and promoting healthy lifestyles to seniors, assessing and identifying disease at early stages, and prescribing and monitoring age adjusted therapies. Lifestyle adjustments are key both prior to diagnosis and as a component of functional disease adaptation. Prevention and intervention can improve senior quality of life and reduce senior and societal health care costs. The emphasis of this chapter is to highlight age differences rather than provide comprehensive reviews of each of the conditions.

Falls

Etiology, Epidemiology, and Clinical Presentation Specific to Geriatrics

Falls and their consequences are serious health issues for seniors since they can decrease quality of life and independence and sometimes result in death. They also create a challenge for health care providers and caregivers because of their multi-factorial nature and complexity. Falls are either provoked (e.g., push, syncope, seizure related, icy walkway) or unintentional/unexpected (e.g., loss of balance, weakness) with the latter type being the main focus of this section. Risk factors include advanced age, female gender, neurological condition (e.g., cognitive impairment, depression, stroke, Parkinson's disease), medications, muscle weakness, gait and balance difficulties, sensory loss (e.g., vision impairments, peripheral neuropathy), mobility limitations (e.g., arthritis, walkers), cardiovascular disease (e.g., syncope, orthostatic hypotension, arrhythmias), decreased activities of daily living, alcohol use, and history of falls.[1-4] Although more women fall, men have the higher mortality after a fall.[5] Most of the medications associated with falls such as antidepressants, benzodiazepines, sedative hypnotics, antipsychotics, anticonvulsants, and pain medications have a central nervous system effect.[6] Medications can also induce falls through effects on blood pressure, glucose concentration, electrolyte disturbances, vision, gait, balance, and muscle weakness. Poly-pharmacy, which is usually defined as four or more medications, is also an independent risk factor.[7] The environment (e.g., throw rugs, poor lighting, and loose electrical cords) and personal extrinsic factors (e.g., ill fitting footwear, inappropriate walking aids, and nocturnal voiding) also create hazards that increase fall risk.

About a third of seniors residing in the community[7] and 50% in institutional care[1] experience a fall every year. About 75% of unintentional falls occur in seniors.[5] In fact, unintentional injury and accidents were the fifth leading cause of mortality in 2006.[8] Falls resulted in about 1.8 million emergency room visits and 500,000 hospitalizations.[2,7] In one study, 40% of nursing home admissions were related to falls.[4] Health expenditures for falls are significant (2000 data: $179 million for fatal falls and $19 million for nonfatal falls).[5]

Injuries from falls range from minor to severe. Moderate to severe injury occurs in about 20–30% of falls, most notably bruises, head trauma, and fractures.[5] Falls resulted in 1.7 million nonfatal injuries (e.g., 5–10% falls result in head trauma, lacerations, and fractures) and 16,000 deaths annually.[2,7] Falls occurring in the nursing home result in serious injury 12% of the time and fracture 4% of the time.[9] After a fall, patients can become fearful of subsequent falls resulting in restricted mobility, social isolation, depression, and further balance and strength deficits.[3,5]

Assessment of patients with falls is complex beginning with a simple history and routine physical examination and progressing to multifactorial assessments and mobility tests. Simple tests such as the Get Up and Go (See Chapter 4),[10] a timed test to get out of a chair and walk a short distance, and observation of gait and balance can easily be done in the clinic whereas other more complex assessments require occupational and or physical therapist assessments.[1] A complete medication assessment including over-the-counter (OTC) medications, herbals, and supplements should be conducted. Patients with osteoporosis are more likely to fracture after a fall, therefore, a dual energy X-ray absorptiometry (DXA) test should be performed for all patients who have risk factors for osteoporosis and who have a reasonable likelihood of achieving benefit from antiresorptive therapy. A 25 (OH) vitamin D level should be ordered to evaluate for vitamin D deficiency-related muscle weakness, gait abnormalities, and decreased strength. Other tests ordered will be specific to evaluating comorbidities and medications.

Summary of Standard Treatment

A new falls guideline has been created by the American Geriatrics Society and the British Geriatrics Society that describes patient assessment, interventions, and education and evaluates quality of available data.[4] Goal 9 of the National Patient Safety Program of the Joint Commission is related to falls reduction including patient assessment, patient harm reduction, and program evaluations; which are applicable to health care practice in many settings such as hospitals and long term care facilities.[11]

KEY POINT: Fall reduction is a goal of the Joint Commission's National Patient Safety Goals program.

Review of Evidence Base Supporting Treatment Recommendations for Elderly Patients

A multifactorial and multidisciplinary approach to evaluate and resolve falls risk utilizing non-pharmacologic and pharmacologic interventions should be employed to prevent falls (Figure 15-1).[3] A multifaceted team with physicians, other health care professionals, and community members (patients, family members, senior centers) can decrease the number of serious falls, pain, immobility, emergency room visits, and health care costs.[12] Each medication should be evaluated for need, lower dose, and/or safer alternatives including nonpharmacologic interventions. Adequacy of vitamin D dietary and supplement intake should be assessed and deficiencies corrected. Some but not all trials document decreased falls when daily vitamin D supplementation is 700 units or more or the 25 (OH) vitamin D concentration is 26 ng/mL or higher.[13,14]

Risk modification and fall prevention strategies can be implemented. Exercises to strengthen muscles and improve balance such as tai chi should be instituted.[15] Seniors should be encouraged to wear their glasses and use their hearing aids. As patients lose weight and/or height, appropriateness of footwear and assistive devices should be re-evaluated, and adjusted or replaced as needed. The patient, family members and/or occupational therapists can do a home safety assessment and make adjustments to correct problems.[16] Although hip protectors do decrease fractures from falls in nursing home residents, adherence with usage is poor.[17,18]

The impact of various fall intervention programs is mixed. In a meta analysis on fall prevention programs that evaluated 14 trials, programs that reduced one risk factor through interventions such as exercise improvement, syncope cor-

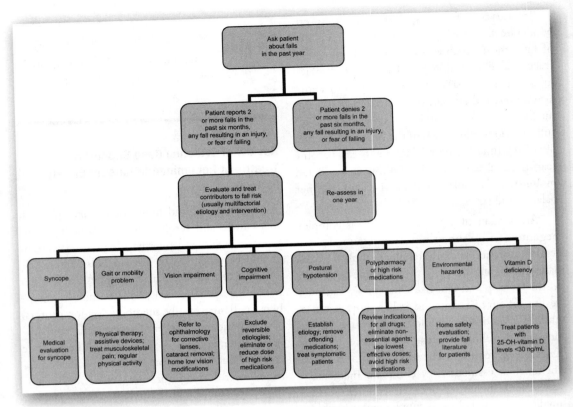

Figure 15-1. Multifactorial approach to minimizing or eliminating falls. *Source:* reference 3.

rection, psychotropic medication withdrawal, or enhanced home safety had a combined fall risk reduction of 23% (0.77 RRR; 95% CI 0.67-0.89) and the multifactorial programs had a combined fall risk reduction of 22% (0.78 RRR; 95% CI 0.68-0.89).[19] In another meta analysis focusing on hospitals and residential care facilities, multifactorial programs were better than single intervention programs to prevent falls.[17] In the largest meta-analysis, interventions decreased falls and nursing home and hospital admissions and improved physical function but had no effect on mortality.[20] A meta-analysis focused solely on injury prevention after falls, also concluded that interventions can decrease injury.[21] In contrast, only one meta-analysis of 19 studies found multifactorial interventions to have no effect on falls and fall related outcomes.[22] Thus population and individual based interventions should be implemented following an approach similar to Figure 15-1.[3] Seniors at high risk for falling might benefit from a referral to a falls clinic or multidisciplinary falls intervention

program. Of note, absolute elimination of falls is often not an achievable goal, and not all intervention programs are practical or cost-effective.[9]

Common Problems Encountered When Treating Elderly Patients with This Condition

Multiple barriers exist to optimal implementation of fall reduction interventions. Adverse medication withdrawal reactions can be precipitated by well meaning medication reduction attempts if the complete history is not considered. Many medications or medication classes, particularly CNS active medications, are common offenders increasing fall risk. However, medication reduction or elimination can be difficult if complete information about medical/medication history is not available to provide perspective on reason for use and patient responsiveness. Determining if the fall risk is from the medication or treated condition can also be difficult. Although decreasing medication use to less than 4 medications is often difficult, sometimes eliminating CNS related medications by slowly tapering them one at a time can be achieved. Careful follow-up observation of the patient's response over weeks or months is required to insure the appropriateness of medication changes.

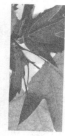 **KEY POINT:** A thorough patient history is required to assess the contribution of medications to fall risk. Medication changes should be made slowly, one drug at a time, followed by careful observation of the results.

Concern exists about using warfarin in seniors with a history of falls and intermediate to high stroke risk.[23] Seniors with intermediate stroke risk (i.e., 65–74 years old without other risk factors) could receive aspirin 325 mg daily instead of warfarin. The benefit risk ratio needs to be determined for seniors with high stroke risk in which case warfarin might be better especially if atrial fibrillation exists. The CHADS score (based on congestive heart failure, hypertension, age, diabetes, and stroke) can be calculated for patients with atrial fibrillation, with warfarin preferred if the score is 2 or greater. Some researchers estimate that the benefits of appropriate anticoagulation far outweigh the bleeding risk associated with falling (see Chapter 7), but falling is nonetheless a fear that leads some prescribers to avoid warfarin. Although a common practice has been to use low dose warfarin in high risk falls patients, subsequent research documented less benefit with equal bleeding risk than standard dosing in patients with atrial fibrillation.[24] Minimizing fall risk and closely monitoring warfarin therapy will help decrease major bleeding risk.

Limited mobility or functional status presents barriers to timely reaction to a fall after it has occurred. Many seniors live alone making it more complicated to seek help after a fall. A senior can wear a device that triggers medical assistance, such as a Lifeline™, that can be pressed after a serious fall to have medical help come to the home.[3] Periodic checks from relatives and friends can also be an informal, yet important, mechanism for insuring continued safety in the home. If a person lies on the floor too long, a pressure ulcer can occur. More serious complications related to delays in medical attention include dehydration, rhabdomyolysis, and renal failure.

Useful patient information on falls and fall prevention are available.[25-27] These websites include general information, statistics, patient education materials such as a fall prevention/safety checklist (also available in Spanish and Chinese), and or patient and health care provider resources. Pharmacists and other health care providers can provide or recommend information from the above websites to patients and caregivers.

Osteoarthritis

Etiology, Epidemiology, and Clinical Presentation Specific to Geriatrics

Osteoarthritis (OA) is damage to joint cartilage that over time causes changes to joint structure. Hands and knees are the most commonly affected joints followed by hips and other smaller joints. Factors that increase the risk for OA include advancing age, increased weight, heredity, over use/repetitive use of a joint, joint injury, lack of physical activity, or nerve injury. Osteoarthritis development can follow injury to a joint as a result of trauma or repetitive use. When obtaining medical histories, health care providers should ask about past events that can lead to OA such as history of contact sports, motor vehicle accidents, and occupations with repetitive joint use and heavy lifting.

Osteoarthritis is the most common joint disorder in adults with prevalence increasing with age. An estimated 26.9 million people have OA.[28] The prevalence of knee OA in adults older than 26 years is 5%[29] increasing to 12% in adults older than 60 years (13.6% in women).[30] Women are more likely to have OA than men.[28] African Americans are more likely than Caucasians to have hand and knee OA.[30] Using Framingham data, the prevalence of symptomatic hand OA was estimated to be over 9 million and knee OA over 13 million adults.

Seniors generally have experienced osteoarthritic pain impacting mobility and have self-medicated before presenting to a provider.[31] Osteoarthritis typically has an asymmetric presentation, as opposed to rheumatoid arthritis, which is symmetrical. Osteoarthritic pain typically worsens with use and improves with rest. Morning stiffness is common, typically lasting less than 30 minutes. Stiffness can also occur with extended inactivity. Pain in the joint at night and joint crepitus are other common signs. Over time, joint instability can develop as can joint enlargement and limited range of motion. These joint changes and instability increase the risk of falls in older patients who often already have several other fall risk factors. No laboratory markers exist for osteoarthritis.

Summary of Standard Treatment

Nonpharmacologic treatment is the cornerstone of OA treatment including weight loss if overweight, aerobic and muscle strengthening exercise, physical therapy with range of motion exercises, appropriate footwear, occupational therapy, joint protection, energy conservation, and appropriate use of assistive ambulation and occupational devices. Extra body weight increases OA risk by stressing weight bearing joints. Even small amounts of weight loss can make a significant difference. In women, an 11 pound weight loss can decrease OA risk in the knee by 50%.[32,33] Muscle strengthening around a joint with OA decreases the workload on the joint and improves joint stability.[34] Physical therapists guide patients in the most appropriate exercises and training routines and are the best resource for assistive devices for ambulation. Occupational therapists help patients find ways to perform daily activities in spite of OA limitations. For instance, adaptive tools can assist with the use of eating utensils, hair brushes, tooth brushes, reaching for items on top shelves, putting on shoes, and many other common daily activities. Such tools can help to maintain an older adult's autonomy, function, independence, and quality of life.

Acetaminophen is the gold standard, first line OA medication in both younger and older adults. When acetaminophen is inadequate or

contraindicated, nonsteroidal anti-inflammatory drugs (NSAIDs) and cyclooxygenase 2 (COX-2) inhibitors are generally used next if no serious gastrointestinal (GI), liver, or kidney disorders are present, especially when soft-tissue inflammation exists from osteophyte formation. Tramadol is an alternative for patients who cannot tolerate or have cardiovascular or GI risk factors precluding NSAID or COX-2 inhibitor use.[35-36] Although tramadol has less abuse potential than opioids, some states have recently given tramadol controlled status, mostly schedule IV-V, due to mounting evidence of abuse potential. Opioids are usually reserved for later stage disease. Temporary relief can be achieved with glucocorticoid or hyaluronic acid joint injections.[37-38] Equal access and optimal OA pain control should be the therapeutic goal for all patients. However, in a Veterans Affairs study, African Americans were less likely to receive prescription strength NSAIDs or COX-2 inhibitors or the same quantity as Caucasians.[39] Additional information about pain management issues among elderly patients can be found in Chapter 14.

Self-care treatments are employed by patients with OA. **Nutraceuticals** for OA prevention and treatment such as glucosamine,[37,40-41] chondroitin,[37-38,41-42] methylsulfonylmethane (MSM),[43] and adenosylmethionine (SAMe)[44-46] as either single agents or combination products have limited efficacy and safety data especially in seniors. The European League Against Rheumatism (EULAR) has given glucosamine and chondroitin 1A ratings indicating beneficial evidence from meta-analyses of randomized controlled trials.[38] Systematic reviews of glucosamine and chondroitin have demonstrated inconsistent efficacy with OA pain and function improvement.[38,40]

Sometimes topical therapies will be used instead or concomitantly since they have decreased systemic absorption and thus fewer adverse effects. Analgesic topicals (e.g., NSAID, salicylates, capsaicin) have limited efficacy. With capsaicin, immediate and thorough hand washing following application is critical to avoid hot pepper contact to sensitive skin and organs such as the eyes. Overuse of salicylate topicals has rarely been linked to salicylate toxicity.[47-49]

Glucocorticoid injections can be effective for treatment of individually affected joints with most data being for the knee. Temporary synovitis can occur but typically has a short duration. No single joint should receive glucocorticoid injections more than 3 times per year to avoid further joint damage. Good aseptic technique is critical to avoid infection. For a patient awaiting knee arthroplasty, glucocorticoid joint injections are a method to provide temporary pain relief while muscle strength is improved through physical therapy to aid in the surgical recovery and rehabilitation process.[49]

Hyaluronic acid injections are a treatment option especially good for patients who cannot take NSAIDs or COX-2 inhibitors and have pain not controlled on acetaminophen. Studies have indicated efficacy similar to NSAIDs.[50] Hyaluronic acid injections are well tolerated with the primary adverse effects being a small incidence of local injection site pain and swelling. The older injectable hyaluronic acid products (i.e, Hyalgan™, Synvisc™) were derived from rooster combs or bovine vitreous humor and thus are contraindicated in patients with avian and egg related allergies whereas the newer products (i.e., Euflexxa™) are formulated through fermented bacteria, which increased yield and decreased production costs but might have more immune response potential with repeated use.[50-53] Data are limited with prolonged use.[49-50,54]

Opioids are reserved for severe OA pain significantly impacting daily function and quality of life for which other treatments have been ineffective.[49] Opioids have significant adverse effect profiles that are especially pertinent in older patients with OA and can increase falls and safety risks. Limited data have been published about intraarticular opioid injections. Propoxyphene has not been demonstrated to be more effective than acetaminophen but carries significantly more risk.[55]

Joint replacement is effective in many patients but is costly, thus typically reserved for failure of nonpharmacologic and pharmacologic interventions. Mounting data support physical therapy and muscle strengthening prior to joint arthroplasty and then resuming activity within a day after the arthroplasty. Data have shown that increased time between surgery and ambulation/physical therapy significantly increased length of stay and recovery times.[56]

Review of Evidence Base Supporting Treatment Recommendations for Elderly Patients

The most recent evidence for OA treatment in seniors focuses on prevention of harm while providing pain relief, maintaining function, and possibly slowing if not reversing some of the joint damage.[49] Acetaminophen is still the gold standard OA medication for seniors because it is effective, relatively safe, and affordable compared to alternate treatments. If liver function is normal and no contraindications exist, acetaminophen on a scheduled basis is the accepted first-line treatment.[49,57]

The nonselective NSAIDs pose GI ulcer formation and bleeding risks, especially in seniors.[58-62] Major risks associated with ulcer formation are age over 65 years, history of peptic ulcer disease or upper GI bleeding, and concomitant medical conditions such as cardiovascular disease, diabetes, and renal or hepatic dysfunction. Concomitant use of glucocorticoids, antiplatelet agents, anticoagulants, tobacco, and ethanol further increases the risk for ulcers and bleeding. Use of proton pump inhibitors (PPIs) with NSAIDs can decrease GI ulcer risk but they also increase therapy costs.[61-64] H_2-antagonists or antacids do not reduce GI ulcer risk. Cardiovascular risks are also major considerations with NSAIDs. NSAIDs can increase blood pressure, worsen heart failure, and increase risk of myocardial infarction through their impact on the renal collecting tubules leading to increased fluid retention.[65]

To minimize the risk of GI toxicity, cost-effectiveness studies have indicated a cost benefit of using COX-2 inhibitors in patients over age 65 years requiring NSAIDs.[65] However, cost is not the only consideration in the use of COX-2 inhibitors. Cardiovascular risk with COX-2 inhibitors appears to be even greater than that of nonselective NSAIDs resulting in some of these agents being pulled from the market.[66-69]

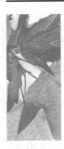

KEY POINT: When evaluating older adults with OA, consider their medical history especially GI and cardiovascular conditions, medication history, and risks before choosing to use a NSAID or a COX-2 inhibitor.

Nutraceuticals are commonly used by seniors for OA but differences in efficacy and safety due to aging are unknown. The glucosamine/chondroitin arthritis intervention trial (GAIT) compared glucosamine hydrochloride (not the more commonly used sulfate salt in the US) 500 mg three times daily, chondroitin sulfate 1200 mg daily, the combination of the two, celecoxib 200 mg daily, and placebo in a largely geriatric sample.[41] Significant improvement in knee OA was not found in this trial, which might be related to the very large placebo effect. A trend of pain improvement was found in patients with moderate to severe knee pain using the glucosamine/chondroitin combination. A follow up radiographic trial, likewise, did not find significant improvement in joint space narrowing with the therapy arms of the trial.[37] A secondary analysis of chondroitin treated patients in GAIT demonstrated improvement in knee swelling for patients with early OA.[42]

Propoxyphene is still commonly prescribed in spite of being on the Beer's list of medications to avoid in seniors.[70] This medication can cause cognitive impairment and falls in seniors. Use has been linked to increased mortality. The addictive potential and euphoria adverse effects might explain senior resistance to stopping it. An FDA advisory committee on January 30, 2009, voted by a narrow margin to recommend that the FDA discontinue marketing propoxyphene products in the US based on safety and efficacy data.[55] However, the final action by the FDA was only a strengthening of the warning language in the product information.

Common Problems Encountered When Treating Elderly Patients with This Condition

Self-medication is common in OA treatment. This can lead to problems of both under and over use of medication to treat OA. Thus when working with seniors, specific questions related to both prescription use obtained through other providers and nonprescription medication therapy should be included in the medication history. The acetaminophen dose from all sources including opioid and OTC combination products needs to be added together to determine safety.

In seniors, nonspecific symptoms and unusual symptom presentations are more common making evaluation of pain control and medication adverse effects even more difficult. Sometimes pain can be expressed as a decrease in eating, more sadness or depression, or behavioral problems, especially in individuals with cognitive impairment. Normal liver function is required to use the maximum acetaminophen dose. Ethanol consumption should be screened prior to recommending high dose chronic acetaminophen use and the dose should be decreased in anyone with reduced hepatic function or with regular and/or binge consumption of ethanol.[71] Some data suggest that concomitant acetaminophen use can extend the half-life of warfarin and thereby elevate INR and increase bleeding risk.[72] Seniors with GI ulcers secondary to NSAIDs do not always have symptoms.[73] Regular evaluation of renal function is also important to monitor for common adverse effects associated with some OA medications. Both OA and OA medications, especially opioids and tramadol, can increase fall risk.

Osteoporosis and Fractures
Etiology, Epidemiology, and Clinical Presentation Specific to Geriatrics

Osteoporosis is a skeletal disease characterized by low bone density, decreased bone strength, and deterioration of bone micro-architecture that results in an increase in bone fragility and risk of fracture.[74] Osteoporosis related to aging is related more to bone formation problems than bone resorption problems whereas the opposite is more common for bone loss associated with estrogen loss during and early after menopause.[75] The risk factors for osteoporosis and osteoporotic fractures [74,76] are similar between middle aged and senior adults, however some of them become more prevalent in seniors. For women osteoporosis is generally related to estrogen deficiency and aging, whereas for men osteoporosis is usually related to secondary causes, aging or hypogonadism.[77] Causes of secondary osteoporosis (e.g., diseases and medications associated with bone loss)[74,76,78] have higher prevalences in seniors. Risk factors for subsequent fractures include older age, cognitive impairment, lower bone mineral density, impaired depth perception, impaired mobility, previous falls, dizziness, and poor or fair self-perceived health.[79]

Osteoporosis and osteoporotic fractures increase with aging. Middle aged women have an osteoporosis prevalence of 4% that increases to 44–52% in women 80 years and older.[38] Whites and Hispanics have the highest incidence of fractures after adjusting for weight, BMD, and other factors.[78] Eighty percent of hip fractures in women occur in senior women.[80] Lifetime hip fracture risk for women is 6–17% and for men 6–11%. More fractures occur in nursing homes than the community.[81] The U.S. hip fracture incidence rate increased significantly as age increased from 65–69 years to 85–100 years for both women (from 21 to 325/10,000 women) and men (from 9 to 236/10,000 men). Hip fractures resulted in 317,000 hospital stays with hospital stays on average 6.3 days and health care costs on average $34,300 per event; making them the 12th top Medicare hospital expenditure. Having a fracture also increases the likelihood of having subsequent fractures.[77]

Fractures can be silent or painful. They can result in decreased height, mobility, functioning, independence, and respiratory and gastrointestinal function (secondary to spine kyphosis) and death. Seniors with cognitive impairment might express their pain differently, such as a decrease in appetite or more behavioral problems. Complications following a hip fracture include fear of falling, thromboembolic events, depression, infection, subsequent fracture, pressure ulcer, poor nutrition and death. Men have a higher mortality rate after fracture (up to 38%) than women.[77] After hip fracture surgery, 9% of patients went home,

24% went to inpatient rehabilitation, 61% went to a skilled nursing facility, 3% went to a nursing home, and 3% died.[82] Long term nursing home care was required for about 20% of patients after a hip fracture.[74] Only 40% of patients with a fracture returned to pre-fracture mobility.

Summary of Standard Treatment in General Adult Population

Current recommendations suggest all women 65 years and older, all men 70 years and older, and patients at high risk for the disease (e.g., fragility fracture, presence of disease and or medications known to decrease bone mass) be evaluated for osteoporosis.[74,77-78] The preferred diagnostic test is the DXA. Bone density ultrasound measurements can be used for screenings to motivate people to seek further medical evaluation. Fracture risk assessment with the **FRAX questionnaire** can be conducted for all people 40–90 years old who are not on osteoporosis prescription medications. FRAX provides 10 year major osteoporotic and hip fracture risks specific to that person.[74,83] If age is above 90 years old, then 90 can be utilized for the age. For FRAX, patients' measured weight and height and race background are required while a DXA femoral neck T-score is optional. Accurate height measurements should be obtained.[84]

The 2010 North American Menopause Society (NAMS) position statement,[78] 2008 revised National Osteoporosis Foundation (NOF) guidelines,[74] the 2008 American College of Physicians guidelines,[85] the 13 potential osteoporosis quality indicators for vulnerable elders,[86] and the 2004 Surgeon General's report[87] on osteoporosis provide the framework for osteoporosis prevention and treatment. Prevention of osteoporosis requires a bone healthy lifestyle that includes adequate calcium and vitamin D intake; exercise to improve bone strength, muscle function, and balance; minimization of alcohol and caffeine intake; no smoking; and fall prevention. For adults 50 years and older, recommended daily intakes for calcium are 1200–1500 mg and for vitamin D 800–1000 units from diet and or supplements. Calcium can decrease bone loss[88] but needs to be combined with sufficient doses of vitamin D to prevent fractures.[89-90] General consensus is the vitamin D dose needs to be at least 800–1000 units and or the 25 (OH) vitamin D concentration needs to be at least 30 ng/mL to have a fracture prevention effect, however all studies do not document this benefit.

The NOF guidelines[74] and NAMS position statement[78] make recommendations for prescription osteoporosis medication use. Any patient with a history of hip or vertebral fracture is eligible for treatment, even without a DXA exam. Patients with osteoporosis, defined as a T-score ≤ -2.5 at femoral neck, total hip <u>or</u> spine by central DXA warrant fracture prevention therapy. Postmenopausal women and men 50 years or older with osteopenia, defined as a T-score between −1 and −2.5, can be treated if the FRAX 10-year all major osteoporosis-related fracture probability is 20% or higher <u>or</u> the 10-year hip fracture probability is 3% or higher. Table 15-1 contains specific information about OTC and prescription medications for osteoporosis prevention and treatment.

Antiresorptive medications (i.e., bisphosphonates, raloxifene, calcitonin) are generally used to treat osteoporosis and prevent fractures before formation medications (i.e., teriparatide) are used.[78] Bisphosphonates are the drugs of choice for osteoporosis treatment based on hip, spine and nonvertebral fracture prevention data and are relatively safe. If oral bisphosphonates cannot be tolerated, quarterly ibandronate or yearly zoledronic acid intravenous therapy can be instituted. Duration of therapy is not known but 7–10 year safety data exist for risedronate and alendronate, respectively.[76]

Other osteoporosis options exist if bisphosphonates are not tolerated or contraindicated.[78] Raloxifene or nasal calcitonin can be used, however these medications have not shown hip and nonvertebral fracture prevention. Infrequently, calcitonin is used for pain management after an acute osteoporotic fracture. Men with osteoporosis and hypogonadism could receive testosterone replacement therapy if they have no current or past prostate cancer.[77] Teriparatide is the only osteoporosis medication that can increase bone architecture and has been documented to decrease spine and nonvertebral fractures but not hip frac-

tures. This medication is reserved for patients with significant bone loss (e.g., T-score < -3.5, or fragility fracture) or patients that cannot use or tolerate antiresorptive medications. Teriparatide is a daily injection for up to two years, which can be challenging for some seniors or cost prohibitive.

Review of Evidence Base Supporting Treatment Recommendations for Elderly Patients

All bisphosphonates are indicated for postmenopausal women but only alendronate, risedronate, and zoledronic acid have indications for male osteoporosis and glucocorticoid-induced osteoporosis. Zoledronic acid is the only osteoporosis medication with secondary fracture prevention data (spine and nonvertebral fractures), which showed it not only decreased fractures but also had a significant decrease in mortality.[91] Bisphosphonates have documented osteoporosis and fracture prevention efficacy in community dwelling seniors less than 75 years old.[81] Effectiveness data in seniors 75 years and older is less but suggestive of vertebral fracture reduction with risedronate, alendronate, and teriparatide and nonvertebral and hip fracture reduction with risedronate for those 70–79 years old.[92] Of note, many studies were underpowered to evaluate fracture risk reduction in older seniors.

Treating osteoporosis in seniors is cost effective. A well designed pharmacoeconomic study showed that treating senior women 65–84 years old with osteoporosis was cost effective and for seniors 85 years and older with osteoporosis demonstrated cost savings.[93-94] For senior men, cost effectiveness could be realized for men 65 years and older with a prior fracture and men 80–85 years old.[95] If osteoporosis treatment is less than $500 annually, treating men 70 years and older with osteoporosis would also be cost effective. The challenges are to get providers to assess and treat seniors for osteoporosis and for seniors to adhere to bone healthy lifestyles and treatment. After a hip fracture, less than 25% of seniors received a DXA or prescription therapy.[80] Only 10–20% of nursing home residents with osteoporosis or a past fracture received osteoporosis treatment.[96]

Table 15-1. Pharmacotherapy for Osteoporosis Prevention and Treatment

Drug	Dose	Advantages	Limitations
Calcium Most common salts used are: carbonate (40% elemental calcium), citrate (21% elemental calcium)	300–500 mg elemental calcium 1–3 times a day to achieve adequate intakes. Carbonate products should be taken with food	Sometimes easier than ingesting foods, especially for those who are lactose intolerant or have dyslipidemia. Alternative formulations– chewable, dissolving tablet, liquid	*Administration* • Citrate tablets are more expensive and more tablets needed to achieve adequate intakes. *Adverse effects* • Constipation, gas, bloating, kidney stones (rare). *Drug interactions* • Proton pump inhibitors can decrease calcium absorption from carbonate salts. • Iron, tetracycline, quinolones, bisphosphonates, phenytoin, and fluoride have decreased absorption with concomitant therapy. *Food interactions* • Oxalates, phytates, sulfates, and fiber (variable) can decrease calcium absorption.
Vitamin D	400–1000 units 1–2 times a day to achieve therapeutic 25 (OH) vitamin D concentrations (≥ 30 ng/mL) 50,000 units weekly to monthly sometimes used for insufficiency until replete 50,000 units 1–2 times weekly for deficiency until replete	More accessible than vitamin D fortified foods	• Inactive compound that must be metabolized in liver to 25 (OH) vitamin D and then in kidneys to 1,25(OH) vitamin D, which is the active moiety for calcium absorption. If severe renal or hepatic failure, different vitamin D analogs are required for therapy. *Adverse effects* • Hypercalcemia (uncommon). *Drug interactions* • Phenytoin, barbiturates, carbamazepine, and rifampin increase vitamin D metabolism. • Cholestyramine, colestipol, orlistat, and mineral oil decrease vitamin D absorption.

(continued)

Table 15-1. **Pharmacotherapy for Osteoporosis Prevention and Treatment (cont'd)**

Drug	Dose	Advantages	Limitations
Bisphosphonates alendronate	5 mg daily, 35 mg weekly (prevention) 10 mg daily, 70 mg tablet, 70 mg tablet with vitamin D 2800 or 5600 units, or 75 mL liquid weekly (treatment)	Reasonably safe, 7–10 year safety data. Much BMD data and hip and spine fracture prevention data.	*Administration* • Check Medicare Part D plan to see what is tier 1 and requirements for intravenous administrations. *Complex oral administration* • Take with a full glass of water not juice, coffee, or tea and on an empty stomach. • Remain upright for at least 30–60 minutes. • Do not take with any other medications.
ibandronate	150 mg monthly, 3 mg intravenous infusion quarterly	Weekly, monthly, quarterly, and yearly administration to improve adherence. Ibandronate has a company sponsored e-mail and postal service reminder system free to patients.	*Contraindications* • Renal function CrCl less than 30–35 mL/min (controversial); some say ok in age related renal dysfunction etiologies until CrCl 15–20 mL/min. • Esophageal disorders or severe gastrointestinal problems (oral). *Adverse effects* • Gastrointestinal: nausea, heartburn, pain, irritation, ulceration, perforation, and bleeding with oral therapy. • Muscle aches and pains (uncommon); discontinue if severe. • Transient flu-like symptoms with intravenous administration, can pretreat. • Osteonecrosis of the jaw (rare) *Drug interactions* • Calcium and minerals decrease its absorption.
risedronate	5 mg daily, 35 mg weekly, 150 mg monthly		
zoledronic acid	5 mg intravenous infusion yearly		
Raloxifene	60 mg daily	Estrogen positive breast cancer prevention indication. Small lipid lowering effect.	*Efficacy* • Only vertebral fracture prevention. *Adverse effects* • Hot flushes, leg cramps, venous thromboembolism, peripheral edema; cataracts and gallbladder disease rare. • Black box warning for fatal stroke.

(continued)

Table 15-1. **Pharmacotherapy for Osteoporosis Prevention and Treatment (cont'd)**

Drug	Dose	Advantages	Limitations
Calcitonin	200 units intranasal daily, alternating nares every other day	Some analgesic effect after a fracture and for metastatic bone pain	*Efficacy* • Only vertebral fracture prevention. • Refrigeration until first use. *Adverse effects* • Rhinitis, epistaxis.
Teriparatide	20 mcg subcutaneously daily for up to 2 years	Only product that builds new bone. Pen device for administration.	*Efficacy* • Limited use for only 24 months. • Expensive; might need prior authorization to use. *Administration* • Daily injection. • Discard pen 28 days after being opened. • Refrigeration required, can complicate travel. • Expensive. *Contraindications* • Bone cancer, Paget's disease, open epiphyses, hypercalciuria or unexplained increased alkaline phosphatase, and prior skeletal radiation. *Adverse effects* • Pain at injection site, nausea, dizziness, leg cramps, increase in uric acid (rare) and calcium.

Source: Modified from reference 20.

Adherence to osteoporosis medications is suboptimal in all age groups.[97-98] Decreased adherence leads to decreased fracture risk reduction.

Common Problems Encountered When Treating Elderly Patients with This Condition

Lack of access and suboptimal osteoporosis care are significant problems. Many seniors are not being evaluated or treated for prevention and treatment of osteoporosis. Only 30% of Medicare recipients have had a DXA exam.[98] Of nursing home residents with either osteoporosis or a recent fracture, only 69% received calcium, 63% received vitamin D, 19% received a bisphosphonate, 14% received calcitonin, 3% received raloxifene, and 0.1% received teriparatide.[81] Seniors who are 80 years old have on average 5.5–9 more years of life, and those 85 years old have on average 4.2–6.8 more years of life. Thus frail elders could be offered osteoporosis prevention and treatment therapies, especially if their lifespan is at least a couple of years and they rate their health at least good quality.[96] However, some comorbidities such as a neurologically limiting stroke, advanced stage dementia, and terminal cancer generally warrant not using osteoporosis medications and even considering stopping them, especially for hospice residents.

Calcium absorption is quite variable and most likely lower in some seniors. With aging some seniors will have decreased gastric acid secretion production that could decrease the disintegration and dissolution of calcium carbonate supplements. Taking the calcium carbonate with food might overcome this problem.[99] Furthermore, seniors have a high prevalence of H_2-blocker and PPI use, which could also decrease calcium absorption from calcium carbonate products.[100] Based on epidemiology studies, PPI use was associated with increased fracture rate.[101] For seniors using PPIs, increasing calcium carbonate daily intake and ensuring its administration with food or using calcium citrate, an acid independent product, might solve this absorption problem.

Vitamin D intake can come from the diet and sun exposure. Because of suboptimal diets, seniors are at increased risk for low vitamin D intake. Seniors might also have minimal sun exposure, especially if they reside in assisted living or nursing homes. Sun screen blocks the essential sunrays. Furthermore, the sun's rays in northern climates in the winter are inadequate to convert skin cholesterol to vitamin D. Thus these deficits generally result in the need for vitamin D supplementation in seniors.

The ability to achieve therapeutic vitamin D concentrations with vitamin D supplements is quite variable in seniors. Although the adequate intake has been increased, one Canadian study documented that a vitamin D intake of 1000 units per day only resulted in 35% of seniors in the therapeutic range (> 30 ng/mL) whereas 4000 units per day resulted in 88% in the therapeutic range.[102] However, no guidelines for monitoring exist nor a consistent relationship of vitamin D concentration to fracture prevention. Since the levels are expensive, a cost saving measure is to draw a 25 (OH) vitamin D level after 800–1000 units vitamin D_3 daily supplement has been used for 3–4 months (i.e., time for biological steady state) without or after prior high dose replacement (e.g., 50,000 units weekly for 12 weeks) to ascertain need for maintenance dosage adjustment. Since inter-assay variability exists, patients should have follow-up vitamin D levels analyzed at the same laboratories until all assays are standardized (i.e., using the standard reference material 972 for vitamin D assay calibrations). Various repletion dosage schedules for vitamin D insufficiency (21–29 ng/mL) exist; ranging from 800–4000 units vitamin D_3 daily to 50,000–100,000 units vitamin D_2 weekly to monthly.[96] For vitamin D deficiency (< 21 ng/mL), repletion dosage schedules are also variable but generally involve using 50,000 units vitamin D_2 1–2 times weekly for 8–12 weeks and then implementing a daily maintenance dose of 800–1000 units or higher as needed.

Prior to initiating bisphosphonate therapy, especially intravenous therapy, a patient's serum calcium should be in the normal range and if not, corrected before administration. Bisphosphonates require the senior to be able to remain upright (seated or standing) for at least 0.5–1 hour after ingestion, which might be difficult for some seniors with stroke, immobility or dementia. Once monthly administration might help decrease pill burden or medication administration workload. For patients with difficulties swallowing or with feeding tubes, alendronate is the only bisphosphonate available in a liquid formulation.

The most common adverse effects of bisphosphonates are GI intolerance (i.e., upset stomach, nausea).[103] Some patients can experience muscle aches and pain. More serious consequences such as GI ulceration, perforation, and bleeding can occur but are uncommon. Weekly and monthly administrations decrease serious but not common GI bisphosphonate adverse effects. Although bisphosphonates are labeled not to use if creatinine clearance is less than 30–35 mL/min,[103] some but not all experts suggest bisphosphonates at a lower dose (e.g., 50% reduction) and for short durations (e.g., 3 years) might be safe for patients who have experienced at least one fragility fracture. This recommendation is not evidence based. This option is only suggested if renal function is decreased secondary to aging rather than chronic kidney disease disorders and creatinine clearance is above 15 mL/min (i.e., CKD stage 4).[96,103-104] Stage 5 chronic kidney disease would require a bone biopsy before bisphosphonate therapy can be initiated.

Adherence might be more compromised in seniors using many other medications due to increased pill burden, cognitive impairments, and limited resources. Directions for safe bisphosphonate use, nasal calcitonin, and teriparatide injections might be too complex for seniors with limited cognitive impairment. Therefore, patient use and understanding of medications should be frequently reassessed.

Due to polypharmacy, seniors are at increased risk for medication induced bone loss. Some of these medications are commonly used in seniors. Glucocorticoids are the most potent bone destroying medications and were common therapies in the past before safer medications existed for diseases such as COPD and rheumatoid arthritis.[76,105] Glucocorticoids decrease GI calcium absorption, increase calcium urinary excretion, alter vitamin D metabolism to more inactive metabolites, increase osteoclast number, function, and lifespan, and decrease osteoblast function and lifespan.[106]

A comprehensive history of current and past glucocorticoid therapy is warranted to assess for increased bone loss. Any glucocorticoid therapy of prednisone 5 mg or more (or equivalent) for more than 3 months throughout a person's life increases bone loss and fracture risk. Although guidelines exist on glucocorticoid-induced osteoporosis prevention and treatment, they are frequently not followed.[107-108] Less than 16% of seniors on a glucocorticoid medication received a prescription medication for osteoporosis prevention, and only 44% took calcium and 24% took vitamin D.[107] For patients starting long-term glucocorticoid therapy (e.g., $\geq$ 5 mg prednisone or equivalent for $\geq$ 3 months), a baseline hip and spine DXA is recommended and then bisphosphonate therapy started if no contraindications.[76,108] If the patient is already on glucocorticoids, bisphosphonate therapy is suggested if the DXA T-score is less than -1.0 (vs. $\leq$-2.5 T-score for patients without glucocorticoid therapy). A bone healthy lifestyle should be implemented at the onset of glucocorticoid therapy. Higher calcium (1500 mg) and vitamin D (800 units or more) intakes are required if on glucocorticoids. The 25 (OH) vitamin D concentration should be at least 30 ng/mL with some recommending higher concentrations (> 80 ng/mL) in patients receiving glucocorticoids.[106] Bisphosphonates can prevent and treat glucocorticoid induced osteoporosis and subsequent fractures, and thus are the drug class of choice over other antiresorptive and formation osteoporosis medications.[85,106,108] Recent trials also support yearly intravenous zoledronic acid[109] and teriparatide,[110] however these therapies might present cost issues to seniors, especially if in or near the coverage gap of their Medicare Part D insurance programs. If hypogonadism is present, hormonal therapy might also be required.

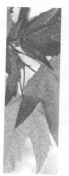

KEY POINT: Most patients receiving long-term glucocorticoid therapy for various indications have not been educated about drug-induced osteoporosis and the various side effects making additional diagnostic, prevention, treatment, and education strategies necessary.

Besides glucocorticoids, many other medications have bone effects. As seniors age, their levothyroxine dosage requirements frequently decrease creating excess concentrations that can increase bone loss if dosage adjustments are not made. Thus yearly thyroxine stimulating hormone (TSH) levels should be drawn. Since TSH concentrations in the lower normal range are associated with bone loss,[111] thyroid replacement doses adjusted to achieve TSH concentrations in the middle to upper normal therapeutic range might be warranted to prevent excessive hormone induced bone loss. Anticonvulsant therapy with medications such as phenytoin and phenobarbital can cause both osteoporosis and osteomalacia due to altered metabolism of vitamin D to more inactive metabolites. With long term use of medications that alter vitamin D metabolism, monitoring 25 (OH) vitamin D concentrations might be helpful to identify and correct any vitamin D deficits. Some of the chemotherapies for prostate and breast cancers such as gonadotrophin releasing hormone (GnRH) agonists (e.g., goserelin, leuprolide) and aromatase inhibitors (e.g., anastrozole) increase bone loss and osteoporosis. Selective serotonin reuptake inhibitors (SSRIs) have been associated with increased fracture risk.[112] The etiology of this association has not been clearly identified, however, monitoring for falls and osteoporosis in these seniors might be warranted.

Polymyalgia Rheumatica and Giant Cell Arteritis

Etiology, Epidemiology, and Clinical Presentation Specific to Geriatrics

Although the exact cause of polymyalgia rheumatica (PMR) and giant cell arteritis (GCA) are unknown, pathophysiology might be related to aging and immune system, genetic, and environmental factors. Various viruses (e.g., common cold, human parvovirus B19, human parainfluenza virus) have been associated with symptoms.[113] Polymyalgia rheumatica predominantly affects older adults (> 50 years old) with average onset at 70 years old.[28] One of every 133 persons older than 50 years old develops PMR with the greatest incidence in seniors 70–80 years old.[111] Women are twice as likely as men and whites more likely than other race groups to develop PMR.[28] The prevalence of PMR and GCA is 739 and 278 patients per 100,000 people, respectively.

Polymyalgia rheumatica symptoms are similar to other conditions. The major symptoms are moderate to severe muscle aches and morning stiffness of the torso (e.g., neck, shoulders, pelvis) and upper and lower extremities that lasts for greater than 30–45 minutes and exists for greater than 2 weeks.[114-115] Patients can experience fatigue, decreased energy, weakness, weight loss, anemia, and sometimes a slight fever and depression. Joints are usually not swollen. Symptoms can begin unilaterally but generally progress to bilateral appearance. Symptoms can be worse in the morning or after extended periods of sitting or lying down. These symptoms can begin quickly or gradually. The disease can remit within one to two years without therapy. About 55% of patients will have a relapse after initial treatment.[116]

Giant cell arteritis (also known as temporal arteritis) can occur concomitantly in 10–20% of patients with PMR.[113-114] Up to 50% of patients with GCA will develop PMR. Symptoms include new headaches, tender scalp, pain with chewing, jaw discomfort, tongue pain, and visual changes. Patients with GCA can also experience swollen and inflamed temple, neck, and or arm arteries. Blindness and strokes sometimes occur as complications. About 31% of patients will have a relapse after initial treatment.[116]

Besides physical examination, some laboratory tests will be helpful to document an inflammatory process and rule out other conditions. In PMR patients, generally the erythrocyte sedimentation rate (ESR > 40–50 mm/hr), platelet count, and C-reactive protein will be elevated; hemoglobin will be decreased with a mild, normochromic, normocytic anemia; and the rheumatoid factor will be negative. A temporal artery biopsy will be obtained to confirm GCA.

Summary of Standard Treatment and Review of Evidence Base Supporting Treatment Recommendations for Elderly Patients

Since this condition occurs mostly in older adults, very few differences exist for treatment of seniors versus middle aged adults. Consensus PMR guidelines were developed in 2007.[115] Nonpharmacologic therapy includes exercise and diet. Regular low impact exercise with stretching should be initiated, gradually increasing with patient use and tolerance. A well balanced diet might help with immune function and can provide the extra calcium and vitamin D needed to prevent glucocorticoid-induced osteoporosis. If diet is insufficient, nutritional supplements should be recommended.

Glucocorticoids are considered first line therapy although treatment might begin with NSAIDs .[115] The NSAIDs usually provide inadequate symptom resolution. The starting prednisone dose for PMR is 10–20 mg daily with some response experienced quickly and the maximum effect achieved within 2 weeks.[114] The ESR can be used to monitor therapy response. Oral glucocorticoids can be tapered by about 1 mg per day or about 2.5 mg per week after the disease has been controlled for 2–4 weeks, however, some prescribers will do a slower taper decreasing the dose by less every month.[114-115] Intramuscular methylprednisolone 120 mg intramuscularly every 3–4 weeks can be used; decreasing by 20 mg every 2–3 months for the taper.[115] Rapid tapering can result in longer duration of therapy. Sometimes symptoms reappear requiring extended duration of treatment for 1–3 years,[114] which results in long term glucocorticoid adverse effects. An uncommon practice is to use steroid sparing agents (e.g., methotrexate, cyclosporine) to decrease the long term steroid dose. Subsequent flare-ups can be treated with the dose that initially controlled the disease.

Quick response to glucocorticoids is a hallmark of this disease. If 70% plus of symptoms remit within 1 week of glucocorticoid initiation and normalization of inflammatory markers, PMR is most likely the diagnosis.[115] If 50–70% symptoms remit within the first week, the prednisone dose can be increased. If less than 50% response, the provider should seek a different diagnosis. However, if the PMR is unresponsive to glucocorticoids, immunotherapy can be tried. Methotrexate has been evaluated for initial and relapse PMR therapy, however the evidence is mixed.[117] In two small trials, no added benefit (i.e., decreasing steroid use or preventing relapse) of combining infliximab with prednisone was documented for newly diagnosed PMR.[116]

The glucocorticoid therapy for GCA is higher (40–60 mg prednisone per day) than PMR.[86] Similar to PMR, after 2–4 weeks of symptom remission, a slow taper is begun. The maintenance dose is usually 7.5–10 mg daily with further dose lowering attempts to completely taper therapy by 2–3 years. Preliminary research has suggested that low dose aspirin might prevent blood clots, strokes, and vision impairment in GCA patients.[118]

Common Problems Encountered When Treating Elderly Patients with This Condition

Glucocorticoids are associated with many adverse effects. They can cause osteoporosis,[76,105] induce myopathies that can increase falls, and can cause hypogonadism that also can increase bone loss, as described previously in the osteoporosis section. Glucocorticoids can also cause, hasten progression, or worsen other comorbidities such as joint pain symptoms in some seniors.[105] Glucocorticoids are associated with wasting/weakening of muscles, ligaments, tendons, and skin, drug-induced Cushing syndrome, and peptic ulcers. With aging, cataracts and glaucoma develop, which are also glucocorticoid adverse effects. They can increase blood glucose and blood pressure, requiring initiation or adjustment of diabetes or hypertension medications. Risk for infection can also increase. Many psychological adverse effects exist with these medications, with some of the negative mood and behavior therapies compounding underlying depression and potentially behavior problems in patients with Alzheimer's disease. Glucocorticoid use can increase GI bleeding risk related to the increased risk of peptic ulcer formation. Additional use of NSAIDs can further compound this risk. If long-term glucocorticoid use is warranted and prescribed with concomitant NSAIDs, a PPI might reduce GI bleeding risk. Careful monitoring of a senior is required to identify and resolve glucocorticoid induced adverse effects.

Rheumatoid Arthritis

Etiology, Epidemiology, and Clinical Presentation Specific to Geriatrics

Rheumatoid arthritis (RA) is a progressive autoimmune disorder of unknown etiology generally starting one to several decades before a person reaches the age generally considered "geriatric". It is a chronic, destructive disease characterized by symmetric, erosive synovitis. As with many medical conditions, especially autoimmune disorders, stress can negatively impact control of the condition.

Rheumatoid arthritis is found in approximately 0.5-1 percent of the population impacting approximately 1.3 million Americans.[119-120] In working age adults the incidence is higher in women. After age 65 years men and women have RA at about the same rate, but evidence in recent years suggests an increase for women.[119] Rheumatoid arthritis can occur at any age, but most commonly presents in the 30s–50s. Rheumatoid arthritis is seldom diagnosed after age 65 years. The average age of those living with RA has gradually increased to 66.8 years based on 1995 data.[120] The mortality rate of people with RA has remained relatively stable between 1965 and 2005 while the mortality rate overall has declined.[121] The average lifespan of someone with RA is shortened by 3-7 years. For those with more aggressive rheumatoid arthritis with extraarticular manifestations, life can be shortened by 10-15 years.[122]

Rheumatoid arthritis affects both joints and other organ systems. Joint destruction can significantly impact daily function. Fatigue is a component of RA that can further limit daily function. Extraarticular manifestations of RA include cardiovascular disease, anemia, interstitial lung disease, osteopenia, osteoporosis, and ocular involvement including scleritis, rheumatoid nodules, Felty's syndrome, and Sjogren's syndrome. The presence of extraarticular manifestations and markers of more active disease such as more involved joints, higher ESR, positive rheumatoid factors, and more functional impairment are all associated with high mortality rates.[119,121,123] The presence of certain genotypes of tumor necrosis factor receptor associated factor 1 (TRAF1)/C5 locus has also been associated with higher mortality rates.[124] Genotyping for predicting RA prognosis and perhaps guiding the assertiveness of therapy might occur in the future.

Summary of Standard Treatment in General Adult Population

Nonpharmacologic therapy is a key part of RA care. Exercise to maintain range of motion and strength, rest, thermal modalities, weight loss if overweight, relaxation techniques, and physical and occupational therapy are all important nonpharmacologic therapy components. Therapists can aid people with RA in the use of joint braces and assistive devices to minimize functional limitations.

The 2008 American College of Rheumatology (ACR) guideline summarized the evidence guiding appropriate use of nonbiologic **disease modifying anti-rheumatic drugs** (**DMARDs** such as methotrexate) and **biologic response modifiers** (**BRMs** such as rituximab).[125] Since 1999 the BRMs have offered a new treatment option for RA. More long-term evidence exists for the DMARDs than for the BRMs. Treatment is dependent on disease activity and duration of medication efficacy. The DMARDs are used singularly or combined depending on disease severity and aggressiveness. Most DMARDs take several weeks before onset of full therapeutic benefit and have relatively short durations of efficacy. To overcome delay in onset, therapies can be overlapped so that one is building to therapeutic efficacy while the other is declining in efficacy. A different strategy initiates therapy with multiple agents and then gradually reduces medications or doses to the minimum effective regimen once RA is controlled.

The ACR guideline provides detailed instruction on RA treatment.[125] Since most geriatric patients will have longer duration of disease, choice of therapy is based on disease activity and individual unique factors. Nonbiologic DMARDs are indicated for low disease activity. Specifically, leflunomide or methotrexate is chosen as first line therapy if no contraindications or past failures with these treatments. For patients with moderate to severe disease activity, triple DMARD therapy with methotrexate, hydroxychloroquine, and sulfasalazine is recommended. For patients with longer disease activity not controlled with methotrexate, anti-tumor necrosis factor alpha (TNFα), a type of BRM, is warranted. Anti-TNFα agents can be added to methotrexate or can replace nonbiologic DMARD therapy. Abatacept is recommended when methotrexate plus anti-TNFα therapy are not effective. Rituximab can be used when patients have poor prognostic factors or have failed other therapies. Combinations of biologic therapies are not supported by current evidence.[125] Glucocorticoids do not alter the disease course of RA, however, they can help manage the pain and inflammation of flares and can help while awaiting full efficacy of a recently started DMARD. Because of the limited time of efficacy for each agent, constant monitoring and therapeutic agent changes are needed over time.

Individual risks and benefits must be considered when choosing appropriate therapy for a patient. DMARDs suppress more of the immune system than BRMs. Both increase infection risk,[126] cause infections to be more difficult to treat, and increase cancer risk. Therefore, prior to initiation of nonbiologic DMARDs or BRMs, guidelines suggest flu and pneumococcal immunization if not current. In addition, for patients with possible exposure or risk, hepatitis B vaccination is warranted. For patients considered for biologic therapy, routine tuberculosis (TB) screening is warranted to screen for latent TB.[125] Genotyping to identify patients at risk of death due to malignancy or sepsis may soon be available.[124]

When nonpharmacologic and pharmacologic therapies are not sufficient, joint replacement is an option. Obvious risks with surgical interventions include risk of infection, blood loss, decreased control of concomitant medical conditions, pain, and the potential for failed recovery (further disability), and death. However, when used appropriately with adequate rehabilitation, joint replacement can help patients maintain autonomy and maintain or regain function.

Review of Evidence Base Supporting Treatment Recommendations for Elderly Patients

The standard RA treatment for seniors is the same as other adults with little data specific to geriatric patients. Because older patients with RA have typically had the condition for many years, the disease is often further progressed with greater impact on function.

Some factors indicate a poorer prognosis to medication therapy. These include advanced age, decreased physical function, extraarticular disease, positive rheumatoid factor, anti-CPP antibodies, and or bony erosions on radiography.[125] Additional poor prognostic factors include female gender, smoking, radiographic progression, early disability, and morbidity such as need for joint replacement. These factors can be greater in seniors and should be considered when determining prognosis and aggressiveness of therapy.

Availability of BRMs has allowed for simpler regimens with fewer systemic adverse effects that might be important in some seniors. Long term efficacy of BRMs in seniors is not yet available. Hopefully prescribing BRMs near the time of diagnosis will lead to greater disease control over time. Theoretically this could lead to less loss of function and joint destruction by the geriatric years for the next generation of seniors with RA.

Treatments might need to be adjusted for age or disease-induced pathophysiologic changes. Leflunomide, methotrexate, and sulfasalazine should be avoided in patients with liver function tests more than 2 times the upper limit of normal. Methotrexate is contraindicated with creatinine clearance less than 30 mL/min.[125] Biologic agents are contraindicated in patients with class III or IV heart failure or chronic hepatitis B or C.[127-128]

Common Problems Encountered When Treating Elderly Patients with This Condition

RA is a progressive disease that leads to loss of muscle tone and function over time, as does aging. So, when flares, fractures, illness, or hospitalization cause weakness, it takes even longer in older patients to regain function. Ability to perform daily tasks, participate in fun activities impacting quality of life, need for personal help, need for assistive devices, and transportation issues contribute to the total picture of RA care.[129]

Several oral health implications exist with both RA and its treatment. The temperomandibular joint is one of the joints that can be impacted by RA. Glucocorticoids and bisphosphonates can increase risk of jaw osteonecrosis. Hand and jaw RA can make it difficult for patients to practice good oral hygiene.[130]

Constipation is a common problem for seniors even without concomitant medical conditions. Decreased physical activity due to RA along with decreased total body water, and altered nutritional and fluid intake associated with aging are just some of the contributing factors. The adverse effects of some RA medications add to this problem. Active management of constipation needs to be part of overall RA care.[131]

Both RA and glucocorticoids are independent risk factors for osteoporosis. Glucocorticoid-induced osteoporosis is well documented but one study found no osteoporosis impact of low-dose, long term glucocorticoid therapy in RA patients.[98] The risk of RA flares outweighed the continued impact on bone health. However, considering risks and benefits in individual patients, prudent care still includes bone density monitoring, higher intakes of calcium (e.g., $\geq$ 1500 mg) and vitamin D (e.g., $\geq$ 800 - 1000 units), and osteoporosis prescription medications as warranted (see osteoporosis section for glucocorticoid use discussion).

With age often comes an accumulation of medical conditions with multiple implications on therapy. For instance, some seniors might not be surgical candidates thus eliminating joint replacement as a therapeutic option. In addition, depression is common with any chronic condition especially with most musculoskeletal disorders. Anemia is a common comorbidity, and the fatigue of RA and anemia further contributes to the difficulties of managing RA and other comorbidities and differentiating causative factors.[129,132]

Pressure Ulcers

Etiology, Epidemiology, and Clinical Presentation Specific to Geriatrics

The older and frailer the patient, the higher the risk for pressure ulcer development. **Pressure**, **shear**, and **friction** are the three major factors in the formation of pressure ulcers. Patients greater than 70 years old are at a greater risk for pressure ulcers. Additional factors, some of which have a higher prevalence in seniors, include altered sensory perception, altered mental state, inability to perceive pressure, comorbidities (e.g., diabetes, malignancy, stroke, heart failure, hypertension, renal failure, anemia, impaired circulation, urinary and fecal incontinence, lymphopenia), infection (sepsis, fever, pneumonia), emergency room stay, longer length of stay in a facility, malnutrition (hypoalbuminemia), male gender, white or black race, current smoking history, physical restraints, dry and scaly skin, excessive skin moisture, friction and shear when being moved, history of pressure ulcers, decreased activity level, immobility or inability to reposition, surgical intervention, and weight loss or low body mass index (BMI).[133-135] Critical care patients are at particularly high risk with a direct relationship with mechanical ventilation.[133-135] The Braden scale[136] and the Norton scale[137] are two common scales used to predict pressure ulcer risk. In addition, laboratory values assessing nutrition status have been used in protocols to determine risk and prevent pressure ulcers.[138-139]

Studies on the epidemiology of pressure ulcers have had widely variable results. In an analysis of available evidence, the incidence rate of pressure ulcers is 0.4 to 38% per year in general acute care, with similar variability in home care and long term care settings.[140] The prevalence was found to be 18% in general acute care, up to 28% in long term care and 29% in home care. The incidence of pressure ulcer formation increases with age, especially after age 65 years. About 70% of pressure ulcers are estimated to occur in seniors.[133]

Pressure ulcers are defined by stages indicating depth and severity. Stages range from I to IV and a category for unstageable (see National

Pressure Ulcer Advisory Panel (NPUAP) website for pictures).[141-142] Staging is based on the amount of tissue loss that has occurred, with stage IV representing full tissue loss to the point of bone, tendon, or muscle exposure. Pressure ulcers are associated with increased mortality.

Summary of Standard Treatment

Pressure ulcer care starts with prevention. The cost of treatment of a stage IV pressure ulcer far exceeds the cost of pressure ulcer prevention and early identification programs. Preventive techniques include avoid/minimize friction when changing positions, change positions regularly, keep skin clean and dry (proper incontinence care is particularly important), and avoid vigorous massage (shear). For those patients that can, position shifts should occur at least every 15 minutes. For those patients who cannot, use of mattresses that redistribute weight is recommended. Many available interventions (such as pneumoboots, elevation of the head of the bed, foam supports with holes or indentations at boney prominences, mattress overlays) are also available to decrease pressure on common pressure points (heels, coccyx, ischium, trochanter, shoulders, knees, ankles, elbows) based on the contour of the human body. Nutrition is another key to pressure ulcer prevention and wound healing. A balanced diet with supplements as needed is the minimum level of intervention required.[143]

A protocol for the treatment of pressure ulcers can be found in Figure 15-2.[144] This protocol involves steps to prevent, identify early, diagnose, monitor, treat, and resolve pressure ulcers. A multifactorial approach such as this plus treatment of concomitant conditions is essential for successful pressure ulcer resolution. The National Pressure Ulcer Advisory Panel (NPUAP) pressure ulcer guidelines were released late 2009,[141] which can be used with information related to pressure ulcers in long term care 2008 guidelines.[145] Treatment involves **debridement**, cleansing, and dressing of the wound. Management of bacterial load is another important element. This should be done with debridement whenever possible, but antibiotics can be considered when debridement alone is not effective.

Wound debridement can be done in several different ways depending on the nature of the wound. For quick debridement, surgical (also known as sharp) debridement is typically used. Wet to dry debridement can be effective but does not differentiate healthy from nonhealthy tissue well. Enzymatic debridement targets and digests the extracellular proteins in the nonhealthy tissue.

The pharmacologic treatment of pressure ulcers is primarily in the dressing phase.[133,135,143,146] The therapeutic goal is to maintain a moist wound environment.[146] More than 300 different products are available including transparent films, hydrocolloids, alginates, foams, hydrogels, and hydrofibers™. The choice of dressing is primarily driven by the moisture status of the wound. Transparent films maintain the moisture already in the wound. Hydrocolloids do not allow moisture to escape the wound. Alginate dressings are absorbent for moderate exudative wounds. Foam dressings are very absorbent. Hydrogels and hydrofibers provide some moisture to the wound and are best in wounds that need only moisture to heal.[146] Gauze based dressings have been a standard. Some evidence documents that the more expensive nongauze dressings can save time with fewer dressing changes.[147-148] They also may have a lower infection rate and speed recovery times.

Pressure ulcer care can be associated with significant discomfort. Therefore, pain control is a key factor in the treatment of pressure ulcers, especially during dressing changes or debridement where pretreatment with an analgesic may be required.

Antibiotics are often used inappropriately for individuals with pressure ulcers. Systemic antibiotics are appropriate if clinical signs of infection exist, such as elevated fever, elevated white blood cell count, or the surrounding tissue is red and swollen. However routine cultures of wound bed do not yield useful results in directing antibiotic selection. Topical antibiotics are usually not recommended.

The seriousness of pressure ulcers and the need to prevent, identify early, and treat effectively have been identified and emphasized by many leading healthcare agencies. The Institute for Healthcare Improvement, Centers for Medicare and Medic-

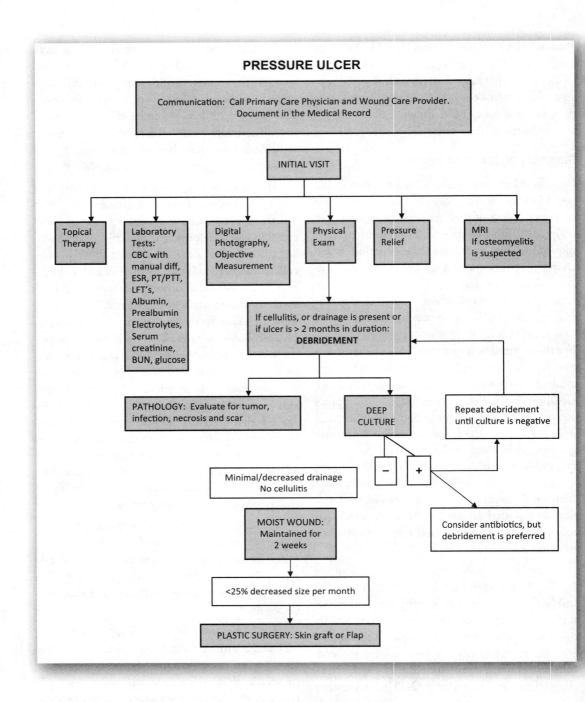

Figure 15-2. Schematic representation of the pressure ulcer protocol.
*Drainage is often a sign of infection, in which case compression is not advisable.
BUN, serum urea nitrogen; CBC, complete blood cell count; ESR, erythrocyte sedimentation rate; LFTs, liver function tests; MRI, magnetic resonance imaging; PT, prothrombin time; PTT, partial thromboplastin time.
Source: Reprinted with permission from reference 144.

aid Services (CMS), the NPUAP, Surgeon General's Healthy People 2010 are a few. The National Quality Forum with CMS has designated some serious and expensive medical errors "never errors," meaning they should never occur.[149] Stage III and IV ulcers acquired in the hospital are on this list.[150] CMS will reduce or not pay for hospital stays due to these hospital-acquired ulcers.

Common Problems Encountered When Treating Elderly Patients with This Condition

Many people over 65 years old have accumulated comorbid conditions and other variables associated with increased pressure ulcer risk. Medications can also decrease mobility, alter perfusion, or negatively impact wound healing. Specific medication classes to avoid or at least carefully monitor in patients with high pressure ulcer risk include glucocorticoids, sedative/hypnotics, opioids, antipsychotics, tricyclic antidepressants, and antihypertensives.

Prevention, identification, and treatment of pressure ulcers have always been a challenge, especially when caring for frail seniors. The prevalence of pressure ulcers in a health care environment is an indicator of care quality. Those who audit or pay for care scrutinize both the frequency of pressure ulcer development as well as the effectiveness of wound healing programs. Pressure ulcer treatment requires addressing all of the many factors frequently requiring interdisciplinary teams. Pharmacist participation on a multidisciplinary team has been demonstrated to contribute to improved patient outcomes.[151]

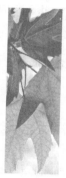

KEY POINT: Since prevention is the first step to pressure ulcer treatment planning, patients should be immediately assessed upon any sort of institutional placement or ambulation change. Nutritional status and skin checks are both essential components of the prevention or treatment plan.

CASE 1: REHABILITATION UNIT OF A SKILLED NURSING FACILITY

Subjective:
BN is a 70-year-old widowed Asian American man in the rehabilitation program after sustaining a hip fracture of the femur neck followed by arthroplasty 2 weeks ago. His postsurgical pain is much improved.

Past Medical History:
Hypothyroidism, incontinence

Medications:
Levothyroxine 100 mcg daily, tolterodine LA 2 mg daily, fondaparinux 2.5 mg daily (for total of 35 days then switch to warfarin for 5 months), aspirin 81 mg daily, Tylenol # 3 1–3 per day prn (no longer using), and calcium chew (Viactiv™) 1 twice a day prn.

Allergies:
No known drug allergies

Social History:
Quit smoking 10 years ago and has a beer a day; Meals on Wheels at home; diet low in dairy products; minimal exercise. Prior to hip fracture he lived independently in his own home. Wife died 3

years ago; two children with families residing nearby

Family History:

Mother died age 68 years due to breast cancer; she had a hip fracture at 65 years old; father died age 83 years from a myocardial infarct; he had osteoarthritis and dyslipidemia. BN has two sisters with osteoporosis.

Objective:

Height 5'6" per stadiometer (past height 5'9"), weight 160 pounds
Blood pressure 160/95 mmHg, Heart rate 80 bpm, temperature 98.6°F, respiratory rate 18 bpm

Physical Exam:

Range of motion improving but still limited. Difficulties with gait and balance. All other aspects within normal limits.

Laboratory:

TSH 0.6 mIU/L (nl 0.4–10 mIU/L), T4 12.2 mcg/dL (nl 4.6–12 mcg/dL), Scr 1.4 mg/dL, BUN 25 mg/dL, 25 (OH) vitamin D 22 ng/mL, albumin 3.1 g/dL (nl 3.4-5.4 g/dL); all other lab values within normal limits

Procedures:

Lunar DXA spine T-score -2.3, nonsurgical hip - femoral neck T-score -2.8, total hip T-score -2.3

Assessment:

BN is a 70-year-old man with poor prior nutrition thus at increased risk for a pressure ulcer, previously undiagnosed and undertreated osteoporosis, and vitamin D insufficiency. A walker is needed for mobility assistance

Plan:

1. Begin alendronate 10 mg weekly; provide adequate patient education and recheck for understanding in a week and upon discharge to home.

2. Until warfarin therapy is completed, switch the Viactiv™ to calcium carbonate 1250 mg with vitamin D 400 units twice daily with food. Increase dairy (after determining no lactose intolerance) and other high calcium content food intake. Provide patient with list of high calcium containing foods. Educate patient on counting calcium intake from foods to try to achieve a daily intake of 1200–1500 mg in divided servings and or supplements.

3. Begin ergocalciferol 50,000 units weekly for 6 weeks, then begin vitamin D supplement 1000 units daily. Reassess 25 (OH) vitamin D level in 4 months and adjust daily supplementation as needed.

4. Decrease levothyroxine dose to 88 mcg daily and reassess TSH in 4–6 months with additional decreases to achieve a TSH concentration in the middle of the normal therapeutic range.

5. Provide patient and caregiver with fall prevention guidelines and a checklist for home safety. If patient or caregiver can not do this assessment, schedule a home visit by the occupational therapist.

6. Assess patient's skin for "hot spots" (i.e., red spots from pressure but without skin breakdown) and pressure ulcers frequently.

Rationale:

1. Patient has had a fragility fracture, which alone warrants osteoporosis treatment and has been found to be cost effective. Based on NOF guidelines, the patient's femoral neck DXA score prior to fracture would have warranted osteoporosis prevention therapy. His estimated Cockcroft Gault creatinine clearance is above 35 mL/min. Since no underlying renal pathophysiology

besides aging safe to use a bisphosphonate. He will require education, with repeated reinforcement, about proper bisphosphonate administration and importance of medication adherence.

2. FRAX calculations are not needed to determine osteoporosis medication therapy but can be
    helpful with patient education and motivation to prescribers to use and for patients to take
    osteoporosis medications. His mother's and his own hip fracture are his risk factors outside of
    age and race. If calculated, FRAX estimations for 10 year major osteoporosis and hip fracture
    risks would be 14% and 7% pre fracture and 21% and 11% post fracture, respectively.

3. Patient has poor nutrition and osteoporosis thus he needs to improve his nutrition and in-
    crease his daily calcium and vitamin D intake to prevent further bone loss and future fractures.
    Improved nutrition will also help prevent pressure ulcers. The Viactiv™ chew contains vitamin
    K and can be problematic with warfarin especially if erratic use but currently is not a problem
    with injectable anticoagulants with direct effects on clotting factors. A dietician can deter-
    mine BN's nutritional needs and suggest a balanced diet. Most likely supplementation will be
    required.

4. His vitamin D concentration is considered insufficient but not deficient. Thus higher dose
    replacement therapy probably is warranted but can be less aggressive than deficiency replace-
    ment requirements. The replacement schedule should replenish his stores and then the NOF
    vitamin D recommendations of 800 - 1000 units daily can be implemented. Since biologic
    feedback and equilibrium of vitamin D takes awhile, follow-up monitoring is usually done 3–6
    months after replenishment and stabilization with a maintenance dose. His follow-up vitamin D
    assessment should be done at the same laboratory as the first assessment until all vitamin D
    assays have been standardized.

5. Excessive levothyroxine replacement can increase bone metabolism. Currently BN's TSH con-
    centration is at the lower end of the normal range and his T4 is at the higher end of the normal
    range, suggesting excessive replacement.

6. BN has osteoporosis and might benefit from a home environment that is not conducive to falls,
    which can be achieved by completing the home safety ideas for falls prevention as described in
    the above suggested websites.

7. Male gender, decreased mobility, advanced age, poor nutrition, and surgical intervention in-
    crease BN's risk for a pressure ulcer, which can be prevented with modifications of risk factors.

Case Summary:

Osteoporosis is common in seniors, and a proactive approach to preventing bone loss and preventing falls is required. Although men are at lower risk, as seen with BN, they still develop osteoporosis
and fractures. Men also have higher mortality after an osteoporotic fracture, so close monitoring of
BN is required. Nutrition is a common problem, especially for seniors who live alone. Pharmacologic
interventions exist to improve BN's quality of life and potentially extend life duration.

CASE 2: MULTIDISCIPLINARY GERIATRIC CLINIC

Subjective:

SB is a 78-year-old African American woman living in an assisted living facility for the last two years since the death of her husband. For the past two days she has experienced a sudden significant increase in joint stiffness, weakness and fatigue.

Past Medical History:

Rheumatoid arthritis for past 22 years with acceptable control past few years, gout with last attack 3 years ago, and hypertension.

Medications:

Methotrexate 7.5 mg weekly, etanercept 50 mg injection weekly, celecoxib 100 mg twice daily, and enalapril 10 mg daily. Occasional Tums. Previous treatments with various combinations of DMARD medications.

Allergies:

No known drug allergies

Social History:

Negative for tobacco and alcohol use. SB has two children and 5 grandchildren living in other states. She worked for 28 years in a hosiery textile mill.

Family History:

Mother died age 61 years after 30 years with rheumatoid arthritis; father died age 82 years from a motor vehicle accident.

Objective:

Height 5'3", weight 173 pounds
Blood pressure 156/76 mmHg, Heart rate 82 bpm, Temperature 98.6 °F, Respiratory rate 16 bpm
Pain today 8/10; average one month ago 4/10.

Physical Exam:

Significant for joint and muscle aches in neck, shoulders with right greater than left, and hips significantly worse in the past 2 days. Patient also describes weakness and lethargy.

Laboratory:

ESR 89 mm/hr

Assessment:

SB is a 78-year-old woman with suspected polymyalgia rheumatica in addition to long standing rheumatoid arthritis.

Plan:

1. Initiate glucocorticoid therapy with prednisone 20 mg daily for 2 weeks then return to clinic. After two weeks, if symptoms are eliminated and the ESR has returned to normal, the prednisone can be tapered by 1 mg per week. If pain persists, wait a month and then reevaluate. If pain returns while tapering, slow the taper schedule to decreasing dose by 1 mg every 2 weeks. Patient might require low dose long-term (i.e., 1–2 years) prednisone therapy to eliminate pain. Assessment of bone density will be necessary with long-term prednisone use. As she does not currently take calcium or vitamin D, these can be recommended and she may be a candidate for osteoporosis antiresorptive therapy as well.

2. Monitor blood pressure during glucocorticoid therapy and adjust enalapril if blood pressure exceeds 180/90 mmHg or if any symptoms of end stage organ impact (e.g., extreme headache, chest pain, altered urine output).

3. Obtain patient's tolerable pain level and use this as therapeutic goal until PMR controlled.

4. Monitor gastrointestinal symptoms. Another option would be to start a PPI in conjunction with the glucocorticoid regimen.

Rationale:

1. Glucocorticoids are the gold standard treatment for PMR. They have the additional benefit of assistance in confirmation of diagnosis. If a patient's symptoms resolve, and ESR and anemia, if present, respond to the therapy, then it is even more likely the patient has PMR. If this patient also had headache, jaw pain, and inflamed arteries in the temples, neck, and arms then GCA could also be considered. Higher glucocorticoid doses are used to treat GCA.

2. Symptom relief is the primary goal of therapy, but the long-term effects of glucocorticoid therapy will have to be managed. Glucocorticoids can decrease bone density and increase blood pressure, so it is important to evaluate this patient for osteoporosis and the need for antiresorptive therapy, monitor blood pressure and adjust hypertensive medication as needed.

3. Sometimes seniors can not describe their pain or have different means of expressing pain such as decreased eating and sleeping and increased aggression. In addition, increased function and quality of life are important goals. SB is already on celecoxib, so a change in NSAID is unlikely to control the PMR pain. The glucocorticoid therapy should help control pain and joint inflammation.

4. Since glucocorticoids and celecoxib can cause GI ulcers, a PPI might prevent GI adverse effects instead of treating them after the fact.

Case Summary:

The sudden increase in pain and stiffness with concomitant fatigue and weakness could indicate polymyalgia rheumatica. This patient's rheumatoid arthritis has been fairly well controlled with her current regimen for over two years making a flare up less likely. The location of the specific pain is not indicative of a gout flare. PMR is quickly responsive to glucocorticoid treatment, and a rapid response helps to confirm the diagnosis. In this senior woman with pre-existing hypertension, all of the potential side effects of glucocorticoids should be monitored.

Chapter Summary

Musculoskeletal conditions have increased prevalence with increased age. Such conditions have a direct negative impact on function and increase fall potential. Through risk factor modification, exercise, healthy nutrition, and good medical care, some of these conditions can be prevented or onset delayed. The care of patients with these conditions requires a patient specific approach taking into consideration all risk factors, concomitant medical conditions and medications, and patient preferences, tolerances, and longevity. The cornerstone of therapy for the musculoskeletal conditions covered is nonpharmacologic therapies. Pharmacologic therapy is one aspect of this care, but carries associated risks and generally does not eradicate the disease. The medications commonly used to treat these conditions have adverse effect profiles that can further negatively impact function, comorbidities, and increase morbidity. Some of these therapies require age related adjustments.

To maximize effectiveness and minimize risk, a health care professional with expertise in pharmacologic therapy is an important part of the health care team. Achieving and maintaining control of these conditions are key for patient function, quality of life, and safety.

Self-Assessment Questions

1. What risk factors for musculoskeletal disease can be modified to prevent disease development?

2. What aspects of daily life could be modified to decrease the development or progression of musculoskeletal diseases?

3. How can you prevent falls, especially related to medication therapies?

4. What information is needed to calculate osteoporotic fracture risks for the FRAX estimation for a senior?

5. Which medications for musculoskeletal disorders require dose adjustments due to age induced decreases in renal or hepatic function?

6. Which medications for musculoskeletal disorders require attention to product selection based on comorbidities?

7. What are the risks of NSAIDs and COX-2 inhibitors in seniors and how can you minimize these?

8. What patient comorbidities can worsen with use of glucocorticoids?

References

1. Morris R. Predicting falls in older women. *Menopause Int.* 2007;13:170–177.

2. Thurman DJ, Stevens JA, Rao JK. Practice parameter: Assessing patients in a neurology practice for risk of falls (an evidence-based review): Report of the quality standards subcommittee of the American Academy of Neurology. *Neurology.* 2008;70:473–479.

3. Moylan KC, Binder EF. Falls in older adults: Risk assessment, management and prevention. *Am J Med.* 2007;120:493.e1–6.

4. American Geriatrics Society and British Geriatric Society. AGS/BGS clinical practice guideline: prevention of falls in older persons. Available at www.american-geriatrics.org/education/prevention_of_falls.shtml. Accessed January 18, 2010.

5. Centers for Disease Control and Prevention. Falls among older adults: An overview. 2008. Available at www.cdc.gov/ncipc/factsheets/adultfalls.htm. Accessed January 18, 2010.

6. Hartikainen S, Lonnroos E, Louhivuori K. Medication as a risk factor for falls: Critical systematic review. *J Gerontol A Biol Sci Med Sci.* 2007;62:1172–1181.

7. Ganz DA, Bao Y, Shekelle PG, et al. Will my patient fall? *JAMA.* 2007;297:77–86.

8. National Center for Health Statistics. LCWK9: Deaths, percent of total deaths, and death rates for the 15 leading causes of death: United States and each state, 1999–2006. 2009. Available at www.cdc.gov/nchs/data/dvs/LCWK9_2006.pdf. Accessed January 18, 2010.

9. Magaziner J, Miller R, Resnick B. Intervening to prevent falls and fractures in nursing homes: Are we putting the cart before the horse? *J Am Geriatr Soc.* 2007;55:464–466.

10. Mathias S, Nayak US, Isaacs B. Balance in elderly patients: The "get-up and go" test. *Arch Phys Med Rehabil.* 1986;67:387–389.

11. The Joint Commission. Accreditation program: hospital national patient safety goals.2008. Available at www.jointcommission.org/NR/rdonlyres/31666E86-E7F4-423E-9BE8-F05BD1CB0AA8/0/HAP_NPSG.pdf. Accessed January 18, 2010.

12. Tinetti ME, Baker DI, King M, et al. Effect of dissemination of evidence in reducing injuries from falls. *N Engl J Med.* 2008;359:252–261.

13. Dawson-Hughes B. Serum 25-hydroxyvitamin D and functional outcomes in the elderly. *Am J Clin Nutr.* 2008;88:537S–540S.

14. Fosnight SM, Zafirau WJ, Hazelett SE. Vitamin D supplementation to prevent falls in the elderly: Evidence and practical considerations. *Pharmacotherapy.* 2008;28:225–234.

15. Harmer PA, Li F. Tai chi and falls prevention in older people. *Med Sport Sci.* 2008;52:124–134.

16. Department of Health and Human Services, Centers for Disease Control and Prevention and National Center for Injury Prevention and Control. Check for safety, a home fall prevention checklist for older adults. Available at cdc.gov/ncipc/pub-res/toolkit/CheckList-ForSafety.htm. Accessed January 18, 2010.

17. Oliver D, Connelly JB, Victor CR, et al. Strategies to prevent falls and fractures in hospitals and care homes and effect of cognitive impairment: Systematic review and meta-analyses. *BMJ.* 2007;334:82.

18. Sawka AM, Boulos P, Beattie K, et al. Hip protectors decrease hip fracture risk in elderly nursing home residents: A Bayesian meta-analysis. *J Clin Epidemiol.* 2007;60:336–344.

19. Campbell AJ, Robertson MC. Rethinking individual and community fall prevention strategies: A meta-regression comparing single and multifactorial interventions. *Age Ageing.* 2007;36:656–662.

20. Beswick AD, Rees K, Dieppe P, et al. Complex interventions to improve physical function and maintain independent living in elderly people: A systematic review and meta-analysis. *Lancet.* 2008;371:725–735.

21. McClure R, Turner C, Peel N, et al. Population-based interventions for the prevention of fall-related injuries in older people. *Cochrane Database Syst Rev.* 2005;CD004441.

22. Gates S, Fisher JD, Cooke MW, et al. Multifactorial assessment and targeted intervention for preventing falls and injuries among older people in community and emergency care settings: Systematic review and meta-analysis. *BMJ.* 2008;336:130–133.

23. Garwood CL, Corbett TL. Use of anticoagulation in elderly patients with atrial fibrillation who are at risk for falls. *Ann Pharmacother.* 2008;42:523–532.

24. Patients with nonvalvular atrial fibrillation at low risk of stroke during treatment with aspirin: Stroke prevention in atrial fibrillation III study. The SPAF III writing committee for the stroke prevention in atrial fibrillation investigators. *JAMA.* 1998;279:1273–1277.

25. Department of Health and Human Services, Centers for Disease Control and Prevention. Preventing falls

among older adults. 2009. Available at: www.cdc. gov/Homeand RecreationalSafety/Falls/preventfalls. html#Compendium. Accessed January 18, 2010.

26. National Council on Aging. Fall prevention. Available at www.healthyagingprograms.com. Accessed January 18, 2010.

27. American Geriatrics Society. Falls in older adults management in primary practice. Available at: www. americangeriatrics.org/education/falls.shtml. Accessed January 18, 2010.

28. Lawrence RC, Felson DT, Helmick CG, et al. Estimates of the prevalence of arthritis and other rheumatic conditions in the United States. Part II. *Arthritis Rheum.* 2008;58:26–35.

29. Felson DT, Naimark A, Anderson J, et al. The prevalence of knee osteoarthritis in the elderly. The Framingham osteoarthritis study. *Arthritis Rheum.* 1987;30:914–918.

30. Dillon CF, Rasch EK, Gu Q, et al. Prevalence of knee osteoarthritis in the United States: Arthritis data from the third national health and nutrition examination survey 1991–94. *J Rheumatol.* 2006;33:2271–2279.

31. Sleath B, Cahoon WD, Jr., Sloane PD, et al. Use of conventional and nonconventional treatments for osteoarthritis in the family medicine setting. *South Med J.* 2008;101:252–259.

32. Messier SP, Gutekunst DJ, Davis C, et al. Weight loss reduces knee-joint loads in overweight and obese older adults with knee osteoarthritis. *Arthritis Rheum.* 2005;52:2026–2032.

33. Felson DT, Zhang Y, Anthony JM, et al. Weight loss reduces the risk for symptomatic knee osteoarthritis in women. The Framingham study. *Ann Intern Med.* 1992;116:535–539.

34. Ettinger WH, Jr., Burns R, Messier SP, et al. A randomized trial comparing aerobic exercise and resistance exercise with a health education program in older adults with knee osteoarthritis. The fitness arthritis and seniors trial (FAST). *JAMA.* 1997;277:25–31.

35. Gibofsky A, Barkin RL. Chronic pain of osteoarthritis: Considerations for selecting an extended-release opioid analgesic. *Am J Ther.* 2008;15:241–255.

36. Vorsanger G, Xiang J, Jordan D, et al. Post hoc analysis of a randomized, double-blind, placebo-controlled efficacy and tolerability study of tramadol extended release for the treatment of osteoarthritis pain in geriatric patients. *Clin Ther.* 2007;29 Suppl:2520–2535.

37. Sawitzke AD, Shi H, Finco MF, et al. The effect of glucosamine and/or chondroitin sulfate on the progression of knee osteoarthritis: A report from the glucosamine/chondroitin arthritis intervention trial. *Arthritis Rheum.* 2008;58:3183–3191.

38. Monfort J, Martel-Pelletier J, Pelletier JP. Chondroitin sulphate for symptomatic osteoarthritis: Critical appraisal of meta-analyses. *Curr Med Res Opin.* 2008;24:1303–1308.

39. Dominick KL, Dudley TK, Grambow SC, et al. Racial differences in health care utilization among patients with osteoarthritis. *J Rheumatol.* 2003;30:2201–2206.

40. Towheed TE, Maxwell L, Anastassiades TP, et al. Glucosamine therapy for treating osteoarthritis. *Cochrane Database Syst Rev.* 2005;CD002946.

41. Clegg DO, Reda DJ, Harris CL, et al. Glucosamine, chondroitin sulfate, and the two in combination for painful knee osteoarthritis. *N Engl J Med.* 2006;354:795–808.

42. Hochberg MC, Clegg DO. Potential effects of chondroitin sulfate on joint swelling: A gait report. *Osteoarthritis Cartilage.* 2008;16 Suppl 3:S22–24.

43. Brien S, Prescott P, Lewith G. Meta-analysis of the related nutritional supplements dimethyl sulfoxide and methylsulfonylmethane in the treatment of osteoarthritis of the knee. *Evid Based Complement Alternat Med.* 2009;

44. Soeken KL, Lee WL, Bausell RB, et al. Safety and efficacy of s-adenosylmethionine (SAMe) for osteoarthritis. *J Fam Pract.* 2002;51:425–430.

45. Najm WI, Reinsch S, Hoehler F, et al. S-adenosyl methionine (SAMe) versus celecoxib for the treatment of osteoarthritis symptoms: A double-blind cross-over trial. *BMC Musculoskelet Disord.* 2004;5:6.

46. di Padova C. S-adenosylmethionine in the treatment of osteoarthritis. Review of the clinical studies. *Am J Med.* 1987;83:60–65.

47. O'Malley P. Sports cream and arthritic rubs: The hidden dangers of unrecognized salicylate toxicity. *Clin Nurse Spec.* 2008;22:6–8.

48. Diclofenac gel for osteoarthritis. *Med Lett Drugs Ther.* 2008;50:31–32.

49. American College of Rheumatology Subcommittee on Osteoarthritis Guidelines. Recommendations for the medical management of osteoarthritis of the hip and knee. *Arthr Rheumatol.* 2000;43:1905-1915.

50. Bellamy N. Hyaluronic acid and knee osteoarthritis. *J Fam Pract.* 2006;55:967–968.

51. Ferring Pharmaceuticals Inc. Euflexxa package insert. Available at: www.euflexxa.com/files/euflexxa_physician.pdf. Accessed January 18, 2010.

52. Onel E, Kolsun K, Kauffman JI. Post-hoc analysis of a head-to-head hyaluronic acid comparison in knee osteoarthritis using the 2004 OMERACT-OARSI responder criteria. *Clin Drug Investig.* 2008;28:37–45.

53. Kirchner M, Marshall D. A double-blind randomized controlled trial comparing alternate forms of high molecular weight hyaluronan for the treatment of osteoarthritis of the knee. *Osteoarthritis Cartilage.* 2006;14:154-162.

54. Waddell DD. Viscosupplementation with hyaluronans for osteoarthritis of the knee: Clinical efficacy and economic implications. *Drugs Aging.* 2007;24:629–642.

55. U.S. Department of Health and Human Services, U.S. Food and Drug Administration. Propoxyphene ques-

tions and answers. 2009. Available at: www.fda.gov/ Drugs/DrugSafety/PostmarketDrugSafetyInformationforPatientsandProviders/ucm170268.htm. Accessed January 18, 2010.

56. Husted H, Holm G, Jacobsen S. Predictors of length of stay and patient satisfaction after hip and knee replacement surgery: Fast-track experience in 712 patients. *Acta Orthop.* 2008;79:168–173.

57. MacLean CH. Quality indicators for the management of osteoarthritis in vulnerable elders. *Ann Intern Med.* 2001;135:711–721.

58. Gabriel SE, Jaakkimainen L, Bombardier C. Risk for serious gastrointestinal complications related to use of nonsteroidal anti-inflammatory drugs. A meta-analysis. *Ann Intern Med.* 1991;115:787–796.

59. Griffin MR, Piper JM, Daugherty JR, et al. Nonsteroidal anti-inflammatory drug use and increased risk for peptic ulcer disease in elderly persons. *Ann Intern Med.* 1991;114:257–263.

60. Griffin MR, Ray WA, Schaffner W. Nonsteroidal anti-inflammatory drug use and death from peptic ulcer in elderly persons. *Ann Intern Med.* 1988;109:359–363.

61. Naesdal J, Brown K. NSAID-associated adverse effects and acid control aids to prevent them: A review of current treatment options. *Drug Saf.* 2006;29:119–132.

62. Lanas A, Ferrandez A. Inappropriate prevention of NSAID-induced gastrointestinal events among long-term users in the elderly. *Drugs Aging.* 2007;24:121–131.

63. Blandizzi C, Tuccori M, Colucci R, et al. Clinical efficacy of esomeprazole in the prevention and healing of gastrointestinal toxicity associated with nsaids in elderly patients. *Drugs Aging.* 2008;25:197–208.

64. Rahme E, Barkun A, Nedjar H, et al. Hospitalizations for upper and lower GI events associated with traditional NSAIDs and acetaminophen among the elderly in Quebec, Canada. *Am J Gastroenterol.* 2008;103:872–882.

65. Feenstra J, Heerdink ER, Grobbee DE, et al. Association of nonsteroidal anti-inflammatory drugs with first occurrence of heart failure and with relapsing heart failure: The Rotterdam study. *Arch Intern Med.* 2002;162:265–270.

66. Solomon SD, Wittes J, Finn PV, et al. Cardiovascular risk of celecoxib in 6 randomized placebo-controlled trials: The cross trial safety analysis. *Circulation.* 2008;117:2104–2113.

67. Caldwell B, Aldington S, Weatherall M, et al. Risk of cardiovascular events and celecoxib: A systematic review and meta-analysis. *J R Soc Med.* 2006;99:132–140.

68. van Staa TP, Smeeth L, Persson I, et al. What is the harm-benefit ratio of COX-2 inhibitors? *Int J Epidemiol.* 2008;37:405–413.

69. Mukherjee D, Nissen SE, Topol EJ. Risk of cardiovascular events associated with selective COX-2 inhibitors. *JAMA.* 2001;286:954–959.

70. Fick DM, Cooper JW, Wade WE, et al. Updating the beers criteria for potentially inappropriate medication use in older adults: Results of a US consensus panel of experts. *Arch Intern Med.* 2003;163:2716–2724.

71. Fink A, Tsai MC, Hays RD, et al. Comparing the alcohol-related problems survey (arps) to traditional alcohol screening measures in elderly outpatients. *Arch Gerontol Geriatr.* 2002;34:55–78.

72. Parra D, Beckey NP, Stevens GR. The effect of acetaminophen on the international normalized ratio in patients stabilized on warfarin therapy. *Pharmacotherapy.* 2007;27:675–683.

73. Larkai EN, Smith JL, Lidsky MD, et al. Gastroduodenal mucosa and dyspeptic symptoms in arthritic patients during chronic nonsteroidal anti-inflammatory drug use. *Am J Gastroenterol.* 1987;82:1153–1158.

74. National Osteoporosis Foundation. Clinician's guide to prevention and treatment of osteoporosis. 2008. Available at www.nof.org/professionals/Clinicians_Guide.htm. Accessed January 18, 2010.

75. Duque G, Troen BR. Understanding the mechanisms of senile osteoporosis: New facts for a major geriatric syndrome. *J Am Geriatr Soc.* 2008;56:935–941.

76. O'Connell MB, Vondracek SF. Osteoporosis and other metabolic bone diseases. In: DiPiro JT, Talbert RL, Yee GC, Matzke GR, Wells BG, Posey LM (eds.) *Pharmacotherapy a pathophysiologic approach*, Seventh ed. New York: McGraw Hill Medical; 2008: 1483–1504.

77. Ebeling PR. Clinical practice. Osteoporosis in men. *N Engl J Med.* 2008;358:1474–1482.

78. The North American Menopause Society. Management of osteoporosis in postmenopausal women: 2010 position statement of The North American Menopause Society. Menopause 10;17:25–54.

79. Egan M, Jaglal S, Byrne K, et al. Factors associated with a second hip fracture: A systematic review. *Clin Rehabil.* 2008;22:272–282.

80. Siris ES. Patients with hip fracture: What can be improved? *Bone.* 2006;38:S8–12.

81. Schneider DL. Management of osteoporosis in geriatric populations. *Curr Osteoporos Rep.* 2008;6:100–107.

82. Nguyen-Oghalai TU, Kuo YF, Zhang DD, et al. Discharge setting for patients with hip fracture: Trends from 2001 to 2005. *J Am Geriatr Soc.* 2008;56:1063–1068.

83. Kanis JA. FRAX WHO fracture risk assessment tool. 2008. Available at www.shef.ac.uk/FRAX/. Accessed January 18, 2010.

84 Health 24. Measure your height. Available at: www.health24.com/dietnfood/Great_diet_guides/15-3089-3242.asp. Accessed January 18, 2008.

85. Qaseem A, Snow V, Shekelle P, et al. Pharmacologic treatment of low bone density or osteoporosis to prevent fractures: A clinical practice guideline from the American College of Physicians. *Ann Intern Med.* 2008;149:404–415.

86. Grossman J, MacLean CH. Quality indicators for the care of osteoporosis in vulnerable elders. *J Am Geriatr Soc.* 2007;55 Suppl 2:S392–402.

87. US Department of Health and Human Services, Office of the Surgeon General. Bone health and osteoporosis: A report of the Surgeon General. 2004. Available at: www.surgeongeneral.gov/library/bonehealth/docs/exec_summ.pdf. Accessed January 18, 2010.

88. Heaney RP. Calcium, dairy products and osteoporosis. *J Am Coll Nutr.* 2000;19:83S–99S.

89. Dawson-Hughes B, Bischoff-Ferrari HA. Therapy of osteoporosis with calcium and vitamin D. *J Bone Miner Res.* 2007;22 Suppl 2:V59–63.

90. Tang BM, Eslick GD, Nowson C, et al. Use of calcium or calcium in combination with vitamin d supplementation to prevent fractures and bone loss in people aged 50 years and older: A meta-analysis. *Lancet.* 2007;370:657–666.

91. Lyles KW, Colon-Emeric CS, Magaziner JS, et al. Zoledronic acid and clinical fractures and mortality after hip fracture. *N Engl J Med.* 2007;357:1799–1809.

92. Inderjeeth CA, Foo AC, Lai MM, et al. Efficacy and safety of pharmacological agents in managing osteoporosis in the old old: Review of the evidence. *Bone.* 2009;44:744–751.

93. Schousboe JT, Ensrud KE, Nyman JA, et al. Universal bone densitometry screening combined with alendronate therapy for those diagnosed with osteoporosis is highly cost-effective for elderly women. *J Am Geriatr Soc.* 2005;53:1697–1704.

94. Schousboe JT, Nyman JA, Kane RL, et al. Cost-effectiveness of alendronate therapy for osteopenic postmenopausal women. *Ann Intern Med.* 2005;142:734–741.

95. Schousboe JT, Taylor BC, Fink HA, et al. Cost-effectiveness of bone densitometry followed by treatment of osteoporosis in older men. *JAMA.* 2007;298:629–637.

96. Warriner AH, Outman RC, Saag KG, et al. Management of osteoporosis among home health and long-term care patients with a prior fracture. *South Med J.* 2009;102:397–404.

97. Siris ES, Selby PL, Saag KG, et al. Impact of osteoporosis treatment adherence on fracture rates in North America and Europe. *Am J Med.* 2009;122:S3–13.

98. Lewiecki EM. Prevention and treatment of postmenopausal osteoporosis. *Obstet Gynecol Clin North Am.* 2008;35:301–315, ix.

99. Recker RR. Calcium absorption and achlorhydria. *N Engl J Med.* 1985;313:70–73.

100. O'Connell MB, Madden DM, Murray AM, et al. Effects of proton pump inhibitors on calcium carbonate absorption in women: A randomized crossover trial. *Am J Med.* 2005;118:778–781.

101. Yang YX. Proton pump inhibitor therapy and osteoporosis. *Curr Drug Saf.* 2008;3:204–209.

102. Vieth R, Chan PC, MacFarlane GD. Efficacy and safety of vitamin D3 intake exceeding the lowest observed adverse effect level. *Am J Clin Nutr.* 2001;73:288–294.

103. Recker RR, Lewiecki EM, Miller PD, et al. Safety of bisphosphonates in the treatment of osteoporosis. *Am J Med.* 2009;122:S22–32.

104. Miller PD. Diagnosis and treatment of osteoporosis in chronic renal disease. *Semin Nephrol.* 2009;29:144–155.

105. Fardet L, Kassar A, Cabane J, et al. Corticosteroid-induced adverse events in adults: Frequency, screening and prevention. *Drug Saf.* 2007;30:861–881.

106. Canalis E, Mazziotti G, Giustina A, et al. Glucocorticoid-induced osteoporosis: Pathophysiology and therapy. *Osteoporos Int.* 2007;18:1319–1328.

107. Solomon DH, Morris C, Cheng H, et al. Medication use patterns for osteoporosis: An assessment of guidelines, treatment rates, and quality improvement interventions. *Mayo Clin Proc.* 2005;80:194–202.

108. Compston JE. Emerging consensus on prevention and treatment of glucocorticoid-induced osteoporosis. *Curr Rheumatol Rep.* 2007;9:78–84.

109. Reid DM, Devogelaer JP, Saag K, et al. Zoledronic acid and risedronate in the prevention and treatment of glucocorticoid-induced osteoporosis (Horizon): A multicentre, double-blind, double-dummy, randomised controlled trial. *Lancet.* 2009;373:1253–1263.

110. Saag KG, Shane E, Boonen S, et al. Teriparatide or alendronate in glucocorticoid-induced osteoporosis. *N Engl J Med.* 2007;357:2028–2039.

111. Morris MS. The association between serum thyroid-stimulating hormone in its reference range and bone status in postmenopausal American women. *Bone.* 2007;40:1128–1134.

112. Ziere G, Dieleman JP, van der Cammen TJ, et al. Selective serotonin reuptake inhibiting antidepressants are associated with an increased risk of nonvertebral fractures. *J Clin Psychopharmacol.* 2008;28:411–417.

113. Mayo Clinic Staff. Polymyalgia rheumatica. 2008. Available at www.mayoclinic.com/health/polymyalgia-rheumtacia/DS00441. Accessed January 18, 2101.

114. Unwin B, Williams CM, Gilliland W. Polymyalgia rheumatica and giant cell arteritis. *Am Fam Physician.* 2006;74:1547–1554.

115. Dasgupta B, Matteson EL, Maradit-Kremers H. Management guidelines and outcome measures in polymyalgia rheumatica (PMR). *Clin Exp Rheumatol.* 2007;25:130–136.

116. Luqmani R. Treatment of polymyalgia rheumatica and giant cell arteritis: Are we any further forward? *Ann Intern Med.* 2007;146:674–676.

117. Stone JH. Methotrexate in polymyalgia rheumatica: Kernel of truth or curse of tantalus? *Ann Intern Med.* 2004;141:568–569.

118. Fraser JA, Weyand CM, Newman NJ, et al. The treatment of giant cell arteritis. *Rev Neurol Dis.* 2008;5:140–152.

119. Gabriel SE, Michaud K. Epidemiological studies in incidence, prevalence, mortality, and comorbidity of the rheumatic diseases. *Arthritis Res Ther.* 2009;11:229.

120. Helmick CG, Felson DT, Lawrence RC, et al. Estimates of the prevalence of arthritis and other rheumatic conditions in the United States. Part I. *Arthritis Rheum.* 2008;58:15–25.

121. Gonzalez A, Maradit Kremers H, Crowson CS, et al. The widening mortality gap between rheumatoid arthritis patients and the general population. *Arthritis Rheum.* 2007;56:3583–3587.

122. Medline Plus. Rheumatoid arthritis. Available at www.nlm.nih.gov/MEDLINEPLUS/ency/article/000431.htm. Accessed January 18, 2010.

123. Gabriel SE, Crowson CS, Kremers HM, et al. Survival in rheumatoid arthritis: A population-based analysis of trends over 40 years. *Arthritis Rheum.* 2003;48:54–58.

124. Panoulas VF, Smith JP, Nightingale P, et al. Association of the traf1/c5 locus with increased mortality, particularly from malignancy or sepsis, in patients with rheumatoid arthritis. *Arthritis Rheum.* 2009;60:39–46.

125. Saag KG, Teng GG, Patkar NM, et al. American College of Rheumatology 2008 recommendations for the use of nonbiologic and biologic disease-modifying antirheumatic drugs in rheumatoid arthritis. *Arthritis Rheum.* 2008;59:762–784.

126. McDonald JR, Zeringue AL, Caplan L, et al. Herpes zoster risk factors in a national cohort of veterans with rheumatoid arthritis. *Clin Infect Dis.* 2009;48:1364–1371.

127. Chung ES, Packer M, Lo KH, et al. Randomized, double-blind, placebo-controlled, pilot trial of inflix-imab, a chimeric monoclonal antibody to tumor necrosis factor-alpha, in patients with moderate-to-severe heart failure: Results of the anti-tnf therapy against congestive heart failure (ATTACH) trial. *Circulation.* 2003;107:3133–3140.

128. Mann DL, McMurray JJ, Packer M, et al. Targeted anticytokine therapy in patients with chronic heart failure: Results of the randomized etanercept worldwide evaluation (renewal). *Circulation.* 2004;109:1594–1602.

129. Mittendorf T, Dietz B, Sterz R, et al. Personal and economic burden of late-stage rheumatoid arthritis among patients treated with adalimumab: An evaluation from a patient's perspective. *Rheumatology (Oxford).* 2008;47:188–193.

130. Kelsey JL, Lamster IB. Influence of musculoskeletal conditions on oral health among older adults. *Am J Public Health.* 2008;98:1177–1183.

131. Grainger M, Castledine G, Wood N, et al. Researching the management of constipation in long-term care. Part 2. *Br J Nurs.* 2007;16:1212–1217.

132. Yount S, Sorensen MV, Cella D, et al. Adalimumab plus methotrexate or standard therapy is more effective than methotrexate or standard therapies alone in the treatment of fatigue in patients with active, inadequately treated rheumatoid arthritis. *Clin Exp Rheumatol.* 2007;25:838–846.

133. O'Neil CK. Prevention and treatment of pressure ulcers. *J Pharm Prac.* 2004;17:137–148.

134. Padula CA, Osborne E, Williams J. Prevention and early detection of pressure ulcers in hospitalized patients. *J Wound Ostomy Continence Nurs.* 2008;35:65–75; discussion 76–68.

135. Lyder CH. Pressure ulcer prevention and management. *JAMA.* 2003;289:223–226.

136. Prevention Plus Home of the Braden scale. Available at www.bradenscale.com/products.htm. Accessed January 18, 2010.

137. The Medical Algorithms Project. Norton scale for predicting risk of pressure ulcer. Available at www.medal.org/visitor/www/Active/ch21/ch21.01/ch21.01.01.aspx. Accessed January 18, 20101.

138. Hatanaka N, Yamamoto Y, Ichihara K, et al. A new predictive indicator for development of pressure ulcers in bedridden patients based on common laboratory tests results. *J Clin Pathol.* 2008;61:514–518.

139. Hengstermann S, Fischer A, Steinhagen-Thiessen E, et al. Nutrition status and pressure ulcer: What we need for nutrition screening. *JPEN J Parenter Enteral Nutr.* 2007;31:288–294.

140. National Pressure Ulcer Advisory Panel Board of Directors. Pressure ulcers in America: Prevalence, incidence, and implications for the future. An executive summary of the National Pressure Ulcer Advisory Panel monograph. *Adv Skin Wound Care.* 2001;14:208–215.

141. National Pressure Ulcer Advisory Panel. Updated staging system. Available at www.npuap.org. Accessed January 18, 2010.

142. National Pressure Ulcer Advisory Panel. Pressure ulcer stages revised by NPUAP. Available at www.npuap.org/pr2.htm. Accessed January 18, 2010.

143. Reddy M, Gill SS, Rochon PA. Preventing pressure ulcers: A systematic review. *JAMA.* 2006;296:974–984.

144. Brem H, Lyder C. Protocol for the successful treatment of pressure ulcers. *Am J Surg.* 2004;188:9–17.

145. American Medical Directors Association. *Pressure ulcers in the long-term care setting. Clinical practice guidelines.* 2008. Available at http://amda.networkats.com/members_online/members/viewitem.asp?item=CPG212&catalog=CPGS&pn=1&af=AMDA. Access January 20, 2010

146. Garcia AD, Thomas DR. Assessment and management of chronic pressure ulcers in the elderly. *Med Clin North Am.* 2006;90:925–944.

147. Xakellis GC, Chrischilles EA. Hydrocolloid versus saline-gauze dressings in treating pressure ulcers: A cost-effectiveness analysis. *Arch Phys Med Rehabil.* 1992;73:463–469.

148. Colwell JC, Foreman MD, Trotter JP. A comparison of the efficacy and cost-effectiveness of two methods of managing pressure ulcers. *Decubitus.* 1993;6:28–36.

149. US Department of Health and Human Services. Eliminating serious, preventable, and costly medical errors—never events. 2006. Available at www.cms.hhs.gov/apps/media/press/release.asp?Counter=1863. Accessed January 18, 2010.

150. National Quality Forum. Serious reportable events. 2008. Available at www.qualityforum.org/Publications/2008/10/Serious_Reportable_Events.aspx. Accessed January 18, 2010.

151. Vu T, Harris A, Duncan G, et al. Cost-effectiveness of multidisciplinary wound care in nursing homes: A

pseudo-randomized pragmatic cluster trial. *Fam Pract.* 2007;24:372–379.

152. Geusens P. Bisphosphonates for postmenopausal osteoporosis: Determining duration of treatment. *Curr Osteoporos Rep.* 2009;7:12–17.

153. O'Connell MB, Patel NP, Hames SL. Bone and musculoskeletal disorders. In: Borgelt L, O'Connell MB, Smith JA, Calis KA, eds. *Women's Health Across the Lifespan: A Pharmacotherapeutic Approach.* Bethesda, MD: American Society of Heath-System Pharmacists; 2010.

16

Hematology and Immunology

SUM LAM, JAMES NAWARSKAS, AND ANGELA CHENG-LAI

Learning Objectives

1. Characterize the common causes and complications of anemia and their prevalence in the elderly patient.

2. For a given patient with anemia, develop a treatment plan which includes pharmacologic and non-pharmacologic therapy.

3. Recognize the epidemiology, pathophysiology, and clinical presentation of herpes zoster.

4. Given a patient case, recommend appropriate pharmacotherapy for acute herpes zoster, as well as monitoring parameters to ensure efficacy and safety.

5. Summarize the current recommendations on immunization for older adults.

6. Given a patient case, recommend appropriate immunization and monitoring parameters to optimize efficacy and safety of vaccination.

7. Describe various cancer screening tests that are recommended for the geriatric population including associated problems and barriers.

8. Describe various cancer prevention measures including medications and vitamin supplements.

Key Terms

ALLODYNIA: Painful response to a usually non-painful stimulus.

BEERS CRITERIA: Widely used consensus criteria created by geriatrician Mark H. Beers for safe medication use in elderly patients. The Beers criteria was last updated in 2003 and provides a list of medications that are generally considered inappropriate in the elderly due to an unfavorable risk:benefit ratio.

CANCER CHEMOPREVENTION: Use of natural, synthetic, or biologic chemical agents to reverse, suppress, or prevent carcinogenic progression to invasive cancer.

ERYTHROPOIESIS: The process of producing red blood cells.

ERYTHROPOIETIN: Protein secreted by the kidneys that stimulates the production of red blood cells.

FERRITIN: Main intracellular iron storage protein in the body.

HEMATOPOIETIC: Relating to the formation and maturation of blood cells and their derivatives.

HEPCIDIN: Hormone produced by the liver which regulates iron hemostasis. Hepcidin inhibits ferroportin, a protein found on enterocytes and macrophages which transports iron out of storage cells. Inhibition of ferroportin prevents iron release from macrophages as well as secretion of iron from the intestines into the hepatic portal system, thereby reducing iron absorption.

HUMORAL: Relating to the fluids of the body.

INTRINSIC FACTOR: Protein produced by the stomach which is necessary for the absorption of vitamin B_{12} in the terminal ileum.

MYELODYSPLASIA: Condition characterized by dysfunctional production of cells in the bone marrow and thereby ineffective hematopoiesis.

TRANSFERRIN: Plasma protein which binds to and transports iron in the body.

Introduction

Diseases of the hematologic and immune system are common in the older adult. In addition, system decline theories of aging focus upon failures with these systems as potential explanations for the frailty seen in many of the very old population. Anemia, cancer, and loss of immune function are common with aging, but have yet to be identified as normal diseases associated with the aging process. Causes of anemia in the elderly patient and its proper treatment are reviewed in the first section of this chapter followed by a section on Herpes zoster. The chapter ends with a focus on immunizations and cancer screenings appropriate for older adults. The tenets of public health provide the necessary prevention of infections and early detection of cancer which will aid older adults to live healthier, longer lives, just as in younger patients.

Anemia

Prevalence, Pathogenesis, and Etiology of Anemia Specific to Geriatrics

Prevalence

Anemia in the elderly has recently been termed a "public health crisis" due to its high prevalence and possibility for adverse consequences.[1] As with many chronic diseases, the prevalence of anemia increases with increasing age (Figure 16-1).[2] The Third National Health and Nutrition Examination Survey (NHANES III) documented an anemia prevalence rate of 10.6% in community-dwelling adults age 65 years or older.[2,3] Other reports have described substantially higher rates of anemia in the homebound elderly (39.6%) and in nursing home residents (48–63%).[4-7]

With regards to gender, there is a crossover in which anemia is more common in females

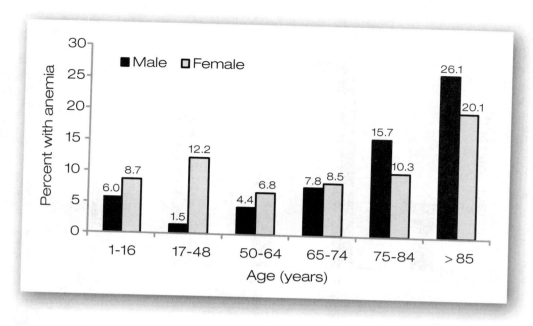

Figure 16-1. Prevalence of anemia in the United States by age and gender. Data are from NHANES III, phases 1 and 2, 1988 to 1994. *Source:* Figure adapted from reference 2.

less than 65 years of age, but is more common in males over 75 years of age (Figure 16-1).[2,3] This may be due to gender-related differences in terms of defining anemia. The diagnosis of anemia most commonly used is that of the World Health Organization (WHO), which defines anemia as a hemoglobin concentration of < 13 g/dL in men and < 12 g/dL in women.[8] While this gender distinction in defining anemia may be reasonable pre-menopause, some have questioned whether this is appropriate for post-menopausal females.[2] If anemia is defined as a hemoglobin concentration of < 13 g/dL regardless of gender, then the rates of anemia in women would likely be consistently higher than men regardless of age.[2,9] Racial differences have also been demonstrated with regards to anemia prevalence in the elderly, with a remarkably higher rate seen in African American individuals (Figure 16-2).[2,3] The racial differences in hemoglobin concentration between African Americans and non-Hispanic Caucasians is believed to be due to genetic mutations that have evolved secondary to environmental pressures in Africa and Europe rather than due to health, nutrition, or behavioral or socioeconomic factors.[2,9] Some have therefore advocated for racial distinc-

tions in defining anemia, which is further supported by recent data demonstrating that a hemoglobin concentration below the current WHO threshold for anemia is associated with increased mortality in African American patients.[9,10]

Pathogenesis

The fundamental cause of most anemias in elderly patients is defective or deficient red blood cell production, otherwise known as diminished **erythropoiesis**.[11] Age-related changes in erythropoiesis may be considered in the context of two broad categories: 1) changes intrinsic to erythroid progenitor or **hematopoietic** stem cells, and 2) changes in **humoral** control mechanisms.[11] With regards to alterations in progenitor and stem cells, morphologic studies have shown a decrease in hematopoietic tissue in the bone marrow of elderly patients, although erythropoietic activity is not necessarily diminished.[11,12] While some studies have shown a decrease in erythroid burst-forming and colony-forming units in anemic elderly patients, other studies have shown no changes.[13-16] One study in particular showed a lower number of CD34+ progenitor cells in the blood of elderly (but not necessarily anemic) individuals with an

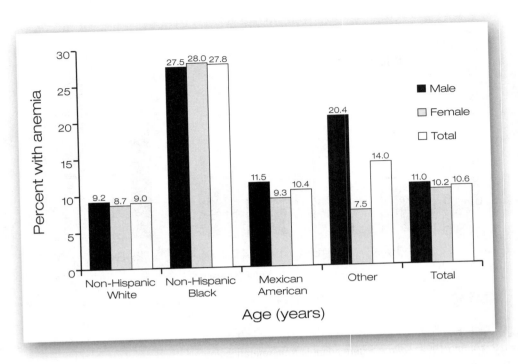

Figure 16-2. Prevalence of anemia in individuals aged 65 or older in the United States by self-declared racial or ethnic group. *Source:* Data from references 2 and 3.

increase in serum stem cell factor concentrations, which may be a compensatory mechanism to stimulate erythroid cell differentiation. In this study, CD34+ cells, in the presence of optimal concentrations of recombinant hematopoietic growth factors, were able to form erythroid burst-forming units and colony-forming units at a rate similar to that seen in young individuals. This would indicate that humoral mechanisms may be more likely responsible for the hematopoietic changes seen in the elderly as opposed to an unresponsiveness of hematopoietic progenitors to growth factors.[16]

From a humoral perspective, **erythropoietin** concentrations generally increase with aging, although studies have shown mixed results in this regard.[11] Confounding this issue is that worsening renal function, which is often present in the elderly, corresponds to a blunted erythropoietin response to anemia and lower erythropoietin concentrations.[17-19] It has been theorized that the increase in erythropoietin concentrations seen with aging is a consequence of a state of relative erythroid resistance to erythropoietin, thereby

resulting in increased erythropoietin secretion. Anemia then develops when this feedback loop is interrupted, which may occur in the presence of renal disease, diabetes, or hypertension.[11] Other humoral links to anemia have been made with testosterone, growth hormone, and inflammatory mediators. The androgenic hormones may play a role in erythropoiesis and their secretion decreases with aging. Associations have been made with low testosterone concentrations and anemia and, independently, growth hormone administration has been shown to reverse anemia in adults with growth hormone deficiency.[20,21] However, direct links between androgen hormone deficiency and the development of anemia are lacking and require further study. Conversely, concentrations of inflammatory mediators are known to be chronically, albeit mildly, elevated in elderly individuals even in the absence of an acute illness or autoimmune disease.[22-25] Concentrations of interleukin (IL)-6, IL-1, tumor-necrosis factor (TNF), and C-reactive protein (CRP) have all been shown to be elevated in elderly patients with anemia compared to non-anemic counterparts.[26,27] However, one study showed elevations in IL-6 and CRP in patients with anemia of chronic disease, but showed significantly lower CRP concentrations in patients with unexplained anemia compared to non-anemic controls along with the lowest concentrations of IL-6, TNF-alpha and CRP of all types of anemia studied (i.e. compared to iron deficiency, nutritional, and anemia of chronic disease). [28] In addition, elevated cytokine concentrations may impede erythropoietin production and impair erythropoiesis. [29,30] Specifically, IL-6 and IL-1 have been shown to increase hepatic synthesis of hepcidin, a polypeptide which inhibits both iron absorption form the gut as well as the release of iron from bone marrow macrophages to erythroid progenitors. [31]

Etiology

Data from NHANES III demonstrate that the etiology of anemia in the elderly is almost evenly split into thirds, with nutrient deficiency, chronic disease, and unexplained anemia each comprising roughly one third of cases (Table 16-1). [2] It is also believed that in 30–50% of elderly anemic patients, multiple etiologies are responsible. [32] Most

cases of anemia in the elderly are mild; about 90% of patients have a hemoglobin of 11 g/dL or greater and about 98% have a hemoglobin of 10 g/dL or greater. [2]

Nutritional Anemias

Most cases of nutritional anemias in the elderly are due to iron deficiency, either alone or in combination with vitamin B12 and/or folate deficiency (Table 16-1). The diagnosis of iron deficiency (typically diagnosed by low serum iron and **ferritin** concentrations and a high total iron binding capacity [TIBC]) in the elderly is complicated by the fact that serum ferritin concentrations rise with advancing age probably as a consequence of low-grade inflammatory processes. [33] Consequently, serum ferritin concentrations below 45 mcg/L are usually indicative of iron deficiency in the elderly, whereas much lower concentrations may define iron deficiency in younger individuals. [33,34] More recently, serum **transferrin** receptor (sTfr) concentrations have been studied as more sensitive estimations of iron stores in the elderly. This receptor is overexpressed on the surface of progenitor cells in response to diminished iron

Table 16-1. **Prevalence of Different Types of Anemia in Individuals Over 65 Years of Age in the United States**

Type of Anemia	Number of Patients	Percentage Based on All Patients with Anemia
Nutrient deficiency	**965,000**	**34.3%**
Iron deficiency	467,000	16.6%
Folate deficiency	181,000	6.4%
B12 deficiency	166,000	5.9%
Folate + B12 deficiency	56,000	2.0%
Iron + folate and/or B12 deficiency	95,000	3.4%
Anemia of chronic disease	**904,000**	**32.2%**
Anemia of chronic inflammation *without* renal insufficiency	554,000	19.7%
Anemia of chronic inflammation *with* renal insufficiency	120,000	4.3%
Anemia of chronic kidney disease	230,000	8.2%
Unexplained anemia	**945,000**	**33.6%**
Total	2,814,000	100.0%

Source: Data from NHANES III, phase 2, 1991 to 1994 (reference 2).

concentrations reaching the cell surface. Elevations of sTfr indicate iron deficiency and the ratio of sTfr to the log of serum ferritin (sTfr index) is believed to be the most predictive tool for estimating iron stores in the elderly.[35] The sTfr index may also help distinguish iron-deficiency anemia from anemia of chronic inflammation. Although classified as a nutritional deficiency, iron deficiency anemia most often results from blood loss in the gastrointestinal tract, either from gastritis, ulcer disease, arterio-venous malformations, colon polyps, colorectal cancer or hemorrhoids. If blood loss cannot be detected, then disorders involving iron absorption and bioavailability should be considered. In the elderly, atrophic gastritis may reduce iron absorption, and this condition is present in 20–48% of the elderly.[33,36,37]

KEY POINT: Iron deficiency anemia is usually a result of blood loss, most often from the gastrointestinal tract.

Pernicious anemia is prevalent in 1.9% of all elderly and is responsible for 76% of cases of vitamin B12-deficiency anemia.[38] It is usually caused by malabsorption and takes years before it manifests. This is due to the relatively large body stores of vitamin B12 (about 2500 mcg) in relation to the daily requirement (1 mcg). The recommended daily allowance of vitamin B12 of 2.4 mcg is to account for the incomplete ability of intrinsic factor to facilitate the absorption of vitamin B12. Individuals with pernicious anemia lack **intrinsic factor** and only absorb about 1.2% of ingested vitamin B12.[33] Of special concern in the elderly is the prevalence of atrophic gastritis, which retards the release of vitamin B12 from food thereby resulting in mild malabsorption and a delayed and often subclinical manifestation of vitamin B12 deficiency.[33] Vitamin B12 deficiency resulting in anemia is due to dysfunctional intrinsic-factor mediated vitamin B12 absorption in 94% of cases.[39] Small bowel disorders comprise 14% of cases and gastric surgery or disorders represent 3% of cases. Inadequate intake of animal-derived foods represents only about 1% of cases.[39]

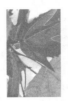

KEY POINT: Vitamin B12 deficiency anemia is the only nutritional anemia with an affinity for the elderly and is usually caused by malabsorption.

Currently, folic acid fortification of dietary sources causes folate-deficiency anemia to be rare in all age groups. In fact, only 0.1% to 0.4% of folate tests ordered by providers demonstrate low folate concentrations.[40,41] Compared to younger adults, older adults have been shown to have higher folate concentrations both before and after the introduction of folic acid fortification.[42,43]

Anemias of Chronic Disease

These anemias broadly refer to any anemia occurring in the presence of chronic illness that cannot be associated with another known etiology. For purposes of this chapter, these anemias will be subjectively categorized as anemia of chronic kidney disease and anemia of chronic inflammation and it is possible for both of these to occur together. Anemia of chronic inflammation has been described as a state of elevated inflammatory cytokines which stimulate the production of **hepcidin** in the liver, leading to a reduction in the intestinal absorption of iron and release of iron from macrophages. This manifests as low concentrations of serum iron in the presence of normal or increased total iron stores.[2] The distinction of anemia of chronic inflammation and iron-deficiency anemia therefore is a diagnostic conundrum in the elderly, especially in the patient with a serum ferritin concentration in the intermediate range (e.g. 20–100 mcg/L) which can be seen with both types of anemia. As mentioned above, the sTfr index may be helpful in distinguishing these types of anemia.

Anemia of chronic kidney disease is due to reduced erythropoietin production in the kidney, which is responsible for about 90% of the production of this hormone. In this setting, the kidney loses the ability to effectively produce erythropoietin in response to decreased oxygenation.[44] In the elderly, anemia associated with chronic kidey disease represents 12.5% of all anemia cases (Table 16-1).[2] In patients over 50 years of age, even mild degrees of renal insufficiency (creatinine clearance of 30–50 mL/min) are associated with anemia and a direct association between degree of renal insufficiency and prevalence of anemia has been documented.[45] The relationship of renal function, erythropoietin, and anemia in the elderly was investigated in the InCHIANTI study, which showed a progressive increase in anemia prevalence and a progressive decrease in renal function and hemoglobin with advancing age.[46] A linear inverse relationship was seen with regards to anemia prevalence and kidney function (i.e., decreased kidney function = increased anemia prevalence) with creatinine clearances of 30 mL/min or lower.[46]

Unexplained Anemia

The term unexplained anemia refers to anemia that cannot be attributed to some other cause. This type of anemia represents about one third of all anemias in the elderly (Table 16-1).[2] Unexplained anemia is usually mild, with hemoglobin concentrations about 1 g/dL lower than the standard set forth by the WHO, likely resulting in underdiagnosis.[47] Unexplained anemia is somewhat of a misnomer, since this type of anemia is more likely due to the interplay of many different causes as opposed to ignorance of the cause. Age-related factors that contribute to unexplained anemia in the elderly are:

   Renal dysfunction leading to a reduced response to erythropoietin,

   Reduction in hematopoietic stem cell proliferative and regenerative function,

   Lower androgen levels, resulting in a decline in hemoglobin concentration of up to 1 g/dL,

   Chronic inflammation and cytokine dysregulation, and

   Myelodysplasia.

Additionally, other comorbidities and medications as well as nutritional deficits and alcohol abuse may further contribute to the etiology of unexplained anemia. As most of these contributors are age-related, the prevalence of unexplained anemia is directly related to age, being most common in the very old and virtually non-existent in those less than 50 years of age.[47]

Summary of Standard Treatment in General Adult Population and Considerations in the Elderly

Nutritional Anemias

In general, the treatment of anemias of nutritional etiology does not differ between elderly patients and younger adults. The treatment of iron deficiency anemia involves iron supplementation. This can be done through diet as well as through iron supplements. Iron supplementation is typically via the oral route, but can also be given parenterally in patients with malabsorption or intolerance to oral preparations. In younger adults, iron-deficiency anemia is treated with a total oral daily dosage of 200 mg elemental iron daily, given in 2–3 divided doses to improve tolerability. Lower dosages are recommended in the elderly patient to improve tolerability with the understanding that iron stores will replenish at a slower rate.[48,49] The most recent **Beers criteria** state that dosages of ferrous sulfate > 325 mg/day do not dramatically increase absorption but do greatly increase the incidence of constipation.[50] Gastrointestinal adverse effects may also be minimized by taking iron products with food, although if taken with meals, the absorption of iron will be reduced by about one half.[48] Acid conditions improve iron absorption, leading to the recommendation to administer iron with a vitamin C-containing food such as orange juice.

Restoration of iron stores and subsequent improvement in hemoglobin may take about 4 months with expected increases in hemoglobin of 1–2 g/dL every couple of weeks.[51] A hemoglobin increase of less than 2 g/dL over a 3-week period warrants evaluation for therapeutic failure. Treatment is continued until iron stores are repleted or chronically with low dosages of oral iron if the anemia is recurrent without a reversible underlying cause (e.g., bleed).[48] Should oral iron therapy fail, parenteral iron may be administered, although this form of therapy is more expensive and cumbersome to administer than oral therapy and possesses a risk of anaphylactic reactions. However, iron stores are not replenished any faster with parenteral versus oral therapy. In severe cases of iron-deficiency anemia, red blood cell transfusion may be necessary.

The treatment of vitamin B12 deficiency anemia is administration of exogenous vitamin B12. This can be obtained through food sources or more efficiently through oral or parenteral supplementation. Oral and intramuscular administrations are equally effective.[52] Given that the majority of cases in the elderly are due to pernicious anemia, chronic therapy is usually necessary and daily oral or monthly subcutaneous/intramuscular injections of 1 mg vitamin B12 are indicated. In these individuals, dietary fortification is usually an insufficient means of restoring vitamin B12 stores due to the malabsorptive nature of the condition.[53] It has been recommended that individuals 50 years of age and older consume vitamin B12 in its crystalline form, which does not require gastric acid or enzymes for digestion.[54] With treatment, reversal of the anemia usually occurs in about 8 weeks.[33]

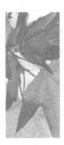

KEY POINT: The treatment of anemia in the elderly patient differs little from treatment in the younger adult, although considerations need to be made for the multiple comorbidities often occurring in the elderly.

Folate-deficiency anemia is treated with oral folic acid or rarely, with parenteral folic acid. The dosage is typically 1 mg daily, but may be as high as 5 mg daily in cases of malabsorption. Given the infrequency of this type of anemia, underlying causes should be considered prior to the initiation of folate therapy. Specifically, malabsorption and alcoholism, which interferes with folate absorption and metabolism, should be ruled out. Drug-induced causes should also be considered. Folate metabolism may be altered by methotrexate, pentamidine, trimethoprim, and triamterene. Azathioprine, 6-mercaptopurine, 5-fluorouracil, hydroxyurea, and reverse transcriptase inhibitors (e.g. stavudine, lamivudine, and zidovudine)

may cause folate deficiency by directly inhibiting DNA synthesis. Cholestyramine, metformin, and sulfasalazine may decrease folate absorption. The anticonvulsants phenytoin, phenobarbital, primidone, and valproic acid may cause folate deficiency through impaired vitamin absorption and/or altered metabolism.[48,55]

Anemias of Chronic Disease and Unexplained Anemia

Anemia of chronic kidney disease is typically treated with a combination of iron supplementation and erythropoietic-stimulating agents (ESAs). The target hemoglobin concentration should be 11–12 g/dL, but no greater than 13 g/dL in dialysis patients and nondialysis patients with CKD who are receiving ESAs.[56] This is largely due to the lack of evidence demonstrating benefit and some evidence of potential harm by achieving higher hemoglobin concentrations with ESA therapy.[56] Oral iron therapy in this situation is often inadequate due to poor absorption and parenteral therapy is often employed. Parenteral iron improves the response to ESAs and also provides a dose-sparing effect for these agents.[56] The use of ESAs for treating chronic kidney disease is based on the need to stimulate erythropoiesis in a condition characterized by low production of this hormone. Epoetin alpha and darbepoetin alpha are the two ESAs approved in the United States for treating anemia of chronic kidney disease.

Anemia of chronic disease and unexplained anemia are treatment challenges due to the multifactorial nature of these conditions. Identifying and treating the underlying causes is the logical approach, but most of these causes have limited treatment options themselves and isolating each cause is a challenge in and of itself. Complicating matters is the lack of clinical trial data to help guide the decision-making process with regards to treatment.[32] To begin, it is recommended to treat any identifiable cause that is amenable to treatment (e.g., nutritional deficiency). Should anemia persist, then ESA therapy may be considered. Two small studies in elderly patients with anemia of chronic disease have demonstrated the benefits of epoetin alfa for treating this condition. In these reports (n = 17 combined), mean hemoglobin increases of 3–4 g/dL were seen in the majority of patients.[57,58]

KEY POINT: Anemia in the elderly has been repeatedly linked to a number of serious complications even with mildly depressed hemoglobin concentrations.

Common Problems Associated with Anemia in the Elderly Patient

Anemia has been shown to be an independent predictor of mortality in elderly in both the community as well as the nursing home settings.[59-61]

Anemia has also been associated with cognitive impairment in the elderly. One case-control study documented an association between anemia and a higher risk of being diagnosed with Alzheimer's disease and another longitudinal study showed an association between anemia and the subsequent diagnosis of dementia.[62,63] Mild anemia (hemoglobin 10–12 g/dL) has also been linked with a reduction in executive function (a set of high-level cognitive abilities involving goal-oriented tasks) in elderly community-dwelling women.[64] More recently, a systematic review documented a significant hazard ratio of 1.94 for the risk of incident dementia in the elderly with anemia. However, the paucity of studies in this area allowed only two studies to be included in this analysis.[65]

Physical function in the elderly is also adversely affected by anemia, even in its milder forms. The Women's Health and Aging Studies (WHAS) showed that even the mildest forms of anemia (i.e., hemoglobin concentrations of 12 g/dL) were associated with mobility difficulties compared with hemoglobin concentrations in the normal range.[66] Frailty has also been shown to more likely with hemoglobin concentrations of 12 g/dL or lower compared with concentrations of 13.5 g/dL.[67] Anemia in the elderly has also been associated with reduced muscle strength, an increased risk of falls, an increased likelihood for hospitalizations, and an increased length of stay once hospitalized.[68-73]

The optimal hemoglobin concentration for elderly patients with anemia is a hotly debated topic. There is evidence of a J-curve phenomenon which shows elevated complication rates with hemoglobin concentrations of 11 and 12 g/dL and > 15 g/dL with lower complication rates in-between these values.[62,74] However, there are no prospective clinical trials which demonstrate that correcting low hemoglobin concentrations to achieve these numbers is beneficial for most elderly patients with anemia. The data with ESA therapy for treating anemia of chronic kidney disease further confuse the issue by thus far showing no benefit for using ESA therapy to achieve hemoglobin concentrations over 13 g/dL in this specific patient population. As such, the target hemoglobin concentration for treating anemias with pharmacologic intervention and the benefits of such intervention remain largely unknown.

Herpes Zoster
Etiology, Epidemiology and Clinical Presentation Specific to Elderly Patients

Herpes zoster (shingles) is a painful localized cutaneous eruption caused by the reactivation of latent varicella zoster, a virus which causes varicella (chickenpox). After the primary varicella infection, the virus is suppressed by cell-mediated immunity and establishes latency in the cranial nerve ganglia and dorsal root. However, it may be reactivated during the decline of cell-mediated immunity caused by advancing age, certain disease and immunosuppressive therapy. It is spread from a single ganglion to the neural tissues of the affected segment and the corresponding cutaneous dermatome. The most common complication associated with zoster is persistent pain after the zoster rash has healed.[75] Zoster pain can last for up to 30 days (acute herpetic pain), for 30–120 days (sub-acute herpetic neuralgia), or persist for at least 120 days (post-herpetic neuralgia) after rash onset.[76,77] The average cost of each zoster-associated hospitalization was $15,583 in 1995.[78] Due to the aging population, zoster infection and post-herpetic neuralgia can potentially create significant burden to the society.

Fifty percent of older adults who are 85 years or older are expected to have zoster at least once in their lifetime.[79] The incidence of zoster among immuno-competent individuals in the community is 1.2–3.4 cases per 1000 person-years; it increases to 3.9–11.8 cases per 1000 person-years among those who are older than 65 years.[75,76] The prevalence of post-herpetic neuralgia is 0.5 to 1.0 million cases in the United States.[76] Advancing age also substantially increases the incidence, severity and duration of post-herpetic neuralgia. The prevalence of acute herpetic pain is 15 times higher among patients who are 50 years or older. Similarly, the prevalence of sub-acute post-herpetic pain is about 30 times higher among patients in their 70s.[76]

The major risk factors for zoster are age, as well as a compromised cellular immune system due to disease or drug treatments. Although zoster can affect immuno-competent individuals of all ages, it occurs much more frequently in immuno-suppressed individuals and older adults. The risk for zoster sharply increases after the age of 50; more than half of all cases are among persons who are 60 years or older.[76] The risk for zoster also increases with HIV infection, hematological malignancies, bone marrow and solid organ transplantation, systemic lupus erythematosus, and immunosuppressive therapy (chemotherapy or steroid treatment). Other risk factors for zoster include physical trauma at the involved dermatome, psychological stress, white race, and possibly being female.[76,78]

The important risk factors for post-herpetic neuralgia are greater acute pain severity, greater rash severity and the presence of a prodrome.[76] Several studies have shown that the risk for post-herpetic neuralgia also increases with age; about 80 to 85% of cases occur in patients who are 50 years or older. Moreover, these patients are 27 times more likely to experience pain for at least 2 months compared to their younger counterparts.[79] Hospitalization rate due to zoster infection is most common in patients who are 85 years or older (1,604.5 per 100,000 persons); 2.5 times higher than in those with ages between 70 and 74 years, and 23 times higher than in those in 30s.[79]

The clinical course of acute zoster is variable. About 70–80% of patients describe a prodrome of pain or abnormal sensations that precede the appearance of the characteristic rash erupting in one or two adjacent dermatomes. Prodromal pain may be constant or intermittent and frequent or sporadic. It is commonly described as "burning," "shooting," "stabbing," or "throbbing." The prodrome may also include fatigue, headache and other flu-like symptoms. It typically begins several days before rash onset and lasts for 2–3 days, but longer duration is not uncommon. The unilateral dermatomal zoster rash usually begins as erythematous and macular, then rapidly progresses to papules, followed by vesicles within 1 or 2 days. The vesicles are usually clustered at the sites of cutaneous sensory nerve branches for several days, and progress to pustules and crusts within 7 to 10 days. Lesion ulceration and crusting typically disappear within 2–4 weeks, but scarring and hypo- or hyper-pigmentation may persist long after the zoster resolves. Systemic symptoms (fever, headache, malaise) can occur in up to 20% of cases. Zoster does not usually cross the midline or involve multiple dermatomes. The rash is usually accompanied by pain and/or pruritus.[75,78] The complications of zoster include post-herpetic neuralgia, super-infection with *Streptococcal* or *staphylococcal* organisms, encephalitis, herpes zoster ophthalmicus, myelitis, retinitis, zoster paresis and post-herpetic itch.[75] Acute zoster pain has been associated with lower physical, social and emotional functioning, which can lead to markedly reduced quality of life.[76]

Post-herpetic neuralgia is often described as continuous burning or throbbing pain, intermittent sharp or electric shock-like pain, and **allodynia**. The pain may last for weeks or months and occasionally persists indefinitely.[75,79,80] It reduces quality of life and functional status among older adults, particularly in those with moderate to severe intensity. It can cause chronic fatigue, anorexia, weight loss, physical inactivity and neuropsychiatric problems (insomnia, depression, difficulty with concentration). It may also interfere with activities of daily living and lead to social withdrawal.[79]

Zoster is usually diagnosed based on clinical features: unilateral, dermatomal, vesicular rash and neuralgic pain in older adults. Other conditions, such as herpes simplex virus, contact dermatitis, burns, fungal infection should be ruled out. Zoster can be diagnosed using laboratory testing on vesicle fluid, which contains abundant varicella zoster virus. Available diagnostic tests include viral culture, immunofluorescence antigen or enzyme immunoassay antigen detection, polymerase chain reaction (PCR) and serology.[81]

Standard Treatment of Acute Herpes Zoster

The principal goals of acute zoster treatment are to reduce acute pain, to prevent post-herpetic neuralgia, and to maintain functional status, mood and quality of life. Appropriate patient education, social support, adequate nutrition should be incorporated in conjunction with the zoster treatment.[75,81]

Antiviral Therapy

Treatment with antiviral agents should be initiated within 72 hours of rash onset, or as soon as possible, particularly when new vesicle formation or zoster complications are present.[78,79] The efficacy of antiviral therapy for zoster has been demonstrated by multiple randomized controlled trials. Acyclovir, famciclovir, and valacyclovir are approved by the Food and Drug Administration for the treatment of zoster in immuno-competent patients. They are phosphorylated by viral thymidine kinase and cellular enzymes to a triphosphate form that inhibits viral replication (Table 16-2). Clinical trials have indicated that these agents when taken orally, reduce the duration of viral shedding and lesion formation, reduce the time to rash healing, and decrease the severity and duration of acute pain from zoster and the risk for progression to post-herpetic neuralgia.[75,79]

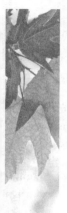

KEY POINT: Systemic antiviral therapy is the first-line treatment for all immuno-competent zoster patients who are 50 years of older, have moderate-severe pain or rash, or have non-truncal involvement. Prompt antiviral therapy can decrease the intensity and duration of acute rash phase of zoster, especially in adults age ≥ 50 years.

The benefits of initiating antiviral therapy after 72 hours of rash onset remain unclear. Such practice is sometimes recommended in patients with advanced age, severe pain, new vesicle formation, and complications (cutaneous, motor, neurologic, or ocular) based on the minimal risk associated with treatment.[75,79,81] Topical antiviral therapy, however, lacks efficacy in zoster treatment.[75] Patients should keep the rash clean and dry, avoid topical antibiotics, and, if possible, keep the rash covered. They should alert their physician if the rash worsens or they have fever, which could indicate bacterial super-infection.

Acyclovir was the first antiviral agent developed to treat zoster and its efficacy has been established in randomized controlled trials.[75,81,82] A meta-analysis suggests that acyclovir significantly reduces the severity of acute zoster-related pain with the greatest effect found in patients who are 50 years or older.[83] Another meta-analysis suggests that acyclovir reduces the incidence of post-herpetic neuralgia.[84] Famciclovir and valacyclovir are pro-drugs of acyclovir with better oral absorption; thus they are currently considered the drugs of choice in treating zoster. Famciclovir has established its efficacy in zoster treatment in several placebo- and acyclovir-controlled studies.[82,85-88] In a randomized, placebo controlled trial, it significantly reduced time to lesion crusting (63 vs. 119 days).[85] Valacyclovir reduced the duration of acute zoster pain faster than acyclovir in older adults (38 vs. 51 days).[89] In a randomized study, it significantly accelerated the resolution of zoster pain within one month from rash onset compared with acyclovir.[90] All of these antiviral agents require dose adjustment based on renal function. It is important to obtain baseline renal function before initiating the therapy, and continue to monitor for efficacy and safety during the course of therapy. While there seems to be no difference between the efficacy of famciclovir and valacyclovir, these new antivirals may be superior to acyclovir in reducing the likelihood of prolonged pain.[82,89,91] Unfortunately, 20 to 30% of treated patients experience pain within 6 months of zoster onset.[81] In a randomized placebo-control trial, 18.5% of zoster patients who were 70 years or older experienced post-herpetic neural-

Table 16-2. Oral Antiviral Medications for Herpes Zoster in the United States

Medication	Normal Dosage	Renal Dosing	Precaution & Contraindications	Notes
Acyclovir	800 mg every 4 hr (5 times daily) for 7–10 days	• CrCl 10–25 mL/min: 800 mg every 8 hr • CrCl <10 mL/min: 800 mg every 12 hr • Hemodialysis: administer dose after hemodialysis	• Dosage adjustment in patients with renal insufficiency • Use with caution with immunocompromised patients • Thrombocytopenic purpura/hemolytic uremic syndrome reported	• Available in generic • Capsules, tablets and oral solution
Famciclovir	500 mg every 8 hr (3 times daily) for 7 days	• CrCl 40–59 mL/min: 500 mg every 12 hr • CrCl 20–39 mL/min: 500 mg every 24 hr • CrCl < 20 mL/min: 250 mg every 24 hr • Hemodialysis: 250 mg after each hemodialysis	• Dosage adjustment in patients with renal insufficiency • Not studied in immunocompromised patients or patients with ophthalmic or disseminated zoster • Tablets contains lactose	• Fewer daily doses than acyclovir • Tablets
Valacyclovir	1000 mg 3 times daily for 7 days	• CrCl 30–49 mL/min: 1 g every 12 hr • CrCl 10–29 mL/min: 1 g every 24 hr • CrCl <10 mL/min: 500 mg every 24 hr • Hemodialysis: administer dose after hemodialysis	• Dosage adjustment in patients with renal insufficiency • Thrombocytopenic purpura/hemolytic uremic syndrome reported with 8000 mg daily in immunocompromised patients	• Fewer daily doses than acyclovir • Caplets

Source: Semla TP, Beizer JL, Higbee MD. *Geriatric Dosage Handbook.* 13th ed. Hudson, OH: LexiComp, Inc. 2008.

gia despite initiation of antiviral therapy within 72 hours of rash onset.[92]

Systemic antiviral therapy is generally well tolerated; nausea, vomiting, headache and diarrhea occur in up to 20% of patients.[75,86,89] The selection of one therapeutic agent over another depends on other factors besides efficacy and tolerability (Table 16-2). Acyclovir is less expensive but requires inconvenient every 5-hour dosing. Famciclovir and valacyclovir are better absorbed and offer much higher and reliable blood levels.[75,81] However, if the zoster erupts in a dermatone that includes the eye, it can lead to blindness. Older adults may have impaired vision from other etiologies. Prompt intravenous treatment with acyclovir for ophthalmic zoster is essential to minimize additional visual damage.[81]

Pain Management

Treatment of zoster-related pain should follow the same principles of general pain management as described in Chapter 14: frequent standardized pain assessment, scheduled regimen for chronic persistent pain, as-needed short-acting analgesics for acute breakthrough pain, as well as close monitoring of pain control and side effects. In general, non-opioid analgesics, such as acetaminophen or non-steroidal anti-inflammatory drugs (NSAIDs) are used to manage mild pain. Long-term use of NSAIDs should be cautioned to avoid strointestinal side effects, bleeds, hypertension, dema and further deterioration of renal function in the elderly. Weak opioids (hydrocodone, codeine, or oxycodone in combination with acetaminophen) can be considered for moderate pain. Strong opioids (oxycodone, fentanyl transdermal patch) should be reserved for severe pain. The goal of pain management is to make the patients comfortable as possible to improve quality of life. There is no ceiling dose for pain regimen although the escalation of analgesic doses are often limited by side effects (nausea, vomiting, sedation, constipation, etc.). Prophylactic laxative therapy should be considered in all patients with chronic opioid therapy. Patients with physical limitations should be closely monitored for falls.[81]

Approximately 20% of zoster patients who received antiviral treatment continue to experience persistent pain, and may require adjuvant agents, such as oral corticosteroids.[75] The addition of corticosteroids to acyclovir diminishes acute zoster pain and reduces the time to cutaneous healing, cessation of analgesic therapy, and return of uninterrupted sleep and normal daily activities.[79] However, it does not shorten the time to pain cessation, nor reduce the incidence or duration of post-herpetic neuralgia. Corticosteroids can cause detrimental side effects (hyperglycemia, dyspepsia, edema, and mental status change), especially in adults who may have preexisting conditions, such as diabetes, gastrointestinal problems, heart failure, hypertension, or psychiatric problems. Its long-term use can lead to reduced bone mineral density, which increases risk for fractures. It is important to note that the use of corticosteroids alone without systemic antiviral therapy is not recommended.[79]

The main treatment goal of post-herpetic neuralgia is to reduce pain and other associated problems (depression, insomnia, and functional impairment).[81] Non-pharmacologic interventions, such as social support, psychological therapy and nerve blocks, should be considered to improve treatment benefits and quality of life. The selection of pharmacologic agents should depend on patient co-morbidities, side effects, cost and patient preferences, generally utilizing agents that target neuropathic pain such as gabapentin or topical lidocaine (see Chapter 14).

Prevention of Herpes Zoster

Recently approved live zoster vaccine has shown to prevent zoster infection. The Centers for Disease Control and Prevention recommends giving zoster vaccines routinely to all persons who are 60 years or older, unless they have contraindications. Persons with chronic medical conditions or a previous episode of zoster can still receive zoster vaccine. Although zoster vaccine is not recommended for persons who have received varicella vaccine, it is not necessary to obtain a history of varicella (chickenpox) or conduct serologic testing for varicella immunity prior to the vaccination.[79] More information on zoster vaccine can be found in the section on immunizations, below.

Immunizations
Influenza

Epidemics of influenza are caused by influenza A (H1N1), influenza A (H3N2), and influenza B viruses, and usually occur annually between late fall and early spring. It has been associated with approximately 36,000 deaths and 226,000 hospitalizations each year in the United States.[93,94] Vaccination is the most effective method to prevent the mortality and morbidity associated with influenza and its complications (pneumonia, secondary infection, exacerbations of chronic diseases and death).[95] Each year at least one or more virus strains in the vaccine might be changed based on global surveillance of the emergence and spread of new strains.[95]

The Advisory Committee on Immunization Practices (ACIP) recommends influenza vaccination early in October or November until the supply is exhausted.[93] The primary target groups are persons with high risk for influenza complications, including all persons aged ≥ 50 years and younger persons with chronic medical conditions. Individuals who are in contact with the high-risk target groups should also be vaccinated to prevent transmission of infection. These include health care personnel, staff of long-term care facilities, assisted living and other residential settings, household contacts and caregivers of high-risk groups who are at risk for severe complications from influenza (Table 16-3). The vaccine has an efficacy of 40–55% among the nursing home residents and 58% in ambulatory elderly.[96-98] A systematic review suggests that the vaccine reduces hospitalizations by 26% and deaths by 42% in long term care facilities.[99] A cohort study indicates a vaccine efficacy of 27% in reducing hospitalization and 48% in reducing death among the community-dwelling elderly.[100] Other studies support the efficacy in older adults with or without high-risk medical conditions.[101-103] The vaccine and its administering fee are covered under Medicare part B. A study suggests a savings of $980 per quality-adjusted life year with influenza vaccination among persons aged ≥ 65.[104]

Adults 50 years of age and older should receive an annual single dose of inactivated influenza vaccination (0.5 mL) intramuscularly in the deltoid muscle. Intranasal live attenuated influenza vaccine is not indicated for this target group. Influ-

Table 16-3. Adult Target Groups for Influenza, Pneumococcal, and Herpes Zoster Vaccinations

Vaccine	Adult Target Groups
Influenza	• Adults age ≥ 50 years • Residents of nursing homes or other long term care and assisted living facilities • Women who will be pregnant during the influenza season • Patients with chronic pulmonary (including asthma), cardiovascular disorders (except hypertension), renal or hepatic, hematological or metabolic disorder (including diabetes mellitus) • Persons who have immunosuppression, including that caused by medications or human immunodeficiency virus (HIV) • Persons who have any conditions that can compromise respiratory function (e.g., cognitive dysfunction, spinal cord injury, or seizure disorder or other neuromuscular disorders); or the handling of respiratory secretions that can increase the risk of aspiration • Healthcare personnel • Household contacts and caregivers of children aged < 5 years and adults age ≥ 50 years, with particular emphasis on vaccinating contacts of children age < 6 months • Household contacts and caregivers of persons with medical conditions that put them at high risk for severe complications from influenza
Pneumococcal	• Age ≥ 65 • Chronic pulmonary disease, excluding asthma • Chronic cardiovascular disease • Diabetes mellitus • Chronic liver disease, including cirrhosis due to alcohol abuse • Chronic alcoholism • Chronic renal failure or nephritic syndrome • Functional or anatomic asplenia (sickle cell disease or splenectomy) • Immunosuppressive conditions • Cochlear implants • Cerebrospinal fluid leaks • Alaska Natives and certain American Indian populations • Residents of nursing homes or other long-term care facilities
Tetanus	• Adults who have completed a primary series and the last vaccination was received ≥ 10 years previously • Wound management
Herpes zoster	• All adults aged ≥ 60 years with no contraindications to vaccines

Source: The Advisory Committee on Immunization Practices. Recommended adult immunization schedule, United States, October 2007–September 2008. *MMWR.* 2007;56:41.

enza vaccination is contraindicated in persons with a previous severe allergic reaction to the vaccine or egg protein. Persons with moderate or severe acute illness should defer receiving the vaccine until symptoms subside.[93] The common side effects are mild and transient (< 2 days) local reactions at the injection site (10–65%). Systemic symptoms (fever, malaise, myalgia, and headache) can occur as with placebo injections.[105-107] Guillain-Barre syndrome is rarely associated with the vaccine (10–20 cases per 1 million adults per year).[95] Influenza single-dose vaccine products contain no or trace amount of preservatives. The vaccine should be stored refrigerated at 35°F–46°F (2°C–8°C), and should be discarded if accidentally frozen. It should not be used in any subsequent seasons as the antigenic components are different each year.[95]

Antiviral chemoprophylaxis is not a substitute for vaccination, but is recommended in persons at high risk during influenza outbreaks (see also Chapter 8). The target groups are persons with immune deficiencies or contraindication to influenza vaccine, persons who received vaccination within 2 weeks or who might not respond to vaccination, and unvaccinated persons with high risk, including staff and residents during an outbreak in a closed institution with residents at high risk for influenza.[95]

Chemoprophylaxis should be continued until the peak influenza activity resolves. A 6-week oseltamivir regimen has a 92% efficacy against influenza illness among nursing home residents, and a 4-week zanamivir regimen is 83% effective among high risk groups in the community.[108-109] Chemoprophylaxis with these agents does not impair the immunologic response to trivalent inactivated influenza vaccine.

Pneumococcal Disease

Invasive pneumococcal disease (pneumonia, bacteremia, meningitis, endocarditis) is caused by Gram-positive, facultative, anaerobic *Streptococcus pneumoniae*. The organism accounts for up to 36% of community-acquired pneumonia cases and 50% of hospital-acquired pneumonia cases in the United States.[110] The incidence of pneumococcal

bacteremia is 15–30 cases per 100,000 persons per year, and increases to 50–83 cases per 100,000 adults who are 65 years or older.[111,112] Vaccination is the most effective strategy for preventing invasive disease caused by the most common serotypes of *Streptococcus pneumoniae*. The Healthy People 2010 initiative aims to reduce the incidence of invasive pneumococcal infection to 42 per 100,000 persons in the elderly.[113]

The ACIP recommends one time pneumococcal vaccination to all persons who are 65 years or older, immunocompromised persons, and residents of nursing homes or other long-term care facilities.[111] One-time revaccination is indicated for certain groups, including an elderly person who was vaccinated at least 5 years previously and was aged < 65 years at the time of primary vaccination. All persons who have unknown vaccination status should receive one dose.[111] The pneumococcal vaccine is 60–70% effective in preventing invasive disease although it has not been shown to provide protection against nonbacteremic pneumonia or common upper respiratory disease.[110,111,114] It is 75% effective in immunocompetent persons with age ≥ 65 years.[115] The vaccination is cost-effective and potentially cost-saving among older adults for prevention of bacteremia, and is covered under Medicare Part B.[116,117]

Persons who are 65 years or older should receive pneumococcal polysaccharide vaccine (PPV23), not the pediatric pneumococcal conjugate vaccine (PCV7).[118,119] PPV 23 contains polysaccharide capsular antigen from 23 types of pneumococcal bacteria. It should be administered intramuscularly or subcutaneously as one 0.5-mL dose, and may be administered at the same time with influenza or tetanus vaccine, provided that they are injected at opposite sites.[111] The most common adverse effects are local site reaction including pain, swelling, and erythema (30–50%), that usually lasts for < 2 days. Moderate systemic reaction (fever and myalgia) occur < 1% of vaccine recipients.[111,118] Persons with a severe allergic reaction to a vaccine component or following a prior dose should avoid further doses. Persons with moderate or severe acute illness should defer receiving the vaccine until the symptoms subside. Minor illness, such as upper respiratory infection, is not a contraindication to receiving the vaccine. The vaccine should be stored under refrigeration at 35°F–46°F (2°C–8°C). Opened multi-dose pneumococcal vaccines may be used until the expiration date if they are not visibly contaminated.[118]

Tetanus

Tetanus is caused by *Clostridium tetani* spores, which are ubiquitous in the environment and enter the body after blunt trauma or deep puncture wounds. Its typical symptoms are trismus (lockjaw), generalized rigidity, painful muscular and impaired respiratory function. Glottic spasm, respiratory failure, and autonomic instability can result in death.[120] It has a reported case-fatality of 18% in the United States.[120,121]

Older adults have a disproportionate burden of illness from tetanus. During 1999 and 2001, approximately 38% of 534 reported cases occurred in persons with age ≥ 65 years in the United States.[120] During 1995 and 1997, the average annual incidence of tetanus among persons who were 60 years or older was 0.33 cases per 1 million population, which was doubled from that among younger persons. The case fatality rate increases with age, most likely due to the lack of adequate immunization. A national population-based study indicates that only 45% of men and 21% of women aged ≥ 70 years had protective levels of antibody to tetanus in the United States during 1988 to 1994.[122]

The ACIP recommends one tetanus booster dose every 10 years for adults who have completed a primary series.[123,124] Adults with uncertain histories of a complete primary vaccination series with tetanus and diphtheria toxoids-containing vaccines should begin or complete a primary 3-dose series (the first and second doses at least 4 weeks apart; the third dose 6–12 months after the second). Tetanus vaccine can be used after an exposure to tetanus under some circumstances, and is covered under Medicare Part B when directly related to the treatment of an injury or direct exposure to a disease or condition.[120]

The tetanus booster has an efficacy of about 65%.[120] Although there is no data on the cost-effectiveness of its use in the elderly, the vaccine should be considered for those who are at risk for wounds or injuries, and for institutionalized elderly who are a significant risk for cutaneous ulcers. Tetanus vaccine can be administered with other indicated vaccines, provided that each vaccine is administered using a separate syringe at a different anatomic site. Contraindications include serious allergic reactions or adverse effects with any tetanus-containing vaccines (Td, DTP, DTap, or DT), moderate or severe illness and pregnancy. The most common adverse effects are pain at the injection site (60–65%), followed by erythema, headache, tiredness, swelling, and generalized body ache.[120]

Herpes Zoster

Herpes zoster infection (shingles) is a localized, painful cutaneous eruption due to the reactivation of latent varicella zoster virus (chickenpox). The risk of zoster infection increases with advancing age. The annual incidence among adults age 50 years is 2.5–5.1 cases per 1,000 persons and increases to 11–14 cases per 1,000 among those at 75 years.[125,126] Zoster infection affects nearly half of persons age ≥ 85 at least once in a lifetime.[127] Older adults are also more likely to experience postherpetic neuralgia, and with increased severity and duration.[128] About 80% of postherpetic neuralgia occurs in zoster patients aged ≥ 50 years, who also report more persistent pain.[129,130] In addition, persons age 70–74 years and ≥ 85 older adults are 9 times and 23 times, respectively, more likely to require hospitalization due to zoster than younger persons.[131] In 1995, each zoster-associated hospitalization costs about $16,000 (see also section on herpes zoster).[131]

The ACIP recommends routine zoster vaccination of all persons aged ≥ 60 years for prevention of zoster infection. The vaccine is not indicated to treat acute zoster, to prevent persons with acute zoster from developing post-herpetic neuralgia, or to treat ongoing post-herpetic neuralgia. Persons with previous episodes of zoster and those with chronic medical conditions can be vaccinated unless those conditions are contraindications or precautions (Table 16-4). One randomized, placebo-controlled, double-blind trial indicates that the vaccine is 51% effective for preventing zoster although efficacy declines with increasing age on or after 70 years. It is 57% effective for reducing severity-by-duration of zoster, and 61% for burden of illness associated with post-herpetic neuralgia. It is associated with better activities of daily living, but does not reduce other complications with zoster.[132,133]

Zoster vaccine is a live attenuated vaccine, and should be administered as a single 0.65-mL dose subcutaneously in the deltoid region of the arm. It may be given at the time of an inactivated vaccine provided that a different anatomic site is used.[133] It should be given at least 4 weeks before or after another live attenuated vaccine.[134] It is contraindicated for persons with a history of anaphylactic reaction to any component of the vaccine, including gelatin and neomycin. A history of contact dermatitis to neomycin is not a contraindication.[134] The vaccine should be stored at a freezer with a separate sealing door at -15°C (+5°F) or colder. It should be reconstituted immediately upon removal from storage and administered or discarded within 30 minutes. The common side effects with the vaccine are injection site reactions (17%), which include mild and transient erythema, pain, swelling, warmth, and pruritus. Headache occurred in 6.3% of vaccine recipients.[134]

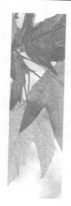

KEY POINT: Zoster vaccine should be offered to older adults (age ≥ 60) even if they had a previous episode of zoster, as long as they do not have contraindications to the vaccine. The vaccine recipients should be educated that the zoster vaccine prevents zoster, but does not treat zoster or post-herpetic neuralgia.

Cancer Screening

Etiology and Epidemiology Specific to the Elderly Population

Despite much advancement we have achieved in technology and medicine, cancer remains one of the worst fears of humans and an important cause for morbidity and mortality in the world. The American Cancer Society (ACS) estimated a total of 1,437,180 new cases of cancer and 565,650 deaths form cancer in the United States in 2008.[135] This translates to one in four deaths

Table 16-4. **Contraindications for Zoster Vaccine**[133,134]

- History of anaphylactic reaction to any component of the vaccine, including gelatin and neomycin
- Leukemia, lymphomas, or other malignant neoplasms affecting the bone marrow or lymphatic system
- AIDS or other clinical manifestations of HIV (persons with CD4+ T-lymphocyte values ≤ 200 per mm³ or ≤15% of total lymphocytes)
- Therapy with high-dose corticosteroids (≥ 20 mg/day of prednisone or equivalent) for ≥ 2 weeks
- Clinical or laboratory evidence of other unspecified cellular immunodeficiency. However, persons with impaired humoral immunity (e.g., hypogammaglobulinemia or dysgammaglobulinemia) can receive zoster vaccine
- Hematopoietic stem cell transplantation
- Therapy with recombinant human immune mediators and immune modulators (adalimumab, infliximab, or etanercept)
- Pregnancy
- Severe acute illness
- Initiation of immunosuppressive therapy within 14 to 30 days
- Therapy with antiviral in the past 24 hr

in the United States due to cancer. Among men, the three most common types of cancers which account for about 50% of all newly diagnosed cases are cancers of the prostate, lung and bronchus, and colon and rectum.[135] In women, cancers of the breast, lung and bronchus, and colon and rectum are the three most commonly diagnosed types of cancers which account for about 50% of cancer cases.[135]

Fortunately, overall death rates from cancer have decreased in recent years. Between 1990/1991 and 2004, death rates from cancer reduced by 18.4% among men and by 10.5% among women.[135] Reductions in death rates from lung, prostate, and colorectal cancers, which account for almost 80% of the total decrease in cancer death rates, was observed among men.[135] In comparison, reductions in death rates from breast and colorectal cancers accounted for 60% of the decrease among women.[135] The decrease in lung cancer death rates among men was largely attributed to a reduction of tobacco use over the last 40 years, while the decrease in death rates for colorectal, female breast, and prostate cancer was credited to improvements in cancer screening and treatment.[135]

Cancer can be caused by both external factors and internal factors. External factors include tobacco, chemicals, radiation, and infectious organisms (such as hepatitis B virus, human papillomavirus, human immunodeficiency virus, *Helicobacter pylori*, and others).[136] Internal factors consist of inherited mutations, hormones, immune conditions, and mutations that occur from metabolism.[136] With increased age, increase exposures to these factors may occur thus increasing the risk of cancer development. In fact, most new cancers and cancer deaths occur in men and women older than 65 years of age.[137,138] According to data derived from the National Cancer Institute Surveillance, Epidemiology, and End Results Program from 1998–2002, 56% of all newly diagnosed cancer patients and 71% of cancer deaths occur in this age group.[138] Specifically, the median ages of cancer patients at death for major malignancies such as lung, colorectal, lymphoma, leukemia, pancreas, stomach, and urinary bladder range from 71 to 77 years.[138] Thus, cancer affects older people to a much greater extent compared

to younger adults and it is important to educate the older as well as the general adult population regarding cancer prevention and screening.

Cancer Prevention Measures Recommended in the Geriatric Population

Cancer Prevention

Cancers caused by cigarette smoking, heavy use of alcohol, obesity, and excessive sun exposures are preventable. Based on evidence from the ACS, approximately one third of the more than 500,000 cancer deaths that occur in the United States each year can be attributed to poor dietary and physical habits and thus could be prevented.[139] In addition, another one-third of these 500,000 cancer deaths is caused by exposure to tobacco products and thus could also be avoided.[139] Cancer prevention measures used in younger adults are also important to apply in geriatric populations and include tobacco avoidance; diet, nutrition and physical activity; sun safety; and decreased exposure to radon.[140-150]

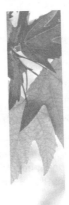

KEY POINT: According to the ACS, two thirds of all cancer deaths can be prevented through healthy dietary and physical habits and by tobacco avoidance. The risk of developing cancer can be substantially reduced by avoiding tobacco and overexposure of sunlight and radon; as well as maintaining a healthy weight through diet and exercise.

Cancer Screening Tests Applicable in the Geriatric Population

Regular cancer screening can prevent cancers of the cervix, colon, and rectum by allowing removal of precancerous tissue before it becomes malignant.[136] Regular screening can also lead to detection of cancers at early stages which increases their chance of being treatable. Malignancies that can be detected in their early stages include cancers of the breast, colon, rectum, cervix, prostate, oral cavity, and skin. For most of these cancers, early detection has been proven to reduce mortality.[136] According to the ACS, cancers that can be prevented or detected earlier by screening account for at least half of all new cancer cases. Thus, there are ample opportunities as well as challenges for health care professionals to make positive impacts on their patients through proper cancer screening procedures. The following paragraphs describe cancer screening tests that are recommended by the ACS and the U.S. Preventive Services Task Force (USPSTF) for the detection of various cancers in the average-risk asymptomatic population.[151,152] Patients with high risk for certain cancers (such as strong family history for colon or breast cancer) may require screening at an earlier time, at more frequent intervals, and/or genetic counseling. Interested readers are referred to the ACS and USPSTF guidelines for these special circumstances.

Breast Cancer Screening

Breast cancer is the most common cancer diagnosed in women in the United States. It is also the second leading cause of cancer death in US women. The ACS guidelines for the early detection of breast cancer in average-risk women consist of clinical breast examination (CBE) and counseling to raise awareness of breast symptoms beginning at age 20 years; an annual mammography beginning at age 40 years is also recommended.[151] Because false-positive results have been associated with breast self-examination (BSE), the ACS no longer recommends this monthly procedure. Instead, women may choose to perform BSE regularly, occasionally, or not at all based on information regarding the potential benefits, limitations, and harms (possibility of a false-positive result) of BSE.

Women should be informed about the potential benefits as well as the potential harms associated with mammographic screening. Regular mammography may help to detect breast cancer in its early stage, thus allowing less aggressive therapy, a greater range of treatment options, and a greater chance for survival. On the contrary, limitations to mammography include false positive result (which may lead to unnecessary biop-

sies, exposures to futile treatment, and emotional distress) and false negative results (the inability to detect about 5% of breast cancer).[137,151] Furthermore, some breast cancer detected with mammography may still have poor prognoses.

Because breast cancer grows faster in younger women compared with older women, the ACS recommend annual screening to women in their forties. However, some data suggest that women 50 and older may be able to wait as long as two years between mammograms.[153] There is no specific upper age at which mammography screening should be discontinued.[151] The decision to stop regular mammography screening should be individualized based on the potential benefits and risks of screening along with considerations of overall health and estimated longevity of the patient.[151] Therefore, a woman should continue to receive regular mammography screening as long as she is in good health and would be a candidate for breast cancer treatment.[151] In contrast to the ACS recommendations, the USPSTF recommends against routine screening mammography in women aged 40–49 years (according to their latest breast cancer screening recommendations from November 2009). In addition, the USPSTF recommends biennial (every 2 years) screening mammography for women 50 to 74 years of age and has no recommendation for women 75 years of age or older.

Colorectal Cancer Screening

Colorectal cancer is the third leading cause of cancer death in the general population in the United States.[135] Fortunately, it is also one of the most preventable cancers. Screening can lead to the detection and removal of adenomatous polyps before they transform into cancers. Colorectal cancers screening (CRC) also detect cancers at earlier stages, increase survival, and reduce mortality rate.[154] Given that 90% of all cases of colon cancer occur after age 50 years, the ACS and the USPSTF both recommend that clinicians screen men and women 50 years of age or older for colorectal cancer.[137,151-152]

CRC screening test are classified into 2 types; there are tests that primarily detect cancer (such as the guaiac-based fecal occult blood tests [gFOBT], fecal immunochemical tests [FIT], and the stool DNA test [sDNA]) and there are tests that can detect cancer and advanced lesions (such as endoscopic and radiographic exams). The ACS has suggested several methods for colorectal screening[151]:

1. Annual gFOBT and FIT, following manufacturer's recommendations for specimen collection.

2. sDNA, for which at this time there is uncertainty in the screening interval.

3. Flexible sigmoidoscopy (FSIG) every 5 years.

4. Colonoscopy every 10 years.

5. Double contrast barium enema (DCBE) every 5 years.

6. Computed tomographic colonography (CTC, or virtual colonoscopy) every 5 years.

7. Annual stool blood testing (gFOBT or FIT) with FSIG every 5 years.

Due to its very low sensitivity for advanced adenomas and cancer, single-panel FOBT in the medical office using a stool sample collected during a digital rectal exam (DRE) is not recommended.[151] Although definitive evidence is lacking, colonoscopy may be superior to other screening methods since this allows one to view the entire colon and to take biopsy specimens immediately.[151,155]

Similar to breast cancer screening, there is no specific upper age limit in screening for colorectal cancer based on clinical or cost analysis data.[137] Clinician should educate patients on the risk, benefit, and proper usage of take home screening tests. For example, in order to maximize the accuracy of the gFOBT or FIT, patients should be advised regarding the importance of commitment to annual at-home testing and adherence to manufacturers' instructions. Patients should also be informed about the potential risks and adverse effects of certain procedures. Although the risk of colon perforation with colonoscopy was less than 0.5% in patients 75 years and older according to a

study that examined 39,286 colonoscopies, it was still four times the risk compared to patients in the 65 to 69 age range.[155,156] Older patients may also have more difficulties tolerating adverse effects such as vomiting, abdominal cramps and diarrhea from bowel preparations. CRC screening in older patients may be individualized by balancing the likelihood of finding polyps and the time for neoplastic transformation of a polyp against the patient's estimated life expectancy.[155] Because few polyps transform into cancer in less than 10 years, patients with a life expectancy less than 7 to 10 years may not benefit from detection and removal of precancerous polyps.[155]

Cervical Cancer Screening

Cervical cancer developed in an estimated 11,150 women and caused 3600 deaths in the United States in 2007.[157] Because screening can prevent cancers of the cervix by allowing removal of precancerous tissue before it becomes malignant, the ACS and the USPSTF recommend screening for cervical cancer in women. Infection with high-risk "oncogenic" types of human papillomavirus (HPV) has been implicated as the cause of 100% of cervical cancer.[157] Due to the long latency between infection and development of cervical cancer, older women with at least two negative Pap smear results and no evidence of HPV infection may be at extremely low risk for cervical cancer.[137] For this reason, the ACS and the USPSTF recommend discontinuation of screening in older women when Pap test results have been normal. At this time, the USPSTF recommends against routine screening of women older than age 65 for cervical cancer if they have had adequate recent screening with normal Pap smears and are not otherwise at high risk for cervical cancer.[152] The ACS recommends screening of healthy women with an intact cervix until the age of 70 years. Thereafter, women may elect to discontinue screening if they have had no abnormal/positive cytology test within the 10-year period before age 70 years and if there is documentation that the 3 most recent Pap tests were technically satisfactory and interpreted as normal.[151] Screening after age 70 years is recommended for women in good health who have not been previously screened, and in women for whom information regarding previous screening is unavailable.[151]

Prostate Cancer Screening

Prostate cancer is the most common non-skin cancer and the second leading cause of cancer-related death in U.S. men.[158,159] Approximately 218,890 men received a new diagnosis of this disease in 2007 and it is estimated that 1 in 6 men will be diagnosed with prostate cancer in their lifetime.[158] Two screening tests, the prostate-specific antigen (PSA) test and the digital rectal examination (DRE), have been used to detect prostate cancer. Although the PSA test is more sensitive than the DRE and it has been used frequently for the screening of prostate cancer, this test is not specific to prostate cancer. Besides prostate cancers, common conditions such as benign prostatic hyperplasia and prostatitis can increase PSA levels.[158] Thus, false positive results can occur from PSA screening tests which may lead to painful experiences through unnecessary prostate biopsy as well as emotional distress.

In men who are diagnosed with prostate cancer, treatment can cause harms such as sexual dysfunction, bowel and bladder incontinence, and death.[159] Furthermore, a proportion of those treated, and possibly harmed, would never have developed cancer symptoms during their lifetime thus leading to unnecessary treatment and associated adverse effects.[158,159] Based on these findings, the USPSTF conclude that there is insufficient evidence to recommend for or against routine prostate cancer screening in men younger than 75 years of age.[159] In addition, the USPSTF does not recommend the routine screening for prostate cancer in men who are 75 years of age or older. In contrast, the ACS recommend offering PSA measurement and DRE to men annually beginning at the age of 50 years provided that they have a life expectancy of at least 10 years.[151] In either case, clinicians should discuss the potential benefits, limitations and known harms of PSA screening with their patients.[151,159] Individualized screening decisions should be made based on shared decision (between clinicians and patients) or patients' preferences.[151,159]

Cancer-related Checkup

At this time, the ACS and the USPSTF endorse population screening for cancers of the cervix, breast, and colon and rectum.[151] There is insufficient evidence to recommend for or against routine screening for other cancers such as cancer of the lung, oral cavity and skin.[152] The USPSTF also recommends against routine screening for bladder cancer, ovarian cancer, pancreatic cancer and testicular cancer due to at least fair evidence that routine screening of these cancers in the general population is ineffective or that harms outweigh benefits.[152]

For the average risk elderly population, the best approach to cancer prevention may be through periodic health evaluations.[160-162] The accessibility of health care through primary care physicians has been associated with a higher rate of early breast, cervical, and colon cancer detection.[160] Regular preventive health examinations provide opportunities for health counseling, cancer screening, and case finding examinations of the thyroid, testicles, ovaries, lymph nodes, oral cavity, and skin.[151] In addition, shared decision making about cancer screening for early cancer for sites where population-based screening is not yet recommended can be explored.[151]

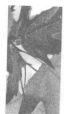 KEY POINT: Periodic health examination provides a good opportunity for health counseling and cancer screening that could lead to prevention and early detection of cancer.

Review of Evidence Base Supporting Screening Recommendations for the Older Population

Guidelines as established by the ACS and the USPSTF note age groups for whom cancer screening recommendations are applicable based upon the best available evidence. For the average risk older population they recommend:

1. Mammography screening for women beginning at the age of 40 according to the ACS.

Mammography screening for women starting at the age of 50 according to the USPSTF.

2. Colorectal cancer screening for men and women beginning at the age of 50.

3. Discontinuation of Pap test in women at the age of 65 or 70 years if they have had normal test results and no other risk factor for cervical cancer.

4. Prostate cancer screening to be offered beginning at the age of 50 for men with a life expectancy of at least 10 years (ACS recommendation).

Common Concerns with Cancer Screening in Elderly Patients

Although the incidence of cancer development is greater in older adults, cancer screening may not always be beneficial due to a number of concerns faced by this population. These concerns include: complications from additional diagnostic procedures due to inaccurate test results, identification and treatment of clinically unimportant cancers, and psychological as well as physical distress from screening.[163] A false positive diagnosis of cancer can lead to pain and emotional stress from additional biopsies and procedures. In the case of prostate cancer screening, men with false-positive PSA test results were more likely to worry specifically about prostate cancer, have a higher perceived risk of prostate cancer, and report problems with sexual function compared with control participants for up to one year after the test.[158] As life expectancy decreases in the elderly, the probability of finding inconsequential cancer increases.[163] Thus, the identification of cancer that would never have caused symptoms in the patient's lifetime could lead to unnecessary treatment and associated adverse effects. Lastly, elderly patients may have cognitive, physical, or sensory dysfunctions that make screening tests and further workup particularly difficult, painful, or frightening.[137,163]

In contrast to the above scenarios, the decision not to screen a particular individual based on health status or life expectancy may lead to a decrease in quality of life.[137,164] The decision to screen elderly people for cancer can be complex and is based on many factors other than survival benefit alone.[164] Clinicians should discuss the benefit, risk, and limitations of each screening test with the patient. Decisions on choosing cancer screening should be individualized based on the life expectancy of the patient, the risk versus benefit associated with screening, and preferences of the patient or his/her caregiver.[137,151]

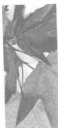

KEY POINT: Some older patients may not benefit from cancer screening tests due to factors such as decreased life expectancy, decreased physical functions, and/or comorbid conditions.

Evidence Supporting Cancer Prevention Medications and Supplements

Cancer chemoprevention is defined as the use of natural, synthetic, or biologic chemical agents to reverse, suppress, or prevent carcinogenic progression to invasive cancer.[165] In an attempt to prevent the development or progression of cancer, substances such as vitamins, pharmaceutical products and herbal remedies have been examined. The following paragraphs briefly describe some of the vitamins and medications that have been tested for the prevention of various cancers. Interested readers are referred to more comprehensive review literature on cancer chemoprevention.[165-167]

Breast Cancer Chemoprevention

Chemoprevention trials in breast cancer have set the standard for other disease types to follow.[165] Tamoxifen is an oral selective antiestrogen agent or selective estrogen receptor modulator (SERM). This medication is most commonly used as a treatment for women with estrogen receptor positive (ER+) breast cancer. In addition, tamoxifen is indicated for risk reduction in women at high risk for breast cancer. Meta-analyses from various trials showed that tamoxifen reduced the rate of contralateral breast cancers by 40–50% in women with ER+ tumors.[165] This beneficial effect was confirmed in a placebo-controlled trial, the Breast Cancer Prevention Trial (BCPT) or NSABP P-1, which studied 13,000 women. This trial was stopped early after an interim analysis showed a significant 49% reduction in incidence of invasive breast cancer in the tamoxifen arm.[165] Similar to findings from earlier meta-analyses, only ER+ tumors were affected (69% decrease) by tamoxifen. With regards to adverse effects, an increased risk of invasive endometrial cancer and thrombotic events (especially in women age 50 and older) were observed. Thus, the use of tamoxifen as chemoprevention for breast cancer should be highly individualized based on the potential risk and benefit to the patient.[165]

Raloxifene is a SERM indicated for the treatment and prevention of osteoporosis in postmenopausal women. It also has an FDA-approved indication for the risk reduction of invasive breast cancer in postmenopausal women with osteoporosis or in women at high risk for invasive breast cancer. In their reports of results from the study of tamoxifen and raloxifene (STAR), researchers stated that tamoxifen and raloxifene lowered the risk of invasive breast cancer to similar extent in 19,747 postmenopausal women who took raloxifene 60 mg or tamoxifen 20 mg daily for 5 years.[168,169] The observed incidence rates of invasive breast cancer were raloxifene 4.4 and tamoxifen 4.3 per 1000 women per year.[169] Women on both drugs had similar risks for strokes and heart attacks. Raloxifene did not protect women from lobular carcinoma in situ (LCIS) and ductal carcinoma in situ (DCIS) as well as did tamoxifen. However, women on raloxifene had fewer uterine cancers and blood clots than women on tamoxifen.[168] At this time, the USPSTF recommends against routine use of tamoxifen or raloxifene for the primary prevention of breast cancer in women at low or average risk. In women at high risk for breast cancer and at low risk for adverse effects of chemoprevention, the USPSTF recommends a discussion of chemoprevention to be initiated with this group of patients.[152]

Phytoestrogens are a group of plant-derived substances that are structurally or functionally similar to estradiol.[170] These substances are thought to have protective effects against breast cancer since a decreased risk of breast cancer was observed in women from countries with high phytoestrogen consumption. Studies show that soy exposure during adolescent appears to be protective. However, results of studies that examine effects of adult exposure to phytoestrogen are conflicting and inconclusive.[170] Furthermore, data on the role of phytoestrogens in the prevention of breast cancer recurrence are scarce and the few studies conducted do not support a protective role.[170] For these reasons, supplemental intake or augmentation of dietary phytoestrogen sources is not recommended.[170] Consumption of naturally occurring soy products such as tofu or soy flour as part of a balanced diet low in saturated fats and high in fruits and vegetables is likely safe and may even be beneficial.[170]

Colon Cancer Chemoprevention

Aspirin is a promising medication for colon cancer chemoprevention and it has been studied in several large randomized trials for the prevention of colon adenomas and cancer. In a randomized double-blind trial conducted by Baron et al., daily aspirin (325 mg or 81 mg) or placebo was given to 1,121 patients with a recent history of colon adenomas.[171] Results showed that low-dose aspirin prevented recurrence of colorectal adenomas to a greater degree compared to the other two regimens (Incidence of one or more adenomas was significant with 47% in placebo, 38% in the aspirin 81 mg group, and 45% in the aspirin 325 mg group).[171] This translated into a relative-risk reduction of 19% in the aspirin 81 mg group and a nonsignificant reduction of 4% in the aspirin 325 mg group. Furthermore, a relative risk reduction of 40% for advanced neoplasms was observed in the aspirin 81 mg group.[171] Aspirin at a daily dose of 300 mg or higher has shown protective effects in the prevention of colorectal adenomas and colorectal cancer in other studies.[172-174] In a recent pooled analysis of 2 large trials (The British Doctors Aspirin Trial and the United Kingdom Transient Ischaemic Attack Aspirin Trial) that involves more than 7,500 patients, the use of 300 mg or more of aspirin daily for about 5 years was found to be effective in the primary prevention of colorectal cancer.[172]

Contrary to the above findings, the US Physician's Health Study, which included 22,071 male physicians with a mean follow-up of 5 years, reported that regular use of low-dose aspirin had no effect on the incidence of polyps or colon cancer.[175] Although aspirin has shown encouraging results in decreasing colorectal adenomas in some trials, this effect was not consistent and the optimal dose for colon protective effect seemed unclear. This suggest that aspirin use cannot be a substitute for colon surveillance and that further studies are needed for effective colon cancer chemoprevention.[165]

Calcium and vitamin D supplementation have been the focus of colorectal cancer prevention in a number of studies.[176-179] Calcium is thought to prevent colorectal carcinoma by binding bile and fatty acids as well as inhibiting the proliferation of colonic epithelial cells.[165,180] Calcium supplementation was shown to reduce colorectal adenomas moderately in some studies.[176-178] However, it is unclear whether calcium supplementation translates into prevention of invasive colorectal cancer and a survival benefit at this time.[165] In addition to maintaining bone health, evidence showed that vitamin D may have a role in colorectal cancer prevention.[181] Low levels of vitamin D have been associated with increased risk of digestive-system cancers in men.[179] In addition, vitamin D was shown to play an important role in promoting the effects of calcium in reducing the risk of colorectal adenoma recurrence.[178] The current intake recommendations for vitamin D, as set by the Institute of Medicine, are 200 international units (IU) daily for children and adults up to 50 years of age; 400 IU for adults 51–70 years of age; and 600 IU for adults 71 years of age and older.[181] It is unclear whether these dosage recommendations as advocated by the Institute of Medicine are sufficient enough to provide the possible cancer protective effect of vitamin D. In fact, many experts have recommended doses of vitamin D as much as 1,000 IU daily for optimal health.[181] At this time, the ACS does not have a recommendation regarding the role of vitamin D in cancer prevention or treatment.[181]

Lung Cancer Chemoprevention

Various agents, such as beta carotene, alpha-tocopherol, aspirin, isotretinoin, and N-acetylcysteine have been tested in lung cancer chemoprevention trials.[165] Unfortunately, no chemoprevention agents have clearly demonstrated clinical benefit in lung cancer to this date.[165] Because fruits and vegetable consumption have been associated with a reduced risk of cancer, attempts have been made to isolate specific nutrient and administer them as supplements for cancer prevention. However, a higher rate of lung cancer was found in cigarette smokers who took high-dose beta carotene supplements in two clinical trials.[182-183] This points to the perception that beta carotene may only be a proxy for other single nutrients or combinations of nutrients found in whole foods, and that taking a single nutrient in large amounts can be dangerous.[139] Thus, consuming fruits and vegetables that contain beta carotene may be beneficial, but high-dose beta carotene supplements should be avoided.[139]

Prostate Cancer Chemoprevention

Finasteride, a steroidal analog of testosterone, has shown some promise in the prevention of prostate cancer. In the Prostate Cancer Prevention Trial, 18,882 men age 55 years or older with a normal digital rectal examination and a PSA level of 3.0 ng per milliliter or lower were randomized to finasteride 5 mg per day or placebo for seven years.[184] This trial reported 18.4% of prostate cancer incidence in the finasteride group compared to 24.4% in the placebo group, for a 24.8% reduction in prevalence over the 7-year period that was statistically significant.[184] Patients who received finasteride also experienced less urinary symptoms compared to the placebo group. However, the prostate cancers that developed in the finasteride group were of higher Gleason grade (7, 8, 9, or 10) and patients who received finasteride also had more adverse sexual side effects.[184] Although finasteride decreased the incidence of prostate cancer, it was associated with more sexual side effects and histologically more aggressive malignancies. Therefore, finasteride as primary prevention for prostate cancer should be considered with caution at this time.[165]

KEY POINT: The decision to use certain medications for chemoprevention should be individualized based on the risk and benefit for each person.

Nutrition may play a role in reducing the risk of prostate cancer. Frequent intake of tomato products which contain lycopene has been associated with a lower risk of prostate cancer.[185] Foods that contain specific antioxidant nutrients, such as vitamin E, selenium, and beta carotene may also have protective effects in prostate cancer.[139] On the contrary, greater consumption of red meat or dairy products may be associated with an increased risk of prostate cancer.[139,186] A high calcium intake, primarily through supplements, has

also been associated with increased risk for more aggressive types of prostate cancer.[187] Base on the data available at this time, the best way to reduce prostate cancer risk may be through consuming five or more servings of a wide variety of fruits and vegetables each day, limiting intake of red meats and dairy products, and maintaining an active lifestyle and healthy weight.[139]

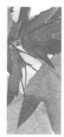

KEY POINT: Consumption of fruits and vegetables that contain certain vitamins such as beta carotene may be beneficial, but high-dose vitamin supplements such as beta carotene should be avoided.

CASE 1: ANEMIA

Setting:
Long-term care nursing facility

Subjective:
RO is a 74-year-old female who has been in a skilled nursing facility for about 18 months. She was originally admitted following an accident in which she slipped on a wet floor and fell and broke her hip. She has been ambulating well with the use of a walker for about the last 6 months as is overall in good spirits with a good appetite. She recently has been complaining of fatigue and lethargy so her physician ordered a complete blood count which showed anemia. Other laboratory was ordered to evaluate the type of anemia and RO's physician asks for you to proceed with treatment as appropriate under your collaborative practice agreement.

Past Medical History:
Type II diabetes, hypothyroidism, osteoarthritis, and chronic kidney disease

Medications:
Glipizide 10 mg once daily, aspirin 81 mg once daily, simvastatin 10 mg once daily, pioglitazone 45 mg once daily, levothyroxine 75 mcg once daily, acetaminophen 500 mg four times daily, geriatric multivitamin with minerals

Allergies:
NKDA

Social History:
Negative for smoking, alcohol, or recreational drugs

Family History:

Non-contributory

Vital Signs:

Height 5'2", weight 118 lb; BP 122/68, HR 72 bpm, temperature 98.0, respiratory rate 14/min, pain 4/10 at both knees

Physical Exam:

Unremarkable other than decreased range of motion and crepitus in her knees. There is no evidence of bleeding.

Laboratory:

BUN 38; serum creatinine 1.6 mg/dL (BUN 30, SCr 1.4 3 months ago); potassium 4.1 mmol/L; hemoglobin 9.5 g/dL; hematocrit 28.5%; MCV 92fL; hemoglobin A_{1c} 7.2%; TSH 1.3 mIU/L; Fe 29 mcg/dL, TIBC 161 %, ferritin 815 ng/mL, folate 5.11 ng/mL, vitamin B-12 791 ng/mL.

Assessment:

RO is a 74-year-old female with diabetes, hypothyroidism, osteoarthritis, and chronic kidney disease who offers new complaints of fatigue and lethargy consistent with anemia. She has no signs of bleeding and her hypothyroidism is well controlled. Her hemoglobin is low, with a normal MCV. Vitamin B-12 and folate are normal. Iron studies are consistent with anemia of chronic kidney disease.

Plan:

1. Initiate epoetin alpha 3000 units subcutaneously three times a week. Adjust dose to achieve a hemoglobin target of 11–12 g/dL.

2. Initiate oral ferrous sulfate 325 mg daily. Consider parenteral iron therapy if response is inadequate based on hemoglobin and iron studies.

3. Repeat hemoglobin twice weekly for dosage adjustments. Measure ferritin in 1 month.

Rationale:

1. ESA is the treatment of choice for anemia of chronic kidney disease, generally initiated at 50–100 units/kg three times weekly. Dosage requires adjustment to maintain the hemoglobin below 12 g/dL.

2. Geriatric multivitamins do not contain iron, and RO's iron and ferritin levels will drop with initiation of ESA. Iron therapy should be initiated in conjunction with ESA to allow for maximal effect. Oral ferrous sulfate is frequently chosen, but doses over 325 mg daily are not recommended due to a significant risk for constipation with higher doses without much more absorption. Parenteral iron therapy is more effective than oral iron therapy for anemia of chronic kidney disease and improves the response to ESAs, so it should be considered if RO does not respond as expected to ESAs.

3. In all forms of anemia, monitoring for therapeutic response requires a complete blood count for hemoglobin and hematocrit. Frequent testing is required with use of ESAs to adjust to the proper dose which will minimize risk for thrombosis and maximize cost effectiveness.

Case Summary:

As in this case, anemia can present very subtly in the elderly patient, with symptoms that many attribute simply to old age. Clinicians must remain vigilant to identify the causes of anemia, as it is not a normal consequence of aging. Anemia of chronic kidney disease is common in older patients as renal function declines, but may occur in combination with nutritional anemias or other anemias of chronic disease. Appropriate therapy addressing the cause or causes of anemia require monitoring, particularly when ESAs are initiated, to avoid the risks of thrombosis and stroke associated with higher hemoglobin levels.

CASE 2: HERPES ZOSTER

Setting:
Ambulatory clinic

Subject:
TJ is a 65-year-old Caucasian man who presents to his primary care physician and complains of 2-day duration of painful vesicular rash on the right side of his neck. He describes the pain as 6 out of 10 on the pain index, "burning" and "throbbing." He is afebrile but complains of chills, fatigue, and headache. He reports experiencing pain and itch in the same area before the rash developed. He recalls no previous episodes of this type of pain and lesion. He does not remember having chicken-pox as a child.

Past Medical History:
Hypertension, dyslipidemia, osteoarthritis, seasonal allergies

Medications:
Hydrochlorothiazide 25 mg daily, aspirin 81 mg daily, simvastatin 20 mg at bedtime, acetaminophen 325 mg every 6 hours, loratadine 10 mg daily as needed.

Allergy:
NKDA

Social History:
Denies tobacco or alcohol use

Family History:
Non-contributory

Vital signs:
BP 120/70, HR 70 bpm, temp 99.5, RR 18, ht 5'6" wt 60 kg

Appearance:
Thin Caucasian man in no acute distress; unilateral redness and clustered blisters erupting at one dermatome on the right side of neck.

Laboratory:
Within normal limits except BUN 45; SCr 2.0

Immunizations:
Influenza and pneumococcal vaccine updated.

Assessment:
TJ is a 65-year-old man who is diagnosed with herpes zoster based on the classical signs and symptoms, including dermatomal pain rash followed by visible lesions within a few days. His pain is not controlled despite a daily dose of acetaminophen 1300 mg.

Plan:
1. Start famciclovir 500 mg once daily or valacyclovir 1 g every 12 hours for 7 days, and monitor for headache and gastrointestinal symptoms.

2. Increase acetaminophen to 500 mg every 4 hours. Start gabapentin 300 mg at bedtime on day 1; 300 mg twice daily on day 2, 300 mg three times daily on day 3. The dose may be titrated as

needed for pain relief; not to exceed 1400 mg daily. Monitor for somnolence, dizziness, peripheral edema, and risk for falls.

3. Patient education about zoster and its complications. Reinforce medication adherence.

Rationale:

1. TJ is diagnosed with herpes zoster based on the clinical signs and symptoms: prodrome of pain, itch, and flu-like symptoms, unilateral dermatomal rash that quickly developed into vesicles with persistent pain. Antiviral therapy should be initiated within 72 hours of rash onset. Famciclovir or valacyclovir are preferred over acyclovir due to more convenient dosing. Both agents required dose reduction as TJ's creatinine clearance is estimated at 30 mL/min.

2. TJ reports constant and moderate nerve pain. It is reasonable to optimize the dosage of acetaminophen (not to exceed 4 g daily), before switching to a weak opioid. The appropriate analgesics for nerve pain include lidocaine patch (once vesicles are healed), antiepileptics and tricyclic antidepressants. Gabapentin is a safe and cost-effective choice for this indication. It requires dose titration and should not exceed 1400 mg per day based on his CrCl of 30 mL/min.

3. Persons older than 60 years who have a previous episode of zoster can be vaccinated unless there are contraindications. It may be prudent to defer vaccine until the complete resolution of the acute infection. TJ should be educated to keep the rash clean and dry, to avoid topical antibiotics, and if possible, to keep the rash covered. Clinicians should stress the importance of completing the full course of antiviral therapy.

Case Summary:

TJ has the most important risk factor for zoster infection (advanced age). He presents with the characteristic clinical symptoms of zoster: prodromal pain, rash and vesicles that occur at a unilateral dermatome. The systemic antiviral therapy can decrease the intensity and duration of acute zoster rash, and should be initiated within 72 hours of rash onset if possible. Appropriate pain management is important to maintain patients' functional status and quality of life.

Clinical Pearls

- *Injectable vitamin B12 is often supplemented in patients for a placebo effect such as a boost in vitality. If the clinical record does not contain a clearly documented vitamin B12 deficiency anemia or serum concentration requiring an injectable route of vitamin replacement it can be cited as an unnecessary medication without supporting indication.*

- *The live zoster vaccine is 14 times more potent than varicella vaccine, and should be stored at a freezer with a separate sealing door. The "dormitory" refrigerator with an open freezer compartment is not appropriate for its storage. Once reconstituted, it must be administered or discarded within 30 minutes. Both the vaccine and its administration fee are covered by Medicare Part D.*

Chapter Summary

The common types of anemias seen in the elderly are nutritional, chronic disease, and unexplained anemia, with these three types seen with almost equal prevalence. Complications due to anemia in older adults are high and can be rather severe even at what many would consider to be very mild reductions in hemoglobin. More research is sorely needed in the elderly anemic population to define an optimal hematologic treatment goal, and help identify optimal treatment regiments that are specific for this population.

Advanced age is a critical risk factor for herpes zoster and post-herpetic neuralgia. The ages of highest risk for zoster and post-herpetic neuralgia are after 50 years and after 60 years, respectively. Due to the aging population, both conditions are expected to cause significant healthcare burden, as well as reduced functioning and quality of life in the geriatric population. Prompt and appropriate antiviral treatment is recommended to reduce zoster-related morbidity. Appropriate analgesic therapy for zoster pain and post-herpetic neuralgia requires close monitoring for efficacy and tolerability.

Elderly persons are at risk for influenza, pneumococcal disease, tetanus and herpes zoster and should receive these vaccines unless contraindications exist. The ACIP recommends strategies to improve vaccination levels, including using reminder/recall systems and standing orders programs, administering vaccines during hospitalization or routine health-care visits; providing vaccines in alternative settings, including pharmacies, and to provide publicity and education to reach potential vaccine recipients.

As our population of older men and women increases, more people will be confronted with cancer as this disease mostly affects individuals over 65 years of age. Fortunately, a number of cancers can be prevented through proper dietary and physical habits. Further, cancer screening can prevent or provide early diagnosis which leads to better prognosis for some cancers. At this time, most positive outcomes from screening are derived from detecting cancers of the cervix, breast, and colon and rectum. In spite of the many potential benefits from cancer screening, certain older individuals may not benefit from cancer screening due to concerns such as decreased life expectancy, decreased physical functions, and comorbid diseases. Thus, the decision on cancer screening should be based on factors such as the benefit, risk, and patient's preference other than survival benefit alone.

Self-Assessment Questions

1. What are the most common causes of anemia in the elderly?

2. What are the standard pharmacologic options (drugs and dosages) for treating nutritional anemias?

3. What is the rationale for the use of erythropoietic-stimulating agents in the treatment of anemia and which anemias are they used to treat?

4. What are some complications that can occur in an elderly patient as a consequence of anemia?

5. What are the clinical features of herpes zoster infection?

6. What are the antiviral treatment options for acute zoster infection? What are the most common side effects?

7. What is the current ACIP recommendation on influenza, pneumococcal, tetanus and zoster vaccines for a 65-year-old person?

8. What are the efficacies and adverse effects of influenza, pneumococcal, tetanus and zoster vaccines?

9. What are contraindications and precautions for live zoster vaccine?

10. What are the various cancer screening tests recommended by the ACS and the USPSTF for the general population?

11. What are the cancer prevention measures that most people can adapt?

12. What are some of the medications that have shown promise in the prevention of cancer?

References

1. Guralnik JM, Ershler WB, Schrier SL, Picozzi VJ. Anemia in the elderly: a public health crisis in hematology. *Hematol Am Soc Hematol Educ Program.* 2005:528–532.

2. Guralnik JM, Eisenstaedt RS, Ferrucci L, Klein HG, Woodman RC. Prevalence of anemia in persons 65 years and older in the United States: evidence for a high rate of unexplained anemia. *Blood.* 2004;104:2263–2268.

3. U.S. Department of Health and Human Services, Center for Disease Control and Prevention, National Center for Health Statistics. Plan and Operation of the Third National Health and Nutrition Examination Survey, 1988–94. *Vital Health Stat.* 1994;32:1–407.

4. Argento V, Roylance J, Skudlarska B, Dainiak N, Amoateng-Adjepong Y. Anemia prevalence in a home visit geriatric population. *J Am Med Dir Assoc.* 2008;9:422–426.

5. Artz AS, Fergusson D, Drinka PJ, Gerald M, Gravenstein S, Lechich A, et al. Prevalence of anemia in skilled-nursing home residents. *Arch Gerontol Geriatr.* 2004;39:201–206.

6. Robinson B, Artz AS, Culleton B, Critchlow C, Sciarra A, Audhya P. Prevalence of anemia in the nursing home: Contribution of chronic kidney disease. *J Am Geriatr Soc.* 2007;55:1566–1570.

7. Landi F, Russo A, Danese P, Liperoti R, Barillaro C, Bernabei R, et al. Anemia status, hemoglobin concentration, and mortality in nursing home older residents. *J Am Med Dir Assoc.* 2007;8:322–327.

8. World Health Organization. Nutritional anemias: report of a WHO scientific group. *World Health Organ Tech Rep Ser.* 1968;405:5–37.

9. Patel KV. Epidemiology of anemia in older adults. *Semin Hematol.* 2008;45:210–217.

10. Beutler E, Waalen J. The definition of anemia: What is the lower limit of normal of the blood hemoglobin concentration? *Blood.* 2006;107:1747–1750.

11. Price EA. Aging and erythropoiesis: current state of knowledge. *Blood Cells Molecules Dis.* 2008;41:158–165.

12. Hartstock RJ, Smith EB, Petty CS. Normal variations with aging of the amount of hematopoietic tissue in bone marrow from the anterior iliac crest. A study made from 177 cases of sudden death examined by necropsy. *Am J Clin Pathol.* 1965;43:326–331.

13. Baraldi-Junkins CA, Beck AC, Rothstein G. Hematopoiesis and cytokines. Relevance to cancer and aging. *Hematol Oncol Clin North Am.* 1000;14:45–61viii.

14. Lipschitz DA, Udupa KB, Milton KY, Thompson CO. Effect of age on hematopoiesis in man. *Blood.* 1984;63:502–509.

15. Hirota Y, Okamura S, Kimura N, et al. Haematopoiesis in the ages as studied by in vitro colony assay. *Eur J Haematol.* 1988;40:83–90.

16. Bagnara GP, Bonsi L, Strippoli P, et al. Hemopoiesis in healthy old people and centenarians: well-maintained responsiveness of CD34+ cells to hemopoietic growth factors and remodeling of cytokine network. *J Gerontol A Biol Sci Med Sci.* 2000;55:B61–66.

17. Adamson JW, Eschbach J, Finch CA. The kidney and erythropoiesis. *Am J Med.* 1968;44:725–733.

18. Radtke HW, Claussner A, Erbes PM, et al. Serum erythropoietin concentration in chronic renal failure: relationship to degree of anemia and excretory renal function. *Blood.* 1979;54:877–884.

19. Artunc F, Risler T. Serum erythropoietin concentrations and responses to anemia in patients with or without chronic kidney disease. *Nephrol Dial Transplant.* 2007;22:2900–2908.

20. Ferrucci L, Maggio M, Bandinelli S, et al. Low testosterone levels and the risk of anemia in older men and women. *Arch Intern Med.* 2006;166:1380–1388.

21. Sohmiya M, Kato Y. Effect of long-term administration of recombinant human growth hormone (rhGH) on plasma erythropoietin (EPO) and haemoglobin levels in anaemic patients with adult GH deficiency. *Clin Endocrinol.* 2001;55:749–754.

22. Bruunsgaard H, Andersen-Ranberg K, Jeune B, et al. A high plasma concentration of TNF-alpha is associated with dementia in centenarians. *J Gerontol A Biol Sci Med Sci.* 1999;54:M357–M364.

23. Paolisso G, Rizzo MR, Mazziotti G, et al. Advancing age and insulin resistance: role of plasma tumor necrosis factor-alpha. *Am J Physiol.* 1998;275:E294–E299.

24. Wei J, Xu H, Davies JL, Hemmings GP. Increase of plasma IL-6 concentration with age in healthy subjects. *Life Sci.* 1992;51:1953–1956.

25. Maggio M, Guralnik JM, Longo DL, Ferrucci L. Interleukin-6 in aging and chronic disease: a magnificent pathway. *J Gerontol A Biol Sci Med Sci.* 2006;61:575–584.

26. Ferrucci L, Guralnik JM, Woodman RC, et al., Proinflammatory state and circulating erythropoietin in persons with and without anemia. *Am J Med.* 2005;118:1288.

27. Penninx BW, Pahor M, Cesari M, et al. Anemia is associated with disability and decreased physical performance and muscle strength in the elderly. *J Am Geriatr Soc.* 2004;52:719–724.

28. Ferrucci L, Guralnik JM, Bandinelli S, et al. Unexplained anaemia in older persons is characterised by low erythropoietin and low levels of pro-inflammatory markers. *Br J Haematol.* 2007;136:849–855.

29. Silva M, Grillot D, Benito A, et al. Erythropoietin can promote erythroid progenitor survival by repressing apoptosis through Bcl-XL and Bcl-2. *Blood.* 1996;88:1576–1582.

30. Spivak JL. The blood in systemic disorders. *Lancet.* 2000;355:1707–1712.

31. Ganz T. Hepcidin-a regulator of intestinal iron absorption and iron recycling by macrophages. *Best Pract Res Clin Haematol.* 2005;18:171–182.

32. Woodman R, Ferrucci L, Guralnik J. Anemia in older adults. *Curr Opin Hematol.* 2005;12:123–128.

33. Carmel R. Nutritional anemias in the elderly. *Semin Hematol.* 2008;45:255–234.

34. Guyatt GH, Patterson C, Ali M, et al. Diagnosis of iron-deficiency anemia in the elderly. *Am J Med.* 1990;88:205–209.

35. Rimon E, Levy S, Sapir A, et al. Diagnosis of iron deficiency anemia in the elderly by transferrin receptor-ferritin index. *Arch Intern Med.* 2002;162:445–449.

36. DuBois S, Kearney DJ. Iron deficiency anemia and *Helicobacter pylori* infection: a review of the evidence. *Am J Gastroenterol.* 2005;100:453–459.

37. Hershko C, Patz J, Ronson A. The anemia of achylia gastric revisited. *Blood Cells Mol Dis.* 2007;39:178–183.

38. Carmel R. Prevalence of undiagnosed pernicious anemia in the elderly. *Arch Intern Med.* 1996;156:1097–1100.

39. Savage DG, Lindenbaum J, Stabler SP, Allen RH. Sensitivity of serum methylmalonic acid and total homocysteine determinations for diagnosing cobalamin and folate deficiencies. *Am J Med.* 1994;96:239–246.

40. Joelson DW, Fiebig EW, Wu AHB. Diminished need for folate measurements among indigent populations in the post folic acid supplementation era. *Arch Pathol Lab Med.* 2007;131:477–480.

41. Ashraf MJ, Cook JR, Rothberg MB. Clinical utility of folic acid testing for patients with anemia or dementia. *J Gen Intern Med.* 2008;23:824–826.

42. Pfeiffer CM, Johnson CL, Jain RB, et al. Trends in blood folate and vitamin B-12 concentrations in the United States, 1988–2004. *Am J Clin Nutr.* 2007; 86:718–727.

43. Wright JD, Bialosotsky K, Gunter EW, et al. Blood folate and vitamin B12: United States, 1988–84. National Center for Health Statistics. *Vital Health Stat.* 1988;11.

44. Hudson JQ. Chronic kidney disease: Management of complications. In: DiPiro JT, Talbert RL, Yee GC, Matzke GR, Wells BG, Posey LM, eds. *Pharmacotherapy: A Pathophysiologic Approach.* 7th ed. New York: McGraw Hill; 2008.

45. Cumming RG, Mitchell P, Craig JC, Knight JF. Renal impairment and anaemia in a population-based study of older people. *Int Med J.* 2004;34:20–23.

46. Ble A, Fink JC, Woodman RC, et al. Renal function, erythropoietin, and anemia of older persons. The InCHIANTI study. *Arch Intern Med.* 2005;165:2222–2227.

47. Makipour S, Kanapuru B, Ershler WB. Unexplained anemia in the elderly. *Semin Hematol.* 2008;45:250–254.

48. Ineck B, Mason BJ, Lyons W. Anemias. In: DiPiro JT, Talbert RL, Yee GC, Matzke GR, Wells BG, Posey LM, eds. *Pharmacotherapy: A Pathophysiologic Approach.* 7th ed. New York: McGraw Hill; 2008.

49. Saffel D. Putting it into practice: strategizing a successful anemia management protocol in the long-term setting. *Consult Pharm.* 2008;23(suppl.A):18–23.

50. Fick DM, Cooper JW, Wade WE, Waller JL, Maclean JR, Beers MH. Updating the Beers criteria for potentially inappropriate medication use in older adults. Results of a U.S. Consensus Panel of Experts. *Arch Intern Med.* 2003;163:2716–2724.

51. Clark SF. Iron deficiency anemia. *Nutr Clin Pract.* 2008;23:128–141.

52. Vidal-Alaball J, Butler CC, Cannings-John R, et al. Oral vitamin B12 versus intramuscular vitamin B12 for vitamin B12 deficiency. *Cochrane Database Syst Rev.* 2005;3:CD004655.

53. Carmel R. Efficacy and safety of fortification and supplementation with vitamin B12: Biochemical and physiological effects. *Food Nutr Bull.* 2008;29(suppl.):S177–S187.

54. Park S, Johnson MA. What is an adequate dose of oral vitamin B12 in older people with poor vitamin B12 status? *Nutr Rev.* 2006;64:373–378.

55. Kaferle J, Strzoda CE. Evaluation of macrocytosis. *Am Fam Physician.* 2009;79:203–208.

56. KDOQI Clinical Practice Guideline and Clinical Practice Recommendations for anemia in chronic kidney disease: 2007 update of hemoglobin target. *Am J Kidney Dis.* 2007;50:471–530.

57. Ershler WB, Artz AS, Kandahari MM. Recombinant erythropoietin treatment of anemia in older adults. *J Am Geriatr Soc.* 2001;49:1396–1397.

58. Grimley CE, Crouch D, Dolan G. Correction of the anaemia of chronic disease (ACD) with small doses of recombinant erythropoietin [abstract]. *Br J Haematol.* 2003;121(suppl 1):95.

59. Izaks GJ, Westendorp RG, Knook DL. The definition of anemia in older persons. *JAMA.* 1999;281:1714–1717.

60. Kikuchi M, Inagaki T, Shinagawa N. Five-year survival of older people with anemia: variation with hemoglobin concentration. *J Am Geriatr Soc.* 2001;49:1226–1228.

61. Chaves PH, Xue QL, Guralnik JM, Ferrucci L, Volpato S, Fried LP. What constitutes normal hemoglobin concentration in community-dwelling disabled older women? *J Am Geriatr Soc.* 2004;52:1811–1816.

62. Beard CM, Kokmen E, O'Brien PC, Ania BJ, Melton LJ. Risk of Alzheimer's disease among elderly patients with anemia: Population-based investigations in Olmstead County, Minnesota. *Ann Epidemiol.* 1997;7:219–224.

63. Atti AR, Palmer K, Volpato S, Zuliani G, Winblad B, Fratiglioni L. Anaemia increases the risk of dementia in cognitively intact elderly. *Neurobiology Aging.* 2006;27:278–284.

64. Chaves PH, Carlson MC, Ferrucci L, Guralnik JM, Semba R, Fried LP. Association between mild anemia and executive function impairment in community-

dwelling older women. The Women's Health Aging Study II. *J Am Geriatr Soc.* 2006;54:1429–1435.

65. Peters R, Burch L, Warner J, Beckett N, Poulter R, Bulpitt C. Haemoglobin, anemia, dementia and cognitive decline in the elderly, a systematic review. *BMC Geriatrics.* 2008;8:18.

66. Chaves PH, Ashar B, Guralnik JM, Fried LP. Looking at the relationship between hemoglobin concentration and prevalent mobility difficulty in older women. Should the criteria currently used to define anemia in older people be reevaluated? *J Am Geriatr Soc.* 2002;50:1257–1264.

67. Chaves PHM, Semba RD, Leng SX, et al. Impact of anemia and cardiovascular disease on frailty status of community-dwelling older women: The Women's Health and Aging Studies I and II. *J Gerontol A Biol Sci Med.* 2005;60:729–735.

68. Penninx BW, Pahor M, Cesari M, et al. Anemia is associated with disability and decreased physical performance and muscle strength in the elderly. *J Am Geriatr Soc.* 2004;52:719–724.

69. Penninx BW, Pluijm SM, Lips P, et al. Late-life anemia is associated with increased risk of recurrent falls. *J Am Geriatr Soc.* 2005;53:2106–2111.

70. Duh MS, Mody SH, Lefebvre P, Woodman RC, Buteau S, Piech CT. Anaemia and the risk of injurious falls in a community-dwelling elderly population. *Drugs Aging.* 2008;25:325–334.

71. Pandya N, Bookhart B, Mody SH, Funk Orsini PA, Reardon G. Study of anemia in long-term care (SALT): prevalence of anemia and its relationship with the risk of falls in nursing home residents. *Curr Med Res Opin.* 2008;24:2139–2149.

72. Dharmarajan TS, Avula S, Norkus EP. Anemia increases risk for falls in hospitalized older adults: an evaluation of falls in 362 hospitalized, ambulatory, long-term care, and community patients. *J Am Med Dir Assoc.* 2006;7:287–293.

73. Dharamrajan TS, Pankratov A, Morris E, et al. Anemia: its impact on hospitalizations and length of hospital stay in nursing home and community older adults. *J Am Med Dir Assoc.* 2008;9:354–359.

74. Culleton BF, Manns BJ, Zhang J, Tonelli M, Klarenbach S, Hemmelgarn BR. Impact of anemia on hospitalization and mortality in older adults. *Blood.* 2006 May 15;107(10):3841–3846.

75. Dworkin RH, Johnson WR, Breuer J, et al. Recommendations for the management of herpes zoster. *CID.* 2007;44(supp 1)S1–26.

76. Schmader KE, Gnann JW, Watson CP. The epidemiological, clinical, and pathological rationale for the herpes zoster vaccine. *J Infect Dis.* 2008;197(Suppl 2):S207–215.

77. Lin F, Hadler JL. Epidemiology of primary varicella and HZ hospitalizations: the pre-varicella vaccine era. *J Infect Dis.* 2000;181:1897–1905.

78. Schmader KE, Dworkin RH. Natural history and treatment of herpes zoster. *J Pain.* 2008;9(1):suppl 1:S3–9.

79. Department of Health and Human Services. Centers for Disease Control and Preventions. Prevention of Herpes Zoster. Recommendations of the Advisory Committee on Immunization Practice. *MMWR.* June 6, 2008;57(05):1–30. Available at www.cdc.gov/mmwr. Accessed May 30th, 2008.

80. Dworkin RH, Gnann JW, Oaklander AL, et al. Diagnosis and assessment of pain associated with herpes zoster and postherpetic neuralgia. *J Pain.* 2008;9:S37–44.

81. Schmader K. Herpes Zoster and postherpetic neuralgia in older adults. *Clin Geriatr Med.* 2007;23:615–632.

82. Degreef H. Famciclovir, a new oral antiherpes drug: results of the first controlled clinical study demonstrating its efficacy and safety in the treatment of uncomplicated herpes zoster in immunocompetent patients. *Int J Antimicrob Agents.* 1994;4:241–246.

83. Wood MJ, Kay R, Dworkin RH, Soong SJ, Whitley RJ. Oral acyclovir therapy accelerates pain resolution in patients with herpes zoster: a meta-analysis of placebo-controlled trials. *Clin Infect Dis.* 1996;22:341–347.

84. Jackson JL, Gibbons R, Meyer G, Inouye L. The effect of treating herpes zoster with oral acyclovir in preventing postherpetic neuralgia: a meta-analysis. *Arch Intern Med.* 1997;157:909–912.

85. Tyring S, Barbarash RA, Nahlik JE, et al. Famciclovir for the treatment of acute herpes zoster: effects on acute disease and postherpetic neuralgia: a randomized, double-blind, placebo-controlled trial. *Ann Intern Med.* 1995;123:89–96.

86. Dworkin RH, Boon RJ, Griffin DR, Phung D. Postherpetic neuralgia: impact of famciclovir, age, rash severity and acute pain in herpes zoster patients. *J Infect Dis.* 1998; 178(Suppl 1):S76–80.

87. Shen MC, Lin HH, Lee SSJ, et al. Double blind, randomized, acyclovir-controlled, parallel-group trial comparing the safety and efficacy of famciclovir and acyclovir in patients with uncomplicated herpes zoster. *J Microbiol Immunol Infect.* 2004; 37:75–81.

88. Shafran SD, Tyring SK, Ashton R, et al. Once, twice, or three times daily famciclovir compared with aciclovir for the oral treatment of herpes zoster in immunocompetent adults: a randomized, multicenter, double-blind clinical trial. *J Clin Virol.* 2004; 29:248–253.

89. Beutner KR, Friedman DJ, Forszpaniak C, Andersen PL, Wood MJ. Valacyclovir compared with acyclovir for improved therapy for herpes zoster in immunocompetent adults. *Antimicrob Agents Chemother.* 1995; 39:1546–1553.

90. Lin WR, Lin HH, Lee SSJ, et al. Comparative study of the efficacy and safety of valacyclovir versus acyclovir in the treatment of herpes zoster. *J Microbiol Immunol Infect.* 2001;34:138–142.

91. Tyring SK, Beutner KR, Tucker BA, Anderson WC, Crooks RJ. Antiviral therapy for herpes zoster: randomized, controlled clinical trial of valacyclovir and famciclovir therapy in immunocompetent patients 50 years and older. *Arch Fam Med.* 2000;9:863–869.

92. Oxman MN, Levin MJ, Johnson GR, et al. A vaccine to prevent herpes zoster and postherpetic neuralgia in older adults. *N Engl J Med.* 2005;352:2271–2284.

93. Recommendation of the Advisory Committee on Immunization Practices (ACIP). Prevention and control of influenza. *MMWR.* 2008;57. Available at: www.cdc.gov/mmwr. Accessed August 23, 2008.

94. Thompson WW, Shay DK, Weintraub E, et al. Influenza-associated hospitalizations in the United States. *JAMA.* 2004;292:1333–1340.

95. Thompson WW, Shay DK, Weintraub E, et al. Mortality associated with influenza and respiratory syncytial virus in the United States. *JAMA.* 2003;289:179–186.

96. Govaert TM, Thijs CT, Masurel N, et al. The efficacy of influenza vaccination in elderly individuals. A randomized double-blind placebo-controlled trial. *JAMA.* 1994;272:1661–1665.

97. Monto AS, Hornbuckle K, Ohmit SE. Influenza vaccine effectiveness among elderly nursing home residents: a cohort study. *Am J Epidemiol.* 2001;154:155–160.

98. Ohmit SE, Arden NH, Monto AS. Effectiveness of inactivated influenza vaccine among nursing home residents during an influenza A (H3N2) epidemic. *J Am Geriatr Soc.* 1999;47:165–171.

99. Jefferson T, Rivetti D, Rudin M, et al. Efficacy and effectiveness of influenza vaccines in elderly people: a systematic review. *Lancet.* 2005;366:1165–1174.

100. Nichol KL, Nordin JD, Nelson DB, et al. Effectiveness of influenza vaccine in the community-dwelling elderly. *N Engl J Med.* 2007;357:1373–1381.

101. Nichol KL, Wuorenma J, von Sternberg T. Benefits of influenza vaccination for low-, intermediate-, and high-risk senior citizens. *Arch Intern Med.* 1998;158:1769–76.

102. Mullooly JP, Bennett MD, Hornbrook MC, et al. Influenza vaccination programs for elderly persons: cost-effectiveness in a health maintenance organization. *Ann Intern Med.* 1994;121:947–952.

103. Nordin J, Mullooly J, Poblete S, et al. Influenza vaccine effectiveness in preventing hospitalizations and deaths in persons 65 years or older in Minnesota, New York, and Oregon: data from 3 health plans. *J Infect Dis.* 2001;184:665–670.

104. Maciosek MV, Solberg LI, Coffield AB, et al. Influenza vaccination health impact and cost-effectiveness among adults aged 50 to 64 and 65 and older. *Am J Prev Med.* 2006;31:72–79.

105. Govaert TM, Dinant GJ, Aretz K, et al. Adverse reactions to influenza vaccine in elderly people: randomised double blind placebo controlled trial. *BMJ.* 1993;307:988–990.

106. Margolis KL, Nichol KL, Poland GA, et al. Frequency of adverse reactions to influenza vaccine in the elderly. A randomized, placebo-controlled trial. *JAMA.* 1990;264:1139–1141.

107. Nichol KL, Margolis KL, Lind A, et al. Side effects associated with influenza vaccination in healthy working adults. A randomized, placebo-controlled trial. *Arch Intern Med.* 1996;156:1546–1550.

108. Peters PH Jr., Gravenstein S, Norwood P, et al. Long-term use of oseltamivir for the prophylaxis of influenza in a vaccinated frail older population. *J Am Geriatr Soc.* 2001;49:1025–1031.

109. LaForce C, Man CY, Henderson FW, et al. Efficacy and safety of inhaled zanamivir in the prevention of influenza in community-dwelling, high-risk adult and adolescent subjects: a 28-day, multicenter, randomized, double-blind, placebo-controlled trial. *Clin Ther.* 2007;29:1579–1590.

110. Pneumococcal disease. Available at: http://www.cdc.gov/vaccines/pubs/pinkbook/downloads/pneumo.pdf. Accessed August 20th 2008.

111. Prevention of Pneumococcal Disease: Recommendations of the Advisory Committee on Immunization Practices (ACIP). *MMWR.* April 04, 1997;46(RR-08);1–24.

112. Plouffe JF, Breiman RF, Facklam RR, Franklin County Pneumonia Study Group. Bacteremia with *Streptococcus pneumoniae* in adults: implications for therapy and prevention. *JAMA.* 1996;275:194–198.

113. The U.S. Department of Health Human Services. Healthy People 2010. http://www.healthypeople.gov/document/htmL/objectives/14-05.htm. Accessed August 18, 2008.

114. Whitney CG. Preventing pneumococcal disease: ACIP recommends pneumococcal polysaccharide vaccine for all adults age ≥65. *Geriatrics.* 2003;58:20–22, 25.

115. Fine MJ, Smith MP, Carson CA, et al. Efficacy of pneumococcal vaccination in adults: a meta-analysis of randomized controlled trials. *Arch Intern Med.* 1994;154:2666–2677.

116. Evers SM, Ament AJ, Colombo GL, et al. Cost-effectiveness of pneumococcal vaccination for prevention of invasive pneumococcal disease in the elderly: an update for 10 Western European countries. *Eur J Clin Microbiol Infect Dis.* 2007 Aug;26(8):531–540.

117. Middleton DB, Lin CJ, Smith KJ, et al. Economic evaluation of standing order programs for pneumococcal vaccination of hospitalized elderly patients. *Infect Control Hosp Epidemiol.* 2008 May;29(5):385–394.

118. Pneumovax 23 (pneumococcal vaccine polyvalent) package insert. Whitehouse Station, NJ: Merck & Co, Inc; January 2008.

119. Product Information: Prevnar(R), Pneumococcal 7-valent conjugate vaccine (Diphtheria CRM197 Protein). Philadelphia: Wyeth Pharmaceuticals Inc.; 2005.

120. Prevention of pertussis, tetanus, and diphtheria among adults: use of tetanus toxoid, reduced diphtheria toxoid and acellular pertussis vaccine (ACIP recommendations). *MMWR.* 2006;55(RR-17). Available at: http://www.cdc.gov/mmwr/PDF/rr/rr5517.pdf

121. CDC. Tetanus surveillance—United States, 1998–2000. *MMWR.* 2003;52:1–8.

122. McQuillan G, Kruszon-Moran D, Deforest A, Chu S, Wharton M. Serologic immunity to diphtheria and tetanus in the United States. *Ann Intern Med.* 2002;136:660–666.

123. Tetanus toxoid absorbed (Ttox) package insert. Swiftwater, PA: Aventis Pasteur, Inc; July 2005. Available at: http://www.fda.gov/cber/label/ttoxave092305LB.pdf

124. Tetanus toxoid, reduced diphtheria toxoid and acellular pertussis vaccine adsorbed (Tdap; Adacel®) package insert. Swiftwater, PA: Sanofi Pasteur, Inc; March 2008. Available at: http://www.fda.gov/cber/label/adacelLB.pdf

125. Wallace MS, Oxman MN. Acute herpes zoster and postherpetic neuralgia. *Anesth Clin North Am.* 1997;15:371.

126. Donahue JG, Choo PW, Manson JE, Platt R. The incidence of herpes zoster. *Arch Intern Med.* 1995;155:1605–1609.

127. Oxman MN, Levin MJ, Johnson GR, et al. A vaccine to prevent herpes zoster and postherpetic neuralgia in older adults. *N Engl J Med.* 2005;352:2271–2284.

128. Helgason S, Petursson G, Gudmundsson S, et al. Prevalence of postherpetic neuralgia after a first episode of herpes zoster: prospective study with long term follow up. *BMJ.* 2000;321:794–796.

129. Yawn BP, Saddier S, Wollan P, Sauver JS, Kurland M, Sy L. A population-based study of the incidence and complications of herpes zoster before zoster vaccine introduction. *Mayo Clin Proc.* 2007;82:1341–1349.

130. Choo PW, Galil K, Donahue JG, Walker AM, Spiegelman D, Platt R. Risk factors for postherpetic neuralgia. *Arch Intern Med.* 1997;157:1217–1224.

131. Lin F, Hadler JL. Epidemiology of primary varicella and HZ hospitalizations: the pre-varicella vaccine era. *J Infect Dis.* 2000;181:1897–905.

132. Schmader K, Saddier P, Johnson G, et al. The effect of a zoster vaccine on interference of herpes zoster with activities of daily living (ADL) [Abstract 859]. 44th Annual Meeting of IDSA, Oct. 12–15, 2006, Toronto.

133. Merck. ZOSTAVAX® Package Insert. 2006. Available at: http://www.merck.com/product/usa/pi_circulars/z/zostavax/zostavax_pi.pdf.

134. Department of Health and Human Services. Centers for Disease Control and Preventions. Prevention of Herpes Zoster. Recommendations of the Advisory Committee on Immunization Practice. *MMWR.* 2008;57(05):1–30. Available at: www.cdc.gov/mmwr. Accessed May 30th, 2008.

125. Jemal A, Siegel R, Ward E, et al. Cancer statistics, 2008. *CA Cancer J Clin.* 2008:58;71–96.

136. Cancer: Basic facts. Cancer facts & figures 2008. Atlanta, GA: American Cancer Society, 2008. Available at: http://www.cancer.org/downloads/STT/2008CAFFfinalsecured.pdf Accessed 8/25/08.

137. Resnick B, McLeskey SW. Cancer screening across the aging continuum. *Am J Manag Care.* 2008;14(5):267–276.

138. Yancik R. Population aging and cancer: a cross-national concern. *Cancer J.* 2005;11(6):437–41.

139. Kushi LH, Byers T, Doyle C, et al. American Cancer Society guidelines on nutrition and physical activity for cancer prevention: reducing the risk of cancer with healthy food choices and physical activity. *CA Cancer J Clin.* 2006;56:254–281.

140. World Health Organization. Cancer prevention. http://www.who.int/cancer/prevention/en/ Accessed 9/3/2008.

141. Demark-Wahneried W. Rock CL, Patrick K, et al. Lifestyle interventions to reduce cancer risk and improve outcomes. *Am Fam Physician.* 2008;77(11):1573–1578.

142. American Cancer Society. ACS report: Half of cancer deaths could be prevented. *CA Cancer J Clin.* 2005;55:209–210.

143. Chao A, Thun MJ, Connell CJ, et al. Meat consumption and risk of colorectal cancer. *JAMA.* 2005;293:172–182.

144. American Cancer Society. More details on red meat, colon cancer link. *CA Cancer J Clin.* 2005;55:143–144.

145. Patel AV, Callel EE, Bernstein L, et al. Recreational physical activity and risk of postmenopausal breast cancer in a large cohort of U.S. women. *Cancer Causes Control.* 2003;14(6):519–529.

146. Slattery ML, Edwards SL, Ma KN, et al. Physical activity and colon cancer: a public health perspective. *Ann Epidemiol.* 1997;7(2):137–145.

147. Zhang Y, Cantor KP, Dosemeci M, et al. Occupational and leisure-time physical activity and risk of colon cancer by subsite. *J Occup Environ Med.* 2006;48(3):236–43.

148. Centers for Disease Control and Prevention. Skin cancer prevention and education initiative. http://www.cdc.gov/cancer/skin/pdf/0607_skin_fs.pdf Accessed 9/3/2008.

149. American Cancer Society. Radon risk for lung cancer back in the spotlight. *CA Cancer J Clin.* 2005;55:139–140.

150. Darby S. Hill D, Auvinen A, et al. Radon in homes and risk of lung cancer: collaborative analysis of individual data from 13 European case-control studies. *BMJ.* 2005;330:223–228.

151. Smith RA, Cokkinides V, Webb BO. Cancer screening in the United States, 2008: A review of current American Cancer Society guidelines and cancer screening issues. *CA Cancer J Clin.* 2008;58:161–179.

152. U.S. Preventive Services Task Force. The guide to clinical preventive services. 2007 http://www.ahrq.gov/clinic/pocketgd07/pocketgd07.pdf Accessed 8/25/08.

153. American Cancer Society. Study questions need for yearly mammograms in women over 50. *CA Cancer J Clin.* 2005;55:141–143.

154. Sarfaty M, Wender R. How to increase colorectal cancer screening rates in practice. *CA Cancer J Clin.* 2007;57:354–366.

155. Losey R, Messinger-Rapport BJ. At what age should we discontinue colon cancer screening in the elderly? *Cleve Clin J Med.* 2007;74(4):269–272.

156. Gatto NM, Frucht H, Sundararajan V, et al. Risk of perforation after colonoscopy and sigmoidos-

copy: a population-based study. *J Natl Cancer Inst.* 2003;95:230–236.

157. Kim JJ, Goldie SJ. Health and economic implications of HPV vaccination in the United States. *N Engl J Med.* 2008;359:821–832.

158. Lin K, Lipsitz R, Miller T, et al. Benefits and harms of prostate-specific antigen screening for prostate cancer: An evidence update for the U.S. Preventive Services Task Force. *Ann Intern Med.* 2008;149:192–199.

159. U.S. Preventive Services Task Force. Screening for prostate cancer: U.S. Preventive Services Task Force recommendation statement. *Ann Intern Med.* 2008;149:185–191.

160. Wender RC. Preserving primary care: the front line in the war against cancer. *CA Cancer J Clin.* 2007;57:4–5.

161. Boulware LE, Marinopoulos S, Phillips KA, et al. Systematic review: the value of the periodic health evaluation. *Ann Intern Med.* 2007;146(4):289–300.

162. Fenton JJ, Cai Y, Weiss NS, et al. Delivery of cancer screening: how important is the preventive health examination? *Arch Intern Med.* 2007 167(6):580–585.

163. Walter LC, Covinsky KE. Cancer screening in elderly patients: a framework for individualized decision making. *JAMA.* 2001;285:2750–2756.

164. Cunningham J, Doerr TD, Walter LC, et al. Discussing cancer screening with elderly patients. *JAMA.* 2001;286:1175–1176.

165. Tsao AS, Kim ES, Hong WK. Chemoprevention of cancer. *CA Cancer J Clin.* 2004;54:150–180.

166. Gray J, Mao JT, Szabo E, et al. Lung cancer chemoprevention: ACCP evidence-based clinical practice guidelines. 2nd ed. *Chest.* 2007;132:56–68.

167. Kelloff GJ, Lippman SM, Dannenberg AJ, et al. Progress in chemoprevention drug development: The promise of molecular biomarkers for prevention of intraepithelial neoplasia and cancer; a plan to move forward. *Clin Cancer Res.* 2006;12(12):3661–3697.

168. American Cancer Society. Raloxifene prevents breast cancer in women at increased risk. *CA Cancer J Clin.* 2006;56:192–194.

169. Evista prescribing information. Eli Lilly and Company, Indianapolis. Revised 12/2007 http://pi.lilly.com/us/evista-pi.pdf Accessed 9/10/2008.

170. Duffy C. Perez K, Partridge A. Implications of phytoestrogen intake for breast cancer. *CA Cancer J Clin.* 2007;57:260–277.

171. Baron JA, Cole BF, Sandler RS, et al. A randomized trial of aspirin to prevent colorectal adenomas. *N Engl J Med.* 2003;348(10):891–899.

172. Flossmann E, Rothwell PM, on behalf of the British Doctors Aspirin Trial and the UK-TIA Aspirin Trial. Effect of aspirin on long-term risk of colorectal cancer: consistent evidence from randomised and observational studies. *Lancet.* 2007;369:1603–13.

173. Sandler RS, Halabi S, Baron JA, et al. A randomized trial of aspirin to prevent colorectal adenomas in patients with previous colorectal cancer. *N Engl J Med.* 2003;348:(10):883–90.

174. Dubé C, Rostom A, Lewin G, et al. for the U.S. Preventive Services Task Force. The use of aspirin for primary prevention of colorectal cancer: a systematic review prepared for the U.S. Preventive Services Task Force. *Ann Intern Med.* 2007;146(5):365–375.

175. Gann PH, Manson JE, Glynn RJ, et al. Low-dose aspirin and incidence of colorectal tumors in a randomized trial. *J Natl Cancer Inst.* 1993;85(15):1220–1224.

176. Baron JA, Beach M, Mandel JS, et al. for the Calcium Polyp Prevention Study Group. Calcium supplements for the prevention of colorectal adenomas. *N Engl J Med.* 1999;340(2):101–107.

177. Bonithon-Kopp C, Kronborg O, Giacosa A et al. Calcium and fibre supplementation in prevention of colorectal adenoma recurrence: a randomized intervention trial. European Cancer Prevention Organisation Study Group. *Lancet.* 2000;356:1300–1306.

178. Grau MV, Baron JA, Sanler RS, et al. Vitamin D, calcium supplementation, and colorectal adenomas: results of a randomized trial. *J Natl Cancer Inst.* 2003;95:1765–1771.

179. Giovannucci E, Liu Y, Rimm EB et al. Prospective study of predictors of vitamin D status and cancer incidence and mortality in men. *J Natl Cancer Inst.* 2006;98:451–459.

180. Lipkin M, Newmark H. Effect of added dietary calcium on colonic epithelial-cell proliferation in subjects at high risk for familial colonic cancer. *N Engl J Med.* 1985;313:1381–1384.

181. American Cancer Society. A call for more vitamin D research. *CA Cancer J Clin.* 2006;56:250–251.

182. The Alpha-Tocopherol, Beta Carotene Cancer Prevention Study Group. The effect of vitamin E and beta carotene on the incidence of lung cancer and other cancers in male smokers. *N Engl J Med.* 1994;330:1029–1035.

183. Omenn GS, Goodman G, Thornquist M, et al. The beta-carotene and retinol efficacy trial (CARET) for chemoprevention of lung cancer in high risk populations: smokers and asbestos-exposed workers. *Cancer Res.* 1994; 54:2038s–2043s.

184. Thompson IM, Goodman PJ, Tangen CM, et al. The influence of finasteride on the development of prostate cancer. *N Engl J Med.* 2003;349:215–224.

185. Giovannucci E, Rimm EB, Liu Y, et al. A prospective study of tomato products, lycopene, and prostate cancer risk. *J Natl Cancer Inst.* 2002;94:391–398.

186. Rodriguez C, McCullough ML, Mondul AM, et al. Meat consumption among Black and White men and risk of prostate cancer in the Cancer Prevention Study II Nutrition Cohort. *Cancer Epidemiol Biomarkers Prev.* 2006;15:211–216.

187. Giovannucci E, Liu Y, Stampfer MJ, et al. A prospective study of calcium intake and incident and fatal prostate cancer. *Cancer Epidemiol Biomarkers Prev.* 2006;15:203–210.

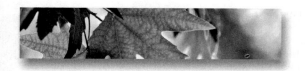

Index

A

Abbreviations, "do not use," 95
Abciximab, 136
Abdominal assessment, 74–75
Absorption changes, 63
Abuse, 37–38
Acamprosate, 354
Acarbose, 236
Access
   to medication, 13–16
   to pharmacy services, 13–16
ACE inhibitor
   cardiovascular disorders, 131–32, 136–37, 141–43, 154
   endocrine disorders, 250
   renal, urologic disorders, 195, 197
Acetaminophen, 19, 44, 45
   adverse drug events, 102
   cardiovascular disorders, 144
   CNS disorders, 326
   endocrine disorders, 248
   gastrointestinal disorders/nutrition, 289
   geriatric assessment, 86, 87
   hematologic and immunologic disorders, 443, 445, 446
   musculoskeletal/connective tissue disorders, 390, 391
   polypharmacy, suboptimal drug use, 111, 118
   psychiatric disorders, 356
   respiratory issues, 184, 219
   sensory issues, 373–74, 376, 377, 382
Acetylcholinesterase, 258
Acute care, 9
Acute coronary syndromes, 127, 135–38
Acyclovir, 429, 430
Adenosylmethionine (SAMe), 390
ADL (activities of daily living), 71, 81–82
Adrenocorticotropic hormone (ACTH), 244
Adult day centers, 10
Advance directives, 33–35, 71, 83, 84
Adverse drug event, 91, 92
   administration/adherence, 97–98
   dispensing, 96–97

identifying, 100
monitoring, 98–99
prescribing, 94–96
prevalence in subgroups, 93–94
reduction of, 100–101
reactions, 28
withdrawal events, 91, 92, 99–100
Adverse health event categories, 92
Age
   strata, 5
   threshold, 4
Aging theories, 54–55
Albumin, 64
Albuterol inhaler, 94–95, 103, 173, 184, 187
Alcohol, 308
   use, 83
   withdrawal assessment, 352
Alendronate, 86, 111, 258, 326, 394, 396, 407
Alfuzosin, 209
Allodynia, 428
Alpha adrenergic blockers, 66, 208, 209, 210
Alpha agonists, 132
Alpha antagonists, 132
Alpha blockers, 278
5–alpha reductase inhibitor, 208, 210, 221
Alpha–glucosidase inhibitors, 233, 234, 236
Alphatocopherol, 442
Alprazolam, 355
Alteplase, 135
Alternative medicine, 33
Alzheimer's disease, 299, 300, 301, 303–4
Alzheimer's Disease Assessment Scale, 79–80
Amantadine, 181–82, 312, 313
American Association of Retired Persons (AARP), 4
American Cancer Society, 75
American Society of Consultant Pharmacists, 8
American Urological Association Symptom Index, 206
Aminoglycoside antibiotics, 63, 262
Amiodarone, 145, 197, 241

Amiodarone–induced thyroid dysfunction, 244
Amitriptyline, 258, 316, 374
Amlodipine, 111, 155, 156, 185
Amoxicillin–clavulanate, 262
Amylin analog, 234
Analgesics, 308
Anastomosis, 257, 262
Androgel, 249
Androgen, 282, 286
Andropause, 246
Anemia, 420–26
Angiotensin receptor blocker (ARB), 136, 142, 143, 195
Angiotensin-converting enzyme inhibitors, 66
Anorexia, 62
Antacids, 281
Anti-aging strategies, 60–61
Antibiotic order, 44–45
Antibiotics, 33, 265, 279, 281, 405
   pneumonia, 177–78
   risk stratification of, 179
Anticholinergic agents, 61, 66
   CNS disorders, 308, 313, 315
   gastrointestinal disorders/nutrition, 258, 264, 275, 278
Anticonvulsants, 66, 197, 239, 281, 308, 373
Antidepressants
   cardiovascular disorders, 149
   gastrointestinal disorders, 274, 275, 281
   psychiatric disorders, 343–44, 345, 358
   renal/urologic disorders, 197
   sensory disorders, 372
Antidiabetic agents, 231–32, 308
Antiepileptic drug, 140, 278, 372, 375
   disease interactions, 322
Antihistamine, 66, 275, 282, 347
Antihypertensive agents, 123, 278
Antimicrobial agents, 214, 269, 308
Antineoplastic agents, 197
Antioxidant therapy, 60
Antioxidants, 370, 443
Anti-Parkinson's agents, 278
Antipsychotic agents